Psychiatric/Mental Health Nursing:
Concepts of Care

Psychiatric/Mental Health Nursing:
Concepts of Care

MARY C. TOWNSEND, RN, MN
Advanced Registered Nurse Practitioner
Clinical Nurse Specialist
Psychiatric/Mental Health Nursing

Nursing Consultant
Private Practice
Wichita, Kansas

Course Coordinator/Clinical Instructor
Psychiatric/Mental Health Nursing
El Dorado, Kansas

 F. A. DAVIS COMPANY • Philadelphia

Printed in the United States of America

Last digit indicates print number: 10 9 8 7 6 5 4 3 2 1

Publisher, Nursing: Robert G. Martone
Production Editor: Gail Shapiro
Cover Design By: Donald B. Freggens, Jr.

As new scientific information becomes available through basic and clinical research, recommended treatments and drug therapies undergo changes. The author(s) and publisher have done everything possible to make this book accurate, up to date, and in accord with accepted standards at the time of publication. The authors, editors, and publisher are not responsible for errors or omissions or for consequences from application of the book, and make no warranty, expressed or implied, in regard to the contents of the book. Any practice described in this book should be applied by the reader in accordance with professional standards of care used in regard to the unique circumstances that may apply in each situation. The reader is advised always to check product information (package inserts) for changes and new information regarding dose and contraindications before administering any drug. Caution is especially urged when using new or infrequently ordered drugs.

Library of Congress Cataloging-in-Publication Data

Townsend, Mary C., 1941–
    Psychiatric/mental health nursing : concepts of care / Mary C.
Townsend.
        p. cm.
    Includes bibliographical references and index.
    ISBN 0-8036-8586-6 (hardbound : alk. paper)
    1. Psychiatric nursing.   I. Title.
    [DNLM: 1. Mental Disorders—nursing.   2. Psychiatric Nursing—
methods.   3. Psychotherapy—nurses' instruction.   WY 160 T749p]
RC440.T693   1993
610.73'68—dc20
DNLM/DLC
for Library of Congress   92-49506
                                                                            CIP

This book is dedicated to:

All of my nursing students, past, present and future. I learn a great deal from you.

Preface

The purpose of this text is to provide nursing students and clinical nurses with a concise, yet comprehensive, relevant, and up-to-date resource to assist with the learning and practice of psychiatric/mental health nursing. The focus is on holistic nursing, and because psychiatric/mental health nursing is applicable to every nurse's individual practice, the concepts discussed in this text may be utilized in all clinical nursing settings.

The idea behind this text was to omit a great deal of extraneous information that is often included in other psychiatric/mental health textbooks and that is most often ignored by students during their short psychiatric nursing rotations. As a psychiatric nursing instructor for 11 years, I have come to understand well the needs and desires of students. I have also come to understand that clinical nurses in psychiatry want a resource that is quick, practical, and relevant to their practice. They want a book that is *usable.* I believe this textbook fulfills the needs in both categories.

This book is based on the conceptual framework of stress-adaptation, largely the work of Lazarus and Selye (see references for Chapter 1). Assessment of the patient has its foundation in predisposing factors (genetic influences, past experiences, and existing conditions) that contribute to the way in which an individual copes with a stressful event. The individual's perception of the event is taken into consideration, along with available strategies for coping with stress. The mental health/mental illness continuum is considered to be dynamic, and it is hypothesized that an individual may assume virtually any position along that continuum at any point in time, based on any of the above considerations. It is also hypothesized that all ill individuals possess some wellness components and all well individuals possess some illness components. Nurses utilize these strengths and limitations in planning care for psychiatric/mental health patients.

The textbook consists of four major units:

Unit I: Basic Concepts in Psychiatric/Mental Health Nursing
Unit II: Therapeutic Approaches in Psychiatric Care
Unit III: Nursing Care of Patients with Alterations in Psychosocial Adaptation
Unit IV: Special Topics in Psychiatric/Mental Health Nursing

The chapters in Unit I provide background information for the textbook. They include a basic overview of the concept of stress, a discussion of the most common psychosocial adaptations to stress, and delineation of the components of personality development as postulated by several major developmental theorists.

Unit II consists of Chapters 3 through 14, which provide information for the practicing nurse regarding various therapies that may be implemented with clients. The role of the nurse in each of these therapies is emphasized, and although the nurse is not likely to be the primary therapist in most instances, therapeutic intervention is well within his or her scope of practice in all of the regimes described in this text.

Unit III comprises the major portion of the text and includes chapters describing psychopathologies that have been identified in the DSM-III-R (1987). Each chapter includes learning objectives; an introduction; pertinent historic and epidemiologic factors; background assessment data, including predisposing factors and symptomatology associated with each disorder; common nursing diagnoses with standardized guidelines for intervention in the care of patients with these disorders; outcome criteria; guidelines for reassessment and evaluation of nursing care; and descriptions of common medical treatment modalities. A unique aspect of this text is the inclusion of critical pathways for nurses working in case management situations. Critical pathways are included for selected diagnoses in which short stays with outcomes pertinent to specific time dimensions are appropriate.

Unit IV includes special topics, such as the aging individual, the individual with HIV/AIDS, victims of violence, and ethical and legal issues in psychiatric/mental health nursing. The topics of aging, AIDS, and victims of violence were selected for inclusion because of their prevalence in society. Nurses in all settings are likely to encounter any or all of these individuals repeatedly and frequently. The final chapter comprises ethical and legal issues as they apply to the practice of psychiatric/mental health nursing.

It is my hope that this text can provide assistance to nurses working with individuals who are experiencing emotional pain and suffering. I believe that psychosocial nursing is the most difficult part of nursing, and I observe that it is often neglected outside the psychiatric nursing specialty area. The practicality of this text makes it a useful tool within both spheres.

I am hopeful that the text will provide students with a positive perspective toward psychiatric nursing. It has been my experience that most students are anxious and somewhat fearful of the unknown when they begin their psychiatric nursing rotations. This text answers the question most frequently asked: "What do psychiatric nurses do?". Hopefully, it will assist students to gain the confidence and skills necessary to practice psychosocial nursing with *all* of their patients, and optimistically, win a few over to psychiatric nursing.

Mary C. Townsend

Acknowledgments

I owe a great deal of thanks to many people who supported me with their time and encouragement throughout this enormous (more so than I ever dreamed!) project. To name a few, I thank:

Ruth DeGeorge, Executive Secretary, F. A. Davis Company, for your bright and cheerful voice on the other end of the phone, and for your never-ending willingness to provide assistance. It seems I only needed to ask.

Robert G. Martone, Publisher, Nursing, F. A. Davis Company, for your sense of humor and continuous optimistic outlook about the outcome of this project.

The nursing educators and clinicians who reviewed the original manuscript and provided valuable input into the final product.

The Administration and Board of Trustees of Butler County College who granted me a semester of sabbatical leave to work on this project.

Patricia Bayles, Division Director, Nursing and Allied Health, Butler County College — my boss and friend, who takes pride in my accomplishments, and tells me so.

My mother, Camalla Welsh, who helped with the "chapter countdown," and is a bright spot in the lives of all who know her.

My daughters, Kerry and Tina, for all the joy you have provided me and all the hope that you instill in me. You keep me young at heart.

My constant companions, Cocoa and Buddy, for the pure pleasure you bring into my life every day that you live.

My husband, Jim, who gives meaning to my life in so many ways. You are the one whose encouragement keeps me motivated, whose support gives me strength, and whose gentleness gives me comfort.

Contents

DSM-III-R Classifications:
Axes 1 and 11 Categories and Codes see pages 27–30.

UNIT 2

UNIT 3

NURSING CARE OF PATIENTS WITH ALTERATIONS IN PSYCHOSOCIAL

15 DISORDERS USUALLY FIRST EVIDENT IN INFANCY, CHILDHOOD, OR ADOLESCENCE

BASIC CONCEPTS IN PSYCHIATRIC/MENTAL HEALTH NURSING

1

AN INTRODUCTION TO THE CONCEPT OF STRESS

OBJECTIVES

After reading this chapter, the student will be able to:
1. Define *adaptation* and *maladaptation*.
2. Identify physiological responses to stress.
3. Explain the relationship between stress and "diseases of adaptation."
4. Describe the concept of stress as an environmental event.
5. Explain the concept of stress as a transaction between the individual and the environment.
6. Discuss adaptive coping strategies in the management of stress.

INTRODUCTION

Psychologists and other health-care professionals have struggled for years to establish an effective definition of the term *stress*. This term is used loosely today and still lacks definitive explanation. As one researcher said, "Stress, in addition to being itself, and the result of itself, is also the cause of itself" (Wallis, 1983). *Adaptation* as a healthy response to stress has been defined as restoration of homeostasis to the internal environmental system (Grinker et al, 1974). This includes responses directed at stabilizing internal biological processes and psychological preservation of self-identity and self-esteem. Roy (1976) defined adaptive response as behavior that maintains the integrity of the individual. Adaptation is viewed as positive and is correlated to a healthy response. When behavior disrupts the integrity of the individual, it is perceived as *maladaptive* (Roy, 1976). Maladaptive responses are negative or unhealthy responses by the individual.

Various researchers of this century have contributed to several different concepts of stress. Three of these concepts include stress as a biological response, stress as an environmental event, and stress as a transaction between the individual and the environment.

STRESS AS A BIOLOGICAL RESPONSE

In 1956, Selye published the results of his research concerning the physiological response of a biological system to a change imposed upon it. Since his initial publication, he has revised his definition of stress to ". . . the state manifested by a specific syndrome which consists of all the nonspecifically-induced changes within a biologic system" (Selye, 1976). This syndrome of symptoms has come to be known as the "fight or flight syndrome." These symptoms are identified specifically in Table 1.1. Selye called this general reaction of the body to stress the *general adaptation syndrome*. He described the reaction in three distinct stages:

1. *Alarm reaction stage.* During this stage, the physiological responses of the "fight or flight" syndrome are initiated.

2. *Stage of resistance.* The individual uses the physiological responses of the first stage as a defense in the attempt to adapt to the stressor. If adaptation occurs, the third stage is prevented or delayed. Physiological symptoms may disappear.

3. *Stage of exhaustion.* This stage occurs when there is a prolonged exposure to the stressor to which the body has become adjusted. The adaptive energy is depleted, and the individual can no longer draw from the resources for adaptation described in the first two stages. Diseases of adaptation (e.g., headaches, mental disorders, coronary artery disease, ulcers, colitis) may occur. Without intervention for reversal, exhaustion and even death ensues (Selye, 1956, 1974).

This "fight or flight" response undoubtedly served our ancestors well. Those Homo sapiens who had to face the giant grizzly bear or the saber-toothed tiger as a facet of their struggle for survival must have used these adaptive resources to their advantage. The response was elicited in the emergency situation, used in the preservation of life, followed by restoration of the compensatory mechanisms to the preemergent condition (homeostasis).

Selye performed his extensive research in a controlled setting with laboratory animals as subjects. He elicited the physiological responses with physical stimuli, such as exposure to heat or frigid temperatures, electric shock, injection of toxic agents, restraint, and surgical injury. Since the publication of Selye's original research, other studies have revealed that the "fight or flight" syndrome of symptoms occurs in response to psychological or emotional stimuli, just as it does to physical stimuli (Lazarus, 1966; Hill et al, 1956; Mason, 1971). The psychological or emotional stressors are often not resolved as rapidly as some physical stressors, and therefore the body may be depleted of its adaptive energy more readily than it is from physical stressors. The "fight or flight" response may be inappropriate, even dangerous, to the life-style of today, in which stress has been described as "a pervasive, chronic and relentless psychosocial situation" (Wallis, 1983). This chronic response, which maintains the body in the aroused condition for extended periods, promotes susceptibility to diseases of adaptation.

Table 1.1 THE "FIGHT OR FLIGHT SYNDROME"

Initial Stress Response:

Physical Component	*Adaptation Response*
Hypothalamus	Sympathetic nervous system (SNS) stimulated
SNS	Adrenal medulla stimulated
Adrenal medulla	Epinephrine and norepinephrine released
Eye	Pupils dilated
Lacrimal glands	Secretion increased
Respiratory system	Bronchioles and pulmonary blood vessels dilated
	Respiration rate increased
Cardiovascular system	Force of cardiac contraction increased
	Cardiac output increased
	Heart rate increased
	Blood pressure increased
Gastrointestinal system	Motility in stomach and intestines decreased
	Secretions decreased
	Sphincters contracted
Liver	Glycogenolysis and gluconeogenesis increased
	Glycogen synthesis decreased
Urinary system	Ureter motility increased
	Bladder muscle contracted
	Bladder sphincter relaxed
Sweat glands	Secretion increased
Fat cells	Lipolysis

Sustained Stress Response:

I. Hypothalamus	Pituitary gland stimulated
A. Pituitary gland releases:	
1. Adrenocorticotropic hormone (ACTH)	Adrenal cortex stimulated
a. Adrenal cortex	Glucocorticoids released
1) Glucocorticoids	Gluconeogenesis increased
	Immune response suppressed
	Inflammatory response suppressed
b. Adrenal cortex	Mineralocorticoids released
2) Mineralocorticoids	Retention of sodium and water increased
2. Vasopressin (antidiuretic hormone)	Blood pressure increased through constriction of blood vessels
	Fluid retention increased
3. Growth hormone	Direct effect on protein, carbohydrate, and lipid metabolism, resulting in increased serum glucose and free fatty acids
4. Thyrotropic hormone (TTH)	Thyroid gland stimulated, resulting in increased Basal Metabolic Rate (BMR)
5. Gonadotropins	Initially, secretion of sex hormones increased; later, with sustained stress, secretion is suppressed, resulting in decreased libido, frigidity, or impotence.

STRESS AS AN ENVIRONMENTAL EVENT

A second concept defines stress as the "thing" or "event" that triggers the adaptive physiological and psychological responses in an individual. The event is one that creates change in the life pattern of the individual, requires significant adjustment in life-style, and taxes available personal resources. The change can be either positive, such as accomplishing an outstanding personal achievement, or negative, such as being fired from a job. The emphasis here is on *change* from the existing steady state of the individual's life pattern.

Holmes and Rahe (1967) developed a method of correlating the effects of life change with illness. They tested their hypotheses with more than 5,000 people. From their research, they devised the Social Readjustment Rating Scale (Table 1.2). Numerical values were assigned to various events, or changes, that are common in people's lives. Holmes and Rahe concluded that the higher the score on the Social Readjustment Rating Scale, the greater the susceptibility of that individual to physical or psychological illness. The score can be interpreted in the following manner:

0–150	No significant possibility of stress-related illness
150–199	Mild life-crisis level—35 percent chance of illness
200–299	Moderate life-crisis level—50 percent chance of illness
300 or more	Major life-crisis level—80 percent chance of illness

Whether stress overload merely predisposes a person to illness or actually precipitates it is unknown, but there does appear to be a causal link (Pelletier, 1977). The Holmes and Rahe Social Readjustment Rating Scale has been criticized because it does not consider the individual's perception of the event. Individuals differ in their reactions to life events, and these variations are related to the degree to which the change is perceived as stressful. The Social Readjustment Rating Scale also fails to consider the individual's coping strategies and available support systems at the time of the life change. Positive coping mechanisms and strong social or familial support can reduce the intensity of a stressful life change and promote a more adaptive response.

Table 1.2 SOCIAL READJUSTMENT RATING SCALE

Life Event	Mean Value
Death of spouse	100
Divorce	73
Marital separation	65
Jail term	63
Death of close family member	63
Personal illness or injury	53
Marriage	50
Fired from work	47
Marital reconciliation	45
Retirement	45
Change in family member's health	44
Pregnancy	40
Sex difficulties	39
Addition to family	39
Business readjustment	39
Change in financial status	38
Death of close friend	37
Change to different line of work	36
Change in number of marital arguments	35
Mortgage or loan more than $10,000	31
Foreclosure of mortgage or loan	30
Change in work responsibilities	29
Son or daughter leaving home	29
Trouble with in-laws	29
Outstanding personal achievement	28
Spouse begins or stops work	26
Starting or finishing school	26
Change in living conditions	25
Revision of personal habits	24
Trouble with boss	23
Change in work hours, conditions	20
Change in residence	20
Change in schools	20
Change in recreational habits	19
Change in church activities	19
Change in social activities	18
Mortgage or loan less than $10,000	17
Change in sleeping habits	16
Change in number of family gatherings	15
Change in eating habits	15
Vacation	13
Christmas season	12
Minor violation of the law	11

Source: Holmes and Rahe (1967) with permission.

STRESS AS A TRANSACTION BETWEEN THE INDIVIDUAL AND THE ENVIRONMENT

This definition of stress emphasizes the *relationship* between the individual and the environment. Personal characteristics as well as the nature of the environmental event are considered (Lazarus & Folkman, 1984). This illustration parallels the modern concept of the etiology of disease. No longer is causation viewed solely as an external organism; whether or not illness occurs depends also on the receiving organism's susceptibility. Similarly, to predict psychological stress as a reaction, the properties of the person in relation to the environment must be considered.

Precipitating Event

Lazarus and Folkman (1984) define stress as a relationship between the person and the environment that is appraised by the person as taxing or exceeding his or her resources and endangering his or her well-being. A precipitating event is a stimulus arising from the internal or external environment and is perceived by the individual in a specific manner. Determination that a particular person/environment relationship is stressful depends on the cognitive appraisal of the situation by the individual. Cognitive appraisal is an individual's evaluation of the personal significance of the event or occurrence. The event "precipitates" a response on the part of the individual, and the response is impacted by the individual's perception of the event. The cognitive response consists of a primary appraisal and a secondary appraisal.

Individual's Perception of the Event

PRIMARY APPRAISAL

Lazarus and Folkman (1984) identify three types of primary appraisal: irrelevant, benign-positive, and stressful. An event is judged *irrelevant* when the outcome holds no significance for the individual. A *benign-positive* outcome is one that is perceived as producing pleasure for the individual. *Stress* appraisals include harm/loss, threat, and challenge. *Harm/loss* appraisals refer to damage or loss already experienced by the individual. Appraisals of a *threatening* nature are perceived as anticipated

harms or losses. When an event is appraised as *challenging*, the individual focuses on potential for gain or growth rather than on risks associated with the event. Challenge produces stress even though the emotions associated with it (eagerness and excitement) are viewed as positive, and coping mechanisms must be called on to face the new encounter. Challenge and threat may occur together when an individual experiences these positive emotions along with fear or anxiety over the possible risks associated with the challenging event.

When stress is produced in response to harm/loss, threat, or challenge, a secondary appraisal is made by the individual.

SECONDARY APPRAISAL

This secondary appraisal is an assessment of skills, resources, and knowledge that the person possesses to deal with the situation. The individual evaluates:

- What coping strategies are available to me?
- Will the option I choose be effective in this situation?
- Do I have the ability to use that strategy in an effective manner?

The interaction between the primary appraisal of the event that has occurred and the secondary appraisal of available coping strategies determines the individual's quality of adaptation response to stress.

Predisposing Factors

A variety of elements influence how an individual perceives and responds to a stressful event. These "predisposing" factors strongly influence whether the response is adaptive or maladaptive. Types of predisposing factors include genetic influences, past experiences, and existing conditions.

Genetic influences are those circumstances of an individual's life that are acquired by heredity. Examples include family history of physical and psychological conditions (strengths and weaknesses) and the individual's temperament (behavioral characteristics present at birth that evolve with development).

Past experiences are occurrences that result in learned patterns that can influence an individual's adaptation response. They include previous exposure to the stressor or other stressors, learned coping responses, and degree of adaptation to previous stressors.

Existing conditions incorporate vulnerabilities that influence the adequacy of the individual's physical, psychological, and social resources for dealing with adaptive demands (Murphy & Moriarty, 1976). Examples include current health status, motivation, developmental maturity, severity and duration of the stressor, financial and educational resources, age, existing coping strategies, and a support system of caring others.

This Transactional Model of Stress/Adaptation will serve as a framework for the process of nursing in this text. A graphic display of the model is presented in Figure 1.1.

STRESS MANAGEMENT*

Stress management has become a multimillion-dollar-a-year business. Stress management involves use of coping strategies in the response to stressful situations. Coping strategies are adaptive when they serve to protect the individual from harm (or additional harm) or to strengthen the individual's ability to meet challenging situations. Adaptive responses help restore homeostasis to the body and impede the development of diseases of adaptation.

Coping strategies are considered maladaptive when the conflict being experienced goes unresolved or intensifies. Energy resources become depleted as the body struggles to compensate for the chronic physiological and psychological arousal being experienced. The effect is a significant vulnerability to physical or psychological illness. (A detailed discussion of the types of diseases of adaptation can be found in Chapter 25.)

Adaptive Coping Strategies

AWARENESS

The initial step in managing stress is awareness —to become aware of the factors that create stress

---

*Techniques of stress management will be discussed in greater length in Unit 2 of this text.

and the feelings associated with a stressful response. Stress can only be controlled when one recognizes that it is being experienced. As one becomes aware of stressors, they can be either omitted, avoided, or accepted.

RELAXATION

Individuals experience relaxation in different ways. Some individuals relax by engaging in large motor activities, such as sports, jogging, and physical exercise. Still others use techniques, such as breathing exercises and progressive relaxation, to relieve stress. (A discussion of relaxation therapy can be found in Chapter 10.)

MEDITATION

Practiced 20 minutes once or twice daily, meditation has been shown to produce a lasting reduction in blood pressure and other stress-related symptoms (Wallis, 1983). Meditation involves assuming a comfortable position, closing the eyes, casting off all other thoughts, and concentrating on a single word, sound, or phrase that has positive meaning to the individual.

INTERPERSONAL COMMUNICATION WITH CARING OTHER

As previously mentioned, the strength of one's available support systems is an existing condition that significantly influences the adaptiveness of coping with stress. Sometimes, just "talking the problem out" with an individual who is empathetic is sufficient to interrupt escalation of the stress response. Writing about one's feelings in a journal or diary can also be very therapeutic.

PROBLEM SOLVING

An extremely adaptive coping strategy is to view the situation in an objective manner (or seek assistance from another individual to accomplish this if anxiety level is too high to concentrate). Following an objective assessment of the situation, the problem-solving/decision-making model can be instituted:

1. Assess the facts of the situation.
2. Formulate goals for resolution of the stressful situation.

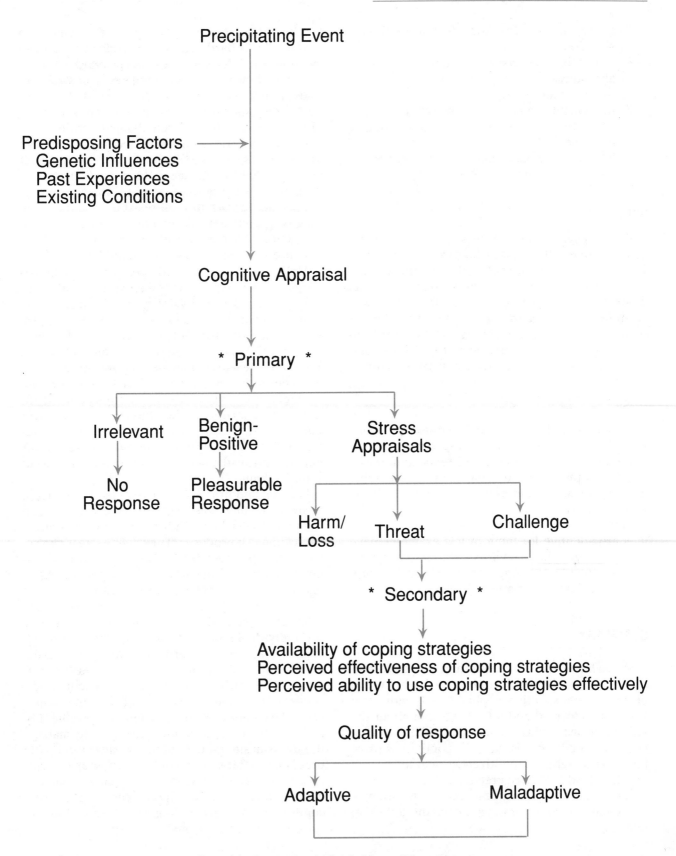

Figure 1.1 Transactional Model of Stress/Adaptation.

3. Study alternatives for dealing with the situation.
4. Determine the risks and benefits of each alternative.
5. Select an alternative.
6. Implement the alternative selected.
7. Evaluate the outcome of the alternative implemented.
8. If the first choice is ineffective, select and implement a second alternative.

PETS

Recent psychological studies have begun to uncover evidence that those who care for pets, especially dogs and cats, are better able to cope with the stressors of life (Leepson, 1984). The physical act of stroking or petting a dog or cat can be therapeutic. It provides the animal with the intuitive knowledge that it is being cared for. It also gives the individual the calming feeling of warmth, affection, and interdependence with a reliable, trusting being.

MUSIC

It is true that music can "soothe the savage beast." Both creating and listening to music stimulate motivation, enjoyment, and relaxation. Music reduces depression and brings about measurable changes in mood and general activity (Feder & Feder, 1981).

Individuals must determine what coping strategies are adaptive for them. A few examples have been presented here. A variety of therapies for assisting individuals to cope adaptively will be presented in Unit 2 of this text.

SUMMARY

Stress has become a chronic and pervasive condition in the United States today. We live in a world of uncertainties, with a sophisticated media that keeps us informed and knowledgeable about the upheavals occurring around the world. In our own country, "life in the fast lane," a continuous drive for advancement, competitiveness, and the search for "the good life" have created a stress epidemic that has individuals, corporations, and health professionals searching for ways to calm the collective masses.

The term *stress* has only recently come into vogue. This is partly due to the persistent lack of an adequate definition for the concept. Selye, who has become known as the founding father of stress research, defined stress as ". . . the state manifested by a specific syndrome which consists of all the nonspecifically-induced changes within a biologic system." He determined that physical beings respond to stressful stimuli with a predictable set of physiological changes. He described the response in three distinct stages: (1) the alarm reaction stage, (2) the stage of resistance, and (3) the stage of exhaustion. Many illnesses, or diseases of adaptation, have their origin in this aroused state, this preparation for "fight or flight."

Holmes and Rahe viewed stress not as the physiological response but as the environmental event that produced the physiological response. Their research centered around the study of life changes, or "events," that trigger the adaptive physiological and psychological responses in an individual. From their research, they devised the Social Readjustment Rating Scale, which is used to determine an individual's vulnerability to stress-related illness. This concept of stress has received criticism based on its lack of consideration of the individual's personal perception of the event, potential for coping, and available support systems at the time of the life change.

Lazarus and others have expanded the concept of stress to encompass more than just change in an individual's existing steady state or the physiological response it produces. They define stress as a relationship between the person and the environment that is appraised by the person as taxing or exceeding his or her resources and endangering his or her well-being. Response to stimuli from the internal or external environment is determined by the individual's perception of the event through cognitive appraisal. A primary appraisal is made, during which the individual determines the personal significance of the event. If the event is perceived as threatening, the individual then makes a secondary appraisal to determine the availability and effectiveness of coping strategies to manage the stressful situation. Another consideration is the predisposing factors that influence how an individual perceives and responds to a stressful event. Genetic influences, past experiences, and existing conditions strongly influence whether the response is adaptive or maladaptive.

Adaptive responses protect the individual from harm (or additional harm) and help restore homeostasis to the body. They impede the development of diseases of adaptation. With maladaptive responses conflict goes unresolved, energy resources become depleted, and the individual becomes vulnerable to physical or psychological illness.

Adaptive coping strategies for stress management are varied and individual. Becoming aware of situations that create stress and the feelings associated with the stress response is an essential foundation in successful stress management.

Relaxation can be achieved by practicing breathing exercises or progressive relaxation techniques. Some individuals relax by engaging in physical exercise, sports, or other large motor activities. *Meditation* for 20 minutes once or twice daily has been shown to be an effective stress-reduction technique for some people. *Interpersonal communica-tion with a caring other* or writing one's feelings in a journal or diary often interrupts escalation of the stress response. Using the *problem-solving/deci-sion-making model* in an objective manner (or seeking assistance in doing so during a crisis situation) is adaptive and gives the individual a feeling of control over his or her life situation. *Pet ownership* has been shown to help individuals better cope with the stressors of life. The reliability and loyalty experienced, along with the giving and receiving of warmth and affection, produce a feeling of security and provide a unique and therapeutic coping strategy for an individual. *Music* is an adaptive coping strategy that has the capacity for stimulating motivation, enjoyment, and relaxation in some people.

Individual requirements for stress reduction vary widely. Nurses are in a unique position to help individuals identify adaptive coping strategies. Stress has reached epidemic proportions in today's society, and efforts aimed at control are essential.

REVIEW QUESTIONS
Self-Examination/Learning Exercise

Test your knowledge of stress-adaptation by answering the following questions:

1. Who is the individual, known as the founding father of stress research, responsible for the recognition of a syndrome of physiological response to stressful stimuli?

2. Discuss physiological changes that occur in the initial stress response to the
   Eye:
   Respiratory system:
   Cardiovascular system:
   Gastrointestinal system
   Urinary system

3. Discuss physiological changes that occur in the sustained stress response as a result of
   Glucocorticoids:
   Mineralocorticoids:
   Vasopressin:
   Growth hormone:
   Thyrotropic hormone:
   Gonadotropins:

4. Determine your own susceptibility to illness by determining your score on the Holmes and Rahe Social Readjustment Rating Scale.

5. Name the three types of predisposing factors.

6. Match each of the following situations to its correct component of the Transactional Model of Stress/Adaptation:

_____ 1. Mr. T. is fixed in a lower level of development.

_____ 2. Mr. T's father had diabetes mellitus.

_____ 3. Mr. T. has been fired from his last five jobs.

_____ 4. Mr. T's baby was stillborn last month.

a. Precipitating stressor
b. Past experiences
c. Existing conditions
d. Genetic influences

7. Match the following types of primary appraisals to their correct definition of the event as perceived by the individual:

_____ 1. Irrelevant

_____ 2. Benign-positive

_____ 3. Harm/loss

_____ 4. Threat

_____ 5. Challenge

a. Perceived as producing pleasure
b. Perceived as anticipated harms or losses
c. Perceived as potential for gain or growth
d. Perceived as no significance to the individual
e. Perceived as damage or loss already experienced

8. Discuss some adaptive coping strategies.

REFERENCES

Feder, E. & Feder, B. (1981). *The expressive arts therapies.* Englewood Cliffs, NJ: Prentice-Hall.
Grinker, R. R. et al. (1974). *Coping and adaptation.* New York: Basic Books.
Hill, S. R. et al. (1956). Studies on adrenocortical and psychological responses to stress in man. *Arch Intern Med 97:*269–298.
Holmes, T. & Rahe, R. (1967). The Social Readjustment Rating Scale. *J Psychosom Res 11:*213–218.
Lazarus, R. S. (1966). *Psychological stress and the coping process.* New York: McGraw-Hill.
Lazarus, R. S. & Folkman, S. (1984). *Stress, appraisal and coping.* New York: Springer Publishing.
Leepson, M. (1984). *The alive and well stress book.* New York: Bantam Books.
Mason, J. W. (1971). A reevaluation of the concept of non-specificity in stress theory. *J Psychiatr Res 8:*323–333.
Murphy, L. B. & Moriarty, A. E. (1976). *Vulnerability, coping, and growth.* New Haven, CT: Yale University Press.
Pelletier, K. R. (1977). *Mind as healer, mind as slayer.* New York: Dell Publishing.
Roy, C. (1976). *Introduction to nursing: An adaptation model.* Englewood Cliffs, NJ: Prentice-Hall.
Selye, H. (1956). *The stress of life.* New York: McGraw-Hill.
Selye, H. (1974). *Stress without distress.* New York: Signet Books.
Selye, H. (1976). *The stress of life* (rev. ed.). New York: McGraw-Hill.
Wallis, C. (1983, June 6). Stress: Can we cope? *Time,* pp. 48–54.

BIBLIOGRAPHY

Bakal, D. A. (1979). *Psychology and medicine — Psychobiological dimensions of health and illness.* New York: Springer Publishing.

Johnson, B. S. (1989). *Psychiatric-mental health nursing — Adaptation and growth.* Philadelphia: JB Lippincott.

Krames Communications. (1985). *A guide to managing stress.* Daly City, CA: Krames Communications.

McCance, K. L. & Huether, S. E. (1990). *Pathophysiology — The biologic basis for disease in adults and children.* St. Louis, MO: CV Mosby.

Phipps, W. J., Long, B. C. & Woods, N. F. (1991). *Medical-surgical nursing — Concepts and clinical practice* (4th ed.). St. Louis, MO: CV Mosby.

Rachman, S. J. & Philips, C. (1980). *Psychology and behavioral medicine.* Cambridge, England: Cambridge University Press.

Stuart, G. W. & Sundeen, S. J. (1991). *Principles and practice of psychiatric nursing* (4th ed.). St. Louis, MO: CV Mosby.

MENTAL HEALTH AND MENTAL ILLNESS

OBJECTIVES

After reading this chapter, the student will be able to:

1. Define *mental health* and *mental illness.*
2. Discuss cultural elements that influence attitudes toward mental health/ mental illness.
3. Describe psychological adaptation responses to stress.
4. Identify correlation of adaptive/maladaptive behaviors to the mental health/mental illness continuum.

MENTAL HEALTH

A number of theorists have attempted to define the concept of mental health. Many of these concepts deal with various aspects of individual functioning. Maslow (1970) emphasized an individual's motivation in the continuous quest for self-actualization. He identified a "hierarchy of needs," the lower ones requiring fulfillment before those at higher levels can be achieved, with self-actualization being fulfillment of one's highest potential. Individuals may reverse their position in the hierarchy from a higher level to a lower level based on life circumstances. For example, an individual facing major surgery who has been working on tasks to achieve self-actualization may become preoccupied, if only temporarily, with the need for physiological safety. A representation of this hierarchy of needs is presented in Figure 2.1.

Maslow described self-actualization as being "psychologically healthy, fully human, highly evolved, and fully mature." He believed that "healthy," or "self-actualized," individuals possess the following characteristics:

1. An appropriate perception of reality
2. The ability to accept one's self, others, and human nature
3. The ability to manifest spontaneity
4. The capacity for focusing concentration on problem solving
5. A need for detachment and desire for privacy
6. Independence, autonomy, and a resistance to enculturation
7. An intensity of emotional reaction
8. A frequency of "peak" experiences that validate the worthwhileness, richness, and beauty of life
9. An identification with humankind
10. The ability to achieve satisfactory interpersonal relationships
11. A democratic character structure and strong sense of ethics
12. Creativeness
13. A degree of nonconformance

Jahoda (1958) has identified a list of six indicators that she suggests are a reflection of mental health:

1. *A positive attitude toward self.* This includes an objective view of self, including knowledge and acceptance of strengths and limitations. The individual feels a strong sense of personal identity and a security within the environment.
2. *Growth, development, and the ability for self-actualization.* This indicator correlates with whether the individual successfully achieves the tasks associated with each level of development (see Erikson, Chapter 3). With successful achievement in each level, the individual gains motivation for advancement to his or her highest potential.
3. *Integration.* Focus is on maintaining an equilibrium or balance among various life processes. Integration includes the ability to adaptively respond to the environment and the development of a philosophy of life, both of which help the individual maintain anxiety at a manageable level in response to stressful situations.
4. *Autonomy.* Refers to the individual's ability to perform in an independent, self-directed manner. The individual makes choices and accepts responsibility for the outcomes.
5. *Perception of reality.* Accurate reality perception is a positive indicator of mental health. This includes perception of the environment without distortion as well as the capacity for empathy and social sensitivity—a respect and concern for the wants and needs of others.
6. *Environmental mastery.* This indicator suggests that the individual has achieved a satisfactory role within the group, society, or environment. He or she is able to love and accept the love of others. Life situations are faced with the ability to strategize, make decisions, change, adjust, and adapt. Life offers satisfaction to the individual who has achieved environmental mastery.

The American Psychiatric Association (APA [1980]) defines mental health as:

". . . simultaneous success at working, loving, and creating with the capacity for mature and flexible resolution of conflicts between instincts, conscience, important other people and reality."

Robinson (1983) has offered the following definition of mental health:

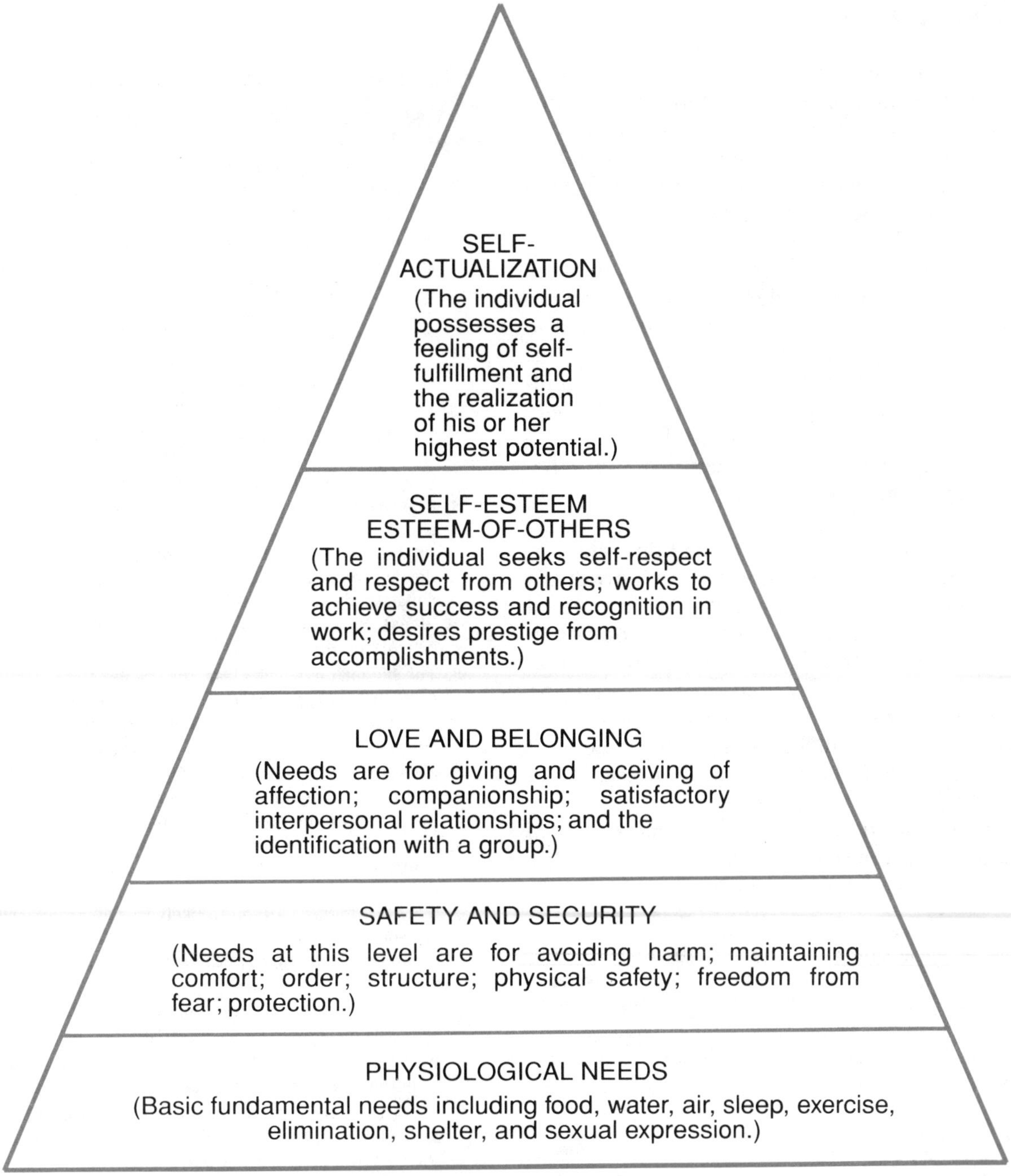

SELF-
ACTUALIZATION
(The individual
possesses a
feeling of self-
fulfillment and
the realization
of his or her
highest potential.)

SELF-ESTEEM
ESTEEM-OF-OTHERS
(The individual seeks self-respect
and respect from others; works to
achieve success and recognition in
work; desires prestige from
accomplishments.)

LOVE AND BELONGING
(Needs are for giving and receiving of
affection; companionship; satisfactory
interpersonal relationships; and the
identification with a group.)

SAFETY AND SECURITY
(Needs at this level are for avoiding harm; maintaining
comfort; order; structure; physical safety; freedom from
fear; protection.)

PHYSIOLOGICAL NEEDS
(Basic fundamental needs including food, water, air, sleep, exercise,
elimination, shelter, and sexual expression.)

Figure 2.1 Maslow's Hierarchy of Needs.

". . . a dynamic state in which thought, feeling, and behavior that is age-appropriate and congruent with the local and cultural norms is demonstrated."

For purposes of this text, and in keeping with the framework of stress/adaptation, a modification of Robinson's definition of mental health will be considered. Thus, *mental health* shall be viewed as "the successful adaptation to stressors from the internal or external environment, evidenced by thoughts, feelings, and behaviors that are age-appropriate and congruent with local and cultural norms."

MENTAL ILLNESS

A universal concept of mental illness is difficult, owing to the cultural factors that influence such a definition. However, certain elements are associated with individuals' perceptions of mental illness, regardless of cultural origin. Horwitz (1982) identifies two of these elements as (1) incomprehensibility and (2) cultural relativity.

Incomprehensibility relates to the inability of the general population to understand the motivation behind the behavior. When observers are unable to find meaning or comprehensibility in behavior, they are likely to label that behavior as mental illness. Horwitz states that, "Observers attribute labels of mental illness when the rules, conventions, and understandings they use to interpret behavior fail to find any intelligible motivation behind an action." The element of *cultural relativity* considers that these rules, conventions, and understandings are conceived within an individual's own particular culture. Behavior that is considered "normal" and "abnormal" is defined by one's cultural or societal norms. Therefore, a behavior that is recognized as mentally ill in one society may be viewed as "normal" in another society and vice versa. Horwitz identified a number of cultural aspects of mental illness, which are presented in Table 2.1.

In the *Diagnostic and Statistical Manual of Mental Disorders*, ed 3, revised (*DSM-III-R* [APA, 1987]) the APA defined mental illness or a mental disorder as:

". . . a clinically significant behavioral or psychological syndrome or pattern that occurs in a person and that is associated with present distress (a painful symptom) or disability (impairment in one or more important areas of functioning), a significantly increased risk of suffering death, pain, disability, or an important loss of freedom, . . . and is not merely an expectable response to a particular event."

For purposes of this text, and in keeping with the framework of stress/adaptation, *mental illness* will be characterized as "maladaptive responses to stressors from the internal or external environment, evidenced by thoughts, feelings, and behaviors that are incongruent with the local and cultural norms, and interfere with the individual's social, occupational, and/or physical functioning."

Table 2.1 CULTURAL ASPECTS OF MENTAL ILLNESS

1. The initial recognition that an individual's behavior deviates from the societal norms usually occurs in the lay community rather than by a psychiatric professional.

2. People who are related to an individual or who are of the same cultural or social group are less likely to label an individual's behavior as mentally ill than someone who is relationally or culturally distant. Relatives (or people of the same cultural or social group) try to "normalize" the behavior—try to find an explanation for the behavior.

3. Psychiatrists see a mentally ill person most often when the family members can no longer deny the illness—often when the behavior is at its worst. The local or cultural norms define pathological behavior.

4. The lowest social class usually displays the highest amount of mental illness symptoms. However, they tend to tolerate a wider range of behaviors that deviate from societal norms and are less likely to consider these behaviors as indicative of mental illness. Mental illness labels are most often applied by psychiatric professionals.

5. The higher the social class, the greater the recognition of mental illness behaviors. Members of the higher social class are likely to be self-labeled or labeled by family members or friends. Psychiatric assistance is sought near the first signs of emotional disturbance.

6. The more highly educated a person is, the greater the recognition of mental illness behaviors. However, even more relevant than *amount* of education is *type* of education. Those individuals in the more humanistic types of professions (lawyers, social workers, artists, teachers, nurses) are more likely to seek psychiatric assistance than professionals such as business executives, computer specialists, accountants, and engineers.

7. In terms of religion, Jewish people are more likely to seek psychiatric assistance than Catholics or Protestants.

8. Women are more likely than men to recognize the symptoms of mental illness and seek assistance.

9. The greater the cultural distance from the *mainstream* of society (i.e., the fewer the ties with *conventional* society), the greater the likelihood of negative response by society to the illness. For example, immigrants have a greater distance from the mainstream than the native born, blacks than whites, bohemians than the bourgeoisie. They are more likely to be subjected to coercive treatment, and involuntary psychiatric commitments are more common.

Source: Horwitz (1982).

PSYCHOLOGICAL ADAPTATION TO STRESS

All individuals exhibit some characteristics associated with both mental health and mental illness at any given point in time. Chapter 1 described how an individual's response to stressful situations is influenced by his or her personal perception of the event as well as a variety of predisposing factors, such as heredity, temperament, learned response patterns, developmental maturity, existing coping strategies, and support systems of caring others.

Anxiety and grief have been described as two major, primary psychological response patterns to stress. A variety of thoughts, feelings, and behaviors are associated with each of these response patterns. Adaptation is determined by the degree to which the thoughts, feelings, and behaviors interfere with an individual's functioning.

Anxiety

Anxiety has been defined as a diffuse apprehension that is vague in nature and is associated with feelings of uncertainty and helplessness (May, 1950). Feelings of anxiety are so common as to almost be considered universal in our society. Low levels of anxiety are adaptive and can provide the motivation required for survival. Anxiety becomes problematic when the individual is unable to prevent the anxiety from escalating to a level that interferes with the ability to meet basic needs.

Peplau (1963) described four levels of anxiety: mild, moderate, severe, and panic. Nurses need to be able to recognize the symptoms associated with each level to plan for appropriate intervention with anxious individuals.

1. *Mild anxiety.* This level of anxiety is seldom a problem for the individual. It is associated with the tension experienced in response to the events of day-to-day living. Mild anxiety prepares people for action. It sharpens the senses and increases motivation for productivity. The perceptual field is increased, resulting in a heightened awareness of the environment. Learning is enhanced and the individual is able to function at his or her optimal level.

2. *Moderate anxiety.* As the level of anxiety increases, the extent of the perceptual field diminishes. The moderately anxious individual is less alert to events occurring within the environment. Attention span and the ability to concentrate decrease, although the individual may still attend to needs with direction. Assistance with problem solving may be required. Increased muscular tension and restlessness are evident.

3. *Severe anxiety.* The perceptual field of the severely anxious individual is so greatly diminished that concentration centers on one particular detail only or on many extraneous details. Attention span is extremely limited, and the individual has much difficulty completing even the most simple task. Physical symptoms (e.g., headaches, palpitations, insomnia) and emotional symptoms (e.g., confusion, dread, horror) may be evident. Discomfort is experienced to the degree that virtually all overt behavior is aimed at relieving the anxiety.

4. *Panic anxiety.* In this most intense state of anxiety, the individual is unable to focus on even one detail within the environment. Misperceptions are common, and a loss of contact with reality may occur. The individual may experience hallucinations or delusions. Behavior may be characterized by wild and desperate actions or extreme withdrawal. Human functioning and communication with others are ineffective. Panic anxiety is associated with a feeling of terror, and individuals often report a "fear of dying or going insane" (APA, 1987). Prolonged panic anxiety can lead to physical and emotional exhaustion and is a life-threatening situation.

A synopsis of the characteristics associated with each of the four levels of anxiety is presented in Table 2.2.

BEHAVIORAL ADAPTATION RESPONSES TO ANXIETY

A variety of behavioral adaptation responses occur at each level of anxiety. Figure 2.2 depicts these behavioral responses on a continuum of anxiety ranging from mild to panic.

Table 2.2 LEVELS OF ANXIETY

Level	Perceptual Field	Ability to Learn	Physical Characteristics	Emotional/Behavioral Characteristics
Mild	Heightened perception (e.g., noises may seem louder; details within the environment are clearer) Increased awareness Increased alertness	Learning is enhanced	Restlessness Irritability	May remain superficial with others Rarely experienced as distressful Motivation is increased
Moderate	Reduction in perceptual field Less alert to environmental events (e.g., someone talking may not be heard; part of the room may not be noticed)	Learning still occurs but not at optimal ability Decreased attention span Decreased ability to concentrate	Increased restlessness Increased heart and respiration rate Increased perspiration Gastric discomfort Increased muscular tension Increase in speech rate, volume, and pitch	A feeling of discontent May lead to a degree of impairment in interpersonal relationships as individual begins to focus on self and the need to relieve personal discomfort
Severe	Greatly diminished Only extraneous details are perceived, or fixation on a single detail may occur May not take notice of an event even when attention is directed by another	Extremely limited attention span Unable to concentrate or problem solve Effective learning cannot occur	Headaches Dizziness Nausea Trembling Insomnia Palpitations Tachycardia Hyperventilation Urinary frequency Diarrhea	Feelings of dread, loathing, and horror Total focus on self and intense desire to relieve the anxiety
Panic	Unable to focus on even one detail within the environment Misperceptions of the environment are common (e.g., a perceived detail may be elaborated and out of proportion)	Learning cannot occur Unable to concentrate Unable to comprehend even simple directions	Dilated pupils Labored breathing Severe trembling Sleeplessness Palpitations Diaphoresis and pallor Muscular incoordination Immobility or purposeless hyperactivity Incoherence or inability to verbalize	Sense of impending doom Terror Bizarre behavior, including shouting, screaming, running about wildly, clinging to anyone or anything from which a sense of safety and security is derived Hallucinations, delusions Extreme withdrawal into the self

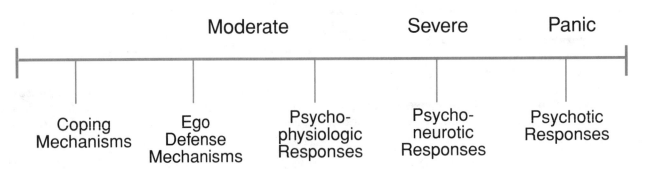

Figure 2.2 Adaptation responses on a continuum of anxiety.

Mild Anxiety At the mild level individuals employ any of a number of coping behaviors that satisfy their needs for comfort. Menninger et al. (1963) described the following types of coping mechanisms that individuals use to relieve anxiety in stressful situations:

- sleeping
- eating
- physical exercise
- smoking
- crying
- pacing
- foot swinging
- fidgeting
- yawning
- drinking
- daydreaming
- laughing
- cursing
- nail biting
- finger tapping
- talking to someone with whom one feels comfortable

Undoubtedly there are many more responses too numerous to mention here, considering that each individual develops his or her own unique ways to relieve anxiety at the mild level. Some of these behaviors are much more adaptive than others.

Mild-to-Moderate Anxiety Sigmund Freud identified the ego as the reality component of the personality that governs problem solving and rational thinking. As the level of anxiety increases, the strength of the ego is tested, and energy is mobilized to confront the threat. Anna Freud (1953) identified a number of defense mechanisms employed by the ego in the face of threat to biological or psychological integrity. Some of these ego defense mechanisms are more adaptive than others, but all are used either consciously or unconsciously as a protective device for the ego in an effort to relieve mild-to-moderate anxiety. They become maladaptive when they are "used to such an extreme degree that they distort reality, interfere with interpersonal relationships, limit one's ability to work productively, and promote ego disintegration instead of self-integrity" (Stuart & Sundeen, 1987). The major ego defense mechanisms identified by Anna Freud are:

1. *Compensation*—covering up a real or perceived weakness by emphasizing a trait one considers more desirable. *Examples:* (a) A handicapped boy who is unable to participate in sports compensates by becoming a great scholar. (b) A young man, the shortest among members of his peer group, views this as a deficiency and compensates by being overly aggressive and daring.
2. *Denial*—refusing to acknowledge the existence of a real situation or the feelings associated with it. *Examples:* (a) A woman is told by her family doctor that she has a lump in her breast, and an appointment is made for her with a surgeon; however, she does not keep the appointment and goes about her activities of daily living with no evidence of concern. (b) Individuals continue to smoke cigarettes even though they have been told of the health risk involved.
3. *Displacement*—transferring feelings from one target to another that is considered less threatening or neutral. *Examples:* (a) A man who is passed over for promotion on his job belittles his son for not making the basketball team. (b) A boy who is teased and hit by the class bully on the playground comes home after school and kicks his dog.
4. *Identification*—attempting to increase self-worth by acquiring certain attributes and characteristics of an individual one admires. *Examples:* (a) A teenage girl emulates the mannerisms and style of dress of a popular female rock star. (b) The young son of a famous civil rights worker adopts his father's attitudes and behaviors with the intent of pursuing similar aspirations.
5. *Intellectualization*—attempting to avoid expressing actual emotions associated with a stressful situation by using the intellectual processes of logic, reasoning, and analysis. *Examples:* (a) A man whose brother is in the critical care unit following a severe myocardial infarction (MI) spends his allotted visiting time in discussion with the nurse analyzing test results and making a reasonable determination about the pathophysiology that may have occurred to induce the MI. (b) A young psychology professor receives a letter from his fiancee breaking off their engagement. He shows no emotion when discussing this with his best friend. Instead he analyzes his fiancee's behavior and tries to reason why the relationship failed.
6. *Introjection*—internalizing the beliefs and values of another individual such that they symbolically become a part of the self to the extent that the feeling of separateness or distinctness is lost. *Examples:* (a) A small child develops his or her conscience by internalizing what the parents believe is right and

wrong. The parents literally become a part of the child. The child says to a friend while playing, "Don't hit people. It's not nice!" (b) A psychiatric patient claims to be the son of God, drapes his/herself in sheet and blanket, "performs miracles" on other patients, and refuses to respond unless addressed as Jesus Christ.

7. *Isolation*—separating thought or a memory from the feeling tone or emotions associated with it (sometimes called *emotional isolation*). *Examples:* (a) A young woman describes being attacked and raped by a street gang. She displays an apathetic expression and no emotional tone. (b) A physician is able to isolate his feelings about the eventual death of a terminally ill cancer patient by focusing his attention instead on the chemotherapy that will be given.

8. *Projection*—attributing feelings or impulses unacceptable to one's self to another person. The individual "passes the blame" for these undesirable feelings or impulses to another, thereby providing relief from the anxiety associated with them. *Examples:* (a) A young soldier who has an extreme fear of participating in military combat tells his sergeant that the others in his unit are "a bunch of cowards." (b) A businessman who values punctuality is late for a meeting. He states, "Sorry I'm late. My secretary forgot to remind me of the time. It's so hard to find good help these days."

9. *Rationalization*—attempting to make excuses or formulate logical reasons to justify unacceptable feelings or behaviors. *Examples:* (a) A young woman is turned down for a secretary's job after a poor performance on a typing test. She claims, "I'm sure I could have done a better job on a word processor. Hardly anyone uses an electric typewriter anymore!" (b) A young man is unable to afford the sports car he wants so desperately. He tells the salesperson, "I'd buy this car, but I'll be getting married soon. This is really not the car for a family man."

10. *Reaction formation*—preventing unacceptable or undesirable thoughts or behaviors from being expressed by exaggerating opposite thoughts or types of behaviors. *Ex-*

amples: (a) The young soldier who has an extreme fear of participating in military combat volunteers for dangerous frontline duty. (b) A secretary is sexually attracted to her boss and feels an intense dislike toward his wife. She treats her boss with detachment and aloofness while performing her secretarial duties and is overly courteous, polite, and flattering to his wife when she comes to the office.

11. *Regression*—retreating to an earlier level of development and the comfort measures associated with that level of functioning. *Examples:* (a) When mother brings his new baby sister home from the hospital, 4-year-old Tommy, who has been toilet trained for more than a year, begins to wet his pants, cry to be held, and suck his thumb. (b) The person who is depressed may withdraw to his or her room, curl up in a fetal position on the bed, and sleep for long periods of time.

12. *Repression*—involuntarily blocking unpleasant feelings and experiences from one's awareness. *Examples:* (a) A woman cannot remember being sexually assaulted when she was 15 years old. (b) A teenage boy cannot remember driving the car that was involved in an accident in which his best friend was killed.

13. *Sublimation*—rechanneling of drives or impulses that are personally or socially unacceptable (e.g., aggressiveness, anger, sexual drives) into activities that are more tolerable and constructive. *Examples:* (a) A teenage boy with strong competitive and aggressive drives becomes the star football player on his high school team. (b) A young unmarried woman with a strong desire for marriage and a family achieves satisfaction and success in establishing and operating a day-care center for preschool children.

14. *Suppression*—voluntarily blocking unpleasant feelings and experiences from one's awareness. *Examples:* (a) Scarlett O'Hara says, "I'll think about that tomorrow." (b) A young woman who is depressed about a pending divorce proceeding tells the nurse, "I just don't want to talk about the divorce. There's nothing I can do about it anyway."

15. *Undoing*—symbolically negating or cancel-

ing out a previous action or experience that one finds intolerable. *Examples:* (a) A man spills some salt on the table, then sprinkles some over his left shoulder to "prevent bad luck." (b) A man who is anxious about giving a presentation at work yells at his wife during breakfast. He stops on his way home from work that evening to buy her a dozen red roses.

Moderate-to-Severe Anxiety Anxiety at the moderate-to-severe level that remains unresolved over an extended period of time can contribute to a number of physiological disorders. The *DSM-III-R* (APA, 1987) describes these disorders as "any physical condition to which psychological factors are judged to be contributory." The physical condition will usually be a physical disorder but in some instances may be only a single symptom, such as vomiting. The condition is initiated or exacerbated by an environmental situation that the individual perceives as stressful. Measurable pathophysiology can be demonstrated.

Common examples of psychophysiologic conditions include but are not limited to tension and migraine headaches, angina pectoris, obesity, anorexia nervosa, bulimia nervosa, rheumatoid arthritis, ulcerative colitis, gastric and duodenal ulcers, asthma, irritable bowel syndrome, nausea and vomiting, gastritis, cardiac arrhythmias, premenstrual syndrome, muscle spasms/pain, sexual dysfunction, and cancer (APA, 1987; Kaplan & Sadock, 1985; LeShan, 1977; Halmi, 1982; Mims & Swensen, 1980). A more comprehensive discussion of specific psychophysiological disorders is presented in Chapter 25.

Severe Anxiety Extended periods of repressed severe anxiety can result in psychoneurotic patterns of behaving. *Neuroses* are no longer a separate category of disorders in the *DSM-III-R* (APA, 1987). However, the term is still used in the *DSM-III-R* to further describe the symptomatology of certain disorders. Neuroses are psychiatric disturbances, characterized by excessive anxiety or depression, disrupted bodily functions, unsatisfying interpersonal relationships, and behaviors that interfere with routine functioning (Kirkham, 1980). People with neuroses:

1. Are aware that they are experiencing distress

2. Are aware that their behaviors are maladaptive
3. Are unaware of any possible psychological causes of the distress
4. Feel helpless to change their situation
5. Experience no loss of contact with reality

The following disorders are examples of psychoneurotic responses to anxiety as they appear in the *DSM-III-R*. They are discussed in this text in Chapters 20, 21, and 22.

1. **Anxiety disorders:** Disorders in which the characteristic features are symptoms of anxiety and avoidance behavior (e.g., phobias, obsessive-compulsive disorder).
2. **Somatoform disorders:** Disorders in which the characteristic features are physical symptoms for which no organic pathology is demonstrable and for which positive evidence or strong implications of psychological conflicts exist (e.g., hypochondriasis, conversion disorder).
3. **Dissociative disorders:** Disorders in which the characteristic feature is a disturbance or alteration in identity, memory, or consciousness (e.g., multiple personality disorder, psychogenic amnesia).

Panic Anxiety At this extreme level of anxiety, an individual is not capable of processing what is happening in the environment and may lose contact with reality. *Psychosis* is defined as a gross disorganization of the personality in which marked disturbance is seen in reality testing (APA, 1987). Psychoses are serious psychiatric disturbances characterized by the presence of delusions or hallucinations and the impairment of interpersonal functioning and relationship to the external world. People with psychoses:

1. Experience minimal distress (emotional tone is flat, bland, or inappropriate)
2. Are unaware that their behavior is maladaptive
3. Are unaware of any psychological problems
4. Are exhibiting a flight from reality into a less stressful world or into one in which they are attempting to adapt

Examples of psychotic responses to anxiety include the schizophrenic, schizoaffective, and delusional disorders. They are discussed at length in Chapter 18.

Grief

Grief is a subjective state of emotional, physical, and social responses to the loss of a valued entity. The loss may be *real*, in which case it can be substantiated by others (e.g., death of a loved one, loss of personal possessions), or it may be *perceived* by the individual alone and unable to be shared or identified by others (e.g., loss of the feeling of femininity following mastectomy). Any situation that creates *change* for an individual can be identified as a loss. *Failure* (either real or perceived) can be viewed as a loss.

The loss, or anticipated loss, of anything of value to the individual can trigger the grief response. This period of characteristic emotions and behaviors is called *mourning*. The "normal" mourning process is adaptive and is characterized by feelings of sadness, guilt, anger, helplessness, hopelessness, and despair. Indeed, an absence of mourning could be considered maladaptive.

STAGES OF GRIEF

Kübler-Ross (1969), in extensive research with terminally ill patients, identified five stages of feelings and behaviors that individuals experience in response to a real, perceived, or anticipated loss:

Stage 1 — Denial This is a stage of shock and disbelief. The response may be one of "No, it can't be true!" The reality of the loss is not acknowledged. Denial is a protective mechanism that allows the individual to cope within an immediate time frame while organizing more effective defense strategies.

Stage 2 — Anger "Why me?" and "It's not fair!" are comments often expressed during the anger stage. Envy and resentment toward individuals not affected by the loss are common. Anger may be directed at the self or displaced on loved ones, caregivers, and even God. There may be a preoccupation with an idealized image of the lost entity.

Stage 3 — Bargaining "If God will help me through this, I promise I will go to church every Sunday and volunteer my time to help others." During this stage, which is generally not visible or evident to others, a "bargain" is made with God in an attempt to reverse or postpone the loss. Some-

times the promise is associated with feelings of guilt for not having performed satisfactorily, appropriately, or sufficiently.

Stage 4 — Depression During this stage, the full impact of the loss is experienced. The sense of loss is intense and feelings of sadness and depression prevail. This is a time of quiet desperation and disengagement from all association with the lost entity. This stage differs from pathological depression in that this is a stage of advancement toward resolution rather than the fixation in an earlier stage of the grief process.

Stage 5 — Acceptance The final stage brings a feeling of peace regarding the loss that has occurred. It is a time of quiet expectation and resignation. Focus is on the reality of the loss and its meaning for the individuals affected by it.

All individuals do not experience each of these stages in response to a loss, nor do they necessarily experience them in this order. Some individuals' grieving behaviors may fluctuate, and even overlap, between stages.

ANTICIPATORY GRIEF

When a loss is anticipated, individuals often begin the work of grieving before the actual loss occurs. Most people re-experience the grieving behaviors once the loss occurs, but having this time to prepare for the loss can facilitate the process of mourning, actually decreasing the length and intensity of the response. Problems arise, particularly in anticipating the death of a loved one, when family members experience anticipatory grieving and the mourning process is completed prematurely. They disengage emotionally from the dying person, who may then experience feelings of being rejected by loved ones at a time when this psychological support is so necessary.

RESOLUTION

The grief response can last from weeks to years. It cannot be hurried, and individuals must be allowed to progress at their own pace. In the loss of a loved one, grief work usually lasts for at least a year, during which the grieving person experiences each significant "anniversary" date for the first time without the loved one present.

Length of the grief process may be prolonged by a number of factors. If the relationship with the lost entity had been marked by ambivalence or if there had been an enduring "love-hate" association, reaction to the loss may be burdened with guilt. Guilt lengthens the grief reaction by promoting feelings of anger toward the self for having committed a wrongdoing or behaved in an unacceptable manner toward that which is now lost, even perhaps to feeling that one's behavior contributed to the loss.

Anticipatory grieving is thought to shorten the grief response in some individuals who are able to work through some of the feelings prior to occurrence of the loss. If the loss is sudden and unexpected, mourning may take longer than it would if individuals were able to grieve in anticipation of the loss.

Length of the grieving process is also affected by the number of recent losses experienced by an individual and whether he or she is able to complete one grieving process before another loss occurs. This is particularly true for elderly individuals who may be experiencing numerous losses, such as spouse, friends, other relatives, independent functioning, home, personal possessions, and pets, in a relatively short period of time. Grief accumulates, and this represents a type of *bereavement overload*, which for some individuals presents an impossible task of grief work.

Resolution of the process of mourning is thought to have occurred when an individual can look back on the relationship with the lost entity and accept both the pleasures and the disappointments (both the positive and the negative aspects) of the association (Bowlby & Parkes, 1970). Disorganization and emotional pain have been experienced and tolerated. Preoccupation with the lost entity has been replaced with energy and desire to pursue new situations and relationships.

MALADAPTIVE GRIEF RESPONSES

Maladaptive responses to loss occur when an individual is not able to satisfactorily progress through the stages of grieving to achieve resolution. Maladaptive responses generally occur when an individual becomes fixed in the denial or anger stages of the grief process. Several types of grief responses have been identified as pathological (Lindemann, 1944; Parkes, 1972; Jackson, 1957). They include responses that are prolonged, delayed/inhibited, or distorted. The *prolonged* response is characterized by an intense preoccupation with

memories of the lost entity for *many years after the loss has occurred*. Behaviors associated with the stages of denial or anger are manifested, and disorganization of functioning and intense emotional pain related to the lost entity are evidenced.

In the *delayed or inhibited* response, the individual becomes fixed in the denial stage of the grieving process. The emotional pain associated with the loss is not experienced, but there may be evidence of anxiety disorders (e.g., phobias, hypochondriasis) or sleeping and eating disorders (e.g., insomnia, anorexia). The individual may remain in denial for many years until the grief response is triggered by a reminder of the loss or even by another unrelated loss.

The individual who experiences a *distorted* response is fixed in the anger stage of grieving. In the distorted response, all the normal behaviors associated with grieving, such as helplessness, hopelessness, sadness, anger, and guilt, are exaggerated out of proportion to the situation. The individual turns the anger inward on the self, is consumed with overwhelming despair, and is unable to function in normal activities of daily living. Pathological depression is a distorted grief response (see Chapter 19).

MENTAL HEALTH/MENTAL ILLNESS CONTINUUM

Anxiety and grief have been described as two major, primary responses to stress. In Figure 2.3, both of these responses are presented on a continuum according to the degree of symptom severity. Disorders as they appear in the *DSM-III-R* are identified at their appropriate placement along the continuum.

THE *DSM-III-R* MULTIAXIAL EVALUATION SYSTEM

The APA endorses case evaluation on a multiaxial system, "to ensure that attention is given to certain types of disorders, aspects of the environment, and areas of functioning that might be overlooked if the focus were on assessing a single presenting problem." Each individual is evaluated on five axes. They are defined by the *DSM-III-R* in the following manner:

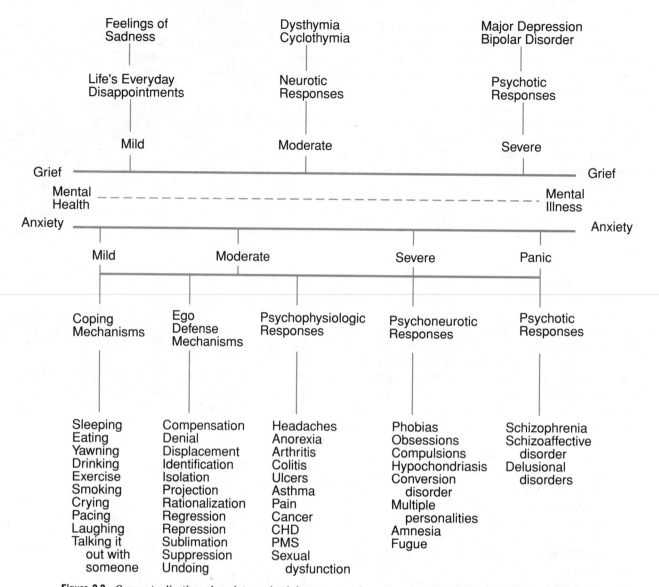

Figure 2.3 Conceptualization of anxiety and grief responses along the mental health/mental illness continuum.

Axis I — clinical syndromes and V codes: Includes all mental disorders (except developmental disorders and personality disorders) and V codes (conditions that are not attributable to a mental disorder but are a focus of attention or treatment)

Axis II — developmental disorders and personality disorders: These disorders generally begin in childhood or adolescence and persist in a stable form into adult life.

Axis III — physical disorders and conditions: Any current physical disorder or condition that is potentially relevant to the understanding or management of the case.

Axis IV — severity of psychosocial stressors: Used in special clinical and research settings, rates overall severity of stressors occurring during the previous year on a scale from 1 to 6 (none to catastrophic).

Axis V — global assessment of functioning: Used in special clinical and research settings, allows the clinician to rate the individual's overall functioning on the Global Assessment of Functioning Scale, which assesses mental health and mental illness.

The *DSM-III-R* outline of Axes I and II categories and codes is presented in Table 2.3.

Table 2.3 *DSM-III-R* CLASSIFICATION: AXES I AND II CATEGORIES AND CODES

DISORDERS USUALLY FIRST EVIDENT IN INFANCY, CHILDHOOD, OR ADOLESCENCE

Developmental Disorders
(NOTE: Coded on Axis II)

Mental Retardation
317.00 Mild mental retardation
318.00 Moderate mental retardation
318.10 Severe mental retardation
318.20 Profound mental retardation
319.00 Unspecified mental retardation

Pervasive Developmental Disorders
299.00 Autistic disorder
299.80 Pervasive developmental disorder NOS*

Specific Developmental Disorders
Academic skills disorders
315.10 Developmental arithmetic disorder
315.80 Developmental expressive writing disorder
315.00 Developmental reading disorder

Language and speech disorders
315.39 Developmental articulation disorder
315.31 Developmental expressive language disorder
315.31 Developmental receptive language disorder†

Motor skills disorder
315.40 Developmental coordination disorder
315.90 Specific developmental disorder NOS

Other Developmental Disorders
315.90 Developmental disorder NOS

Disruptive Behavior Disorders
314.01 Attention-deficit hyperactivity disorder
Conduct Disorder
312.20   Group type
312.00   Solitary aggressive type
312.90   Undifferentiated type
313.81 Oppositional defiant disorder

Anxiety Disorders of Childhood or Adolescence
309.21 Separation anxiety disorder
313.21 Avoidant disorder of childhood or adolescence
313.00 Overanxious disorder

Eating Disorders
307.10 Anorexia nervosa
307.51 Bulimia nervosa
307.52 Pica
307.53 Rumination disorder of infancy
307.50 Eating disorder NOS

Gender Identity Disorders
302.60 Gender identity disorder of childhood
302.50 Transsexualism (specify) asexual, homosexual, heterosexual, unspecified
302.85 Gender identity disorder of adolescence or adulthood, nontranssexual type (specify) asexual, homosexual, heterosexual, unspecified
302.85 Gender identity disorder NOS

Tic Disorders
307.23 Tourette's disorder
307.22 Chronic motor or vocal tic disorder
307.21 Transient tic disorder
307.20 Tic disorder NOS

Elimination Disorders
307.70 Functional encopresis
307.60 Functional enuresis

Speech Disorders Not Elsewhere Classified
307.00 Cluttering
307.00 Stuttering

Other Disorders of Infancy, Childhood, or Adolescence
313.23 Elective mutism
313.82 Identity disorder
313.89 Reactive attachment disorder of infancy or early childhood
307.30 Stereotypy/habit disorder
314.00 Undifferentiated attention-deficit disorder

ORGANIC MENTAL DISORDERS

Dementias Arising in the Senium and Presenium
Primary degenerative dementia of the Alzheimer type, senile onset
290.30 With delirium
290.20 With delusions
290.21 With depression
290.00 Uncomplicated

Primary degenerative dementia of the Alzheimer type, presenile onset
290.11 With delirium
290.12 With delusions
290.13 With depression
290.10 Uncomplicated

Multi-infarct dementia
290.41 With delirium
290.42 With delusions
290.43 With depression
290.10 Uncomplicated

290.00 Senile dementia NOS
290.10 Presenile dementia NOS

Psychoactive Substance-Induced Organic Mental Disorders
Alcohol
303.00 Intoxication
291.40 Idiosyncratic intoxication
291.80 Uncomplicated withdrawal
291.00 Withdrawal delirium
291.30 Hallucinosis
291.10 Amnestic disorder
291.20 Demenia

Amphetamine or similarly acting sympathomimetic
305.70 Intoxication
292.00 Withdrawal
292.81 Delirium
292.11 Delusional disorder

(continued)

Table 2.3   CONTINUED

Psychoactive Substance-Induced Organic Mental Disorders
(*Continued*)
Caffeine
305.90 Intoxication

Cannabis
305.20 Intoxication
292.11 Delusional disorder

Cocaine
305.60 Intoxication
292.00 Withdrawal
292.81 Delirium
292.11 Delusional disorder

Hallucinogen
305.30 Hallucinosis
292.11 Delusional disorder
292.84 Mood disorder
292.89 Posthallucinogen perception disorder

Inhalant
305.90 Intoxication

Nicotine
292.00 Withdrawal

Opioid
305.50 Intoxication
292.00 Withdrawal

Phencyclidine (PCP) or similarly acting arylcyclohexylamine
305.90 Intoxication
292.81 Delirium
292.11 Delusional disorder
292.84 Mood disorder
292.90 Organic mental disorder NOS

Sedative, hypnotic, or anxiolytic
305.40 Intoxication
292.00 Uncomplicated withdrawal
292.00 Withdrawal delirium
292.83 Amnestic disorder

Other or unspecified psychoactive substance
305.90 Intoxication
292.00 Withdrawal
292.81 Delirium
292.82 Dementia
292.83 Amnestic disorder
292.11 Delusional disorder
292.12 Hallucinosis
292.84 Mood disorder
292.89 Anxiety disorder
292.89 Personality disorder
292.90 Organic mental disorder NOS

Organic Mental Disorders Associated with Axis III Physical Disorders or Conditions, or Whose Etiology Is Unknown
293.00 Delirium
294.10 Dementia
294.00 Amnestic disorder
293.81 Organic delusional disorder
293.82 Organic hallucinosis
293.83 Organic mood disorder (specify) manic, depressed, mixed

294.80 Organic anxiety disorder
310.10 Organic personality disorder
294.80 Organic mental disorder NOS

PSYCHOACTIVE SUBSTANCE USE DISORDERS
Alcohol
303.90 Dependence
305.00 Abuse

Amphetamine or similarly acting sympathomimetic
304.40 Dependence
305.70 Abuse

Cannabis
304.30 Dependence
305.20 Abuse

Cocaine
304.20 Dependence
305.60 Abuse

Hallucinogen
304.50 Dependence
305.30 Abuse

Inhalant
304.60 Dependence
305.90 Abuse

Nicotine
305.10 Dependence

Opioid
304.00 Dependence
305.50 Abuse

Phencyclidine (PCP) or similarly acting arylcyclohexylamine
304.50 Dependence
305.90 Abuse

Sedative, hypnotic, or anxiolytic
304.10 Dependence
305.40 Abuse

304.90 Polysubstance dependence
304.90 Psychoactive substance dependence NOS
305.90 Psychoactive substance abuse NOS

SCHIZOPHRENIA
(Code in fifth digit: 1 = subchronic, 2 = chronic,
3 = subchronic with acute exacerbation, 4 = chronic with
acute exacerbation, 5 = in remission, 0 = unspecified.)

Schizophrenia
295.2x Catatonic,_____
295.1x Disorganized,_____
295.3x Paranoid,_____
295.9x Undifferentiated,_____
295.6x Residual,_____

DELUSIONAL (PARANOID) DISORDERS
297.10 Delusional (paranoid) disorder
    Specify type: erotomanic
         grandiose
         jealous
         persecutory
         somatic
         unspecified

(*continued*)

Table 2.3   CONTINUED

PSYCHOTIC DISORDERS NOT ELSEWHERE CLASSIFIED

298.80 Brief reactive psychosis
295.40 Schizophreniform disorder
295.70 Schizoaffective disorder
         Specify: bipolar type or depressive type
297.30 Induced psychotic disorder
298.90 Psychotic disorder NOS (Atypical psychosis)

MOOD DISORDERS

Code current state of major depression and bipolar disorder
in fifth digit:

  1 = mild
  2 = moderate
  3 = severe, without psychotic features
  4 = with psychotic features
  5 = in partial remission
  6 = in full remission
  0 = unspecified

Bipolar Disorders

         Bipolar Disorder
296.6x   mixed,_____
296.4x   manic,_____
296.5x   depressed,_____
301.13 Cyclothymia
296.70 Bipolar disorder NOS

Depressive Disorders

         Major Depression
296.2x   single episode,_____
296.3x   recurrent,_____
300.40 Dysthymia (depressive neurosis)
311.00 Depressive disorder NOS

ANXIETY DISORDERS

         Panic disorder
300.21   With agoraphobia
300.01   Without agoraphobia
300.22 Agoraphobia without history of panic disorder
300.23 Social phobia
300.29 Simple phobia
300.30 Obsessive compulsive disorder
309.89 Post-traumatic stress disorder
300.02 Generalized anxiety disorder
300.00 Anxiety disorder NOS

SOMATOFORM DISORDERS

300.70 Body dysmorphic disorder
300.11 Conversion disorder
300.70 Hypochondriasis
300.81 Somatization disorder
307.80 Somatoform pain disorder
300.70 Undifferentiated somatoform disorder
300.70 Somatoform disorder NOS

DISSOCIATIVE DISORDERS

300.14 Multiple personality disorder
300.13 Psychogenic fugue
300.12 Psychogenic amnesia
300.60 Depersonalization disorder
300.15 Dissociative disorder NOS

SEXUAL DISORDERS

Paraphilias
302.40 Exhibitionism
302.81 Fetishism
302.89 Frotteurism
302.20 Pedophilia
302.83 Sexual masochism
302.84 Sexual sadism
302.30 Transvestic fetishism
302.82 Voyeurism
302.90 Paraphilia NOS

Sexual Dysfunctions

Sexual desire disorders
302.71 Hypoactive sexual desire disorder
302.79 Sexual aversion disorder
302.72 Female sexual arousal disorder
302.72 Male erectile disorder

Orgasm disorders
302.73 Inhibited female orgasm
302.74 Inhibited male orgasm
302.75 Premature ejaculation

Sexual pain disorders
302.76 Dyspareunia
306.51 Vaginismus
302.70 Sexual dysfunction NOS

Other Sexual Disorders

302.90 Sexual disorder NOS

SLEEP DISORDERS

Dyssomnias

         Insomnia disorder
307.42   Related to another mental disorder (nonorganic)
780.50   Related to known organic factor
307.42 Primary insomnia

         Hypersomnia disorder
307.44   Related to another mental disorder (nonorganic)
780.50   Related to known organic factor
780.54 Primary hypersomnia
307.45 Sleep-wake schedule disorder
307.40 Dyssomnia NOS

Parasomnias

307.47 Dream anxiety disorder (nightmare disorder)
307.46 Sleep terror disorder
307.46 Sleepwalking disorder
307.40 Parasomnia NOS

FACTITIOUS DISORDERS

         Factitious disorder
301.51   With physical symptoms
300.16   With psychological symptoms
300.19 Factitious disorder NOS

IMPULSE CONTROL DISORDERS NOT ELSEWHERE CLASSIFIED

312.34 Intermittent explosive disorder
312.32 Kleptomania
312.31 Pathological gambling

(continued)

Table 2.3   CONTINUED

IMPULSE CONTROL DISORDERS NOT ELSEWHERE CLASSIFIED (*Continued*)
312.33 Pyromania
312.39 Trichotillomania
312.39 Impulse control disorder NOS

ADJUSTMENT DISORDER

Adjustment disorder
309.24 With anxious mood
309.00 With depressed mood
309.30 With disturbance of conduct
309.40 With mixed disturbance of emotions and conduct
309.28 With mixed emotional features
309.82 With physical complaints
309.83 With withdrawal
309.23 With work (or academic) inhibition
309.90 Adjustment disorder NOS

PSYCHOLOGICAL FACTORS AFFECTING PHYSICAL CONDITION
316.00 Psychological factors affecting physical condition
(specify physical condition on Axis III)

PERSONALITY DISORDERS
(Note: Coded on Axis II)

Cluster A
301.00 Paranoid
301.20 Schizoid
301.22 Schizotypal

Cluster B
301.70 Antisocial
301.83 Borderline
301.50 Histrionic
301.81 Narcissistic

Cluster C
301.82 Avoidant
301.60 Dependent
301.40 Obsessive-compulsive
301.84 Passive aggressive
301.90 Personality disorder NOS

V CODES FOR CONDITIONS NOT ATTRIBUTABLE TO A MENTAL DISORDER THAT ARE A FOCUS OF ATTENTION OR TREATMENT
V62.30 Academic problem
V71.01 Adult antisocial behavior
V40.00 Borderline intellectual functioning (Note: coded on Axis II)
V71.02 Childhood or adolescent antisocial behavior
V65.20 Malingering
V61.10 Marital problem
V15.81 Noncompliance with medical treatment
V62.20 Occupational problem
V61.20 Parent-child problem
V62.81 Other interpersonal problem
V61.80 Other specified family circumstances
V62.89 Phase of life problem or other life circumstance problem
V62.82 Uncomplicated bereavement

ADDITIONAL CODES
300.90 Unspecified mental disorder
V71.09 No diagnosis or condition on Axis I
799.90 Diagnosis deferred on Axis I
V71.09 No diagnosis or condition on Axis II
799.90 Diagnosis deferred on Axis II

---

*NOS = Not Otherwise Specified
†Some codes appear more than once to maintain compatability with the ICD-9-CM.
Source: From APA, 1987, pp. 3–10.

SUMMARY

Various definitions of mental health and mental illness from the literature were presented. For purposes of this text, mental health is defined as "the successful adaptation to stressors from the internal or external environment, evidenced by thoughts, feelings, and behaviors that are age-appropriate and congruent with local and cultural norms." Mental illness is defined as "maladaptive responses to stressors from the internal or external environment, evidenced by thoughts, feelings, and behaviors that are incongruent with the local and cultural norms, and interfere with the individual's social, occupational, and/or physical functioning."

Most cultures label behavior as mental illness on the basis of *incomprehensibility* and *cultural relativity*. When observers are unable to find meaning or comprehensibility in behavior, they are likely to label that behavior as mental illness. The meaning of behaviors is determined within individual cultures.

Anxiety and *grief* have been identified as the two major, primary responses to stress. Peplau (1963) defined anxiety by levels of symptom severity: mild, moderate, severe, and panic. Behaviors associated with levels of anxiety include coping mechanisms, ego defense mechanisms, psychophysiological responses, psychoneurotic responses, and psychotic responses.

Grief is described as a response to loss of a valued entity. Stages of normal mourning as identified by Kübler-Ross (1969) are denial, anger, bargaining, depression, and acceptance. Anticipatory grief is grief work that is begun, and sometimes completed, prior to the occurrence of the loss. Resolution is thought to occur when an individual is able to remember and accept both the positive and negative aspects associated with the lost entity. Griev-

ing is thought to be maladaptive when the mourning process is prolonged, delayed/inhibited, or becomes distorted and exaggerated out of proportion to the situation. Pathological depression is considered to be a distorted reaction. The behaviors and associated disorders of anxiety and grief were presented on the mental health/mental illness continuum.

The *DSM-III-R* multiaxial system of diagnostic classification was explained and an outline of Axes I and II categories and codes was presented.

REVIEW QUESTIONS
Self-Examination/Learning Exercise

Test your knowledge of the concepts of mental health and mental illness by completing the following exercises:

1. Define *mental health.*
2. Define *mental illness.*
3. Describe how *incomprehensibility* and *cultural relativity* influence the labeling of behaviors as mental illness.
4. Match the following definitions with the correct level of anxiety:

   _____ 1. Mild

   _____ 2. Moderate

   _____ 3. Severe

   _____ 4. Panic

   a. Perceptual field greatly diminished; concentrates on one detail only; limited attention span; all behavior aimed at relief.

   b. Increased awareness; sharpened senses; increased motivation for productivity; learning is enhanced.

   c. Unable to focus on even one detail; misperceptions of the environment; loss of contact with reality; ineffective functioning.

   d. Decreased attention span, although may still attend to needs with direction; needs assistance with problem solving; increased muscular tension and restlessness.

5. Match the following defense mechanisms to the appropriate situation.

_____ 1. Compensation

_____ 2. Denial

_____ 3. Displacement

_____ 4. Identification

_____ 5. Intellectualization

_____ 6. Introjection

_____ 7. Isolation

_____ 8. Projection

_____ 9. Rationalization

_____ 10. Reaction formation

_____ 11. Regression

_____ 12. Repression

_____ 13. Sublimation

_____ 14. Suppression

_____ 15. Undoing

a. Tommy, who is small for his age, is teased at school by the older boys. When he gets home from school, he yells at and hits his little sister.

b. Johnny is in a wheelchair due to paralysis of the lower limbs. Before his accident, he was the star athlete on the football team. Now he obsessively strives to maintain a 4.0 grade point average in his courses.

c. Nancy and Sally are 4 years old. While playing with their dolls, Nancy says to Sally, "Don't hit your dollie. It's not nice to hit people!"

d. Jackie is 4 years old. He has wanted a baby brother very badly, yet when his mother brings the new sibling home from the hospital, Jackie cries to be held when the baby is being fed and even starts to soil his clothing, although he has been toilet trained for 2 years.

e. A young man is late for class. He tells the professor, "Sorry I'm late, but my stupid wife forgot to set the alarm last night!"

f. Nancy was emotionally abused as a child and hates her mother. However, when she talks to others about her mother, she tells them how wonderful she is and how much she loves her.

g. Pete grew up in a rough neighborhood where fighting was a way of coping. He is tough and aggressive and is noticed by the football coach, who makes him a member of the team. Within the year, he becomes the star player.

5. (cont'd)

h. Fred stops at the bar every night after work and has several drinks. During the past 6 months, he has been charged twice with driving under the influence, both times while driving recklessly after leaving the bar. Last night, he was stopped again. The judge ordered rehabilitation services. Fred responded, "I don't need rehab. I can stop drinking anytime I want to!"

i. Mary tried on a beautiful dress she saw in the store window. She discovered that it cost more than she could afford. She said to the salesperson, "I'm not going to buy it. I really don't look good in this color."

j. Janice is extremely upset when her boyfriend of 2 years breaks up with her. Her best friend tries to encourage her to talk about the breakup, but Janice says, "No need to talk about him anymore. He's history!"

k. While jogging in the park, Linda was kidnapped and taken as a hostage by two men who had just robbed a bank. She was held at gunpoint for 2 days until she was able to escape from the robbers. In her account to the police, she speaks of the encounter with no display of emotion whatsoever.

l. While Mark was on his way to work, a black cat ran across the road in front of his car. Mark turned the car around, drove back in the direction from which he had come, and took another route to work.

5. (cont'd)

    m. Fifteen-year-old Zelda has always wanted to be a teacher. Ms. Fry is Zelda's history teacher. Zelda admires everything about Ms. Fry and wants to be just like her. She changes her hair and style of dress to match that of Ms. Fry.

    n. Bart is turned down for a job he desperately wanted. He shows no disappointment when relating the situation to his girlfriend. Instead, he reviews the interview and begins to systematically analyze why the interaction was ineffective for him.

    o. Eighteen-year-old Jennifer can recall nothing related to an automobile accident in which she was involved 8 years ago and in which both of her parents were killed.

6. Identify the five stages of grief as described by Kübler-Ross.

7. Define *anticipatory grief.*

8. When is resolution of grief thought to have occurred? Describe some factors that influence the length of the grief response.

9. Name and describe three maladaptive grief responses.

10. In pathological depression, the individual is fixed in the _____ stage of the grief process. This is considered to be a maladaptive grief response that is _____.

REFERENCES

American Psychiatric Association. (1980). *A psychiatric glossary* (5th ed.). Washington, DC: American Psychiatric Press.

American Psychiatric Association. (1987). *Diagnostic and statistical manual of mental disorders* (3rd ed., rev.). Washington, DC: American Psychiatric Association.

Bowlby, J. & Parkes, C. M. (1970). Separation and loss. In E. J. Anthony & C. Koupernik (Eds.), *International yearbook for child psychiatry and allied disciplines: The child and his family* (Vol. 1). New York: John Wiley & Sons.

Freud, A. (1953). *The ego and mechanisms of defense.* New York: International Universities Press.

Freud, S. (1961). The ego and the id. In *Standard edition of the complete psychological works of Freud, Vol XIX.* London: Hogarth Press.

Halmi, K. A. (1982). Pragmatic information on eating disorders. *Psychiatr Clin North Am* 5(2):371–377.

Horwitz, A. V. (1982). *The social control of mental illness.* New York: Academic Press.

Jackson, E. N. (1957). *Understanding grief: Its roots, dynamics and treatment.* Nashville: Abingdon.

Jahoda, M. (1958). *Current concepts of positive mental health.* New York: Basic Books.

Kaplan, H. I. & Sadock, B. J. (1985). *Comprehensive textbook of psychiatry* (4th ed.). Baltimore: Williams & Wilkins.

Kirkham, A. K. (1980). Neuroses. In J. Lancaster (Ed.), *Adult psychiatric nursing.* Garden City, NY: Medical Examination Publishing.

Kübler-Ross, E. (1969). *On death and dying.* New York: Macmillan.

LeShan, R. (1977). *You can fight for your life.* New York: M. Evans and Co.

Lindemann, E. (1944). Symptomatology and management of acute grief. *Am J Psychiatry, 101*:141.

Maslow, A. (1970). *Motivation and personality* (2nd ed.). New York: Harper & Row.

May, R. (1950). *The meaning of anxiety.* New York: Ronald Press.

Menninger, K. (1963). *The vital balance.* New York: Viking Press.

Mims, F. H. & Swensen, M. (1980). *Sexuality: A nursing perspective.* New York: McGraw-Hill.

Parkes, C. M. (1972). *Bereavement: Studies of grief in adult life.* New York: International Universities Press.

Peplau, H. (1963). A working definition of anxiety. In S. Burd & M. Marshall (Eds.), *Some clinical approaches to psychiatric nursing.* New York: Macmillan.

Robinson, L. (1983). *Psychiatric nursing as a human experience* (3rd ed.). Philadelphia: WB Saunders.

Stuart, G. & Sundeen, S. (1987). *Principles and practice of psychiatric nursing* (3rd ed.). St. Louis, MO: CV Mosby.

BIBLIOGRAPHY

Carter, F. M. (1981). *Psychosocial nursing* (3rd ed.). New York: Macmillan.

Maslow, A. (1968). *Towards a psychology of being* (2nd ed.). New York: D. Van Nostrand.

3

THEORIES OF PERSONALITY DEVELOPMENT

KEY TERMS
personality
temperament
id
ego
superego
symbiotic
cognitive
libido

OBJECTIVES

After reading this chapter, the student will be able to:

1. Define *personality.*
2. Identify the relevance of knowledge associated with personality development to nursing in the psychiatric/mental health setting.
3. Discuss the major components of the following developmental theories:
   a. Psychoanalytic theory — Freud
   b. Interpersonal theory — Sullivan
   c. Theory of psychosocial development — Erikson
   d. Theory of object relations development — Mahler
   e. Cognitive development theory — Piaget
   f. Theory of moral development — Kohlberg

The *Diagnostic and Statistical Manual of Mental Health, ed 3, revised* (*DSM-III-R*) (American Psychiatric Association [APA] 1987) defines *personality* as "deeply ingrained patterns of behavior, which include the way one relates to, perceives, and thinks about the environment and oneself."

Nurses must have a basic knowledge of human personality development to understand maladaptive behavioral responses commonly seen in psychiatric patients. Developmental theories identify behaviors associated with various *stages* through which individuals pass, thereby specifying what is appropriate or inappropriate at each developmental level.

Specialists in child development have historically believed that infancy and early childhood are the major life periods for the origin and occurrence of developmental change (Clunn, 1991). Specialists in life-cycle development believe that people continue to develop and change throughout life, thereby suggesting the possibility for renewal and growth in adults (Schaie, 1984).

Developmental stages are identified by age. Behaviors can then be evaluated by whether or not they are recognized as age-appropriate. Ideally, an individual successfully fulfills all the tasks associated with one stage before moving on to the next stage (at the appropriate age). Realistically, however, this seldom happens. One reason is related to temperament. Temperament refers to inborn personality characteristics that influence an individual's manner of reacting to the environment and ultimately that individual's developmental pro-

gression (Chess & Thomas, 1986). The environment may also influence one's developmental pattern. Individuals who are reared in a dysfunctional family system often have retarded ego development. According to specialists in life-cycle development, behaviors from an unsuccessfully completed stage can be modified and corrected in a later stage.

Stages overlap, and an individual may be working on tasks associated with several stages at one time. When an individual becomes fixed in a lower level of development, with age-inappropriate behaviors focused on fulfillment of those tasks, psychopathology may become evident. Only when personality traits are inflexible and maladaptive and cause either significant functional impairment or subjective distress do they constitute "personality disorders" as identified in *DSM-III-R* (APA, 1987). These disorders are discussed in Chapter 26.

PSYCHOANALYTIC THEORY

Freud (1961), who has been called the father of psychiatry, is credited as the first to identify development by stages. He considered the first 5 years of a child's life to be the most important, as he believed that an individual's basic character had been formed by age 5.

Freud categorized his personality theory according to structure, dynamics, and development.

Structure of the Personality

Freud organized the structure of the personality into three major components: the id, ego, and superego. They are distinguished by their unique functions and different characteristics.

Id

The id is the locus of instinctual drives — the "pleasure principle." Present at birth, it endows the infant with instinctual drives that seek to satisfy needs and achieve immediate gratification. Id-driven behaviors are impulsive and may be irrational.

EGO

The ego, also called the "rational self" or the "reality principle," begins to develop between ages 4 and 6 months. The ego experiences the reality of the external world, adapts to it, and responds to it. As the ego develops and gains strength, it seeks to bring the influences of the external world to bear upon the id, to substitute the reality principle for the pleasure principle (Kaplan & Sadock, 1985). A primary function of the ego is that of mediator, that is, to maintain harmony between the external world, the id, and the superego.

SUPEREGO

If the id is identified as the pleasure principle, and the ego the reality principle, the superego might be referred to as the "perfection principle." The superego, which develops between ages 3 and 6, internalizes the values and morals set forth by primary caregivers. Derived out of a system of rewards and punishments, the superego is comprised of two major components: the *ego-ideal* and the *conscience*. When a child is consistently rewarded for "good" behavior, self-esteem is enhanced and the behavior becomes part of the ego-ideal; that is, it is internalized as part of his or her value system. The conscience is formed when the child is consistently punished for "bad" behavior. The child learns from feedback received from parental figures and from society or culture what is considered morally right or wrong. When moral and ethical principles or even internalized ideals and values are disregarded, the conscience generates a feeling of guilt within the individual. The superego is important in the socialization of the individual as it assists the ego in the control of id impulses. When the superego becomes rigid and punitive, problems with low self-confidence and low self-esteem arise.

Dynamics of the Personality

Freud believed that *psychic energy* is the force or impetus required for mental functioning. Originating in the id, it instinctually fulfills basic physiological needs. As the child matures, psychic energy is diverted from the id to form the ego and then from the ego to form the superego. Psychic energy is distributed within these three personality components, with the ego retaining the largest share to maintain a balance between id impulsive behavior and the idealistic behaviors of the superego. If an excessive amount of psychic energy is stored in one of these personality components, behavior will reflect that part of the personality. For instance, impulsive behavior will prevail when excessive psychic energy is stored in the id. Overinvestment in the ego will reflect self-absorbed, or narcissistic, behaviors, and an excess within the superego will result in rigid, self-deprecating behaviors.

Freud used the terms *cathexis* and *anticathexis* to describe the forces within the id, ego, and superego that are used to invest psychic energy in external sources to satisfy needs. Cathexis is the process by which the id invests energy into an object in an attempt to achieve gratification. An example is the individual who instinctively turns to alcohol to relieve stress. Anticathexis is the use of psychic energy by the ego and the superego to control id impulses. In the example cited, the ego would attempt to control the use of alcohol with rational thinking, such as, "I already have ulcers from drinking too much. I will call my AA counselor for support. I will not drink." The superego would exert control with, "I shouldn't drink. If I drink, my family will be hurt and angry. I should think of how it affects them. I'm such a weak person." Freud believed that an imbalance between cathexis and anticathexis resulted in internal conflicts, producing tension and anxiety within the individual. Freud's daughter Anna devised a comprehensive list of defense mechanisms believed to be used by the ego as a protective device against anxiety in mediating between the excessive demands of the id and the excessive restrictions of the superego (see Chapter 2).

Freud's Stages of Personality Development

Freud described formation of the personality through five stages of *psychosexual* development. He placed much emphasis on the first 5 years of life and believed that characteristics developed during these early years bore heavily on one's adaptation patterns and personality traits in adulthood. Fixation in an early stage of development will almost certainly result in psychopathology. An outline of these five stages is presented in Table 3.1.

ORAL STAGE: BIRTH TO 18 MONTHS

During this stage, behavior is directed by the id, and the goal is immediate gratification of needs. The focus of energy is the mouth. Behaviors include sucking, chewing, and biting. The infant feels a sense of attachment and is unable to differentiate the self from the person who is providing the mothering. This includes feelings such as anxiety, so that a pervasive feeling of anxiety on the part of the mother may be passed on to her infant, leaving the child vulnerable to similar feelings of insecurity. With the beginning of development of the ego at age 4 to 6 months, the infant starts to view the self as separate from the mothering figure. A sense of security and the ability to trust others is derived out of gratification from fulfillment of basic needs during this stage.

ANAL STAGE: 18 MONTHS TO 3 YEARS

The major tasks in this stage are gaining independence and control, with particular focus on the excretory function. Freud believed that the manner in which the parents and other primary caregivers approach the task of toilet training may have long-term effects on the child in terms of values and personality characteristics. When toilet training is strict and rigid, the child may choose to retain the feces, becoming constipated. Adult retentive personality traits influenced by this type of training include stubbornness, stinginess, and miserliness. An alternate reaction to strict toilet training is for the child to expel feces in an unacceptable manner or at inappropriate times. Far-reaching effects of this behavior pattern include malevolence, cruelty to others, destructiveness, disorganization, and untidiness.

Toilet training that is more permissive and accepting attaches the feeling of importance and desirability to feces production. The child becomes extroverted, productive, and altruistic.

PHALLIC STAGE: 3 TO 6 YEARS

In this stage, the focus of energy shifts to the genital area. Discovery of differences between genders results in a heightened interest in the sexuality of self and others. This interest may be manifested in sexual self-exploratory or group-exploratory play. Freud proposed that the development of the Oedipus complex occurred during this stage of development. He described this as the child's unconscious desire to eliminate the parent of the same sex and to possess the parent of the opposite sex

Age	Stage	Major Developmental Tasks
Birth–18 months	Oral	Relief from anxiety through oral gratification of needs
18 months–3 years	Anal	Learning independence and control, with focus on the excretory function
3–6 years	Phallic	Identification with parent of same sex; development of sexual identity; focus is on genital organs
6–12 years	Latency	Sexuality is repressed; focus is on relationships with same-sex peers
13–20 years	Genital	Libido is reawakened as genital organs mature; focus is on relationships with members of the opposite sex

Table 3.1 STAGES OF SEXUAL DEVELOPMENT IN FREUD'S PSYCHOANALYTIC THEORY

for himself or herself. Guilt feelings result with the emergence of the superego during these years. Resolution of this internal conflict occurs when the child develops a strong identification with the parent of the same sex and that parent's attitudes, beliefs, and value system are subsumed by the child.

LATENCY STAGE: 6 TO 12 YEARS

During the elementary school years, the focus changes from egocentrism to one in which there is more interest in group activities, learning, and socialization with peers. Sexuality is not absent during this period, but remains obscure and imperceptible to others. The preference is homosexual; children of this age show a distinct preference for same-sex relationships, even rejecting members of the opposite sex.

GENITAL STAGE: 13 TO 20 YEARS

In the genital stage, there is a reawakening of the libidinal drive with the maturing of the genital organs. The focus is on relationships with members of the opposite sex and preparations for selecting a mate. The development of sexual maturity evolves from self-gratification to behaviors that have been deemed acceptable by societal norms. Interpersonal relationships are based on genuine pleasure derived from the interaction rather than the more self-serving implications of childhood associations.

INTERPERSONAL THEORY

Sullivan (1953) believed that individual behavior and personality development are the direct result of interpersonal relationships. Prior to the development of his own theoretical framework, Sullivan embraced the concepts of Freud. Later, he changed the focus of his work from the *intrapersonal* view of Freud to one with more *interpersonal* flavor in which human behavior could be observed in social interactions with others. His ideas, which were not universally accepted at the time, have only been integrated into the practice of psychiatry through publication since his death in 1949. Sullivan's major concepts include:

Anxiety—a feeling of emotional discomfort, toward the relief or prevention of which all behavior is aimed. Sullivan believed that anxiety is the "chief disruptive force in interpersonal relations and the main factor in the development of serious difficulties in living." It arises out of one's inability to satisfy needs or achieve interpersonal security.

Satisfaction of needs—fulfillment of all requirements associated with an individual's physicochemical environment. Sullivan identified examples of these requirements as oxygen, food, water, warmth, tenderness, rest, activity, sexual expression—virtually anything that, when absent, produces discomfort in the individual.

Interpersonal security—the feeling associated with relief from anxiety. When all needs have been met, one experiences a sense of total well-being, which Sullivan termed *interpersonal security*. He believed individuals have an innate need for interpersonal security.

Self-system—a collection of experiences, or security measures, adopted by the individual to protect against anxiety. Sullivan identified three components of the self-system, which are based upon interpersonal experiences early in life:

- *The "good me"*—the part of the personality that develops in response to positive feedback from the primary caregiver. Feelings of pleasure, contentment, and gratification are experienced. The child learns which behaviors elicit this positive response as it becomes incorporated into the self-system.
- *The "bad me"*—the part of the personality that develops in response to negative feedback from the primary caregiver. Anxiety is experienced, eliciting feelings of discomfort, displeasure, and distress. The child learns to avoid these negative feelings by altering certain behaviors.
- *The "not me"*—the part of the personality that develops in response to situations that produce intense anxiety in the child. Feelings of horror, awe, dread, and loathing are expe-

rienced in response to these situations, leading the child to deny these feelings in an effort to relieve anxiety. These feelings, having then been denied, become "not me," but someone else. This withdrawal from emotions has serious implications for mental disorders in adult life.

Sullivan's Stages of Personality Development

INFANCY: BIRTH TO 18 MONTHS

During this beginning stage, the major developmental task for the child is the gratification of needs. This is accomplished around activity associated with the mouth, such as crying, nursing, and thumb sucking.

CHILDHOOD: 18 MONTHS TO 6 YEARS

At this age, the child learns that interference with fulfillment of personal wishes and desires may result in delayed gratification. He or she learns to accept this and feel comfortable with it, recognizing that delayed gratification often results in parental approval, a more lasting type of reward. Tools of this stage include the mouth, language, the anus, experimentation, manipulation, and identification.

JUVENILE: 6 TO 9 YEARS

The major task of this stage is formation of satisfactory relationships within the peer group. This is accomplished through the use of competition, cooperation, and compromise.

PREADOLESCENCE: 9 TO 12 YEARS

The tasks at this level focus on developing relationships with persons of the same sex. One's ability to collaborate with and show love and affection for another person begins at this stage.

EARLY ADOLESCENCE: 12 TO 14 YEARS

During early adolescence, the child is struggling with developing a sense of identity, separate and independent from the parents. The major task is formation of satisfactory relationships with members of the opposite sex. Sullivan saw the emergence of lust in response to biological changes as a major force occurring during this period.

LATE ADOLESCENCE: 14 TO 21 YEARS

The late adolescent period is characterized by tasks associated with the endeavor to achieve interdependence within the society and the formation of a lasting, intimate relationship with a selected member of the opposite sex. The genital organs are the major developmental focus of this stage.

An outline of the stages of personality development according to Sullivan's interpersonal theory is presented in Table 3.2.

THEORY OF PSYCHOSOCIAL DEVELOPMENT

Erikson (1963) studied the influence of social processes on the development of the personality. He described eight stages of the life cycle during

Table 3.2 STAGES OF DEVELOPMENT IN SULLIVAN'S INTERPERSONAL THEORY		
Age	**Stage**	**Major Developmental Tasks**
Birth–18 months	Infancy	Relief from anxiety through oral gratification of needs
18 months–6 years	Childhood	Learning to experience a delay in personal gratification without undo anxiety
6–9 years	Juvenile	Learning to form satisfactory peer relationships
9–12 years	Preadolescence	Learning to form satisfactory relationships with persons of same sex; the initiation of feelings of affection for another person
12–14 years	Early adolescence	Learning to form satisfactory relationships with persons of the opposite sex; developing a sense of identity
14–21 years	Late adolescence	Establishing self-identity; experiencing satisfying relationships; working to develop a lasting, intimate opposite-sex relationship

Table 3.3 STAGES OF DEVELOPMENT IN ERIKSON'S PSYCHOSOCIAL THEORY

Age	Stage	Major Development Tasks
Infancy (Birth–18 months)	Trust vs. Mistrust	To develop a basic trust in the mothering figure and be able to generalize it to others
Early childhood (18 months–3 years)	Autonomy vs. Shame and doubt	To gain some self-control and independence within the environment
Late childhood (3–6 years)	Initiative vs. Guilt	To develop a sense of purpose and the ability to initiate and direct own activities
School age (6–12 years)	Industry vs. Inferiority	To achieve a sense of self-confidence by learning, competing, performing successfully, and receiving recognition from significant others, peers, and acquaintances.
Adolescence (12–20 years)	Identity vs. Role confusion	To integrate the tasks mastered in the previous stages into a secure sense of self
Young adulthood (20–30 years)	Intimacy vs. Isolation	To form an intense, lasting relationship or a commitment to another person, a cause, an institution, or a creative effort.
Adulthood (30–65 years)	Generativity vs. Stagnation	To achieve the life goals established for oneself, while also considering the welfare of future generations.
Old age (65 years–death)	Ego integrity vs. Despair	To review one's life and derive meaning from both positive and negative events, while achieving a positive sense of self-worth

which individuals struggle with developmental "crises." Specific tasks associated with each stage must be completed for resolution of the crisis and for emotional growth to occur. An outline of Erikson's stages of psychosocial development is presented in Table 3.3.

Erikson's Stages of Personality Development

TRUST VS. MISTRUST: BIRTH TO 18 MONTHS

Major developmental task: To develop a basic trust in the mothering figure and be able to generalize it to others.

- Achievement of the task results in self-confidence, optimism and faith in the gratification of needs and desires, and hope for the future. The infant learns to trust when basic needs are consistently met.
- Nonachievement results in emotional dissatisfaction with the self and others, suspiciousness, and difficulty with interpersonal relationships. The task remains unresolved when primary caregivers fail to respond to the infant's distress signal promptly and consistently.

AUTONOMY VS. SHAME AND DOUBT: 18 MONTHS TO 3 YEARS

Major developmental task: To gain some self-control and independence within the environment.

- Achievement of the task results in a sense of self-control and the ability to delay gratification, and a feeling of self-confidence in one's ability to perform. Autonomy is achieved when parents encourage and provide opportunities for independent activities.
- Nonachievement results in a lack of self-confidence, a lack of pride in the ability to perform, a sense of being controlled by others, and a rage against the self. The task remains unresolved when primary caregivers restrict independent behaviors, both physically and verbally, or set the child up for failure with unrealistic expectations.

INITIATIVE VS. GUILT: 3 TO 6 YEARS

Major developmental task: To develop a sense of purpose and the ability to initiate and direct one's own activities.

- Achievement of the task results in the ability to

exercise restraint and self-control of inappropriate social behaviors. Assertiveness and dependability increase, and the child enjoys learning and personal achievement. The conscience develops, thereby controlling the impulsive behaviors of the id. Initiative is achieved when creativity is encouraged and performance is recognized and positively reinforced.

- Nonachievement results in feelings of inadequacy and a sense of defeat. Guilt is experienced to an excessive degree, even to the point of accepting liability in situations for which one is not responsible. The child may view him- or herself as evil and deserving of punishment. The task remains unresolved when creativity is stifled and parents continually expect a higher level of achievement than the child produces.

INDUSTRY VS. INFERIORITY: 6 TO 12 YEARS

Major developmental task: To achieve a sense of self-confidence by learning, competing, performing successfully, and receiving recognition from significant others, peers, and acquaintances.

- Achievement of the task results in a sense of satisfaction and pleasure in the interaction and involvement with others. The individual masters reliable work habits and develops attitudes of trustworthiness. He or she is conscientious, feels pride in achievement, and enjoys play but desires a balance between fantasy and "real world" activities. Industry is achieved when encouragement is given to activities and responsibilities in the school and community, as well as those within the home, and recognition is given for accomplishments.
- Nonachievement results in difficulty in interpersonal relationships due to feelings of personal inadequacy. The individual is unable to cooperate and compromise with others in group activities, and is unable to problem solve or complete tasks successfully. He or she may become passive and meek, or may become overly aggressive to cover up for feelings of inadequacy. If this occurs, the individual may manipulate or violate the rights of others to satisfy his or her own needs or desires; he or

she may become a workaholic with unrealistic expectations for personal achievement. This task remains unresolved when parents set unrealistic expectations for the child, when discipline is harsh and tends to impair self-esteem, and when accomplishments are consistently met with negative feedback.

IDENTITY VS. ROLE CONFUSION: 12 TO 20 YEARS

Major developmental task: To integrate the tasks mastered in the previous stage into a secure sense of self.

- Achievement of the task results in a sense of confidence, emotional stability, and a view of the self as a unique individual. Commitments are made to a value system, to the choice for a career, and to relationships with members of both sexes. Identity is achieved when adolescents are allowed to experience independence by making decisions that influence their lives. Parents should be available to offer support when needed but should gradually relinquish control to the maturing individual in an effort to encourage the development of an independent sense of self.
- Nonachievement results in a sense of self-consciousness, doubt, and confusion about one's role in life. Personal values or goals for one's life are absent. Commitments to relationships with others are nonexistent, but instead are superficial and brief. A lack of self-confidence is often expressed by delinquent and rebellious behavior. Entering adulthood, with its accompanying responsibilities, may be an underlying fear. This task can remain unresolved for many reasons. Examples include: when independence is discouraged by the parents, and the adolescent is nurtured in the dependent position; when discipline within the home has been overly harsh, inconsistent, or absent; and when there has been parental rejection or frequent shifting of parental figures.

INTIMACY VS. ISOLATION: 20 TO 30 YEARS

Major developmental task: To form an intense, lasting relationship or a commitment to another person, a cause, an institution, or a creative effort (Murray & Zentner, 1975).

- Achievement of the task results in the capacity for mutual love and respect between two people and the ability of an individual to pledge a total commitment to another. The intimacy goes far beyond the sexual contact between two people. It describes a commitment in which personal sacrifices are made for another, be it another person or, if one chooses, a career or other type of cause or endeavor to which an individual elects to devote his or her life. Intimacy is achieved when an individual has developed the capacity for giving of oneself to another. This is learned when one has been the recipient of this type of giving within the family unit.
- Nonachievement results in withdrawal, social isolation, and aloneness; the individual is unable to form lasting, intimate relationships, often seeking intimacy through numerous superficial, sexual contacts. No career is established; he or she may have a history of occupational changes (or may fear change and thus remain in an undesirable job situation). The task remains unresolved when love in the home has been deprived or distorted through the younger years (Murray & Zentner, 1975). One fails to achieve the ability to give of the self without having been the recipient early on from primary caregivers.

GENERATIVITY VS. STAGNATION OR SELF-ABSORPTION: 30 TO 65 YEARS

Major developmental task: To achieve the life goals established for oneself, while also considering the welfare of future generations.

- Achievement of the task results in a sense of gratification from personal and professional achievements, and from meaningful contributions to others. The individual is active in the service of and to society. Generativity is achieved when the individual expresses satisfaction with this stage in life and demonstrates responsibility for leaving the world a better place in which to live.
- Nonachievement results in lack of concern for the welfare of others and total preoccupation with the self. He or she becomes withdrawn, isolated, and highly self-indulgent, with no capacity for giving of the self to others. The task remains unresolved when earlier developmental tasks are not fulfilled and the individual does not achieve the degree of maturity required to derive gratification out of a personal concern for the welfare of others.

EGO INTEGRITY VS. DESPAIR: 65 YEARS TO DEATH

Major developmental task: To review one's life and derive meaning from both positive and negative events, while achieving a positive sense of self at this stage in life.

- Achievement of the task results in a sense of self-worth and self-acceptance as one reviews life goals, accepting that some were achieved and some were not. The individual derives a sense of dignity from his or her life experiences and does not fear death, rather viewing it as another phase of development. Ego integrity is achieved when individuals have successfully completed the developmental tasks of the other stages and would have little desire to make major changes in how their lives have progressed.
- Nonachievement results in a sense of self-contempt and disgust with how life has progressed. The individual would like to start over and have a second chance at life. He or she feels worthless and helpless to change. Anger, depression, and loneliness are evident. The focus may be on past failures or perceived failures. Impending death is feared or denied, or ideas of suicide may prevail. The task remains unresolved when earlier tasks are not fulfilled: self-confidence, a concern for others, and a strong sense of self-identity were never achieved.

THEORY OF OBJECT RELATIONS

Mahler (Mahler, Pine, & Bergman, 1975) has formulated a theory that describes the separation-individuation process of the infant from the maternal figure (primary caregiver). She describes this process as progressing through three major phases. She further deliniates phase 3, the separation-individuation phase, into four subphases. Mahler's developmental theory is outlined in Table 3.4.

Table 3.4 STAGES OF DEVELOPMENT IN MAHLER'S THEORY OF OBJECT RELATIONS		
Age	**Phase/Subphase**	**Major Developmental Tasks**
Birth–1 month	I. Normal autism	Fulfillment of basic needs for survival and comfort
1–5 months	II. Symbiosis	Developing awareness of external source of need fulfillment
	III. Separation-Individuation	
5–10 months	a. Differentiation	Commencement of a primary recognition of separatness from the mothering figure
10–16 months	b. Practicing	Increased independence through locomotor functioning; increased sense of separateness of self
16–24 months	c. Rapprochement	Acute awareness of separateness of self; learning to seek "emotional refueling" from mothering figure to maintain feeling of security
24–36 months	d. Consolidation	Sense of separateness established; on the way to object constancy: able to internalize a sustained image of loved object/person when it is out of sight; resolution of separation anxiety

Phase I: The Autistic Phase (Birth to 1 Month)

In this phase, also called *normal autism*, the infant exists in a half-sleeping, half-waking state and does not perceive the existence of other people or an external environment. The fulfillment of basic needs for survival and comfort is the focus and is merely accepted as it occurs. Fixation in this phase predisposes the child to autistic disorder.

Phase II: The Symbiotic Phase (1 to 5 Months)

In this phase there is a type of "psychic fusion" of mother and child. The child views the self as an extension of the mother, but with a developing awareness that it is she who fulfills his or her every need. Mahler suggests that absence of, or rejection by, the maternal figure at this phase can lead to symbiotic psychosis, which is described as pervasive developmental disorder in the *DSM-III-R*.

Phase III: Separation-Individuation (5 to 36 Months)

This third phase represents what Mahler calls the "psychological birth" of the child. *Separation* is defined as the physical and psychological attainment of a sense of personal distinction from the mothering figure. *Individuation* occurs with a strengthening of the ego and an acceptance of a sense of "self," with independent ego boundaries.

Four subphases through which the child evolves in his or her progression from a symbiotic extension of the mothering figure to a distinct and separate being are described.

Subphase 1 — Differentiation (5 to 10 months): Begins with the child's initial physical movements away from the mothering figure. A primary recognition of separateness commences.

Subphase 2 — Practicing (10 to 16 months): With advanced locomotor functioning, the child experiences feelings of exhilaration from increased independence. He or she is now able to move away from, and return to, the mothering figure. A sense of omnipotence is manifested.

Subphase 3 — Rapprochement (16 to 24 months): This third subphase is extremely critical to the child's healthy ego development. During this time, the child becomes increasingly aware of his or her separateness from the mothering figure, while at the same time the sense of fearlessness and omnipotence diminishes. The child, now recognizing mother as a separate individual, wishes to reestablish closeness with her but shuns the total re-engulfment of the symbiotic stage. The need is for the mothering figure to be available to provide "emotional refueling" on demand.

Critical to this subphase is the mothering figure's response to the child. If she is available to fulfill emotional needs as they are required, the child develops a sense of security in the knowledge that he or she is loved and will not be abandoned. However, if emotional needs are inconsistently met or if the mother rewards clinging, dependent behaviors and withholds nurturing when the child demonstrates independence, feelings of rage and a fear of abandonment develop and often persist into adulthood.

Subphase 4 — Consolidation (24 to 36 months): With achievement of this subphase, a definite individuality and sense of separateness of self are established. Objects are represented as whole, with the child having the ability to integrate both "good" and "bad." A degree of object constancy is established as the child is able to internalize a sustained image of the mothering figure as enduring and loving, while maintaining the perception of her has a separate person in the outside world.

COGNITIVE DEVELOPMENT THEORY

Piaget (Piaget & Inhelder, 1969) has been called the father of child psychology. His work concerning cognitive development in children is based on the premise that human intelligence is an extension of biological adaptation — or one's ability for psychological adaptation to the environment. He believed that human intelligence progresses through a series of stages that are related to age, demonstrating at each successive stage a higher level of logical organization than at the previous stages.

From his extensive studies of cognitive development in children, Piaget discovered four major stages, each of which he believed to be a necessary prerequisite for the one that follows. An outline is presented in Table 3.5.

Stage 1: Sensorimotor (Birth to 2 Years)

From the beginning, the child is concerned only with satisfying basic needs and comforts. The self is not differentiated from the external environment. As the sense of differentiation occurs, with increasing mobility and awareness, the mental system is expanded. The child develops a greater understanding regarding objects within the external environment and their effects upon him or her. Knowledge is gained regarding the ability to manipulate objects and experiences within the environment. The sense of *object permanence*, the notion that an object will continue to exist when it is no longer present to the senses, is initiated.

Stage 2: Preoperational (2 to 6 Years)

Piaget believed that preoperational thought is characterized by egocentrism. Personal experiences are thought to be universal, and the child is unable to accept the differing viewpoints of others. Language development progresses, as does the ability to attribute special meaning to symbolic gestures (e.g., bringing a story book to mother is a symbolic invitation to have a story read). Reality is often given to inanimate objects. Object permanence culminates in the ability to conjure up mental representations of objects or people.

Table 3.5	PIAGET'S STAGES OF COGNITIVE DEVELOPMENT	
Age	**Stage**	**Major Development Tasks**
Birth–2 years	Sensorimotor	With increased mobility and awareness, develops a sense of self as separate from the external environment; the concept of object permanence emerges as the ability to form mental images evolves
2–6 years	Preoperational	Learning to express self with language; develops understanding of symbolic gestures; achievement of object permanence
6–12 years	Concrete operations	Learning to apply logic to thinking; develops understanding of reversibility and spatiality; learning to differentiate and classify; increased socialization and application of rules
12–15+ years	Formal operations	Learning to think and reason in abstract terms; makes and tests hypotheses; logical thinking and reasoning ability expand and are refined; cognitive maturity achieved

Stage 3: Concrete Operations (6 to 12 Years)

The ability to apply logic to thinking begins in this stage; however, "concreteness" still predominates. An understanding of the concepts of reversibility and spatiality is developed. For example, the child recognizes that changing the shape of objects does not necessarily change the amount, weight, volume, or the ability of the object to return to its original form. Another achievement of this stage is the ability to classify objects by any of their several characteristics. For example, he or she can classify all poodles as dogs but recognizes that all dogs are not poodles.

The concept of a lawful self is developed at this stage as the child becomes more socialized and rule conscious. Egocentrism decreases, the ability to cooperate in interactions with other children increases, and understanding and acceptance of established rules grow.

Stage 4: Formal Operations (12 to 15+ Years)

At this stage, the individual is able to think and reason in abstract terms. He or she is capable of making and testing hypotheses with a logical and orderly problem-solving ability. Current situations and reflections of the future are idealized, and a degree of egocentrism returns during this stage. There may be some difficulty reconciling idealistic hopes with more rational prospects. Formal operations, however, enable individuals to distinguish between the ideal and the real. Piaget's theory suggests that most individuals achieve *cognitive maturity*, the capability to perform all mental operations needed for adulthood, in middle to late adolescence.

THEORY OF MORAL DEVELOPMENT

Kohlberg's (1968) stages of moral development are not closely tied to specific age groups. Research was conducted with males ranging in age from 10 to 28 years. Kohlberg believes that each stage is necessary and basic to the next stage and that all individuals must progress through each stage sequentially. He defined three major levels of moral development, each of which is further subdivided into two stages each. Most people do not progress through all six stages. An outline of Kohlberg's developmental stages is presented in Table 3.6.

Table 3.6 KOHLBERG'S STAGES OF MORAL DEVELOPMENT

Level/Age*	Stage	Developmental Focus
I. Preconventional (common from ages 4–10 years)	1. Punishment and obedience orientation	Behavior is motivated by fear of punishment
	2. Instrumental relativist orientation	Behavior is motivated by egocentrism and concern for self
II. Conventional (common from ages 10–13 years and into adulthood)	3. Interpersonal concordance orientation	Behavior is motivated by the expectations of others; strong desire for approval and acceptance
	3. Law and order orientation	Behavior is motivated by respect for authority
III. Postconventional (can occur from adolescence on)	5. Social contract legalistic orientation	Behavior is motivated by respect for universal laws and moral principles, and guided by an internal set of values
	6. Universal ethical principle orientation	Behavior is motivated by internalized principles of honor, justice, and respect for human dignity and guided by the conscience

*Ages in Kohlberg's theory are not well-defined. The stage of development is determined by the motivation behind the individual's behavior.

Level I: Preconventional Level (Prominent from Ages 4 to 10 Years)

Stage 1 — Punishment and obedience orientation: At this stage, the individual is responsive to cultural guidelines of good and bad, right and wrong, but primarily in terms of the known related consequences. Fear of punishment is likely to be the incentive for conformity (e.g., "I'll do it, because if I don't I can't watch TV for one week.")

Stage 2 — Instrumental relativist orientation: Behaviors of this stage are guided by egocentrism and concern for self. There is an intense desire to satisfy one's own needs, but occasionally the needs of others are considered. For the most part, decisions are based upon personal benefits derived (e.g., "I'll do it if I get something in return," or occasionally, ". . . because you asked me to.")

Level II: Conventional Level (Prominent from Ages 10 to 13 Years and into Adulthood)*

Stage 3 — Interpersonal concordance orientation: Behavior at this stage is guided by the expectations of others. Approval and acceptance within one's societal group provide the incentive to conform (e.g., "I'll do it because you asked me to," or ". . . because it will help you," or ". . . because it will please you.")

Stage 4 — Law and order orientation: There is a personal respect for authority. Rules and laws are required and override personal principles and group mores. The belief is that all individuals and groups are subject to the same code of order, and no one shall be exempt (e.g., "I'll do it because it is the law.")

Level III. Postconventional Level (Can Occur from Adolescence On)

Stage 5 — Social contract legalistic orientation: The belief is that there are certain inherent human rights to which all individuals are enti-

tled. Individuals who reach stage 5 have developed a system of values and principles that determine for them what is right or wrong; behaviors are acceptably guided by this value system provided they do not violate the human rights of others. The individual at stage 5 lives according to universal laws and principles; however, he or she holds the idea that the laws are subject to scrutiny and change as needs within society evolve and change (e.g., "I'll do it because it is the moral and legal thing to do, even though it is not my personal choice.")

Stage 6 — Universal ethical principle orientation: Behavior at this stage is directed by internalized principles of honor, justice, and respect for human dignity. Laws are abstract and unwritten, such as the "Golden Rule," "equality of human rights," and "justice for all," not the concrete rules established by society. The conscience is the guide, and when one fails to meet the self-expected behaviors, intense guilt is the personal consequence. The allegiance to these ethical principles is so strong that the individual will stand by them even knowing that negative consequences will result (e.g., "I'll do it because I believe it is the right thing to do, even though it is illegal and I will be imprisoned for doing it.")

SUMMARY

Growth and development are unique with each individual and continue throughout the life span. With each stage, there evolves an increasing complexity in the growth of the personality. This chapter has provided a description of the theories of Freud, Sullivan, Erikson, Mahler, Piaget, and Kohlberg. These theorists together provide a multifaceted approach to personality development, encompassing cognitive, psychosocial, and moral aspects.

Nurses must have basic knowledge of human personality development to understand maladaptive behavioral responses commonly seen in psychiatric patients. Knowledge of the appropriateness of behaviors at each developmental level is vital to the planning and implementation of quality nursing care.

---

*80 percent of adults are fixed in Level II, with a majority of women in stage 3 and a majority of men in stage 4.

REVIEW QUESTIONS
Self-Examination/Learning Exercise

Test your knowledge of personality development by answering the following questions:

1. Define *personality*.

2. Read the situation below and answer the questions relating to theories of personality development that follow.

   Mr. J. is 35 years old. He has been admitted to the psychiatric unit for observation and evaluation following his arrest on charges that he robbed a convenience store and sexually assaulted the store clerk. Mr. J. was the illegitimate child of a teenage mother who deserted him when he was 6 months old. He was shuffled from one relative to another until it was clear that no one wanted him. Social services placed him in foster homes, from which he continuously ran away. During his teenage years, he was arrested several times for stealing, vandalism, arson, and various other infractions of the law. He was shunned by his peers and to this day has little interaction with others. On the unit, he appears anxious, paces back and forth, and darts his head from side to side in a continuous scanning of the area. He is unkempt and unclean. He has refused to eat, making some barely audible comment related to "being poisoned." He has shown no remorse for his misdeeds.

   a. Theoretically, in which level of psychosocial development (according to Erikson) would you place Mr. J?
   b. According to the same theory, where would you place him behaviorally?
   c. Give the rationale for your answer in b.
   d. At what level of moral development would you assess Mr. J? Give the rationale.
   e. According to Mahler's theory, Mr. J. did not receive the critical "emotional refueling" required during the rapprochement phase of development. What are the consequences of this deficiency?
   f. In what stage of development is Mr. J. fixed according to Sullivan's interpersonal theory? Give the rationale.
   g. Which of the following describes the psychoanalytic structure of Mr. J's personality?

      I. Weak id, strong ego, weak superego
      II. Strong id, weak ego, weak superego
      III. Weak id, weak ego, punitive superego

3. In planning care for Mr. J., which of the following would be the primary focus for nursing?

   a. To decrease anxiety and develop trust
   b. To set limits on his behavior
   c. To ensure that he gets to group therapy
   d. To attend to his hygiene needs

REFERENCES

American Psychiatric Association (1987). *Diagnostic and statistical manual of mental disorders* (3rd ed., rev.). Washington, DC: American Psychiatric Association.

Chess & Thomas (1986). *Temperament in clinical practice.* New York: The Guilford Press.

Clunn, P. (1991). *Child psychiatric nursing.* St. Louis, MO: Mosby-Year Book.

Erikson, E. (1963). *Childhood and society* (2nd ed.) New York: WW Norton.

Freud, S. (1961). The ego and the id. In *Standard edition of the complete psychological works of Freud, Vol XIX.* London: Hogarth Press.

Kaplan, H. I. & Sadock, B. J. (1989). *Comprehensive textbook of psychiatry* (5th ed.). Baltimore: Williams & Wilkins.

Kohlberg, L. (1968). Moral development. In *International encyclopedia of social science.* New York: Macmillan.

Mahler, M., Pine, F. & Bergman, A. (1975). *The psychological birth of the human infant.* New York: Basic Books.

Murray, R. & Zentner, J. (1975). *Nursing assessment and health promotion through the life span.* Englewood Cliffs, NJ: Prentice-Hall.

Piaget, J. & Inhelder, B. (1969). *The psychology of the child.* New York: Basic Books.

Schaie, K. (1984). Historical time and cohort effects. In K. McClusky & H. Reese (Eds.), *Life-span developmental psychology.* New York: Academic Press.

Sullivan, H. S. (1953). *The interpersonal theory of psychiatry.* New York: WW Norton.

BIBLIOGRAPHY

Chapman, A. H. (1976). *Harry Stack Sullivan, his life and his work.* New York: GP Putnam's Sons.

Kernberg, O. (1976). *Object relations theory and clinical psychoanalysis.* New York: Jason Aronson.

Kohlberg, L. (1975, November). The cognitive-developmental approach to moral judgment. *Phi Delta Kappan, 56*:571–577.

Kohlberg, L. (1977). *Recent research in moral development.* New York: Holt, Rinehart and Winston.

Mahler, M. (1968). *On human symbiosis and the vicissitudes of individuation.* New York: International Universities Press.

Piaget, J. (1952). *The origin of intelligence in children.* New York: International Universities Press.

Piaget, J. (1963). *The psychology of intelligence.* Patterson, NJ: Littlefield Adama.

THERAPEUTIC APPROACHES IN PSYCHIATRIC CARE

RELATIONSHIP DEVELOPMENT

KEY TERMS
rapport
concrete thinking
confidentiality
unconditional positive regard
genuineness
empathy
sympathy

OBJECTIVES

After reading this chapter, the student will be able to:
1. Describe the relevance of a therapeutic nurse-patient relationship.
2. Discuss the dynamics of a therapeutic nurse-patient relationship.
3. Discuss goals of the nurse-patient relationship.
4. Identify and discuss essential conditions for a therapeutic relationship to occur.
5. Describe the phases of relationship development and the tasks associated with each phase.

ROLE OF THE PSYCHIATRIC NURSE

What is a nurse? Undoubtedly, this question would elicit as many different answers as the number of people to whom it was presented. Nursing as a *concept* has probably existed since the beginning of the civilized world, with the provision of "care" to the ill or infirm by anyone in the environment who took the time to administer to those in need. The emergence of nursing as a *profession* only began in the late 1800s, however, with the graduation of Linda Richards from the New England Hospital for Women and Children in Boston, upon achievement of the diploma in nursing. Since that time, the nurse's role has evolved from that of custodial caregiver and physician's handmaiden to being recognized as a unique, independent member of the professional health-care team.

Peplau (1957) has identified several subroles within the role of the nurse. These subroles include:

1. *The mother-surrogate.* In this subrole, the nurse fulfills needs associated with mothering — basic needs, such as bathing, feeding, dressing, toileting, warning, disciplining, and approving.
2. *The technician.* Focus is on the competent, efficient, and correct performance of technical procedures.
3. *The manager.* In this subrole, the nurse manages and manipulates the environment to improve conditions for patient recovery.
4. *The socializing agent.* The major function is participating in social activities with the patient.
5. *The health teacher.* In this subrole, the nurse identifies learning needs and provides information required by the patient or family to improve the health situation.
6. *The counselor or psychotherapist.* The nurse uses "interpersonal techniques" to assist patients to learn to adapt to difficulties or changes in life experiences.

Peplau (1962) believes that the emphasis in psychiatric nursing is on the counseling or psychotherapeutic subrole. How then does this emphasis influence the role of the nurse in the psychiatric setting? Many sources define the *nurse therapist* as having graduate preparation in psychiatric/mental health nursing. He or she has developed skills through intensive supervised educational experiences to provide helpful individual, group, or family therapy.

Peplau suggests that it is essential for the *staff nurse working in psychiatry* to have a general knowledge of basic counseling techniques. A therapeutic or "helping" relationship is established through use of these interpersonal techniques and based upon a knowledge of theories of personality development and human behavior.

Sullivan (1953) believed that emotional problems stem from difficulties with interpersonal relationships. Interpersonal theorists, such as Peplau and Sullivan, emphasize the importance of relationship development in the provision of emotional care. Through the establishment of a satisfactory nurse-patient relationship, individuals learn to generalize the ability to achieve satisfactory interpersonal relationships to other aspects of their lives.

DYNAMICS OF A THERAPEUTIC NURSE-PATIENT RELATIONSHIP

Travelbee (1971), who expanded upon Peplau's theory of interpersonal relations in nursing, has stated that it is only when each individual in the interaction perceives the other as a human being that a relationship is possible. She refers, not to a nurse-patient relationship, but rather to a human-to-human relationship, which she describes as a "mutually significant experience"; that is, both the nurse and the recipient of care have needs met when each views the other as a unique human being, not as "an illness," or "a room number," or "all nurses" in general.

Therapeutic relationships are goal oriented. Ideally, the nurse and patient decide together what the goal of the relationship will be. Most often the goal is directed at learning and growth promotion, in an effort to bring about some type of change in the patient's life. In general, the goal of a therapeutic relationship may be based on a problem-solving model.

Example

Goal: The patient will demonstrate more adaptive coping strategies for dealing with (specific life situation).

Interventions:

1. Identify what is troubling the patient at this time.
2. Encourage patient to discuss changes he or she would like to make.
3. Discuss with patient which changes are possible and which are not possible.
4. Have patient explore feelings about aspects which cannot be changed, and alternative ways of coping more adaptively.
5. Discuss alternative strategies for creating changes patient desires to make.
6. Weigh benefits and consequences of each alternative.
7. Assist patient to select an alternative.
8. Encourage patient to implement the change.
9. Provide positive feedback for patient's attempts to create change.
10. Assist patient to evaluate outcomes of the change and make modifications as required.

Therapeutic Use of Self

Travelbee (1971) described the instrument for delivery of the process of interpersonal nursing as the *therapeutic use of self*, which she defined as:

"the ability to use one's personality consciously and in full awareness in an attempt to establish relatedness and to structure nursing interventions."

Use of the self in a therapeutic manner requires that the nurse have a great deal of self-awareness and self-understanding; that he or she has arrived at a philosophical belief about life, death, and the overall human condition. The nurse must understand that the ability and extent to which one is able to effectively help others in time of need is strongly influenced by this internal value system—a combination of intellect and emotions.

CONDITIONS ESSENTIAL TO DEVELOPMENT OF A THERAPEUTIC RELATIONSHIP

Several theorists have identified characteristics that enhance the achievement of a therapeutic relationship (Rogers et al., 1967; Travelbee, 1971; Peplau, 1969; Carkhuff, 1968). These concepts are highly significant to the use of self as the therapeutic tool in interpersonal relationship development.

Rapport

Getting acquainted and establishing rapport is the primary task in relationship development. Rapport implies special feelings on the part of both the patient and the nurse based on acceptance, warmth, friendliness, common interest, a sense of trust, and a nonjudgmental attitude. Establishing rapport may be accomplished by discussing non-health-related topics. Travelbee (1971) states:

"(To establish rapport) is to create a sense of harmony based on knowledge and appreciation of each individual's uniqueness. It is the ability to be still and experience the other as a human being—to appreciate the unfolding of each personality one to the other. The ability to truly care for and about others is the core of rapport."

Trust

To trust another, one must feel confidence in that person's presence, reliability, integrity, veracity, and sincere desire to provide assistance when requested. As previously discussed, trust is the initial developmental task described by Erikson. When this task has not been achieved, this component of relationship development becomes more difficult. That is not to say that trust cannot be established, but only that additional time and patience may be required on the part of the nurse.

It is imperative for the nurse to convey an aura of trustworthiness, which requires that he or she possess a sense of self-confidence. Confidence in the self is derived out of knowledge gained through achievement of personal and professional goals, as well as the ability to integrate these roles and to function as a unified whole.

Trust cannot be presumed; it must be earned. Trustworthiness is demonstrated through nursing interventions that convey a sense of warmth and caring to the patient. These interventions are initiated simply and concretely, and directed toward activities that address the patient's basic needs for physiological and psychological safety and security. Many psychiatric patients experience *concrete thinking*, which focuses their thought processes on specifics rather than generalities and immediate issues rather than eventual outcomes. Examples of nursing interventions that would promote trust in an individual who is thinking concretely include:

- Providing a blanket when the patient is cold.
- Providing food when the patient is hungry.
- Keeping promises.
- Being honest, for example, saying "I don't know the answer to your question, but I'll try to find out," then following through.
- Simply and clearly providing reasons for certain policies, procedures, and rules.
- Providing a written, structured schedule of activities.
- Attending activities with the patient if he or she is reluctant to go alone.
- Being consistent in adhering to unit guidelines.
- Taking the patient's preferences, requests, and opinions into consideration when possible in decisions concerning his or her care.
- Ensuring *confidentiality*; providing reassurance that what is discussed will not be repeated outside the boundaries of the health-care team.

Trust is the basis of a therapeutic relationship. The nurse working in psychiatry must perfect the skills that foster the development of trust. Without the establishment of trust, the helping relationship will not progress beyond the level of mechanical provision for tending to superficial needs (Sundeen, Stuart, Rankin, & Cohen, 1985).

Respect

To show respect is to believe in the dignity and worth of an individual regardless of his or her unacceptable behavior. Rogers (1951) called this *unconditional positive regard*. The attitude is nonjudgmental, and the respect is unconditional in that it does not depend on the behavior of the patient to meet certain standards. The nurse, in fact, may not approve of the patient's life-style or pattern of behaving. However, with unconditional positive regard, the patient is accepted and respected for no other reason than that he or she is considered to be a worthwhile and unique human being.

Many psychiatric patients have little self-respect due to the fact that, because of their behavior, they have been rejected by others in the past. Recognition that they are being accepted and respected as unique individuals on an unconditional basis can serve to elevate feelings of self-worth and self-respect. The nurse can convey an attitude of respect by:

- Calling the patient by name (and title, if the patient prefers).
- Spending time with the patient.
- Allowing for sufficient time to answer the patient's questions and concerns.
- Promoting an atmosphere of privacy during therapeutic interactions with the patient or when the patient may be undergoing physical examination or therapy.
- Always being open and honest with the patient even when the truth may be difficult to discuss.
- Taking the patient's ideas, preferences, and opinions into consideration when planning care.
- Striving to understand the motivation behind the patient's behavior, regardless of how unacceptable it may seem.

Genuineness

The concept of genuineness refers to the nurse's ability to be open, honest, and "real" in interactions with the patient. To be "real" is to be aware of what one is experiencing internally and to allow the quality of this inner experiencing to be apparent in the therapeutic relationship (Meador & Rogers, 1979). When one is genuine, there is *congruence* between what is felt and what is being expressed. The nurse who possesses the quality of genuineness responds to the patient with truth and honesty, rather than with responses he or she may consider are more "professional" or those that merely reflect the "nursing role."

Genuineness may call for a degree of *self-disclosure* on the part of the nurse. This is not to say that the nurse must disclose to the patient *everything* he or she is feeling or *all* personal experiences that may relate to what the patient is going through. Indeed, care must be taken when using self-disclosure that the roles of the nurse and patient do not become transposed.

When the nurse uses self-disclosure, a quality of "humanness" is revealed to the patient, creating a role for the patient to model in similar situations. The patient may then feel more comfortable revealing personal information to the nurse.

Most individuals have an uncanny ability to detect artificiality on the part of others. When the nurse does not bring the quality of genuineness to the relationship, a reality base for trust cannot be established. These qualities are essential if the actualizing potential of the patient is to be released and for change and growth to occur (Meador & Rogers, 1979).

Empathy

Empathy is a process wherein an individual is able to see beyond outward behavior and sense accurately another's inner experience at a given point in time (Travelbee, 1971). With empathy, the nurse is able to accurately perceive and understand the meaning and relevance of the patient's thoughts and feelings. The nurse must also be able to communicate this perception to the patient. This is done by attempting to translate words and behaviors into feelings.

It is not uncommon for the concept of empathy to be confused with that of sympathy. The major difference is that with *empathy* the nurse "accurately perceives or understands" what the patient is feeling and encourages the patient to explore these feelings. With *sympathy*, the nurse actually "shares" what the patient is feeling and experiences a need to alleviate distress.

Empathy is considered to be one of the most important characteristics of a therapeutic relationship. Accurate empathic perceptions on the part of the nurse assist the patient to identify feelings that may have been suppressed or denied. Positive emotions are generated as the patient realizes that he or she is truly understood by another. As the feelings surface and are explored, the patient learns aspects about self of which he or she may have been unaware. This contributes to the process of personal identification and the promotion of positive self-concept.

With empathy, while understanding the patient's thoughts and feelings, the nurse is able to maintain sufficient objectivity to allow the patient to achieve problem resolution with minimal assistance. With sympathy, the nurse actually feels what the patient is feeling, objectivity is lost, and the nurse may become focused on relief of personal distress rather than on assisting the patient to resolve the problem at hand. Following is an example of an empathic and a sympathetic response to the same situation.

Situation: BJ is a patient on the psychiatric unit with a diagnosis of dysthymic disorder. She is 5′5″ tall and weighs 295

lb. BJ has been overweight all her life. She is single, has no close friends, and has never had an intimate relationship with another person. It is her first day on the unit, and she is refusing to come out of her room. When she appeared for lunch in the dining room following admission, she was embarrassed when several patients laughed out loud and called her "fatso."

Sympathetic response: Nurse: "I can certainly identify with what you are feeling. I've been overweight most of my life, too. I just get so angry when people act like that. They are so insensitive! It's just so typical of skinny people to act that way. You have a right to want to stay away from them. We'll just see how loud they laugh when *you* get to choose what movie is shown on the unit after dinner tonight."

Empathic response: Nurse: "You feel angry and embarrassed by what happened at lunch today." As tears fill BJ's eyes, the nurse encourages her to cry if she feels like it and to express her anger at the situation. She stays with BJ but does not dwell on her *own* feelings about what happened. Instead, she focuses on BJ and what the patient perceives are her most immediate needs at this time.

PHASES OF A THERAPEUTIC NURSE-PATIENT RELATIONSHIP

Psychiatric nurses use interpersonal relationship development as the primary intervention with patients in various psychiatric/mental health settings. This is congruent with Peplau's (1962) identification of *counseling* as the major subrole of nursing in psychiatry. If what Sullivan (1953) believed is true, that is, that all emotional problems stem from difficulties with interpersonal relationships, then this role of the nurse in psychiatry becomes especially meaningful and purposeful. It becomes an integral part of the total therapeutic regimen.

The therapeutic interpersonal relationship is the means by which the nursing process is implemented. Through the relationship, problems are identified and resolution is sought. Tasks of the relationship have been categorized into four phases: the preinteraction phase, the orientation (introductory) phase, the working phase, and the termination phase. Although each phase is presented as specific and distinct from the others, there may be some overlapping of tasks, particularly when the interaction is limited.

The Preinteraction Phase

The preinteraction phase involves preparation for the first encounter with the patient. Tasks include:

1. Obtaining available information about the patient from the chart, significant others, or other health-team members. From this information, the initial assessment is begun. From this initial information, the nurse may also become aware of personal responses to knowledge about the patient.
2. Examining one's feelings, fears, and anxieties about working with a particular patient. For example, the nurse may have been reared in an alcoholic family and have ambivalent feelings about caring for a patient who is alcohol dependent. All individuals bring attitudes and feelings from prior experiences to the clinical setting. The nurse needs to be aware of how these preconceptions may affect his or her ability to care for individual patients.

The Orientation (Introductory) Phase

During the orientation phase, the nurse and patient become acquainted. Tasks include:

1. Creating an environment for the establishment of trust and rapport.
2. Establishing a contract for intervention that details the expectations and responsibilities of both the nurse and patient.
3. Gathering assessment information to build a strong patient data base.
4. Identifying the patient's strengths and limitations.
5. Formulating nursing diagnoses.
6. Setting goals that are mutually agreeable to the nurse and patient.
7. Developing a plan of action that is realistic for meeting the established goals.

8. Exploring feelings of both the patient and nurse in terms of the introductory phase. Introductions are often uncomfortable, and the participants may experience some anxiety until a degree of rapport has been established. Interactions may remain on a superficial level until anxiety subsides. Several interactions may be required to fulfill the tasks associated with this phase.

The Working Phase

The therapeutic work of the relationship is accomplished during this phase. Tasks include:

1. Maintaining the trust and rapport that was established during the orientation phase.
2. Promoting the patient's insight and perception of reality.
3. Problem solving using the model presented earlier in this chapter.
4. Overcoming resistance behaviors on the part of the patient as the level of anxiety rises in response to discussion of painful issues.
5. Continuously evaluating progress toward goal attainment.

The Termination Phase

Termination of the relationship may occur for a variety of reasons: the mutually agreed-upon goals may have been reached, the patient may be discharged from the hospital, or in the case of a student nurse, it may be the end of a clinical rotation. Termination can be a difficult phase for both the patient and nurse. Tasks include:

1. Bringing a therapeutic conclusion to the relationship. This occurs when:
   a. Progress has been made toward attainment of mutually set goals.
   b. A plan for continuing care or for assistance during stressful life experiences is mutually established by the nurse and patient.
   c. Feelings about termination of the relationship are recognized and explored. Both the nurse and patient may experience feelings of sadness and loss. The nurse should share his or her feelings with the patient. Through these interactions, the patient learns that it is acceptable to undergo these feelings at a time

of separation. Through this knowledge, the patient experiences growth during the process of termination.

NOTE: When the patient feels sadness and loss, behaviors to delay termination may become evident. If the nurse experiences the same feelings, he or she may allow the patient's behaviors to delay termination. For therapeutic closure, the nurse must establish the reality of the separation and resist being manipulated into repeated delays by the patient.

The major nursing goals during each phase of the nurse-patient relationship are listed in Table 4.1.

SUMMARY

Nurses who work in the psychiatric/mental health field use special skills, or "interpersonal techniques," to assist patients in adapting to difficulties or changes in life experiences. A therapeutic or "helping" relationship is established through use of these interpersonal techniques and based on a knowledge of theories of personality development and human behavior.

Therapeutic nurse-patient relationships are goal oriented. Ideally, the goal is mutually agreed on by the nurse and patient, and is directed at learning and growth promotion. The problem-solving model is used in an attempt to bring about some

Table 4.1 PHASES OF RELATIONSHIP DEVELOPMENT AND MAJOR NURSING GOALS

Phase	Goals
1. Preinteraction	Explore self-perceptions
2. Orientation (introductory)	Establish trust
	Formulate contract for intervention
3. Working	Promote patient change
4. Termination	Evaluate goal attainment
	Ensure therapeutic closure

type of change in the patient's life. The instrument for delivery of the process of interpersonal nursing is the therapeutic use of self, which requires that the nurse possess a strong sense of self-awareness and self-understanding.

A number of characteristics that enhance the achievement of a therapeutic relationship have been identified. They include rapport, trust, respect, genuineness, and empathy.

The tasks associated with the development of a therapeutic interpersonal relationship have been categorized into four phases: the preinteraction phase, the orientation (introductory) phase, the working phase, and the termination phase.

The concepts and tasks presented herein can facilitate the promotion of a helping relationship and effective nursing care for patients requiring psychosocial intervention.

REVIEW QUESTIONS
Self-Examination/Learning Exercise

Test your knowledge of therapeutic nurse-patient relationships by answering the following questions:

1. Name the six subroles of nursing identified by Peplau.

2. Which subrole is emphasized in psychiatric nursing?

3. Why is relationship development so important in the provision of emotional care?

4. In general, what is the goal of a therapeutic relationship? What method is recommended for intervention?

5. What is the instrument for delivery of the process of interpersonal nursing?

6. Several characteristics that enhance the achievement of a therapeutic relationship have been identified. Match the therapeutic concept with the corresponding definition.

_____ 1. Rapport

_____ 2. Trust

_____ 3. Respect

_____ 4. Genuineness

_____ 5. Empathy

a. The feeling of confidence in another person's presence, reliability, integrity, and desire to provide assistance.

b. Congruence between what is felt and what is being expressed.

c. The ability to accurately sense what another person is feeling at a given time.

d. Special feelings between two people based on acceptance, warmth, friendliness, and a shared common interest.

e. Unconditional acceptance of an individual as a worthwhile and unique human being.

7. Describe major tasks of each phase of relationship development:

   a. Preinteraction phase:
   b. Orientation (introductory) phase:
   c. Working phase:
   d. Termination phase:

REFERENCES

Carkhuff, R. (1968). *Helping and human relations* (Vols. 1–2). New York: Holt, Rinehart & Winston.

Meador, B. D. & Rogers, C. R. (1979). Person-centered therapy. In R. J. Corsini (Ed.), *Current psychotherapies* (2nd ed.). Itasca, IL: FE Peacock Publishers.

Peplau, H. E. (1957). Therapeutic concepts. In *The league exchange.* New York: National League for Nursing.

Peplau, H. E. (1962). Interpersonal techniques: The crux of psychiatric nursing. *Am J Nursing,* 62(6):50–54.

Peplau, H. E. (1969). *Basic principles of patient counseling* (2nd ed.). Philadelphia: Smith, Kline, and French Laboratories.

Rogers, C. R. (1951). *Client-centered therapy.* Boston: Houghton Mifflin.

Rogers, C. R. Gendlin, E.T., Kiesler, D.J., and Louax, C. (1967). *The therapeutic relationship and its impact.* Madison, WI: University of Wisconsin Press.

Sullivan, H.S. (1953). *The interpersonal theory of psychiatry.* New York: WW Norton.

Sundeen, S. J., Stuart, G. W., Rankin, E. D., & Cohen, S. A. (1985). *Nurse-client interaction— Implementing the nursing process.* St. Louis, MO: CV Mosby.

Travelbee, J. (1971). *Interpersonal aspects of nursing* (2nd ed.). Philadelphia: FA Davis.

BIBLIOGRAPHY

Cormier, L. S., Cormier, W. H., & Weisser, R. J., Jr. (1984). *Interviewing and helping skills for health professionals.* Monterey, CA: Wadsworth Health Sciences Division.

Duldt, B. W., Giffin, K., & Patton, B. R. (1984). *Interpersonal communication in nursing.* Philadelphia: FA Davis.

Maloney, E. (1962, June). Does the psychiatric nurse have independent functions? *Am J Nursing,* 62(6):61–63.

Northouse, P. G. & Northouse, L. L. (1985). *Health communication, A handbook for health professionals.* Englewood Cliffs, NJ: Prentice-Hall.

Peplau, H. E. (1952). *Interpersonal relations in nursing.* New York: G.P. Putnam's Sons.

Rogers, C. R. (1957). The necessary and sufficient conditions of therapeutic personality change. *J Consult Psychol, 21*:95–103.

Rogers, C. R. (1961). *On becoming a person.* Boston: Houghton Mifflin.

THERAPEUTIC COMMUNICATION

OBJECTIVES

After reading this chapter, the student will be able to:
1. Discuss the transactional model of communication.
2. Identify types of preexisting conditions that influence the outcome of the communication process.
3. Define *territoriality, density,* and *distance* as components of the environment.
4. Identify components of nonverbal expression.
5. Describe therapeutic and nontherapeutic verbal communication techniques.

6. Describe active listening.
7. Discuss therapeutic feedback.

INTRODUCTION

The development of the *therapeutic interpersonal relationship* was described in Chapter 4 as the process by which nurses provide care for patients in need of psychosocial intervention. *Therapeutic use of self* was identified as the instrument for delivery of care. The focus of this chapter will be on *techniques*, or more specifically, *interpersonal communication techniques*, to facilitate the delivery of that care.

Hays and Larson (1963) have stated, "To relate therapeutically with a patient it is necessary for the nurse to understand his or her role and its relationship to the patient's illness." They describe the role of the nurse as providing the patient with the opportunity to:

1. Identify and explore problems in relating to others.
2. Discover healthy ways of meeting emotional needs.
3. Experience a satisfying interpersonal relationship.

This is accomplished through use of interpersonal communication techniques (both verbal and nonverbal). The nurse must be aware of the therapeutic or nontherapeutic value of the communication techniques used with the patient, as they are the "tools" of psychosocial intervention.

WHAT IS COMMUNICATION?

It has been said, "You cannot not communicate." Every word that is spoken and every movement that is made gives a message to someone. Interpersonal communication is a *transaction* between the sender and the receiver. In the transactional model of communication, both persons are participating simultaneously. They are mutually perceiving each other, simultaneously listening to each other, and simultaneously and mutually engaged in the process of creating meaning in a relationship (Smith & Williamson, 1981). The transactional model is illustrated in Figure 5.1.

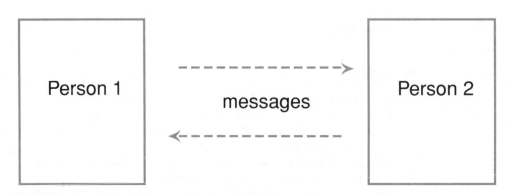

Figure 5.1 The Transactional Model of Communication.

THE IMPACT OF PREEXISTING CONDITIONS

In all interpersonal transactions, both the sender and receiver bring certain preexisting conditions to the exchange that influence both the intended message and the way in which it is interpreted. Examples of these conditions include one's value system, internalized attitudes and beliefs, culture or religion, social status, gender, background knowledge and experience, and age or developmental level. The type of environment in which the communication takes place may also influence the outcome of the transaction. Figure 5.2 shows how these influencing factors are positioned on the transactional model.

Values, Attitudes, and Beliefs

Values, attitudes, and beliefs are learned ways of thinking. By and large, children adopt the value systems and internalize the attitudes and beliefs of their parents. Children may retain this way of thinking into adulthood or develop a different set of attitudes and values as they mature.

Attitudes and beliefs can influence communication in numerous ways. For example, prejudice is expressed verbally through negative stereotyping.

One's value system may be communicated with behaviors that are more symbolic in nature. For example, an individual who values youth may dress and behave in a manner that is characteristic of one who is much younger. A person who values freedom and the American way of life may fly the U.S. flag in front of his or her home each day. In each of these situations, a message is being communicated.

Culture or Religion

Communication has its roots in culture. Cultural mores, norms, ideas, and customs provide the basis for our way of thinking. Cultural values are learned and differ from society to society. For example, in some European countries (e.g., Italy, Spain, and France), men may greet each other with hugs and kisses. These behaviors are appropriate in these cultures but would communicate a different message in America or Great Britain.

Religion can influence communication as well. Priests and ministers who wear clerical collars publicly communicate their mission in life. The collar may also influence the way in which others relate to them, either positively or negatively. Other symbolic gestures, such as wearing a cross around the neck or hanging a crucifix on the wall, communicate an individual's religious beliefs.

Social Status

Mehrabian (1972) conducted studies of nonverbal indicators of social status or power. He reports that high-status persons are associated with ges-

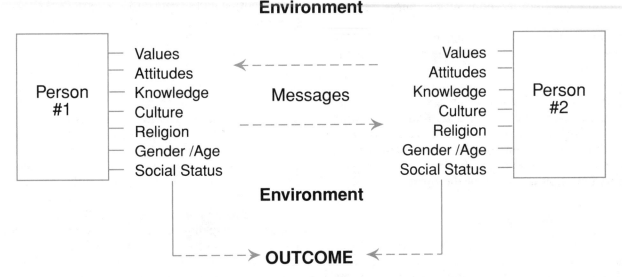

Figure 5.2 Factors Influencing the Transactional Model of Communication.

tures that communicate their higher-power position. For example, they use less eye contact, a more relaxed posture, louder voice pitch, more frequent use of hands on hips, power dressing, greater height, and more distance when communicating with individuals considered to be of lower social status.

Gender

Gender influences the manner in which individuals communicate. Each culture has *gender signals* that are recognized as either masculine or feminine and provide a basis for distinguishing between members of each sex (Smith & Williamson, 1981). Examples include differences in posture, both standing and sitting, between American men and women. Men stand with thighs 10° to 15° apart, the pelvis rolled back, and the arms slightly away from the body. Women are seen with legs close together, the pelvis tipped forward, and the arms close to the body. When sitting, men may lean back in the chair with legs apart or may rest the ankle of one leg over the knee of the other. Women tend to sit more upright in the chair with legs together, perhaps crossed at the ankles, or one leg crossed over the other at thigh level.

Roles have traditionally been identified as either male or female. For example, in America masculinity has been traditionally communicated through such roles as husband, father, breadwinner, doctor, lawyer, or engineer. Traditional female roles include wife, mother, homemaker, nurse, teacher, or secretary.

Gender signals are changing in American society as sexual roles become less distinct. Behaviors that have been considered typically masculine or feminine in the past may now be generally acceptable in both sexes. Words such as "unisex" communicate a desire by some individuals to diminish the distinction between the sexes and minimize the discrimination of either. Gender roles are changing as both women and men enter professions that were once dominated by members of the opposite sex.

Age or Developmental Level

Age influences communication, and it is never more evident than during adolescence. In their struggle to separate from parental confines and es-

tablish their own identity, adolescents generate a pattern of communication that is unique and changes from generation to generation. Words such as awesome, groovy, and cool, have had special meaning for certain generations of adolescents.

Developmental influences on communication may relate to physiological alterations. One example is American Sign Language, the system of unique gestures used by many people who are deaf or hearing impaired. Individuals who are blind at birth never learn the subtle nonverbal gesticulations that accompany language and can totally change the meaning of the spoken word.

Environment in Which the Transaction Takes Place

The place where the communication occurs influences the outcome of the interaction. Some individuals who feel uncomfortable and refuse to speak during a group therapy session may be open and willing to discuss problems privately on a one-to-one basis with the nurse.

Territoriality, density, and *distance* are aspects of environment that communicate messages. *Territoriality* is the innate tendency to own space. Individuals lay claim to areas around them as their own. This influences communication when an interaction takes place in the territory "owned" by one or the other. Interpersonal communication can be more successful if the interaction takes place in a "neutral" area. For example, with the concept of territoriality in mind, the nurse may choose to conduct the psychosocial assessment in an interview room rather than in his or her office or in the patient's room.

Density refers to the number of people within a given environmental space and has been shown to influence interpersonal interaction. Some studies indicate that a correlation exists between prolonged high-density situations and certain behaviors, such as aggression, stress, criminal activity, hostility toward others, and a deterioration of mental and physical health (Knapp, 1980).

Distance is the means by which various cultures use space to communicate. Hall (1966) identified four kinds of spatial interaction, or distances, that people maintain from each other in their interpersonal interactions and the kinds of activities in which people engage at these various distances. *In-*

timate distance is the closest distance that individuals will allow between themselves and others. In America, this distance, which is restricted to interactions of an intimate nature, is 0 to 18 inches. *Personal distance* is approximately 18 to 40 inches and reserved for interactions that are personal in nature, such as close conversations with friends or colleagues. Our *social distance* is about 4 to 12 feet away from the body. Interactions at this distance include conversations with strangers or acquaintances, such as at a cocktail party or in a public building. *Public distances* are those which exceed 12 feet. Examples include speaking in public or yelling to someone some distance away. This distance is considered public space, and communicants are free to move about in it during the interaction.

NONVERBAL COMMUNICATION

Some aspects of nonverbal expression have been discussed in the previous section on preexisting conditions that influence communication. Other components of nonverbal communication include physical appearance and dress, body movement and posture, touch, facial expressions, eye behavior, and vocal cues or paralanguage. These nonverbal messages vary from culture to culture.

Physical Appearance and Dress

Physical appearance and dress are part of the total nonverbal stimuli that influence interpersonal responses—and under some conditions, they are the primary determiners of such responses (Knapp, 1980). Body coverings—both dress and hair—are manipulated by the wearer in a manner that conveys a distinct message to the receiver. Dress can be formal or casual, stylish or sloppy. Hair can be long or short, and even the presence or absence of hair conveys a message about the person. Other body adornments that are also considered potential communicative stimuli include tattoos, masks, cosmetics, badges, jewelry, and eyeglasses. Some jewelry worn in specific ways can give special messages. For example, a gold band or diamond ring worn on the fourth finger of the left hand, a boy's class ring worn on a chain around a girl's neck, or a pin bearing Greek letters worn on the lapel. Some individuals convey a specific message with the total absence of any type of body adornment.

Body Movement and Posture

The way in which an individual positions his or her body communicates messages regarding self-esteem, gender identity, status, and interpersonal warmth or coldness. The individual whose posture is slumped, with head and eyes pointed downward, conveys a message of low self-esteem. Specific ways of standing or sitting are considered to be either feminine or masculine within a defined culture. To stand straight and tall with head high and hands on hips indicates a superior status over the person being addressed. Reece and Whitman (1962) identified response behaviors that were used to designate individuals as either "warm" or "cold" persons. Individuals who were perceived as "warm" responded to others with a shift of posture toward the other person, a smile, direct eye contact, and hands that remained still. Individuals who responded to others with a slumped posture, by looking around the room, drumming fingers on the desk, and not smiling were perceived as "cold."

Touch

Touch is a powerful communication tool. It can elicit both negative and positive reactions, depending on the people involved and the circumstances of the interaction. Touch is a very basic and primitive form of communication, and the appropriateness of its use is culturally determined.

Touch can be categorized according to the message communicated (Knapp, 1980):

1. **Functional-professional:** This type of touch is impersonal and businesslike. It is used to accomplish a task. *Examples:* a tailor who is measuring a customer for a suit or a physician examining a patient.
2. **Social-polite:** This type of touch is still rather impersonal, but it conveys an affirmation or acceptance of the other person. *Example:* a handshake.
3. **Friendship-warmth:** Touch at this level indicates a strong liking for the other person, a feeling that he or she is a friend. *Example:* Laying one's hand upon the shoulder of another.

4. **Love-intimacy:** This type of touch conveys an emotional attachment or attraction for another person. *Example:* to engage in a strong, mutual embrace.
5. **Sexual arousal:** Touch at this level is an expression of physical attraction only. *Example:* Touching another in the genital region.

Some cultures encourage more touching of various types than others. The nurse should understand the cultural meaning of touch before using this method of communication in specific situations.

Facial Expressions

Next to human speech, facial expression is the primary source of communication. Facial expressions primarily reveal an individual's emotional states, such as happiness, sadness, anger, fear, and surprise. The face is a complex, multimessage system. Facial expressions serve to complement and qualify other communication behaviors, and at times even take the place of verbal messages.

Eye Behavior

Smith and Williamson (1981) identified behaviors by which individuals communicate with their eyes: eye contact and gazing/staring. Eyes have been called the "windows of the soul." It is through eye contact that individuals view and are viewed by others in a revealing way. An interpersonal connectedness occurs through eye contact. In American culture, eye contact conveys a personal interest in the other person. Eye contact indicates that the communication channel is open and is often the initiating factor in verbal interaction between two people.

Patterns of gazing/staring are regulated by social rules. These rules dictate where we can look, when we can look, for how long we can look, and at whom we can look (Smith & Williamson, 1981). Staring is often used to register disapproval of the behavior of another. People are extremely sensitive to being looked at, and if the gazing/staring behavior violates social rules, they often assign meaning to it, such as the following statement implies: "He kept staring at me, and I began to wonder if I was dressed inappropriately or had mustard on my face!"

Verbal Cues or Paralanguage

Paralanguage is the gestural component of the spoken word. It consists of pitch, tone, and loudness of spoken messages, the rate of speaking, expressively placed pauses, and emphasis assigned to certain words. These vocal cues greatly influence the way individuals interpret verbal messages. A normally soft-spoken individual whose pitch and rate of speaking increase may be perceived as being anxious or tense.

Different vocal emphases can alter interpretation of the message.

For Example:

1. "I felt SURE you would notice the change." *Interpretation:* I was SURE you would, but you didn't.
2. "I felt sure YOU would notice the change." *Interpretation:* I thought YOU would, even if nobody else did.
3. "I felt sure you would notice the CHANGE. *Interpretation:* Even if you didn't notice anything else, I thought you would notice the CHANGE.

Verbal cues play a major role in determining responses in human communication situations. *How* a message is verbalized can be as important as *what* is verbalized.

THERAPEUTIC COMMUNICATION TECHNIQUES

Hays and Larson (1963) have identified a number of techniques to assist the nurse in interacting more therapeutically with patients. These are the "technical procedures" carried out by the nurse working in psychiatry and should serve to enhance development of a therapeutic nurse-patient relationship. Table 5.1 includes a list of these techniques, a short explanation of their usefulness, and examples of each.

NONTHERAPEUTIC COMMUNICATION TECHNIQUES

Several approaches are considered to be barriers to open communication between the nurse and patient. Hays and Larson (1963) identified a number

Table 5.1 THERAPEUTIC COMMUNICATION TECHNIQUES

Technique	Explanation/Rationale	Examples
Using silence	Gives the patient the opportunity to collect and organize thoughts, to think through a point, or to consider introducing a topic of greater concern than the one being discussed.	
Accepting	Conveys an attitude of reception and regard	"Yes, I understand what you said." Eye contact; nodding
Giving recognition	Acknowledging; indicating awareness. Better than complimenting, which reflects the nurse's judgment.	"Hello, Mr. J. I noticed that you made a ceramic ash tray in OT." "I see you made your bed."
Offering self	Making oneself available on an unconditional basis increases patient's feelings of self-worth.	"I'll stay with you a while." "We can eat our lunch together." "I'm interested in you."
Giving broad openings	Allows the patient to take the initiative in introducing the topic. Emphasizes the importance of the patient's role in the interaction.	"What would you like to talk about today?" "Tell me what you are thinking."
Offering general leads	Offers the patient encouragement to continue.	"Yes, I see." "Go on." "And after that?"
Placing the event in time or sequence	Clarifies the relationship of events in time so that the nurse and patient can view them in perspective.	"What seemed to lead up to . . .?" "Was this before or after . . .?" "When did this happen?"
Making observations	Verbalizing what is observed or perceived. This encourages the patient to recognize specific behaviors and compare perceptions with the nurse.	"You seem tense." "I notice you are pacing a lot." "You seem uncomfortable when you . . ."
Encouraging description of perceptions	Asking the patient to verbalize what is being perceived. Often used with patients experiencing hallucinations.	"Tell me what is happening now." "Are you hearing the voices again?" "What do the voices seem to be saying?"
Encouraging comparison	Asking patient to compare similarities and differences in ideas, experiences, or interpersonal relationships. Helps patient recognize life experiences that tend to recur as well as those aspects of life that are changeable.	"Was this something like . . .?" "How does this compare to the time when . . .?" "What was your response the last time this situation occurred?"
Restating	The main idea of what the patient has said is repeated. Lets the patient know whether or not an expressed statement has been understood and gives him or her the chance to continue or to clarify if necessary.	Pt: "I can't study. My mind keeps wandering." Ns: "You have difficulty concentrating." Pt: "I can't take that new job. What if I can't do it?" Ns: "You're afraid you will fail in this new position."
Reflecting	Questions and feelings are referred back to the patient so that they may be recognized and accepted, and so that the patient may recognize that his or her point of view has value. A good technique to use when patient asks nurse for advice.	Pt: "What do you think I should do about my wife's drinking problem?" Ns: "What do *you* think you should do?" Pt: "My sister won't help a bit toward my mother's care. I have to do it all!" Ns: "You feel angry when she doesn't help."
Focusing	Taking notice of a single idea or even a single word. Works especially well with a patient who is moving rapidly from one thought to another. This technique is *not* therapeutic, however, with the patient who is very anxious. Focusing should not be pursued until the anxiety level has subsided.	"This point seems worth looking at more closely. Perhaps you and I can discuss it together."

(continued)

Table 5.1 CONTINUED

Technique	Explanation/Rationale	Examples
Exploring	Delving further into a subject, idea, experience, or relationship. Especially helpful with patients who tend to remain on a superficial level of communication. However, if the patient chooses not to disclose further information, the nurse should refrain from pushing or probing in an area that obviously creates discomfort.	"Please explain that situation in more detail." "Tell me more about that particular situation."
Seeking clarification and validation	Striving to explain that which is vague or incomprehensible and searching for mutual understanding. Clarifying the meaning of what has been said facilitates and increases understanding for both patient and nurse.	"I'm not sure that I understand. Would you please explain." "Tell me if my understanding agrees with yours." "Do I understand correctly that you said . . .?"
Presenting reality	When the patient has a misperception of the environment, the nurse defines reality or indicates his or her perception of the situation for the patient.	"I understand that the voices seem real to you, but I do not hear any voices." "There is no one else in the room but you and me."
Voicing doubt	Expressing uncertainty as to the reality of the patient's perceptions. Often used with patients experiencing delusional thinking.	"I find that hard to believe." "That seems rather doubtful to me."
Verbalizing the implied	Putting into words what the patient has only implied or said indirectly. Can also be used with the patient who is mute or is otherwise experiencing impaired verbal communication. Clarifies that which is *implicit* rather than *explicit*.	Pt: "It's a waste of time to be here. I can't talk to you or anyone." Ns: "Are you feeling that no one understands?" Pt: (Silence) Ns: "It must have been very difficult for you when your husband died in the fire."
Attempting to translate words into feelings	When feelings are expressed only indirectly, the nurse tries to "desymbolize" what has been said and find clues to the underlying meaning.	Pt: "I'm way out in the ocean." Ns: "You must be feeling very lonely now."
Formulating a plan of action	When a patient has a plan in mind for dealing with what is considered to be a stressful situation, it may serve to prevent anger or anxiety from escalating to an unmanageable level.	"What could you do to let your anger our harmlessly?" "Next time this comes up, what might you do to handle it more appropriately?"

Source: From Hays and Larson (1963).

of these techniques, which are presented in Table 5.2. The nurse should recognize and eliminate the use of these patterns in his or her relationships with patients. Avoiding these communication barriers will maximize the effectiveness of communication and enhance the nurse-patient relationship.

ACTIVE LISTENING

To listen actively is to be attentive to what the patient is saying, both verbally and nonverbally. Attentive listening creates a climate in which the patient can communicate (Bernstein & Bernstein, 1980). With active listening, the nurse communicates acceptance and respect for the patient, and trust is enhanced. A climate is established within the relationship that promotes openness and honest expression.

Several nonverbal behaviors have been designated as facilitative skills for attentive listening. Those listed here can be identified by the acronym SOLER.

S—Sit squarely facing the patient. This gives the message that the nurse is there to listen and interested in what the patient has to say.
O—Observe an open posture. Posture is consid-

Table 5.2 NONTHERAPEUTIC COMMUNICATION TECHNIQUES

Technique	Explanation/Rationale	Examples
Giving reassurance	Indicates to the patient that there is no cause for anxiety, thereby devaluing the patient's feelings. May discourage the patient from further expression of feelings if he or she believes they will only be downplayed or ridiculed.	"I wouldn't worry about that if I were you." "Everything will be all right." **Better to say:** "We will work on that together."
Rejecting	Refusing to consider or showing contempt for the patient's ideas or behavior. This may cause the patient to discontinue interaction with the nurse for fear of further rejection.	"Let's not discuss . . ." "I don't want to hear about . . ." **Better to say:** "Let's look at that a little closer."
Giving approval or disapproval	Sanctioning or denouncing the patient's ideas or behavior. Implies that the nurse has the right to pass judgment on whether the patient's ideas or behaviors are "good" or "bad," and that the patient is expected to please the nurse. The nurse's acceptance of the patient is then seen as conditional, depending on the patient's behavior.	"That's good. I'm glad that you . . ." "That's bad. I'd rather you wouldn't . . ." **Better to say:** "Let's talk about how your behavior invoked anger in the other patients at dinner."
Agreeing/ disagreeing	Indicating accord with or opposition to the patient's ideas or opinions. Implies that the nurse has the right to pass judgment on whether the patient's ideas or opinions are "right" or "wrong." Agreement prevents the patient from later modifying his or her point of view without admitting error. Disagreement implies inaccuracy, provoking the need for defensiveness on the part of the patient.	"That's right. I agree." "That's wrong. I disagree." "I don't believe that." **Better to say:** "Let's discuss what you feel is unfair about the new community rules."
Giving advice	Telling the patient what to do or how to behave implies that the nurse knows what is best and that the patient is incapable of any self-direction. Nurtures the patient in the dependent role by discouraging independent thinking.	"I think you should . . ." "Why don't you . . ." **Better to say:** "What do **you** think you should do?"
Probing	Persistent questioning of the patient. Pushing for answers to issues the patient does not wish to discuss. Causes the patient to feel used and valued only for what is shared with the nurse. Places the patient on the defensive.	"Tell me how your mother abused you when you were a child." "Tell me how you feel toward your mother now that she is dead." **Better technique:** The nurse should be aware of the patient's response and discontinue the interaction at the first sign of discomfort.
Defending	Attempting to protect someone or something from verbal attack. To defend what the patient has criticized is to imply that he or she has no right to express ideas, opinions, or feelings. Defending does not change the patient's feelings and may cause the patient to think the nurse is taking sides with those being criticized and against the patient.	"No one here would lie to you." "You have a very capable physician. I'm sure he only has your best interests in mind." **Better to say:** "I will try to answer your questions and clarify some issues regarding your treatment."
Requesting an explanation	Asking the patient to provide the reasons for thoughts, feelings, behavior, and events. Asking "Why?" a patient did something or feels a certain way can be very intimidating and implies that the patient must defend his or her behavior or feelings.	"Why do you think that?" "Why do you feel this way?" "Why did you do that?" **Better to say:** "Describe what you were feeling just prior to that occurrence."

(continued)

Table 5.2 CONTINUED

Technique	Explanation/Rationale	Examples
Indicating the existence of an external source of power	Attributing the source of thoughts, feelings, and behavior to others or to outside influences. This encourages the patient to project blame for his or her thoughts or behaviors upon others rather than accepting the responsibility personally.	"What makes you say that?" "What made you do that?" "What made you so angry last night?" **Better to say:** "You became angry when your brother insulted your wife."
Belittling feelings expressed	When the nurse misjudges the degree of the patient's discomfort, a lack of empathy and understanding may be conveyed. The nurse may tell the patient to "perk up" or "snap out of it." This causes the patient to feel insignificant or unimportant. When one is experiencing discomfort, it is no relief to hear that others are or have been in similar situations.	Pt: "I have nothing to live for. I wish I were dead." Ns: "Everybody gets down in the dumps at times. I feel that way myself sometimes." **Better to say:** "You must be very upset. Tell me what you are feeling right now."
Making stereotyped comments	Clichés and trite expressions are meaningless in a nurse-patient relationship. For the nurse to make empty conversation is to encourage a like response from the patient.	"I'm fine, and how are you?" "Hang in there. It's for your own good." "Keep your chin up." **Better to say:** "The therapy must be difficult for you at times. How do you feel about your progress at this point?"
Using denial	When the nurse denies that a problem exists, he or she blocks discussion with the patient and avoids helping the patient identify and explore areas of difficulty.	Pt: "I'm nothing." Ns: "Of course you're something. Everybody is somebody." **Better to say:** "You're feeling like no one cares about you right now."
Interpreting	With this technique the therapist seeks to make conscious that which is unconscious, to tell the patient the meaning of his experience.	"What you really mean is . . ." "Unconsciously you're saying . . ." **Better technique:** The nurse must leave interpretation of the patient's behavior to the psychiatrist. The nurse has not been prepared to perform this technique, and in attempting to do so, may endanger other nursing roles with the patient.
Introducing an unrelated topic	Changing the subject causes the nurse to take over the direction of the discussion. This may occur in order to get to something that the nurse wants to discuss with the patient or to get away from a topic that he or she would prefer not to discuss.	Pt: "I don't have anything to live for." Ns: "Did you have visitors this weekend?" **Better technique:** The nurse must remain open and free to hear the patient, to take in all that is being conveyed, both verbally and nonverbally.

Source: From Hays and Larson (1963).

ered "open" when arms and legs remain uncrossed. This suggests that the nurse is "open" to what the patient has to say. With a "closed" position, the nurse can convey a somewhat defensive stance, possibly invoking a similar response in the patient.

L—Lean forward toward the patient. This con-

veys to the patient that you are involved in the interaction, interested in what is being said, and making a sincere effort to be attentive.

E—Establish eye contact. Direct eye contact is another behavior that conveys the nurse's involvement and willingness to listen to what the patient has to say. The absence of eye contact, or constantly shifting eye contact, gives the message that the nurse is not really interested in what is being said. **Note:** Ensure that eye contact conveys warmth and is accompanied by smiling and intermittent nodding of the head, and that it does not come across as "staring" or "glaring," which can create intense discomfort in the patient.

R — Relax. Whether sitting or standing during the interaction, the nurse should communicate a sense of being relaxed and comfortable with the patient. Restlessness and fidgeting communicate a lack of interest and a feeling of discomfort that are likely to be transferred to the patient.

FEEDBACK

Feedback is a method of communication for helping the patient consider a modification of behavior. Feedback gives information to patients about how they are being perceived by others. It should be presented in a manner that discourages defensiveness on the part of the patient. Feedback can be useful to the patient if presented with objectivity by a trusted individual.

Some criteria about useful feedback include:

1. **Feedback is descriptive rather than evaluative and focuses on the behavior rather than on the patient.** Avoiding evaluative language reduces the need for the patient to react defensively. An objective description allows the patient to take the information and use it in whatever way he or she chooses. When the focus is on the patient, the nurse makes judgments about the patient.

Examples

Descriptive and focused on behavior	"Jane was very upset in group today when you called her 'fatty' and laughed at her in front of the others."
Evaluative	"You were very rude and inconsiderate to Jane in group today."
Focus on patient	"You are a very insensitive person."

2. **Feedback should be specific rather than general.** Information that gives details about the patient's behavior can be used more easily than a generalized description for modifying the behavior.

Examples

General:	"You just don't pay attention."
Specific:	"You were talking to Joe when we were deciding on the issue. Now you want to argue about the outcome."

3. **Feedback should be directed toward behavior that the patient has the capacity to modify.** To provide feedback about a characteristic or situation that the patient cannot change will only provoke frustration.

Examples

Can modify:	"I noticed that you did not want to hold your baby when the nurse brought her to you."
Cannot modify:	"Your baby daughter is mentally retarded because you took drugs when you were pregnant."

4. **Feedback should impart information rather than offering advice.** Giving advice fosters dependence and may convey the message to the patient that he or she is not capable of making decisions and solving problems independently. It is the patient's right and privilege to be as self-sufficient as possible.

Examples

Imparting information:	"There are various methods of assistance for people who want to lose weight, such as Overeaters Anonymous, Weight Watchers, regular visits to a dietitian, the Physicians Weight Loss Program. You can decide what is best for you."
Giving advice:	"You obviously need to lose a great deal of weight. I think the Physicians Weight Loss Program would be best for you."

5. **Feedback should be well-timed.** Feedback is most useful when given at the earliest appropriate opportunity following the specific behavior.

Examples

Prompt response:	"I saw you hit the wall with your fist just now when

Delayed response:

you hung up the phone from talking to your mother."

"You need to learn some more appropriate ways of dealing with your anger. Last week after group I saw you pounding your fist against the wall."

SUMMARY

Interpersonal communication is a transaction between the sender and the receiver. In all interpersonal transactions, both the sender and receiver bring certain preexisting conditions to the exchange that influence both the intended message and the way in which it is interpreted. Examples of these conditions include one's value system, internalized attitudes and beliefs, culture or religion, social status, gender, background knowledge and experience, age or developmental level, and the type of environment in which the communication takes place.

Nonverbal expression is a primary communication system in which meaning is assigned to various gestures and patterns of behavior. Some components of nonverbal communication include physical appearance and dress, body movement and posture, touch, facial expressions, eye behavior, and vocal cues or paralanguage. The meaning of each of these nonverbal components is culturally determined.

Hays and Larson (1963) have described various techniques of communication that can facilitate interaction between the nurse and patient. They have also identified a number of barriers to communication that can interfere with a satisfactory nurse-patient interaction. Examples of both were presented in this chapter.

Active listening is described as being attentive to what the patient is saying, both verbally and nonverbally. Facilitative skills for attentive listening include sitting squarely facing the patient, observing an open posture, leaning forward toward the patient, establishing eye contact, and relaxing. They can be identified by the acronym SOLER.

Feedback is a method of communication for helping the patient consider a modification of behavior. It is most useful when it:

1. Is descriptive rather than evaluative.
2. Focuses on behavior rather than on the person.
3. Is specific rather than general.
4. Is directed toward behavior that the patient can change.
5. Imparts information rather than gives advice.
6. Is well-timed.

The nurse must be aware of the therapeutic or nontherapeutic value of the communication techniques used with the patient, as they are the "tools" of psychosocial intervention.

REVIEW QUESTIONS
Self-Examination/Learning Exercise

Test your knowledge about the concept of communication by answering the following questions:

1. Describe the transactional model of communication.
2. List eight types of preexisting conditions that can influence the outcome of the communication process.
3. Define *territoriality*. How does it affect communication?
4. Define *density*. How does it affect communication?
5. Identify four types of spacial distance and give an example of each.
6. Identify six components of nonverbal communication that convey special messages and give an example of each.

7. Describe five facilitative skills for active or attentive, listening that can be identified by the acronym SOLER.

Identify the correct answer in each of the following questions. Provide explanation where requested. Identify the technique used (both therapeutic and nontherapeutic) in all choices given.

8. A patient states: "I refuse to shower in this room. I must be very cautious. The FBI has placed a camera in here to monitor my every move." Which is the most appropriate response by the nurse?
   a. "That's not true."
   b. "I have a hard time believing that is true."

9. Nancy, a depressed patient who has been unkempt and untidy for weeks, today comes to group therapy wearing a clean dress, makeup, and having washed and combed her hair. Which of the following responses by the nurse is most appropriate? Give the rationale.
   a. "Nancy, I see you have put on a clean dress and combed your hair."
   b. "Nancy, you look wonderful today!"

10. Dorothy was involved in an automobile accident while under the influence of alcohol. She swerved her car into a tree and narrowly missed hitting a child on a bicycle. She is in the hospital with multiple abrasions and contusions. She is talking about the accident with the nurse. Which of the following statements by the nurse is most appropriate? Identify the therapeutic or nontherapeutic technique in each.
    a. "Now that you know what can happen when you drink and drive, I'm sure you won't let it happen again. I'm sure everything will be okay."
    b. "That was a terrible thing you did. You could have killed that child!"
    c. "Now I guess you'll have to buy a new car. Can you afford that?"
    d. "What made you do such a thing?"
    e. "Tell me how you are feeling about what happened."

11. Judy has been in the hospital for 3 weeks. She has used Valium "to settle my nerves" for the past 15 years. She was admitted by her psychiatrist for safe withdrawal from the drug. She has passed the physical symptoms of withdrawal at this time, but states to the nurse, "I don't know if I will make it without Valium after I go home. I'm already starting to feel nervous. I have so many personal problems." Which is the most appropriate response by the nurse? Identify the technique in each.
    a. "Why do you think you have to have drugs to deal with your problems?"
    b. "You'll just have to pull yourself together. Everybody has problems, and everybody doesn't use drugs to deal with them. They just do the best that they can."
    c. "I don't want to talk about that now. Look at that sunshine. It's beautiful outside. You and I are going to take a walk!"
    d. "Starting today you and I are going to think about some alternative ways for you to deal with those problems — things that you can do to decrease your anxiety without resorting to drugs."

12. Mrs. S. asks the nurse, "Do you think I should tell my husband about my affair with my boss?" Give one therapeutic response and one

nontherapeutic response, your rationale, and identify the technique used in each response.

13. Carol, an adolescent, just returned from group therapy and is crying. She says to the nurse, "All the other kids laughed at me! I try to fit in, but I always seem to say the wrong thing. I've never had a close friend. I guess I never will." Which is the most appropriate response by the nurse? Identify each technique used.
    a. "You're feeling pretty down on yourself right now."
    b. "Why do you feel this way about yourself?"
    c. "What makes you think you will never have any friends?"
    d. "The next time they laugh at you, you should just get up and leave the room!"
    e. "I'm sure they didn't mean to hurt your feelings."
    f. "Keep your chin up and hang in there. Your time will come."

REFERENCES

Bernstein, L. & Bernstein, R. (1980). *Interviewing: A guide for health professionals.* New York: Appleton-Century-Crofts.

Hall, E.T. (1966). The hidden dimension. Garden City, NY: Doubleday.

Hays, J. S. & Larson, K. H. (1963). *Interacting with patients.* New York: Macmillan.

Knapp, M. L. (1980). *Essentials of nonverbal communication.* New York: Holt, Rinehart and Winston.

Mehrabian, A. (1972). *Nonverbal communication.* Chicago: Aldine-Atherton.

Reece, M. & Whitman, R. (1962). Expressive movements, warmth, and verbal reinforcement. *J Abnorm Soc Psychol, 64:*234–236.

Smith, D. R. & Williamson, L. K. (1981). *Interpersonal communication* (2nd ed.). Dubuque, IA: WC Brown Co, Publishers.

BIBLIOGRAPHY

Cormier, L. S., Cormier, W. H., & Weisser, R. J., Jr. (1984). *Interviewing and helping skills for health professionals.* Monterey, CA: Wadsworth Health Sciences Division.

Duldt, B. W., Giffin, K., & Patton, B. R. (1984). *Interpersonal communication in nursing.* Philadelphia: FA Davis.

Egan, G. (1977). *You and me.* Monterey, CA: Brooks/Cole.

Fritz, P. A., Russell, C.G., Wilcox, E.M., and Shirk, F.I. (1984). *Interpersonal communication in nursing.* Norwalk, CT: Appleton-Century-Crofts.

Hein, E. C. (1980). *Communication in nursing practice* (2nd ed.). Boston: Little, Brown & Co.

Northouse, P. G. & Northouse, L. L. (1985). *Health communication—A handbook for health professionals.* Englewood Cliffs, NJ: Prentice-Hall.

Sundeen, S. J. et al. (1985). *Nurse-client interaction—Implementing the nursing process* (3rd ed.). St. Louis, MO: CV Mosby.

Watzlawick, P., Beavin, J., and Jackson, D.D. (1967). *The pragmatics of human communication.* New York: WW Norton.

6

THE NURSING PROCESS IN PSYCHIATRIC/MENTAL HEALTH NURSING

KEY TERMS
nursing process
nursing diagnosis
case management
critical pathways of care
diagnostic-related group
interdisciplinary
problem-oriented recording
Focus Charting®
PIE charting

OBJECTIVES

After reading this chapter, the student will be able to:

1. Define *nursing process.*
2. Identify five steps of the nursing process and describe nursing actions associated with each.
3. Describe the benefits of using nursing diagnosis.
4. Discuss the list of nursing diagnoses approved by the North American Nursing Diagnosis Association (NANDA).
5. Apply the five steps of the nursing process in the care of a patient within the psychiatric setting.
6. Document patient care that validates use of the nursing process.

THE NURSING PROCESS

Definition

The nursing process has for many years provided a systematic framework for the delivery of nursing care. It consists of five steps and uses a problem-solving approach that has come to be accepted as nursing's scientific methodology. It is goal directed, with the objective being delivery of quality patient care.

Nursing process is dynamic, not static. It is an ongoing process that continues for as long as the nurse and patient have interactions directed toward change in the patient's physical or behavioral responses. Figure 6.1 presents a schematic of the ongoing nursing process.

Steps of the Nursing Process

The five steps of the nursing process include:

1. **Assessment.** In this first step, information is gathered from which to establish a data base for determining the best possible care for the patient. Information for this data base is gathered from a variety of sources, including interviewing the patient or family, observing the patient and his or her environment, consulting other health-team members, reviewing the patient's records, and conducting a nursing physical examination. A biopsychosocial assessment tool based on the stress-adaptation framework is included in Table 6.1.

2. **Analysis.** In the analysis step, data gathered during the assessment are analyzed. From this data analysis, the nurse then

   - Selects the appropriate nursing diagnoses for the patient.
   - Writes measurable goals of care for each nursing diagnosis identified.

3. **Planning.** The care plan is developed during this step of the nursing process. For each nursing diagnosis identified, the most appropriate nursing interventions for meeting the goals are selected. Priorities for delivery of nursing care are determined.

4. **Implementation.** In this step, the interventions selected during the planning stage are exe-

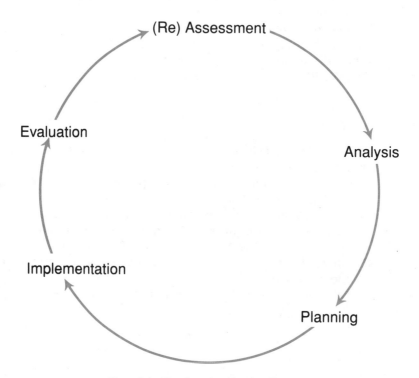

Figure 6.1 The Ongoing Nursing Process.

Table 6.1 NURSING HISTORY AND ASSESSMENT TOOL

I. General Information

Patient name: _____

Room number: _____

Doctor: _____

Age: _____

Sex: _____

Race: _____

Dominant language: _____

Marital status: _____

Chief complaint: _____

_____

_____

Allergies: _____

Diet: _____

Height/weight: _____

Vital signs: TPR/BP _____

Name and phone no. of
    significant other: _____

_____

City of residence: _____

Diagnosis (admitting and current):

_____

_____

Conditions of admission:

Date _____   Time _____

Accompanied by _____

Route of admission _____ (wheelchair, ambulatory, cart)

Admitted from _____

II. Predisposing Factors

A. *Genetic Influences*

1. Family configuration (use genograms):

    Family of origin: Present family:

    Family dynamics (describe significant relationships between family members): _____

    _____

    _____

    _____

    _____

2. Medical/psychiatric history:

    a. Patient: _____

    _____

    _____

    b. Family members: _____

    _____

    _____

3. Other GENETIC influences affecting present adaptation. This might include effects specific to gender, race, appearance, such as genetic physical defects, or any other factor related to genetics that is affecting the patient's adaptation that has not been mentioned elsewhere in this assessment.

    _____

    _____

    _____

    _____

    _____

(continued)

Table 6.1 CONTINUED

B. *Past Experiences*
  1. Cultural and social history:
      a. Environmental factors (family living arrangements, type of neighborhood, special working conditions): _____
      _____
      _____

      b. Health beliefs and practices (personal responsibility for health, special self-care practices): _____
      _____
      _____

      c. Religious beliefs and practices: _____
      _____
      _____

      d. Educational background: _____
      _____
      _____

      e. Significant losses/changes (include dates): _____
      _____
      _____

      f. Peer/friendship relationships: _____
      _____
      _____

      g. Occupational history: _____
      _____
      _____

      h. Previous pattern of coping with stress: _____
      _____
      _____

      i. Other life-style factors contributing to present adaptation: _____
      _____
      _____

C. *Existing Conditions*
  1. Stage of development (Erikson)
      a. Theoretically: _____
      b. Behaviorally: _____
      c. Rationale: _____
      _____
      _____

  2. Support systems: _____
  _____

  3. Economic security: _____
  _____

  4. Avenues of productivity/contribution:
      a. Current job status: _____
      _____

      b. Role contributions and responsibility for others: _____
      _____

(continued)

Table 6.1   CONTINUED

III. Precipitating Event
Describe the situation or events that precipitated this illness/hospitalization. _____
_____
_____

IV. Patient's Perception of the Stressor
Patient's or family member's understanding or description of stressor/illness and expectations of hospitalization: _____
_____
_____
_____

V. Adaptation Responses

A. *Psychosocial*

1. Anxiety level (circle level and check the behaviors that apply):   mild   moderate   severe   panic
   calm _____   friendly _____   passive _____   alert _____   perceives environment correctly _____
   cooperative _____   impaired attention _____   "jittery" _____   unable to concentrate _____
   hypervigilant _____   tremors _____   rapid speech _____   withdrawn _____   confused _____
   disoriented _____   fearful _____   hyperventilating _____   misinterpreting the environment _____
   (hallucinations/delusions) depersonalization _____   obsessions _____   compulsions _____
   somatic complaints _____   excessive hyperactivity _____   other _____
   _____

2. Mood/affect (circle as many as apply):   happiness   sadness   dejection   despair   elation   euphoria
   suspiciousness   apathy (little emotional tone)   anger/hostility

3. Ego defense mechanisms (describe how used by patient):
   Projection _____
   Suppression _____
   Undoing _____
   Displacement _____
   Intellectualization _____
   Rationalization _____
   Denial _____
   Repression _____
   Isolation _____
   Regression _____
   Reaction formation _____
   Splitting _____
   Religiosity _____
   Sublimation _____
   Compensation _____

4. Level of self-esteem (circle one):   low   moderate   high
   Things patient likes about self _____
   _____
   Things patient would like to change about self _____
   _____

(continued)

Table 6.1   CONTINUED

V. Adaptation Responses (cont'd)

    Objective assessment of self-esteem:

      Eye contact _____

      General appearance _____

      _____

      Personal hygiene _____

      Participation in group activities and interactions with others _____

      _____

5. Stage and manifestations of grief (circle one):

    denial   anger   bargaining   depression   acceptance

    Describe patient's behaviors that are associated with this stage of grieving in response to loss or change.

    _____

    _____

    _____

6. Thought processes (circle as many as apply):   clear   logical   easy to follow   relevant   confused

    blocking   delusional   rapid flow of thoughts   slowness in thought association   suspicious

    recent memory: loss   intact;   remote memory: loss   intact

    other _____

    _____

7. Communication patterns (circle as many as apply):   clear   coherent   slurred speech   incoherent

    neologisms   loose associations   flight of ideas   aphasic   perseveration

    rumination   tangential speech   loquaciousness   slow, impoverished speech

    speech impediment (describe) _____

    other _____

8. Interaction patterns (describe patient's pattern of interpersonal interactions with staff and peers on the unit; e.g., manipulative, withdrawn, isolated, verbally or physically hostile, argumentative, passive, assertive, aggressive, passive-aggressive, other): _____

    _____

    _____

    _____

9. Reality orientation (check those that apply):

    Oriented to: time _____   person _____

                place _____   situation _____

10. Ideas of destruction to self/others?   Yes   No

    If yes, consider plan; available means _____

    _____

    _____

    _____

B. *Physiological*

1. Psychosomatic manifestations (describe any somatic complaints that may be stress-related): _____

    _____

    _____

    _____

(continued)

Table 6.1   CONTINUED

2. Drug history and assessment:
   Use of prescribed drugs:

NAME	DOSAGE	PRESCRIBED FOR	RESULTS

   Use of over-the-counter drugs:

NAME	DOSAGE	USED FOR	RESULTS

   Use of street drugs or alcohol:

NAME	AMOUNT USED	HOW OFTEN USED	WHEN LAST USED	EFFECTS PRODUCED

3. Pertinent physical assessments:
   a. Respirations: normal _____   labored _____
      Rate _____   Rhythm _____
   b. Skin: warm _____   dry _____   moist _____   cool _____
      clammy _____   pink _____   cyanotic _____
      poor turgor _____   edematous _____
      Evidence of: rash _____   bruising _____
      needle tracks _____   hirsutism _____
      loss of hair _____   other _____

   c. Musculoskeletal status: weakness _____   tremors _____
      Degree of range of motion (describe limitations) _____

      Pain (describe) _____
      Skeletal deformities (describe) _____
      Coordination (describe limitations) _____

   d. Neurologic status:
      History of (check all that apply):   seizures _____
      (describe method of control) _____
      headaches (describe location and frequency) _____

      fainting spells _____   dizziness _____
      tingling/numbness (describe location) _____

(continued)

Table 6.1 CONTINUED

e. Cardiovascular: B/P _____ Pulse _____
    History of (check all that apply):
        hypertension _____ palpitations _____
        heart murmur _____ chest pain _____
        shortness of breath _____ pain in legs _____
        phlebitis _____ ankle/leg edema _____
        numbness/tingling in extremities _____
        varicose veins _____

f. Gastrointestinal:
    Usual diet pattern: _____
    Food allergies: _____
    Dentures? _____ upper _____ lower _____
        Any problems with chewing or swallowing? _____
        Any recent change in weight? _____
        Any problems with:
        indigestion/heartburn? _____
          relieved by _____
        nausea/vomiting? _____
          relieved by _____
        loss of appetite? _____
    History of ulcers? _____
    Usual bowel pattern _____
        Constipation? _____ Diarrhea? _____
        Type of self-care assistance provided for either of the above problems _____

g. Genitourinary/reproductive:
    Usual voiding pattern _____
    Urinary hesitancy? _____ frequency _____
    Nocturia? _____ Pain/burning? _____
    Incontinence? _____
    Any genital lesions? _____
        Discharge? _____ Odor? _____
    History of venereal disease? _____ If yes, explain:
    _____
    Any concerns about sexuality/sexual activity? _____
    _____
    _____
    Method of birth control used _____
    Females:
        Date of last menstrual cycle _____
        Length of cycle _____
        Problems associated with menstruation? _____
    _____
        Breasts: pain/tenderness? _____
          Swelling? _____ Discharge? _____
          Lumps? _____ Dimpling? _____

(continued)

Table 6.1 CONTINUED

Practice breast self-examination? _____

Frequency? _____

Males:

Penile discharge? _____

Prostate problems? _____

h. Eyes:

	YES	NO	EXPLAIN
Glasses?	_____	_____	_____
Contacts?	_____	_____	_____
Swelling?	_____	_____	_____
Discharge?	_____	_____	_____
Itching?	_____	_____	_____
Blurring?	_____	_____	_____
Double vision?	_____	_____	_____

i. Ears:

	YES	NO	EXPLAIN
Pain?	_____	_____	_____
Drainage?	_____	_____	_____
Difficulty hearing?	_____	_____	_____
Hearing aid?	_____	_____	_____
Tinnitus?	_____	_____	_____

j. Medication side effects:

What symptoms is the patient experiencing that may be attributed to current medication usage? _____
_____
_____

k. Altered lab values and possible significance: _____
_____
_____

l. Activity/rest patterns:

Exercise (amount, type, frequency) _____
_____

Leisure-time activities: _____
_____

Patterns of sleep: Number of hours per night _____

Use of sleep aids? _____

Pattern of awakening during the night? _____
_____

Feel rested upon awakening? _____

m. Personal hygiene/activities of daily living:

Patterns of self-care: independent _____

Requires assistance with: mobility _____

hygiene _____

toileting _____

feeding _____

dressing _____

other _____

(*continued*)

Table 6.1 CONTINUED

Statement describing personal hygiene and general appearance _____

_____

_____

n. Other pertinent physical assessments: _____

_____

_____

VI. Summary of Initial Psychosocial/Physical Assessment

KNOWLEDGE DEFICITS IDENTIFIED:

NURSING DIAGNOSES INDICATED:

Source: From Townsend (1991).

cuted. The care plan serves as a blueprint for delivery of nursing care.

5. **Evaluation.** During the evaluation step, the nurse measures the success of the interventions in meeting the stated goals. Care is documented, validating use of the nursing process in the delivery of care. The plan of care is reviewed and modified as need is determined by the evaluation.

WHY NURSING DIAGNOSIS?

The concept of nursing diagnosis is not new. For centuries, nurses have identified specific patient responses for which nursing interventions were employed in an effort to improve quality of life. Therefore, it is not surprising to hear some nurses who have been in practice for many years ask, "What is this thing called nursing diagnosis? Why must we make changes if what we are doing works?" Historically lacking in the provision of nursing care was the autonomy of practice to which nurses were entitled by virtue of their licensure. Nursing was described as a set of tasks, and nurses were valued as "handmaidens" for the physician (Gordon, 1987).

The term *diagnosis* in relation to nursing first began to appear in the literature in the early 1950s. The formalized organization of the concept, however, was only initiated in 1973 with the convening of the First National Conference on Nursing Diagnosis. The National Task Force for Classification of Nursing Diagnoses was developed during this conference. These individuals were charged with the task of identifying and classifying nursing diagnoses.

Also in the 1970s, the American Nurses' Association (ANA) began to write standards of practice around the five steps of the nursing process, of which nursing diagnosis is an inherent part (ANA, 1973). This format encompasses both the general and specialty standards outlined by the ANA. The standards of psychiatric/mental health nursing practice are presented in Table 6.2.

From this progression, a statement of policy was published in 1980 and included a definition of nursing. The ANA defined nursing as ". . . the diagnosis and treatment of human responses to actual or potential health problems" (ANA, 1980).

Table 6.2 STANDARDS OF PSYCHIATRIC/MENTAL HEALTH NURSING PRACTICE

Standard I. Theory.
The nurse applies appropriate theory that is scientifically sound as a basis for decisions regarding nursing practice.

Standard II. Data Collection.
The nurse continuously collects data that are comprehensive, accurate, and systematic.

Standard III. Diagnosis.
The nurse uses nursing diagnoses or standard classification of mental disorders to express conclusions supported by recorded assessment data and current scientific premises.

Standard IV. Planning.
The nurse develops a nursing care plan with specific goals and interventions delineating nursing actions unique to each client's needs.

Standard V. Intervention.
The nurse intervenes as guided by the nursing care plan to implement nursing actions that promote, maintain, or restore physical and mental health, prevent illness, and effect rehabilitation.

Standard V-A. Intervention: Psychotherapeutic Interventions.
The nurse uses psychotherapeutic interventions to assist clients in regaining or improving their previous coping abilities and to prevent further disability.

Standard V-B. Intervention: Health Teaching.
The nurse assists clients, families, and groups to achieve satisfying and productive patterns of living through health teaching.

Standard V-C. Intervention: Activities of Daily Living.
The nurse uses the activities of daily living in a goal-directed way to foster adequate self-care and physical and mental well-being of clients.

Standard V-D. Intervention: Somatic Therapies.
The nurse uses knowledge of somatic therapies and applies related clinical skills in working with clients.

Standard V-E. Intervention: Therapeutic Environment.
The nurse provides, structures, and maintains a therapeutic environment in collaboration with the client and other health-care providers.

Standard V-F. Intervention: Psychotherapy.
The nurse uses advanced clinical expertise in individual, group, and family psychotherapy; child psychotherapy; and other treatment modalities to function as a psychotherapist, and recognizes professional accountability for nursing practice.

Standard VI. Evaluation.
The nurse evaluates client responses to nursing actions in order to revise the data base, nursing diagnoses, and nursing care plans.

Standard VII. Peer Review.
The nurse participates in peer review and other means of evaluation to assure quality of nursing care provided for clients.

Standard VIII. Continuing Education.
The nurse assumes responsibility for continuing education and professional development and contributes to the professional growth of others.

Standard IX. Interdisciplinary Collaboration.
The nurse collaborates with other health-care providers in assessing, planning, implementing, and evaluating programs and other mental health activities.

Standard X. Utilization of Community Health Systems.
The nurse participates with other members of the community in assessing, planning, implementing, and evaluating mental health services and community systems that include the promotion of the broad continuum of primary, secondary, and tertiary prevention of mental illness.

Standard XI. Research.
The nurse contributes to nursing and the mental health field through innovations in theory and practice and participation in research.

Source: Adapted from American Nurses' Association, Division of Psychiatric/Mental Health Nursing Practice (1982).

A number of states have incorporated the five-step nursing process, including nursing diagnosis, into the scope of nursing practice described in their nurse practice acts. Decisions regarding professional negligence are made based on the standards of practice defined by the ANA and the individual state nurse practice acts. As these guidelines become more widely accepted, it will be the legal duty of the nurse to show that nursing process and nursing diagnosis were accurately implemented in the delivery of nursing care.

The North American Nursing Diagnosis Association (NANDA) evolved from the National Task Force for Classification of Nursing Diagnoses. The major purpose of NANDA is to provide a forum for discussion about the development, refinement, and promotion of a taxonomy of nursing diagnostic terminology (Lancour, 1990). As of the Tenth National NANDA conference held in April, 1992, 109 nursing diagnoses have been approved for use and for testing (Table 6.3). This list is by no means exhaustive or all-inclusive. For purposes of this text, however,

Table 6.3 NURSING DIAGNOSES APPROVED BY NANDA

Through 10th National Conference, April 1992

Activity Intolerance
Activity Intolerance, high risk for
Adjustment, impaired
Airway Clearance, ineffective
Anxiety (specify level)
Aspiration, high risk for

Body Image Disturbance
Body Temperature, altered, high risk for
Bowel Incontinence
Breastfeeding, effective
Breastfeeding, ineffective
Breastfeeding, interrupted *
Breathing Pattern, ineffective

Cardiac output, decreased
Caregiver Role Strain *
Caregiver Role Strain, High Risk for *
Communication, impaired verbal
Constipation
Constipation, colonic
Constipation, perceived

Decisional Conflict (specify)
Defensive Coping
Denial, ineffective
Diarrhea
Disuse Syndrome, high risk for
Diversional Activity Deficit
Dysreflexia

Family Coping, compromised, ineffective
Family Coping, disabling, ineffective
Family Coping, potential for growth
Family Processes, altered
Fatigue
Fear
Feeding Pattern, Infant: ineffective *
Fluid Volume Deficit
Fluid Volume Deficit, high risk for
Fluid Volume Excess

Gas Exchange, impaired
Grieving, anticipatory
Grieving, dysfunctional
Growth and Development, altered

Health Maintenance, altered
Health-Seeking Behaviors (specify)
Home Maintenance Management, impaired
Hopelessness
Hyperthermia
Hypothermia

Incontinence, functional
Incontinence, reflex
Incontinence, stress
Incontinence, total
Incontinence, urge
Individual Coping, ineffective
Infection, high risk for
Injury, high risk for

Knowledge Deficit (specify)

Management of Therapeutic Regimen, Ineffective *
Noncompliance (specify)
Nutrition, altered: less than body requirements
Nutrition, altered: more than body requirements
Nutrition, altered: high risk for more than body requirements

Oral Mucous Membrane, altered

Pain
Pain, chronic
Parental Role Conflict
Parenting, altered
Parenting, altered, high risk for
Peripheral Neurovascular Dysfunction, high risk for *
Personal Identity Disturbance
Physical Mobility, impaired
Poisoning, high risk for
Post-trauma Response
Powerlessness
Protection, altered

Rape-Trauma Syndrome
Rape-Trauma Syndrome: compound reaction
Rape-Trauma Syndrome: silent reaction
Relocation stress syndrome *
Role Performance, altered

Self-Care Deficit,
    bathing/hygiene,
    dressing/grooming,
    feeding,
    toileting
Self-esteem, chronic low
Self-esteem disturbance
Self-esteem, situational low
Self-mutilation, high risk for *
Sensory/Perceptual Alterations: visual, auditory, kinesthetic,
    gustatory, tactile, olfactory
Sexual Dysfunction
Sexuality Patterns, altered
Skin Integrity, impaired
Skin Integrity, impaired, high risk for
Sleep Pattern Disturbance
Social Interaction, impaired
Social Isolation
Spiritual Distress
Suffocation, high risk for
Swallowing, impaired

Thermoregulation, ineffective
Thought Processes, altered
Tissue Integrity, impaired
Tissue Perfusion, altered (specify type); renal, cerebral,
    cardiopulmonary, gastrointestinal, peripheral
Trauma, high risk for

Unilateral Neglect
Urinary Elimination, altered patterns
Urinary Retention

Ventilation, Spontaneous: Inability to sustain *
Ventilatory Weaning Response, Dysfunctional *
Violence, high risk for: self-directed of directed at others

*Newly approved NANDA Diagnoses/April, 1992.

the existing list will be used in an effort to maintain a common language within nursing and to encourage clinical testing of what is available.

An official definition of *nursing diagnosis* was presented to the membership at the Ninth National NANDA Conference in 1990. The definition is as follows:

"Nursing diagnoses are clinical judgments about individual, family, or community responses to actual and potential health problems/life processes. Nursing diagnoses provide the basis for selection of nursing interventions to achieve outcomes for which the nurse is accountable." (Carroll-Johnson, 1990).

The use of nursing diagnosis affords a degree of autonomy that historically has been lacking in the practice of nursing. Nursing diagnosis describes the patient's condition, prescribes interventions, and establishes parameters for outcome criteria based upon what is uniquely nursing. The ultimate benefit is to the patient, who receives effective and consistent nursing care based on knowledge of the problems that the patient is experiencing and of the most beneficial nursing interventions for resolution (Miller, 1989).

NURSING CASE MANAGEMENT

With the advent of diagnosis-related groups and shorter hospital stays, the concept of case management has evolved. Case management is an innovative model of care delivery than can result in improved patient care. The ANA describes nursing case management as ". . . a health care delivery process whose goals are to provide quality health care, decrease fragmentation, enhance the client's quality of life and contain costs" (ANA, 1988). Case management involves having a "case manager" who coordinates the patient's care from admission to discharge and, in many cases, following discharge. Nursing case management is the nursing process expanded in scope and made operational (Faherty, 1990).

Critical pathways have emerged as the tools for provision of care in a case management system. A critical pathway is a type of abbreviated plan of care that provides outcome-based guidelines for goal achievement within a designated length of stay. Critical pathways of care have been included in this text for selected psychiatric diagnoses.

APPLYING THE NURSING PROCESS IN THE PSYCHIATRIC SETTING

Based upon the definition of mental health set forth in Chapter 2, the role of the nurse in psychiatry focuses on assisting the patient to successfully adapt to stressors within the environment. Goals are directed toward change in thoughts, feelings, and behaviors that are age-appropriate and congruent with local and cultural norms.

Therapy within the psychiatric setting is very often team, or interdisciplinary, oriented. Therefore, it is important to delineate nursing's involvement in the treatment regimen. Nursing is indeed a valuable member of the team. Having progressed beyond the role of custodial caregiver in the psychiatric setting, nurses now provide services that are defined within the scope of nursing. Nursing diagnosis is helping to define these nursing boundaries, providing the degree of autonomy and professionalism that has for so long been unrealized.

For example, the treatment team may determine that a newly admitted patient with the medical diagnosis of schizophrenia has the following problems: paranoid delusions, auditory hallucinations, social withdrawal, and developmental regression. These have been evidenced by the patient's inability to trust others, verbalizing hearing voices, refusing to interact with staff and peers, expressing a fear of failure, and poor personal hygiene. Team goals would be directed toward reducing suspiciousness, terminating auditory hallucinations, and increasing feelings of self-worth. From this team assessment, nursing may identify the following nursing diagnoses:

1. Altered thought processes
2. Sensory-perceptual alteration (auditory)
3. Self-esteem disturbance
4. Self-care deficit (hygiene)

Nursing in psychiatry, regardless of the setting —hospital (inpatient or outpatient), office, home, community—is goal-directed care. The goals are patient oriented, measurable, and focus on resolution of the problem if realistic or on a more short-term outcome if resolution is unrealistic. For example, in the previous situation, goals for the identified nursing diagnoses might be:

1. Patient will demonstrate trust in one staff member within 5 days.
2. Patient will verbalize understanding that the voices are not real (not heard by others) within 10 days.
3. Patient will complete one simple craft project within 7 days.
4. Patient will take responsibility for own self-care and perform activities of daily living independently by discharge.

Nursing's contribution to the interdisciplinary treatment regimen will focus on establishing trust on a one-to-one basis, reducing the level of anxiety that is promoting hallucinations, giving positive feedback for small day-to-day accomplishments in an effort to build self-esteem, and assisting with/encouraging independent self-care. These interventions describe *independent nursing* actions and goals that are evaluated apart from, while also being directed toward achievement of, the *team's* treatment goals.

In this manner of collaboration with other team members, nursing provides a service that is unique and based on sound knowledge of psychopathology, scope of practice, and legal implications of the role. While there is no dispute that "following doctor's orders" continues to be accepted in the priority of care, nursing intervention that enhances achievement of the overall goals of treatment is being recognized for its important contribution. The nurse who administers a medication prescribed by the physician to decrease anxiety may also choose to stay with the anxious patient and offer reassurance of safety and security, thereby providing an independent nursing action that is distinct from, yet complementary to, the medical treatment.

DOCUMENTATION TO THE NURSING PROCESS

Equally important as using the nursing process in the delivery of care is the written documentation that it has been used. Some contemporary nursing leaders are advocating that with solid standards of practice and procedures in place within the institution, nurses need only chart when there has been a deviation in the care as outlined by that standard. However, many legal decisions are still based on the precept that "if it was not charted, it was not done."

Because nursing process and nursing diagnosis are mandated by some nurse practice acts, documentation of their use is being considered in those states as evidence in determining certain cases of negligence by nurses. Certain health-care organization accrediting agencies also require that nursing process be reflected in the delivery of care. Therefore, documentation must bear written testament to the use of the nursing process.

A variety of documentation methods can be used to reflect use of the nursing process in the delivery of nursing care. Three examples follow: problem-oriented recording (POR), Focus Charting®, and the PIE (problem, intervention, evaluation) system of documentation.

Problem-Oriented Recording

Problem-oriented recording (POR) follows the subjective, objective, assessment, plan, implementation, and evaluation (SOAPIE) format. It has as its basis a list of problems. When it is used by nursing, the problems (nursing diagnoses) are identified on a written plan of care with appropriate nursing interventions described for each.

Documentation written in the SOAPIE format includes:

S = Subjective data: information gathered from what the patient, family, or other source has said or reported.

O = Objective data: information gathered by direct observation of the person doing the assessment. May include a physiologic measurement, such as blood pressure, or a behavioral response, such as affect.

A = Assessment: the nurse's interpretation of the subjective and objective data.

P = Plan: the actions or treatments to be carried out (may be omitted in daily charting if the plan is clearly explained in the written nursing care plan and no changes are expected).

I = Intervention: those nursing actions that were actually carried out.

E = Evaluation of the problem following nursing intervention. (Some nursing interventions cannot be evaluated immediately, so this section may be an optional entry.)

Table 6.4   VALIDATION OF THE NURSING PROCESS WITH PROBLEM-ORIENTED RECORDING

Problem-Oriented Recording	What Is Recorded	Nursing Process
S and O (Subjective and Objective data)	Verbal reports to, and direct observation and examination by, the nurse.	Assessment
A (Assessment)	Nurse's interpretation of S and O	Analysis
P (Plan) Omitted in charting if written plan describes care to be given.	Description of appropriate nursing actions to resolve the identified problem.	Planning
I (Intervention)	Description of nursing actions actually carried out.	Implementation
E (Evaluation)	A reassessment of the situation to determine results of nursing actions implemented.	Evaluation

Table 6.4 shows how POR corresponds to the steps of the nursing process. Following is an example of a three-column documentation in the POR format.

Example

Date/Time	Problem	Progress Notes
6-22-92 1000	Social isolation	**S:** States he doesn't want to sit with or talk to others; "they frighten me." **O:** Stays in room alone unless strongly encouraged to come out; no group involvement; at times listens to group conversations from a distance but does not interact; some hypervigilance and scanning noted. **A:** Inability to trust; panic level of anxiety; delusional thinking **I:** Initiated trusting relationship by spending time alone with patient. Discussed his feelings regarding interactions with others. Accompanied patient to group activities. Provided positive feedback for voluntarily participating in assertiveness training.

Focus Charting

Another type of documentation that reflects use of the nursing process is Focus Charting. Focus Charting differs from POR in that the main perspective has been changed from "problem" to "focus," and DAR, or data, action, and response, has replaced SOAPIE.

Lampe (1985) suggests that a focus for documentation can be a:

1. Nursing diagnosis
2. Current patient concern or behavior
3. Significant change in the patient status or behavior
4. Significant event in the patient's therapy

The focus cannot be a medical diagnosis.

The documentation is organized in the format of DAR. These categories are defined as follows:

Data: Information that supports the stated focus or describes pertinent observations about the patient.

Action: Immediate or future nursing actions that address the focus, and evaluation of the present care plan along with any changes required.

Response: Description of patient responses to any part of the medical or nursing care.

Table 6.5 shows how Focus Charting corresponds to the steps of the nursing process. Following is an example of a three-column documentation in the DAR format.

Table 6.5 VALIDATION OF THE NURSING PROCESS WITH FOCUS CHARTING

Focus Charting	What Is Recorded	Nursing Process
D (Data)	Information that supports the stated focus or describes pertinent observations about the patient.	Assessment
Focus	A nursing diagnosis; current patient concern or behavior; significant change in patient status; significant event in the patient's therapy.	Analysis
A (Action)	Immediate or future nursing actions that address the focus; evaluation of the care plan along with any changes required.	Plan/implementation
R (Response)	Description of patient responses to any part of the medical or nursing care.	Evaluation

Example

Date/Time	Focus	Progress Notes
6-22-92 1000	Social isolation related to mistrust, panic anxiety, delusions	**D:** States he doesn't want to sit with or talk to others; they "frighten" him. Stays in room alone unless strongly encouraged to come out; no group involvement; at times listens to group conversations from a distance but does not interact; some hypervigilance and scanning noted. **A:** Initiated trusting relationship by spending time alone with patient. Discussed his feelings regarding interactions with others. Accompanied patient to group activities. Provided positive feedback for voluntarily participating in assertiveness training. **R:** Cooperative with therapy; still acts uncomfortable in the presence of a group of people; accepted positive feedback from nurse.

The PIE Method

PIE, or more specifically "APIE" (assessment, problem, intervention, evaluation) is a systematic method of documenting to nursing process and nursing diagnosis. A problem-oriented system, PIE uses accompanying flow sheets that are individualized by each institution. Criteria for documentation are organized in the following manner:

Assessment (A): A complete patient assessment is conducted at the beginning of each shift. Results are documented under this section in the progress notes. Some institutions elect instead to use a daily patient assessment sheet designed to meet specific needs of the unit. Explanation of any deviation from the norm is included in the progress notes.

Problem (P): A problem list, or list of nursing diagnoses, is an important part of the APIE method of charting. The name or number of the problem being addressed is documented in this section.

Intervention (I): Nursing actions are performed, directed at resolution of the problem.

Evaluation (E): Outcomes of the implemented interventions are documented, including an evaluation of patient responses to determine the effectiveness of nursing interventions and the presence or absence of progress toward resolution of a problem.

Table 6.6 shows how APIE charting corresponds to the steps of the nursing process. Following is an

Table 6.6 VALIDATION OF THE NURSING PROCESS WITH APIE METHOD

APIE Charting	What Is Recorded	Nursing Process
A (Assessment)	Results of patient assessment every shift.	Assessment
P (Problem)	Name or number of nursing diagnosis being addressed from written problem list.	Analysis
I (Intervention)	Nursing actions performed, directed at resolution of the problem.	Plan/implementation
E (Evaluation)	Outcomes of the implemented interventions. Evaluation of patient responses to determine effectiveness of nursing interventions.	Evaluation

example of a three-column documentation in the APIE format.

Example

Date/Time	Problem	Progress Notes
6-22-92 1000	Social isolation	**A:** States he doesn't want to sit with or talk to others; they "frighten" him. Stays in room alone unless strongly encouraged to come out; no group involvement; at times listens to group conversations from a distance, but does not interact; some hypervigilance and scanning noted. **P:** Social isolation related to inability to trust, panic level of anxiety, and delusional thinking. **I:** Initiated trusting relationship by spending time alone with patient. Discussed his feelings regarding interactions with others. Accompanied patient to group activities. Provided positive feedback for voluntarily participating in assertiveness training.

Date/Time	Problem	Progress Notes
		E: Cooperative with therapy; still uncomfortable in the presence of a group of people; accepted positive feedback from nurse.

SUMMARY

The nursing process provides a methodology by which nurses may deliver care using a systematic, scientific approach. The focus is goal directed and based on a decision-making or problem-solving model. It consists of five steps: assessment, analysis, planning, implementation, and evaluation.

Nursing diagnosis is inherent within the nursing process. The concept of nursing diagnosis is not new, but has only become formalized with the organization of NANDA in the 1970s. Nursing diagnosis defines the scope and boundaries for nursing, thereby offering a degree of autonomy and independence so long restricted within the practice of nursing. Nursing diagnosis also provides a common language for nursing and assists nurses to provide consistent, quality care for their patients based on an increase in the body of nursing knowledge through research. As of the Tenth National NANDA Conference held in April, 1992, 109 nursing diagnoses have been approved for use and testing.

The psychiatric nurse uses the nursing process

to assist patients to successfully adapt to stressors within the environment. Goals are directed toward change in thoughts, feelings, and behaviors that are age-appropriate and congruent with local and cultural norms. The nurse serves as a valuable member of the multidisciplinary treatment team, working both independently and cooperatively with other team members. Nursing diagnosis, in its ability to define the scope of nursing, is facilitating nursing's role in the psychiatric setting by differentiating that which is specifically nursing from interventions associated with other disciplines.

Nursing in psychiatry is goal-directed care. These goals are evaluated apart from, while also being directed toward achievement of, the team's treatment goals.

Nurses must document that the nursing process has been used in the delivery of care. Its use is mandated in some states by the nurse practice act and is also required by some health-care organization accrediting agencies. Three methods of documentation, POR, Focus Charting, and the PIE system, were presented with examples to demonstrate how they reflect use of the nursing process.

REVIEW QUESTIONS
Self-Examination/Learning Exercise

Test your knowledge of nursing process by supplying the information requested.

1. Name the five steps of the nursing process.
2. Identify the step of the nursing process to which each of the following nursing actions applies:
   a. Obtains short-term contract from patient to seek out staff if feeling suicidal
   b. Identifies nursing diagnosis: potential for self-directed violence
   c. Determines if nursing actions have been appropriate to achieve desired results
   d. Patient's family reports recent suicide attempt
   e. Prioritizes necessity for maintaining a safe environment for the patient
3. S.T. is a 15-year-old girl who has just been admitted to the adolescent psychiatric unit with a diagnosis of anorexia nervosa. She is 5'5" tall and weighs 82 lbs. She was elected to the cheerleading squad for the fall, but states that she is not as good as the others on the squad. The treatment team has identified the following problems: refusal to eat, occasional purging, refusing to interact with staff and peers, and fear of failure.

   Identify three nursing diagnoses and three goals that, as a part of the treatment team, nursing could use to contribute both independently and cooperatively to the team treatment plan.
4. Review various methods of documentation that reflect delivery of nursing care via the nursing process. Practice making entries using the various methods.

REFERENCES

American Nurses' Association (1973). Standards of nursing practice. Kansas City, MO: American Nurses' Association

American Nurses' Association (1980). *Nursing—A social policy statement*. Kansas City, MO: American Nurses' Association.

American Nurses' Association (1988). *Nursing case management*. Kansas City, MO: American Nurses' Association.

Carroll-Johnson, R. M. (1990). Reflections on the ninth biennial conference. *Nursing Diagnosis*, *1*(2):49–50.

Faherty, B. (1990, July) Case management: The latest buzzword—What it is, and what it isn't. *CARING*, pp. 20–22.

Gordon, M. (1987). *Nursing diagnosis—Process and application* (2nd ed.). New York: McGraw-Hill.

Lampe, S. S. (1985). Focus Charting: Streamlining documentation. *Nursing Management, 16*(7), 43–46.

Lancour, J. (1990). President's Message. *Nursing Diagnosis, 1*(1), 4.

McHugh, M. K. (1987, August). Has nursing outgrown the nursing process? *Nursing 87*, pp. 50–51.

Miller, E. (1989). *How to make nursing diagnosis work*. Norwalk, CT: Appleton & Lange.

BIBLIOGRAPHY

Alfaro, R. (1990). *Applying nursing diagnosis and nursing process* (2nd ed.). Philadelphia: JB Lippincott.

American Nurses' Association, Division on Psychiatric/Mental Health Nursing Practice. (1982). *Standards of psychiatric-mental health nursing practice*. Kansas City, MO: American Nurses' Association.

Atkinson, L. D. & Murray, M. E. (1990). *Understanding the nursing process* (4th ed.). New York: Macmillan.

Buckley-Womack, C. & Gidney, S. (1987, October) A new dimension in documentation: The PIE method. *Journal of Neuroscience Nursing*, pp. 256–260.

Doenges, M. E. & Moorhouse, M. F. (1990). *Nurse's clinical pocket manual: Nursing diagnoses, care planning, and documentation*. Philadelphia: FA Davis.

Doenges, M. E. & Moorhouse, M. F. (1992). Application of Nursing Process and Nursing Diagnosis: An Interactive Text. Philadelphia: FA Davis.

Doenges, M. E., Townsend, M. C., & Moorhouse, M. F. (1989). *Psychiatric care plans, Guidelines for client care*. Philadelphia: FA Davis.

Eggland, E. T. (1988, November). Charting: How and why to document your care daily—and fully. *Nursing 88*, pp. 76–84.

Hickey, P. W. (1990). *Nursing process handbook*. St. Louis: CV Mosby.

Iyer, P. W. (1991, January). New trends in charting. *Nursing 91*, pp. 48–50.

Iyer, P. W., Taptich, B. J., & Bernocchi-Losey, D. (1991). *Nursing process and nursing diagnosis*. 2nd ed. Philadelphia: WB Saunders.

LaMonica, E. L. (1979). *The nursing process—a humanistic approach*. Menlo Park, CA: Addison-Wesley.

North American Nursing Diagnosis Association. (1989). *Taxonomy I* (rev. ed.). St. Louis: North American Nursing Diagnosis Association.

Pinnell, N. N. & deMeneses, M. (1986). *The nursing process—Theory, application, and related processes*. Norwalk CT: Appleton-Century-Crofts.

Siegrist, L., Dettor, R.E., and Stocks, B. (1985, June). The PIE system: Complete planning and documentation of nursing care. *Quality Review Bulletin*, pp. 186–189.

Townsend, M. C. (1991). *Nursing diagnoses in psychiatric nursing* (2nd ed.). Philadelphia: FA Davis.

Yura, H. & Walsh, M. B. (1988). *The nursing process* (5th ed.). Norwalk, CT: Appleton & Lange.

7

THERAPEUTIC GROUPS

OBJECTIVES

After reading this chapter, the student will be able to:
1. Define a *group.*
2. Discuss eight functions of a group.
3. Identify various types of groups.
4. Describe physical conditions that influence groups.
5. Discuss "curative factors" that occur in groups.
6. Describe the phases of group development.
7. Identify various leadership styles in groups.
8. Identify various roles that members assume within a group.
9. Discuss psychodrama and family therapy as specialized forms of group therapy.
10. Describe the role of the nurse in group therapy.

THE GROUP, DEFINED

A *group* is defined as "a collection of individuals whose association is founded upon shared commonalities of interest, values, norms, or purpose." Membership in a group is generally by chance (born into the group), by choice (voluntary affiliation), or by circumstance (the result of life-cycle events over which individuals may or may not have control).

FUNCTIONS OF A GROUP

Sampson and Marthas (1990) have outlined eight functions that groups serve for their members. They contend that groups may serve more than one function and generally serve different functions for different members of the group. The eight functions are:

1. *Socialization.* The cultural group into which we are born begins the process of teaching social norms. This is continued throughout our lives by members of other groups with which we become affiliated.
2. *Support.* One's fellow group members are available in time of need. Individuals derive a feeling of security from group involvement.
3. *Task Completion.* Group members provide assistance in endeavors that are beyond the capacity of one individual alone or when results can be achieved more effectively as a team.
4. *Camaraderie.* Members of a group provide the joy and pleasure that individuals seek from interactions with significant others.
5. *Informational.* Learning takes place within groups. Explanations regarding world events occur in groups. Knowledge is gained by individual members who learn how others within the group have experienced situations similar to those they are currently struggling to resolve.
6. *Normative.* This function relates to the ways in which groups enforce the established norms.
7. *Empowerment.* Groups help to bring about improvement in existing conditions by providing support to individual members who seek to bring about change. Groups have power that individuals alone do not possess.
8. *Governance.* An example of the governing function is that of rules being made by committees within a larger organization.

TYPES OF GROUPS

The functions of a group will vary depending on the reason for which the group was formed. Clark (1987) identifies three types of groups in which nurses most often participate: task groups, teaching groups, and supportive/therapeutic groups.

Task Groups

The function of a task group is to accomplish a specific outcome or task. The focus is on solving problems and making decisions to achieve this outcome. Often a deadline is placed on completion of the task, and such importance is placed on a satisfactory outcome that conflict within the group may be smoothed over or ignored to focus on the priority at hand.

Teaching Groups

Teaching, or educational, groups exist to convey knowledge and information to a number of individuals. Nurses can be involved in teaching groups of many varieties, such as medication education, childbirth education, breast self-examination, and effective parenting classes. These groups generally have a set time frame or a set number of meetings. Members learn from each other as well as from the designated instructor. The objective of teaching groups is verbalization or demonstration by the learner of the material presented by the end of the designated period.

Supportive/Therapeutic Groups

The primary concern of support groups is to prevent future upsets by teaching participants effective ways of dealing with emotional stress arising from situational or developmental crises (Clark, 1987).

For the purposes of this text, it is important to differentiate between "therapeutic groups" and "group therapy." Leaders of group therapy generally have advanced degrees in psychology, social work, nursing, or medicine. They often have additional training or experience under the supervision of an accomplished professional in conducting group psychotherapy based on various theoretical frameworks, such as psychoanalytic, psychodynamic, interpersonal, or family dynamics. Approaches based on these theories are used by the group therapy leaders to encourage improvement in the ability of group members to function on an interpersonal level.

Therapeutic groups, on the other hand, are based to a lesser degree in theory. Focus is more on group relations, interactions between group members, and the consideration of a selected issue. Like group therapists, individuals who lead therapeutic groups must be knowledgeable in *group process*, that is, the *WAY* in which group members interact with each other. Interruptions, silences, judg-

ments, glares, and scapegoating are examples of group processes (Clark, 1987). They must also have thorough knowledge of *group content*, the topic or issue being discussed within the group, and the ability to present the topic in language that can be understood by all group members. Many nurses who work in psychiatry lead supportive/therapeutic groups.

PHYSICAL CONDITIONS

Seating

The physical conditions for the group should be set up so that there is no barrier between the members. For example, a circle of chairs is better than chairs set around a table. Members should be encouraged to sit in different chairs each meeting. This openness and change creates an uncomfortableness that encourages anxious and unsettled behaviors that can then be explored within the group.

Size

Various authors have suggested different ranges of size as ideal for group interaction: 5 to 10 (Lego, 1987), 2 to 15 (Sampson & Marthas, 1990), and 4 to 12 (Clark, 1987). Group size does make a difference in the interaction among members. The larger the group, the less time there is available to devote to each member. In fact, in larger groups, the more aggressive individuals are most likely to be heard, while quieter members may be left out of the discussions altogether. On the other hand, larger groups provide more opportunities for individuals to learn from other members. The wider range of life experiences and knowledge provides a greater potential for effective group problem solving. Studies have indicated that seven or eight members provides a favorable climate for optimal group interaction and relationship development.

Membership

Whether the group is open- or closed-ended is another condition that influences the dynamics of group process. Open-ended groups are those in which members leave and others join at any time during the existence of the group. The continuous movement of members in and out of the group creates the type of uncomfortableness described previously that encourages unsettled behaviors in individual members and fosters the exploration of feelings. These are the most common types of groups held on short-term inpatient units, although they are used in outpatient and long-term care facilities as well. Closed-ended groups usually have a predetermined, fixed time frame. All members join at the time the group is organized and terminate at the end of the designated period. Closed-ended groups are often comprised of individuals with common issues or problems they wish to address.

CURATIVE FACTORS

Why are therapeutic groups helpful? Yalom (1985) identified 11 curative factors that individuals can achieve through interpersonal interactions within the group. Some of the factors are present in most groups in varying degrees. The curative factors identified by Yalom include:

1. *The instillation of hope.* By observing the progress of others in the group with similar problems, a group member garners hope that his or her problems can also be resolved.
2. *Universality.* Individuals come to realize that they are not alone in the problems, thoughts, and feelings they are experiencing. Anxiety is relieved by the support and understanding of others in the group who share similar experiences.
3. *The imparting of information.* Knowledge is gained through formal instruction as well as the sharing of advice and suggestions among group members.
4. *Altruism.* Individuals gain self-esteem through mutual sharing and concern. Providing assistance and support to others creates a positive self-image and promotes self-growth.
5. *The corrective recapitulation of the primary family group.* Group members are able to re-experience early family conflicts that remain unresolved. Attempts at resolution are promoted through feedback and exploration.
6. *The development of socializing techniques.* Through interaction with and feedback from other members within the group, individuals are able to correct maladaptive social behaviors and learn and develop new social skills.
7. *Imitative behavior.* In this setting, one who has mastered a particular psychosocial skill or developmental task can be a valuable role model for others. Individuals may imitate selected behaviors that they wish to develop in themselves.
8. *Interpersonal learning.* The group offers many and varied opportunities for interacting with other people. Insight is gained regarding how one perceives and is being perceived by others.
9. *Group cohesiveness.* Members develop a sense of belonging that separates the individual ("I am") from the group ("we are"). Out of this alliance emerges a common feeling that both individual members and the total group are of value to each other.
10. *Catharsis.* Within the group, members are able to express both positive and negative feelings—perhaps feelings that have never been expressed before—in a nonthreatening atmosphere.
11. *Existential factors.* The group is able to help individual members take direction of their own lives and to accept responsibility for the quality of their existence.

It may be helpful for a group leader to explain these curative factors to members of the group. Boyer (1982) stated that positive responses were experienced by group members who understood and were able to recognize curative factors as they occurred within the group.

PHASES OF GROUP DEVELOPMENT

Groups, like individuals, move through phases of life-cycle development. Ideally, groups will progress from the phase of infancy to advanced maturity in an effort to fulfill the objectives set forth by the membership. Unfortunately, as with individuals, some groups become fixed in early developmental levels and never progress, or experience periods of regression in the developmental process. Three phases of group development will be discussed.

Phase I. Initial or Orientation Phase

GROUP ACTIVITIES

Leader and members work together to establish the rules that will govern the group (when and where meetings will occur, the importance of confidentiality, how meetings will be structured). Goals of the group are established. Members are introduced to each other.

LEADER EXPECTATIONS

The leader is expected to orient members to specific group processes, encourage members to participate without disclosing too much too soon, promote an environment of trust, and ensure that rules established by the group do not interfere with fulfillment of the goals.

MEMBER BEHAVIORS

In Phase I, members have not yet established trust and will respond to this lack of trust by being overly polite. There is a fear of not being accepted by the group. They may try to "get on the good side" of the leader with compliments and conforming behaviors. A power struggle may ensue as members compete for their position in the "pecking order" of the group.

Phase II. Middle or Working Phase

GROUP ACTIVITIES

Ideally, during the working phase, cohesiveness has been established within the group. This is the time when the productive work toward completion of the task is undertaken. Problem solving and decision making occur within the group. In the mature group, cooperation prevails, and differences and disagreements are confronted and resolved.

LEADER EXPECTATIONS

The role of leader diminishes and becomes more one of facilitator during the working phase. Some leadership functions are shared by certain members of the group as they progress toward resolution. The leader helps to resolve conflict and continues to foster cohesiveness among the members, while ensuring that they do not deviate from the in-tended task or purpose for which the group was organized.

MEMBER BEHAVIORS

Trust has been established among the members. They turn more often to each other and less often to the leader for guidance. They accept criticism from each other, using it in a constructive manner to create change. Occasionally, subgroups will form in which two or more members will conspire with each other to the exclusion of the rest of the group. To maintain group cohesion, these subgroups must be confronted and discussed by the entire membership. Conflict is managed by the group with minimal assistance from the leader.

Phase III. Final or Termination Phase

GROUP ACTIVITIES

The longer a group has been in existence, the more difficult termination is likely to be for the members. Termination should be mentioned from the outset of group formation. It should be discussed in depth for several meetings prior to the final session. A sense of loss that precipitates the grief process may be in evidence, particularly in groups that have been successful in their stated purpose.

LEADER EXPECTATIONS

In the termination phase, the leader encourages the group members to reminisce about what has occurred within the group, to review the goals and discuss the actual outcomes, and to encourage members to provide feedback to each other about individual progress within the group. The leader encourages members to discuss feelings of loss associated with termination of the group.

MEMBER BEHAVIORS

Members may express surprise over the actual materialization of the end. This represents the grief response of denial, which may then progress to anger. Anger toward other group members or directed at the leader may express feelings that reflect, "You are all abandoning me" (Sampson & Marthas, 1990). These feelings may lead to individual members' discussions of previous losses for which similar emotions were experienced. Successful termination of the group may help members develop the skills needed when losses occur in other dimensions of their lives.

LEADERSHIP STYLES

Three of the most common group leadership styles have been described by Lippitt and White (1958). They include *autocratic*, *democratic*, and *laissez-faire*.

Autocratic

Autocratic leaders have personal goals for the group. They withhold information from group members, particularly issues that may interfere with achievement of their own objectives. The message that is conveyed to the group is: "We will do it my way. My way is best." The focus in this style of leadership is on the leader. Members are dependent on the leader for problem solving, decision making, and permission to perform. The approach of the autocratic leader is one of persuasion, striving to persuade others in the group that his or her ideas and methods are superior. Productivity is high with this type of leadership, but often morale within the group is low due to lack of member input and creativity.

Democratic

The democratic leadership style has its focus on the members of the group. Information is shared with members in an effort to allow them to make decisions regarding achieving the goals for the group. Members are encouraged to participate fully in problem solving of issues that relate to the group, including taking action to effect change. The message that is conveyed to the group is: "Decide what must be done, consider the alternatives, make a selection, and proceed with the actions required to complete the task." The leader provides guidance and expertise as needed. Productivity is lower than it is with autocratic leadership, but morale is much higher due to the extent of input allowed all members of the group and the potential for individual creativity.

Laissez-Faire

This leadership style allows people to do as they please. There is no direction from the leader. In fact, the laissez-faire leader's approach is noninvolvement. Goals for the group are undefined. No decisions are made, no problems are solved, and no action is taken. Members become frustrated and confused, and productivity and morale are low.

Table 7.1 shows an outline of similarities and differences among the three leadership styles.

Table 7.1 LEADERSHIP STYLES—SIMILARITIES AND DIFFERENCES			
Characteristics	**Autocratic**	**Democratic**	**Laissez-Faire**
1. Focus	Leader	Members	Undetermined
2. Task strategy	Members are persuaded to adopt leader ideas	Members engage in group problem solving	No defined strategy
3. Member participation	Limited	Unlimited	Inconsistent
4. Individual creativity	Stifled	Encouraged	Not addressed
5. Member enthusiasm and morale	Low	High	Low
6. Group cohesiveness	Low	High	Low
7. Productivity	High	High (may not be as high as autocratic)	Low
8. Individual motivation and commitment	Low (tend to work only when leader is present to urge them to do so)	High (satisfaction derived from personal input and participation)	Low (feelings of frustration from lack of direction or guidance)

MEMBER ROLES

Benne and Sheats (1948) identified three major types of roles that individuals play within the membership of the group. These are roles that serve to:

1. Complete the task of the group.
2. Maintain or enhance group processes.
3. Fulfill personal or individual needs.

Task roles and maintenance roles contribute to the success or effectiveness of the group. Personal roles satisfy needs of the individual members, sometimes to the extent of interfering with the effectiveness of the group.

Table 7.2 presents an outline of specific roles within these three major types and the behaviors associated with each.

PSYCHODRAMA

A specialized type of therapeutic group, called *psychodrama*, was introduced by J. L. Moreno, a Viennese psychiatrist. Moreno's method employs a dramatic approach in which patients become "actors" in life-situation scenarios.

The group leader is called the *director*, group members are the *audience*, and the *set*, or *stage*, may be specially designed or may just be any room or part of a room selected for this purpose. Actors are members from the audience who agree to take part in the "drama" by role playing a situation about which they have been informed by the director. Usually the situation is an issue with which one individual patient has been struggling. The patient plays the role of himself or herself and is called the *protagonist*. In this role, the patient is able to express true feelings toward individuals (represented by group members) with whom he or she has unresolved conflicts.

In some instances, the group leader may ask for a patient to volunteer to be the protagonist for that session. The patient may choose a situation he or she wishes to enact and select the audience members to portray the roles of others in the life situation.

The psychodrama setting provides the patient with a safer and less threatening atmosphere than the real situation in which to express true feelings. Resolution of interpersonal conflicts is facilitated.

Table 7.2 MEMBER ROLES WITHIN GROUPS

Role	Behaviors
Task Roles	
Coordinator	Clarifies ideas and suggestions that have been made within the group; brings relationships together to pursue common goals.
Evaluator	Examines group plans and performance, measuring against group standards and goals.
Elaborator	Explains and expands upon group plans and ideas.
Energizer	Encourages and motivates group to perform at its maximum potential.
Initiator	Outlines the task at hand for the group and proposes methods for solution.
Orienter	Maintains direction within the group.
Maintenance Roles	
Compromiser	Serves to relieve conflict within the group by assisting members to reach a compromise agreeable to all.
Encourager	Offers recognition and acceptance of others' ideas and contributions.
Follower	Listens attentively to group interaction; is passive participant.
Gatekeeper	Encourages acceptance of, and participation by, all members of the group.
Harmonizer	Minimizes tension within the group by intervening when disagreements produce conflict.
Individual (Personal) Roles	
Aggressor	Expresses negativism and hostility toward other members. May use sarcasm in effort to degrade the status of others.
Blocker	Resists group efforts. Demonstrates rigid and sometimes irrational behaviors that impede group progress.
Dominator	Manipulates others to gain control. Behaves in authoritarian manner.

(continued)

Table 7.2 CONTINUED	
Role	**Behaviors**
Help seeker	Uses the group to gain sympathy from others. Seeks to increase self-confidence from group feedback. Lacks concern for others or for the group as a whole.
Monopolizer	Maintains control of the group by dominating the conversation.
Mute or silent member	Does not participate verbally. Remains silent for a variety of reasons. May feel uncomfortable with self-disclosure or may be seeking attention through silence.
Recognition seeker	Talks about personal accomplishments in an effort to gain attention for self.
Seducer	Shares intimate details about self with group. Is the least reluctant of the group to do so. May frighten others in the group and inhibit group progress with excessive premature self-disclosure.

Source: From Benne and Sheats (1948).

When the drama has been completed, group members from the audience discuss the situation they have observed, offer feedback, express their feelings, and relate their own similar experiences. In this way, all group members benefit from the session, either directly or indirectly.

Nurses often serve as actors, or role players, in psychodrama sessions. Leaders of psychodrama have graduate degrees in psychology, social work, nursing, or medicine with additional training in group therapy and specialty preparation to become a psychodramatist.

THE FAMILY AS A GROUP

Family therapy is broadly defined as "the attempt to modify the relationships in a family to achieve harmony" (Foley, 1979). A basic assumption of family therapy is that there are certain human behavior patterns that can help people grow and live creatively, while there are others that lead to dysfunction and noncommunicative action that result in emotional illness in the family (Barash, 1979).

In family therapy, the family is viewed as a *system* in which the members are interdependent; a change in one part (member) within the system affects or creates change in all the other parts (members). The focus is not on an individual, identified patient but rather on the family as a whole. The basic concept of this form of treatment is that it is more logical, faster, more satisfactory, and more economical to treat all members of a system of relationships than to concentrate on the person who is supposed to be in need of treatment (Foley, 1979).

Since the major goal of family therapy is to bring about positive change in relationships, the therapist ideally conducts the initial assessment with the entire family. If this is not possible, information is gathered from the patient who has sought treatment and an appointment is scheduled to meet with the family at a later date. The initial assessment is not complete until the therapist has had the opportunity to observe the interactions among all family members. Some family therapists favor the use of genograms in the study of multigenerations within families. Genograms offer the convenience of a great deal of information in a small amount of space. They can also be used as teaching tools with the family itself. An overall picture of the life of the family over several generations can be conveyed, including roles that various family members play as well as emotional distance between specific individuals. Areas for change can be easily identified. A sample genogram is presented in Figure 7.1.

Once the assessment has been completed and problems identified, family members establish goals for change with guidance from the therapist. Change occurs through open, honest communication among all family members. The family therapist's role is to facilitate this type of interaction. As goals are achieved and change occurs, family members will demonstrate the ability to communicate effectively, the ability to resolve conflicts adaptively, and the ability for each to function both independently and interdependently in a healthy manner.

Nurses who conduct family therapy are expected to possess a graduate degree with considerable knowledge of family theory. However, it is within the realm of the generalist nurse in psychiatry to

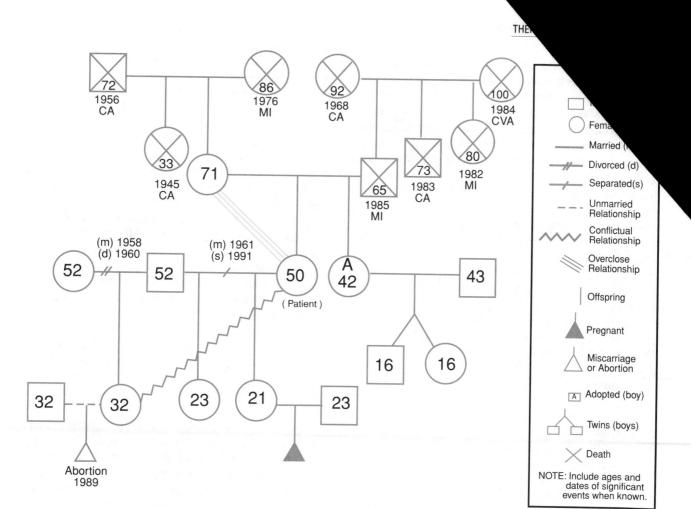

Figure 7.1 Sample genogram.

contribute to the assessment and planning phases of family therapy, as well as ongoing observation and evaluation. Family consideration in individual patient care is also essential. Nurses should have a basic understanding of family dynamics and the ability to distinguish between functional and dysfunctional behaviors within a family system.

THE ROLE OF THE NURSE IN GROUP THERAPY

Nurses participate in group situations on a daily basis. Within health-care settings, nurses serve on or lead task groups that create policy, describe procedures, plan patient care, as well as a variety of other groups aimed at the institutional effort of serving the consumer. Nurses are encouraged to use the steps of the nursing process as a framework for task group leadership.

In psychiatry, nurses may lead various types of therapeutic groups, such as patient education, assertiveness training, support, parent, and transition to discharge groups, among others. To function effectively in the leadership capacity for these groups, nurses need to be able to recognize various processes that occur in groups, such as the phases of group development, the various roles that people play within group situations, and the motivation behind the behavior, and to be able to select the most appropriate leadership style for the type of group being led. Generalist nurses may develop these skills as part of their undergraduate education, or they may pursue additional study while serving and learning as the co-leader of a group with a more experienced nurse leader.

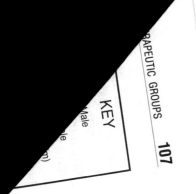

try rarely serve as
ps. Guidelines set
ssociation (ANA)
roup psychother-
a master's degree
riteria that have
l preparation in
as a group co-
sion of an experi-
participation in group
py on an experiential level. Additional specialist training is required beyond the master's
level to prepare nurses to become family therapists
or psychodramatists.

Leading therapeutic groups is within the realm of
nursing practice. Because group work is such a
common therapeutic approach in the discipline of
psychiatry, nurses working in this field must continually strive to expand their knowledge and use of
group process as a significant psychiatric nursing
intervention.

SUMMARY

A *group* is defined as "a collection of individuals
whose association is founded upon shared commonalities of interest, values, norms, or purpose."
Groups serve various functions for their members.
Eight group functions were defined by Sampson
and Marthas (1990). They include *socialization,
support, task completion, camaraderie, informational, normative, empowerment,* and *governance.*

Three types of groups were identified: (1) task
groups, whose function it is to solve problems,
make decisions, and achieve a specific outcome;
(2) teaching groups, in which knowledge and information are conveyed to a number of individuals;
and (3) supportive/therapeutic groups, whose
function it is to educate people to deal effectively
with emotional stress in their lives.

Group therapy is differentiated from *therapeutic
groups* by degree of educational preparation of the
leader. Group psychotherapists have advanced degrees in psychology, social work, medicine, or
nursing. The focus of group psychotherapy is more
theoretically based than it is in therapeutic groups.

Certain physical conditions, such as placement
of the seating and size of the group, influence group
interaction. Whether the group is open-ended or
closed-ended can also affect group performance. In
an *open-ended* group members leave and others
join at any time during the existence of the group.
Closed-ended groups have a predetermined, fixed
time frame. All members join the group at the same
time and leave at the end of the designated period.

Yalom (1985) identified a number of benefits that
individuals derive from participation in therapeutic groups. He called these benefits curative factors.
They include the instillation of hope, universality,
the imparting of information, altruism, the corrective recapitulation of the primary family group, the
development of socializing techniques, imitative
behavior, interpersonal learning, group cohesiveness, catharsis, and existential factors.

Groups progress through three major phases of
development. In the initial (orientation) phase,
members are introduced to each other, rules and
goals of the group are established, and a trusting
relationship is initiated. In the second phase, called
the middle or working phase, the actual work of the
group takes place. As the group matures, trust is established and members cooperate in decision making and problem solving. The leader serves more as
a facilitator during this phase. The final or termination phase can be difficult, particularly if the group
has been together for a long time. A sense of loss
can trigger the grief response, and it is essential
that members confront these feelings and work
through them before the final session.

Group leadership styles may vary. The *autocratic*
leader concentrates on fulfillment of his or her own
objectives for the group. This is achieved through
persuasive selling of personal ideas to the group.
Productivity is high with this type of leader, but morale and motivation are low. With a *democratic*
leader, group members are encouraged to participate fully in the decision-making process. The
leader provides guidance and expertise as needed.
Productivity is lower than with autocratic leadership, but morale and motivation are much higher.
In a group with *laissez-faire* leadership, the members receive no direction at all. Goals are not established, decisions are not made, everyone does as
he or she pleases, and confusion prevails. Productivity, morale, and motivation are low.

Members play various roles within groups.
These roles are categorized according to task *roles,
maintenance roles,* and *personal roles.* Task roles
and maintenance roles contribute to the success or

effectiveness of the group. Personal roles satisfy needs of the individual members, sometimes to the extent of interfering with the effectiveness of the group.

Psychodrama is identified as a specialized type of group therapy. It employs a dramatic approach in which patients become "actors" in life-situation scenarios. The psychodrama setting provides the patient with a safer and less threatening atmosphere than the real situation in which to express and work through unresolved conflicts.

Family therapy brings together some or all members of the family in a group situation. The major goal is to bring about positive cha[...] ships. The therapist helps family me[...] tify problems, establish goals for chang[...] toward achievement of those goals thro[...] honest communication.

Nurses lead various types of therapeutic gr[...] in the psychiatric setting. Knowledge of human b[...] havior in general and group process in particular is essential to effective group leadership.

Specialized training, in addition to a master's degree, is required for nurses to serve as group psychotherapists, psychodramatists, and family therapists.

REVIEW QUESTIONS
Self-Examination/Learning Exercise

Test your knowledge of group process by supplying the information requested.

1. Define a *group*.

2. Identify the type of group and leadership style in each of the following situations:

   a. NJ is the nurse leader of a childbirth preparation group. Each week she shows various films and sets out various reading materials. She expects the participants to use their time on a topic of their choice or practice skills they have observed on the films. Two couples have dropped out of the group, stating, "This is a big waste of time."

   Type of group _____

   Style of leadership _____

   b. MK is a psychiatric nurse who has been selected to lead a group for women who desire to lose weight. The criteria for membership is that they must be at least 20 lb overweight. All have tried to lose weight on their own many times in the past without success. At their first meeting, MK provides suggestions as the members determine what their goals will be and how they plan to go about achieving those goals. They decided how often they wanted to meet and what they planned to do at each meeting.

   Type of group _____

   Style of leadership _____

   c. JJ is a staff nurse on a surgical unit. He has been selected as leader of a newly established group of staff nurses organized to determine ways to decrease the number of medication errors occurring on the unit. JJ has definite ideas about how to bring this about. He has also applied for the position of Head Nurse on the unit and believes that if he is successful in leading the group toward achievement of its goals, he can also facilitate his chances for promotion. At each meeting, he addresses the group in an effort to convince he members to adopt his ideas.

ype of group _____

tyle of leadership _____

h the situation on the right to the curative factor or benefit it ibes on the left.

_____ 1. Instillation of hope

_____ 2. Universality

_____ 3. Imparting of information

_____ 4. Altruism

_____ 5. Corrective recapitulation of the primary family group

_____ 6. Development of socializing techniques

_____ 7. Imitative behavior

_____ 8. Interpersonal learning

_____ 9. Group cohesiveness

_____ 10. Catharsis

_____ 11. Existential factors

a. Sam admires the way Jack stands up for what he believes. He decides to practice this himself.

b. Nancy sees that Jane has been a widow for 5 years now and has adjusted well. Maybe she can too.

c. Susan has come to realize that she has the power to shape the direction of her life.

d. John is able to have a discussion with another person for the first time in his life.

e. Linda now understands that her mother really did love her, although she was not able to show it.

f. Alice has come to feel as though the other group members are like a family to her. She looks forward to the meetings each week.

g. Tony talks in the group about the abuse he experienced as a child. He has never told anyone about this before.

h. Sandra felt so good about herself when she left group tonight. She had provided both physical and emotional support to Judy, who shared for the first time her experience of being raped.

i. Judy appreciated Sandra's support as she expressed her feelings related to the rape. She had come to believe that no one else felt as she did.

j. Paul knew that people did not

want to be his f
his violent temper
group, he has learne
control his temper and
satisfactory interpersona
relationships with others.

k. Henry learned about the effect
   of alcohol on the body when a
   nurse from the chemical
   dependency unit spoke to the
   group.

4. Match the individual on the right to the role he or she is playing within the group.

_____ 1. Aggressor

_____ 2. Blocker

_____ 3. Dominator

_____ 4. Help seeker

_____ 5. Monopolizer

_____ 6. Mute or silent member

_____ 7. Recognition seeker

_____ 8. Seducer

a. Nancy talks incessently in group. When someone else tries to make a comment, she refuses to allow them to speak.

b. On the first day the group met, Valerie shared the intimate details of her incestuous relationship with her father.

c. Colleen listens with interest to everything the other members say, but she does not say anything herself in group.

d. Violet is obsessed with her physical appearance. Although she is beautiful, she has little self-confidence and needs continuous positive feedback. She states, "Maybe if I became a blond my boyfriend would love me more."

e. Larry states to Violet, "Listen, dummy, you need more than blond hair to keep the guy around. A bit more in the brains department would help!"

f. At the beginning of the group meeting, Dan says, "All right now, I have a date tonight. I want this meeting over on time! I'll keep track of the time and let everyone know when their time is up. When I say you're done, you're done, understand?"

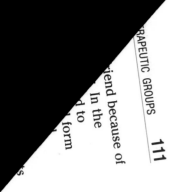

g. Joyce says, "I won my first beauty contest when I was 6 months old. Can you imagine? And I've been winning them ever since. I was prom queen when I was 16, Miss Rose Petal when I was 19, Miss Silver City at 21. And next I go to the state contest. It's just all so exciting!"

h. Joe, an RN on the care-planning committee says, "What a stupid suggestion. Nursing Diagnosis!?! I won't even discuss the matter. We have been doing our care plans this way for 20 years. I refuse to even consider changing."

REFERENCES

Barash, D. A. (1979). Dynamics of the pathological family system. *Perspect Psychiatr Care*, *XVII*(1), 17–25.

Benne, K. B. & Sheats, P. (1948, Spring). Functional roles of group members. *Journal of Social Issues*, *4*(2), 42–49.

Boyer, V. B. (1982). Process and content: Distinctions and implications. In E.H. Janosik & L.B. Phipps (Eds.), *Life cycle group work in nursing*. Monterey, CA: Wadsworth Health Sciences.

Clark, C. C. (1987). *The nurse as group leader* (2nd ed.). New York: Springer Publishing Company.

Foley, V. D. (1979). Family therapy. In R. J. Corsini (Ed.), *Current psychotherapies* (2nd ed.). Itasca, IL: FE Peacock Publishers.

Lego, S. (1987). Group psychotherapy. In Haber, J., Hoskins, P. P., Leach, A. M., and Sidelau, B. F. (Eds.), *Comprehensive psychiatric nursing* (3rd ed.). New York: McGraw-Hill.

Lippitt, R. & White, R. K. (1958). An experimental study of leadership and group life. In Maccoby, E. E., Newcomb, T. M., and Hartley, E. L. (Eds.), *Readings in social psychology* (3rd ed.). New York: Holt, Rinehart and Winston.

Sampson, E. E. & Marthas, M. (1990). *Group process for the health professions* (3rd ed.). Albany, NY: Delmar Publishers Inc.

Yalom, I. (1985). *The theory and practice of group psychotherapy* (3rd ed.). New York: Basic Books.

BIBLIOGRAPHY

Fine, L. J. (1979). Psychodrama. In R. J. Corsini (Ed.), *Current psychotherapies* (2nd ed.). Itasca, IL: FE Peacock Publishers.

Hare, A. P. (1952). A study of interaction and consensus in different sized groups. *Am Sociol Rev, 17,* 261–267.

Larson, M. L. & Williams, R. A. (1978, August). How to become a better group leader? *Nursing78,* pp. 65–72.

MILIEU THERAPY—THE THERAPEUTIC COMMUNITY

KEY TERMS
milieu
milieu therapy
therapeutic community

OBJECTIVES

After reading this chapter, the student will be able to:
1. Define *milieu therapy*.
2. Explain the goal of therapeutic community/milieu therapy.
3. Identify seven basic assumptions of a therapeutic community.
4. Discuss conditions that characterize a therapeutic community.
5. Identify the various therapies that may be included within the program of therapeutic community and the health-care workers that make up the interdisciplinary treatment team.
6. Describe the role of the nurse on the interdisciplinary treatment team.

MILIEU, DEFINED

The word *milieu* is French for "middle." The English translation of the word is "surroundings or environment." In psychiatry, therapy involving the milieu, or environment, may be called milieu therapy, therapeutic community, or therapeutic environment. In this context, it is defined as "a scien-tific structuring of the environment in order to effect behavioral changes and to improve the psychological health and functioning of the individual" (Skinner, 1979). Thus, the goal of milieu therapy is to manipulate the patient's environment so that all aspects of the patient's hospital experience are considered therapeutic. Within this therapeutic community setting, the patient is expected to learn adaptive coping, interaction, and relationship

113

skills that can be generalized to other aspects of his or her life.

BASIC ASSUMPTIONS

Skinner (1979) outlined seven basic assumptions upon which a therapeutic community is based:

1. *The health in each individual is to be realized and encouraged to grow.* All individuals are considered to have strengths as well as limitations. These healthy aspects of the individual are identified and serve as a foundation for growth in the personality and in the ability to function more adaptively and productively in all aspects of life.

2. *Every interaction is an opportunity for therapeutic intervention.* Within this structured setting, it is virtually impossible to avoid interpersonal interaction. The ideal situation exists for patients to improve communication and relationship development skills. Learning occurs from immediate feedback of personal perceptions.

3. *The patient owns his own environment.* Patients make decisions and solve problems related to government of the unit. In this way, personal needs for autonomy as well as needs that pertain to the group as a whole are fulfilled.

4. *Each patient owns his behavior.* Each individual within the therapeutic community is expected to take responsibility for his or her own behavior.

5. *Peer pressure is a useful and a powerful tool.* Behavioral group norms are established through peer pressure. Feedback is direct and frequent, so that behaving in a manner acceptable to the other members of the community becomes essential.

6. *Inappropriate behaviors are dealt with as they occur.* Individuals examine the significance of their behavior, how it affects other people, and discuss more appropriate ways of behaving in certain situations.

7. *Restrictions and punishment are to be avoided.* Destructive behaviors can usually be controlled with group discussion. However, if an individual requires external controls, temporary isolation is preferred over lengthy restriction or other harsh punishment.

CONDITIONS THAT PROMOTE A THERAPEUTIC COMMUNITY

In a therapeutic community setting, everything that happens to the patient, or within the patient's environment, is considered to be part of the treatment program. The community setting is the foundation for the program of treatment. Community factors, such as social interactions, the physical structure of the unit, and schedule of activities, may generate negative responses from some patients. These stressful experiences are used as examples to help the patient learn how to manage stress more adaptively in real-life situations.

Under what conditions, then, is a hospital environment considered therapeutic? A number of criteria have been identified.

1. *Basic physiological needs are fulfilled.* As Maslow (1968) has suggested, individuals do not move to higher levels of functioning until the basic biological needs for food, water, air, sleep, exercise, elimination, shelter, and sexual expression have been met.

2. *The physical facilities are conducive to achievement of the goals of therapy.* Space is provided so that each patient has sufficient privacy, as well as physical space for therapeutic interaction with others. Furnishings are arranged to present a homelike atmosphere, usually in spaces that accommodate communal living, dining, and activity areas, for facilitation of interpersonal interaction and communication.

3. *A democratic form of self-government exists.* In the therapeutic community, patients participate in the decision making and problem solving that affect the management of the unit. This is accomplished through regularly scheduled community meetings. These meetings are attended by staff and patients, and all individuals have equal input into the discussions. At these meetings, unit norms and rules and behavioral limits are set forth. This reinforces the democratic posture of the unit, as these are expectations that affect all patients on an equal basis. An example might be the unit rule that no patient may enter the room of a patient of the opposite sex. Consequences of violating the rules are explained.

Other issues that may be discussed at the community meetings include those with which certain patients have some disagreements. A decision is then made by the entire group in a democratic manner. For example, several patients may disagree with the hours that have been designated for patients to watch TV on a weekend night. They may elect to bring up this issue at a community meeting and suggest an extension in TV viewing time. After discussion by the group, a vote will be taken, and patients and staff agree to abide by the expressed preference of the majority.

Meetings are usually held each morning right after breakfast. Some therapeutic communities elect officers (usually a president and a secretary) who serve for a week or even for a few days. The president calls the meeting to order, conducts the business of discussing old and new unit issues, and asks for volunteers (or makes appointments, alternately so that all patients have a turn) to accomplish the daily tasks associated with community living, for example, cleaning the tables after each meal and watering plants on the unit. New assignments are made each morning.

The secretary reads the minutes of yesterday's meeting and takes minutes of the current meeting. Minutes are important in the event that patients have a disagreement about issues that were discussed at various meetings. Minutes provide written evidence of decisions made by the group.

On units whose patients have short attention spans or disorganized thinking, meetings are brief. Business is generally limited to introductions and expectations of the here and now. Discussions also may include comments about a recent occurrence on the unit or something that has been bothering a member and about which he or she has some questions. These meetings are usually conducted by staff, although all patients have equal input into the discussions.

All patients are expected to attend the meetings each morning. Exceptions are made when aspects of therapy interfere (e.g., scheduled testing, x-rays, electroencephalograms). An explanation is made to patients present so that false perceptions of danger are not generated by another patient's absence. All staff, with the exception of those required to manage the unit and provide necessary care for patients, are expected to attend the daily meetings.

4. ***Unit responsibilities are assigned according to patient capabilities.*** Increasing self-esteem is an ultimate goal of the therapeutic community. Therefore, a patient should not be set up for failure by being assigned a responsibility that is beyond his or her level of ability. By assigning patients responsibilities that promote achievement, self-esteem is enhanced. Consideration must also be given to time during which the patient will show some regression in the treatment regimen. Adjustments in assignments should be made in a way that preserves self-esteem and provides for progression to greater degrees of responsibility as the patient returns to previous level of functioning.

5. ***A structured program of social and work-related activities is scheduled as part of the treatment program.*** Each patient's therapeutic program consists of group activities in which interpersonal interaction and communication with other individuals are emphasized. Time is also devoted to personal problems. Various group activities may be selected for patients with specific needs, for example, an exercise group for a person who expresses anger inappropriately, an assertiveness group for a person who is passive-aggressive, or a stress-management group for a person who is anxious. A structured schedule of activities is the major focus of a therapeutic community. Through these activities, change in the patient's personality and behavior can be effected. New coping strategies are learned and social skills are developed. In the group situation, the patient is able to practice what he or she has learned to prepare for transition to the general community.

6. ***Community and family are included in the program of therapy in an effort to facilitate discharge from the hospital.*** An attempt is made to include family members, as well as certain aspects of the community that affect the patient, in the treatment program. It is important to keep as many links to the patient's life outside the hospital as possible. Family members are invited to participate in specific therapy groups and, in some instances, to share meals with the patient in the communal dining room.

Connection with community life may be maintained through patient group activities, such as shopping, picnicking, attending movies, bowling, and visiting the zoo. Patients may also be awarded passes to visit family or may participate in work-related activities, the length of time being determined by the activity and the patient's condition. These connections with family and community facilitate the discharge process and may also help to prevent the patient from becoming too dependent on hospitalization.

THE PROGRAM OF THERAPEUTIC COMMUNITY

Care for patients in the therapeutic community is directed by an interdisciplinary treatment (IDT) team. An initial assessment is made by the admitting psychiatrist, nurse, or other designated admitting agent who establishes a priority of care. The IDT team meets within 48 hours of admission to determine a comprehensive treatment plan and goals of therapy and to assign intervention responsibilities. All members sign the treatment plan and meet weekly to update the plan as needed. Depending on the size of the institution and scope of the treatment program, members representing a variety of disciplines may participate in the promotion of a therapeutic community. For example, an IDT team may include a psychiatrist, clinical psychologist, psychiatric clinical nurse specialist, psychiatric nurse, mental health technician, psychiatric social worker, occupational therapist, recreational therapist, art therapist, music therapist, psychodramatist, dietitian, and chaplain. Table 8.1 provides an explanation of responsibilities and educational preparation required for these members of the IDT team.

THE ROLE OF THE NURSE

The Standards of Psychiatric/Mental Health Nursing Practice, developed by the American Nurses' Association (ANA), Division of Psychiatric and Mental Health Nursing Practice, clearly specify that the nurse has a role in the therapeutic milieu of a psychiatric unit. Standard V-E, *Intervention: Therapeutic Environment*, states:

"The nurse provides, structures, and maintains a therapeutic environment in collaboration with the client and other health care providers." (ANA, 1982)

Nurses are generally the only members of the IDT treatment team who spend time with the patients on a 24-hour basis. They assume responsibility for management of the therapeutic milieu, and accomplish this through use of the nursing process. An ongoing assessment, analysis, planning, implementation, and evaluation of the environment is necessary for the successful management of a therapeutic milieu. Nurses are involved in all day-to-day activities that pertain to patient care. Suggestions and opinions of nursing staff are given serious consideration in the planning of care for individual patients. Information from the initial nursing assessment is used to create the IDT plan. Nurses have input into the goals of therapy and participate in the weekly updates and modification of the treatment plans.

In some institutions, a separate nursing care plan is required in addition to the IDT plan. When this is the case, the nursing care plan must reflect diagnoses that are specific to nursing and include problems and interventions from the IDT plan that have been assigned specifically to the discipline of nursing.

In the therapeutic milieu, nurses have the responsibility for ensuring that patients' physiological needs are met. Patients must be encouraged to perform as independently as possible in fulfilling activities of daily living. However, the nurse must make ongoing assessments to provide assistance for those who require it. Assessing physical status is an important nursing responsibility that must not be overlooked on the psychiatric unit that emphasizes holistic care.

Reality orientation for patients who have disorganized thinking, are disoriented, or are confused is important in the therapeutic milieu. Clocks with large hands and numbers, calendars that give the day and date in large print, and orientation boards that discuss daily activities and news happenings can help keep patients oriented to reality. Nurses ensure that patients have written schedules of activities to which they are assigned and that they arrive at those activities on schedule. Some patients

Table 8.1 THE INTERDISCIPLINARY TREATMENT TEAM IN PSYCHIATRY		
Team Member	**Responsibilities**	**Education Required**
Psychiatrist	Serves as the leader of the team. Responsible for diagnosis and treatment of mental disorders. Performs psychotherapy; prescribes medication and other somatic therapies.	Medical degree with residency in psychiatry and license to practice medicine.
Clinical psychologist	Conducts individual, group, and family therapy. Administers, interprets, and evaluates psychological tests that assist in the diagnostic process.	Ph.D. in clinical psychology with 2–3 year internship supervised by a licensed clinical psychologist. State license is required to practice.
Psychiatric clinical nurse specialist	Conducts individual, group, and family therapy. Presents educational programs for nursing staff. Provides consultation services to nurses who require assistance in the planning and implementation of care for individual patients.	Registered nurse with minimum of a master's degree in psychiatric nursing.
Psychiatric nurse	Provides ongoing assessment of patient condition, both mentally and physically. Manages the therapeutic milieu on a 24-hour basis. Administers medications. Assists patients with all therapeutic activities as required. Focus is on one-to-one relationship development.	Registered nurse with hospital diploma, associate degree, or baccalaureate degree.
Mental health technician (also called psychiatric aide or assistant, or psychiatric technician)	Functions under the supervision of the psychiatric nurse. Provides assistance to patients in the fulfillment of their activities of daily living. Assists activity therapists as required in the conduct of their groups. May also participate in one-to-one relationship development.	Varies from state to state. Requirements include high school education, with additional vocational education or on-the-job training. Some hospitals hire individuals with B.S. in psychology in this capacity. Some states require a license exam to practice.
Psychiatric social worker	Conducts individual, group, and family therapy. Is concerned with patient's social needs, such as placement, financial support, and community requirements. Conducts in-depth psychosocial history on which the needs assessment is based. Works with patient and family to ensure that requirements for discharge are fulfilled and needs can be met by appropriate community resources.	Minimum of a master's degree in Social Work (MSW).
Occupational therapist	Works with patients to help develop (or redevelop) independence in performance of activities of daily living. Focus is on rehabilitation and vocational training where patients learn to be productive, thereby enhancing self-esteem. Creative activities and therapeutic relationship skills are used.	Baccalaureate or master's degree in occupational therapy.

(*continued*)

Table 8.1 CONTINUED		
Team Member	**Responsibilities**	**Education Required**
Recreational therapist	Uses recreational activities to promote patients to redirect their thinking or to rechannel destructive energy in an appropriate manner. Patients learn skills that can be used during leisure time and during times of stress following discharge from the hospital. Examples include bowling, volleyball, exercises, and jogging. Some programs include activities such as picnics, swimming, and even group attendance at the state fair when it is in session.	Baccalaureate or master's degree in recreational therapy.
Art therapist	Uses the patient's creative abilities to encourage expression of emotions and feelings through artwork. Helps patients to analyze their own work in an effort to recognize and resolve underlying conflict.	Graduate degree with specialty in art therapy.
Music therapist	Encourages patients in self-expression through music. Patients listen to music, play instruments, sing, dance, and even compose songs that help them get in touch with feelings and emotions that they may not be able to experience in any other way.	Graduate degree with specialty in music therapy.
Psychodramatist	Directs patients in the creation of a "drama" that portrays real-life situations. Individuals select problems they wish to enact, and other patients play the roles of significant others in the situations. Some patients are able to "act" out problems that they are unable to work through in a more traditional manner. All members benefit through intensive discussion that follows.	Graduate degree in psychology, social work, nursing, or medicine with additional training in group therapy and specialty preparation to become a psychodramatist.
Dietitian	Plans nutritious meals for all patients. Works on consulting basis for patients with specific eating disorders, such as anorexia nervosa, bulimia nervosa, obesity, pica, and rumination.	Baccalaureate or master's degree with specialty in dietetics.
Chaplain	Assesses, identifies, and attends to the spiritual needs of patients and their family members. Provides spiritual support and comfort as requested by patient or family. May provide counseling if educational background includes this type of training.	College degree with advanced education in theology, seminary, or rabbinical studies.

may require an identification sign on their door to remind them which room is theirs. All of these determinations are made from ongoing nursing assessments.

Nurses are responsible for the management of medication administration. On some psychiatric units, patients are expected to accept the responsibility and request their medication at the appropriate time. While ultimate responsibility lies with the nurse, he or she must encourage patients to be self-reliant. Nurses must work with the patients to determine methods that result in achievement and provide positive feedback for successes.

A major focus of nursing in the therapeutic milieu is the one-to-one relationship, which grows out of a developing trust between patient and nurse. Many patients with psychiatric disorders have never achieved the ability to trust. If this can be accomplished in a relationship with the nurse, the trust may be generalized to other relationships in the patient's life. Developing trust means keeping promises that have been made. It means total acceptance of the individual as a person, separate from behavior that is unacceptable. It means responding to the patient with concrete behaviors that are understandable to him or her (e.g., "If you are frightened, I will stay with you"; "If you are cold, I will bring you a blanket"; "If you are thirsty, I will bring you a drink of water.") Within an atmosphere of trust, the patient is encouraged to express feelings and emotions and discuss unresolved issues that are creating problems in his or her life.

The nurse is responsible for setting limits on unacceptable behavior in the therapeutic milieu. This requires stating to the patient in understandable terminology what behaviors are not acceptable and what the consequences will be should the limits be violated. These limits must be established, written, and carried out by all staff on all shifts. Consistency in carrying out the consequences of violation of the established limits is essential if the learning is to be reinforced.

The role of patient teacher is important in the psychiatric area, as it is in all areas of nursing. Nurses must be able to assess learning readiness in individual patients. Do they want to learn? What is their level of anxiety? What is their level of ability to understand the information being presented? Topics for patient education in psychiatry include information about the patient's medical diagnosis,

the side effects of medication, the importance of continuing to take one's medication, stress management, among others. Some topics must be individualized for specific patients, while others may be taught in group situations. Table 8.2 outlines various topics of nursing concern for patient education in psychiatry.

Devine (1981) has stated:

"It would appear that the role of the nurse is all-encompassing in a therapeutic environment. The nurse must be supportive and encourage the patient to become self-reliant. Normal natural social relationships must be fostered, and a consistent,

Table 8.2 THE THERAPEUTIC MILIEU—TOPICS FOR PATIENT EDUCATION

1. Ways to increase self-esteem
2. Ways to deal with anger appropriately
3. Stress-management techniques
4. How to recognize signs of increasing anxiety and intervene to stop progression
5. Normal stages of grieving and behaviors associated with each stage
6. Assertiveness techniques
7. Relaxation techniques
   a. Progressive relaxation
   b. Tense and relax
   c. Deep breathing
   d. Autogenics
8. Medications (specify)
   a. Harmless side effects
   b. Side effects to report to physician
   c. Importance of taking regularly
   d. Importance of not stopping abruptly
9. Effects of (substance) on the body
   a. Alcohol
   b. Other depressants
   c. Stimulants
   d. Hallucinogens
   e. Narcotics
   f. Cannabinols
10. Problem-solving skills
11. Thought-stopping/thought-switching techniques
12. Sex education
    a. Structure and function of the reproductive system
    b. Contraceptives
    c. Sexually transmitted diseases
13. The essentials of good nutrition
14. (For parents/guardians)
    a. Signs and symptoms of substance abuse
    b. Effective parenting techniques

positive outlook is the primary tool with which to practice milieu therapy."

SUMMARY

In psychiatry, milieu therapy, or a therapeutic community, constitutes a manipulation of the environment in an effort to create behavioral changes and to improve the psychological health and functioning of the individual. The goal of therapeutic community is for the patient to learn adaptive coping, interaction, and relationship skills that can be generalized to other aspects of his or her life. The community environment itself serves as the primary tool of therapy.

According to Skinner (1979), a therapeutic community is based upon seven basic assumptions:

1. The health in each individual is to be realized and encouraged to grow.
2. Every interaction is an opportunity for therapeutic intervention.
3. The patient owns his own environment.
4. Each patient owns his behavior.
5. Peer pressure is a useful and a powerful tool.
6. Inappropriate behaviors are dealt with as they occur.
7. Restrictions and punishment are to be avoided.

Since the goals of milieu therapy relate to helping the patient learn to generalize that which is learned to other aspects of his or her life, the conditions that promote a therapeutic community in the hospital setting are similar to the types of conditions that exist in real-life situations. They include:

1. The fulfillment of basic physiological needs.
2. Physical facilities that are conducive to achievement of the goals of therapy.
3. The existence of a democratic form of self-government.
4. The assignment of unit responsibilities according to patient capabilities.
5. A structured program of social and work-related activities.
6. The inclusion of community and family in the program of therapy in an effort to facilitate discharge from the hospital.

The program of therapy on the milieu unit is conducted by the IDT team. The team includes some, or all, of the following disciplines, and may include others that are not specified here: psychiatrist, clinical psychologist, psychiatric clinical nurse specialist, psychiatric nurse, mental health technician, psychiatric social worker, occupational therapist, recreational therapist, art therapist, music therapist, psychodramatist, dietitian, and chaplain.

Nurses play a crucial role in the management of a therapeutic milieu. They are involved in the assessment, analysis, planning, implementation, and evaluation of all treatment programs. They have significant input into the IDT plans that are developed for all patients. They are responsible for ensuring that patients' basic needs are fulfilled, for continual assessment of physical and psychosocial status, for medication administration, for the development of trusting relationships, for setting limits on unacceptable behaviors, for patient education, and ultimately, for helping patients, within the limits of their capability, become productive members of society.

REVIEW QUESTIONS
Self-Examination/Learning Exercise

Test your knowledge of milieu therapy by supplying the information requested.

1. Define *milieu therapy*.
2. What is the goal of milieu therapy/therapeutic community?

*Select the **best** response in each of the following questions.*

3. In prioritizing care within the therapeutic environment, which of the following nursing interventions would receive the highest priority?

    a. Ensuring that the physical facilities are conducive to achievement of the goals of therapy.

    b. Scheduling a community meeting for 8:30 AM each morning.

    c. Attending to the nutritional and comfort needs of all patients.

    d. Establishing contacts with community resources.

4. In the community meeting, which of the following actions is most important for reinforcing the democratic posture of the unit?

    a. Allowing each person a specific equal amount of time to talk.

    b. Reviewing unit rules and behavioral limits that apply to all patients.

    c. Reading the minutes from yesterday's meeting.

    d. Waiting until all patients are present before initiating the meeting.

5. One of the goals of therapeutic community is for patients to become more independent and accept self-responsibility. Which of the following approaches by staff best encourages fulfillment of this goal?

    a. Including patient input and decisions in the treatment plan.

    b. Insisting that each patient take a turn as "president" of the community meeting.

    c. Making decisions for the patient regarding plans for treatment.

    d. Requiring that the patient be bathed, dressed, and attend breakfast on time each morning.

6. Patient teaching is an important nursing function on the milieu unit. Which of the following statements by the patient indicates the need for knowledge and a readiness to learn?

    a. "Get away from me with that medicine! I'm not sick!"

    b. "I don't belong on the psych unit. It's my migraine headaches that I need help with."

    c. "I've taken Valium every day of my life for the past 20 years. I'll stop when I'm good and ready!"

    d. "The doctor says I have bipolar disorder. What does that really mean?"

7. Match the following activities with the responsible therapist from the IDT team.

_____ 1. Psychiatrist

_____ 2. Clinical psychologist

_____ 3. Psychiatric social worker

_____ 4. Psychiatric clinical nurse specialist

_____ 5. Psychiatric nurse

_____ 6. Mental health technician

_____ 7. Occupational therapist

_____ 8. Recreational therapist

_____ 9. Music therapist

a. Helps patients plan, shop for, and cook a meal

b. Locates half-way house and arranges living conditions for patient being discharged from the hospital

c. Helps patients get to know themselves better by having them describe what they feel when they hear a certain song

d. Helps patients to recognize their own beliefs so that they may draw comfort from those beliefs in time of spiritual need

e. Accompanies patients on community trip to the zoo

_____ 10. Art therapist

_____ 11. Psychodramatist

_____ 12. Dietitian

_____ 13. Chaplain

f. Diagnoses mental disorders, conducts psychotherapy, and prescribes somatic therapies

g. Manages the therapeutic milieu on a 24-hour basis

h. Conducts group and family therapies and administers and evaluates psychological tests that assist in the diagnostic process

i. Conducts group therapies and provides consultation and education to staff nurses

j. Assists staff nurses in the management of the milieu

k. Encourages patients to express painful emotions by drawing pictures on paper

l. Assesses needs, establishes, monitors, and evaluates a nutritional program for a patient with anorexia nervosa

m. Directs a group of patients in acting out a situation that is otherwise too painful for a patient to discuss openly

REFERENCES

American Nurses' Association, Division on Psychiatric/Mental Health Nursing Practice. (1982). _Standards of psychiatric/mental health nursing practice._ Kansas City, MO: American Nurses' Association.

Devine, B. A. (1981, March). Therapeutic milieu/milieu therapy: An overview. _J Psychiatr Nurs_, pp. 20–24.

Maslow, A. (1968). _Towards a psychology of being_ (2nd ed.). New York: D. Van Nostrand Co.

Skinner, K. (1979, August). The therapeutic milieu: Making it work. _J Psychiatr Nurs_, pp. 38–44.

BIBLIOGRAPHY

Canter, D. & Canter, S. (Eds.). (1979). _Designing for therapeutic environments, A review of research._ Chichester, England: John Wiley & Sons.

Carser, D. L. (1981, February). Primary nursing in the milieu. _J Psychiatr Nurs_, pp. 35–41.

Hinds, P. S. (1980, June). Music: A milieu factor with implications for the nurse therapist. _J Psychiatr Nurs_, pp. 28–33.

Hinshelwood, R. D. & Manning, N. (Eds.). (1979). _Therapeutic communities: Reflections and progress._ London: Routledge and Kegan Paul.

Jansen, E. (1980). _The therapeutic community._ London: Croom Helm.

Jones, M. (1953). _The therapeutic community._ New York: Basic Books.

Sharp, V. (1975). _Social control in the therapeutic community._ Westmead, England: Saxon House, D.C. Heath Ltd.

CRISIS INTERVENTION

KEY TERMS
crisis
crisis intervention

OBJECTIVES

After reading this chapter, the student will be able to:
1. Define *crisis*.
2. Describe four phases in the development of a crisis.
3. Identify types of crises that occur in people's lives.
4. Discuss the goal of crisis intervention.
5. Describe the steps in crisis intervention.
6. Identify the role of the nurse in crisis intervention.

CRISIS, DEFINED

The term *crisis* was defined by Caplan (1964) as the

". . . psychological disequilibrium in a person who confronts a hazardous circumstance that for him constitutes an important problem which he can for the time being neither escape nor solve with his customary problem-solving resources."

Certain characteristics have been identified by various individuals who have studied crisis theory (Caplan, 1964; Geissler, 1984; France, 1982) that can be viewed as assumptions upon which the concept of crisis is based. They include:

1. Crisis occurs in all individuals at one time or another and is not necessarily equated with psychopathology.
2. Crises are precipitated by specific identifiable events.
3. Crises are personal by nature. What may be considered a crisis situation by one individual may not be so for another.
4. Crises are acute, not chronic, and will be resolved in one way or another within a brief period.
5. A crisis situation contains the potential for psychological growth or deterioration.

Individuals who are in crisis feel helpless to change. They do not believe they have the resources to deal with the precipitating stressor. Levels of anxiety rise to the point that the individual becomes nonfunctional, thoughts become obsessional, and all behavior is aimed at relief of the anxiety being experienced. The feeling is overwhelming and may affect the individual physically as well as psychosocially.

PHASES IN THE DEVELOPMENT OF A CRISIS

The development of a crisis situation follows a relatively predictable course. Caplan (1964) has outlined four specific phases through which individuals progress in response to a precipitating stressor and which culminate in the state of acute crisis.

Phase 1. The individual is exposed to a precipitating

stressor. Anxiety increases. Previous problem-solving techniques are employed.

Phase 2. When previous problem-solving techniques do not relieve the stressor, anxiety increases further. The individual begins to feel a great deal of discomfort at this point. Coping techniques that have worked in the past are attempted, only to create feelings of helplessness when they are not successful. Feelings of confusion and disorganization prevail.

Phase 3. All possible resources, both internal and external, are called upon to resolve the problem and relieve the discomfort. The individual may try to view the problem from a different perspective or even to overlook certain aspects of it. New problem-solving techniques may be employed, and if effectual, resolution may occur at this phase, with the individual returning to higher, lower, or previous level of premorbid functioning.

Phase 4. If resolution does not occur in previous phases, Caplan states, ". . . the tension mounts beyond a further threshold or its burden increases over time to a breaking point. Major disorganization of the individual with drastic results often occurs." Anxiety may reach panic levels. Cognitive functions are disordered, emotions are labile, and behavior may reflect the presence of psychotic thinking.

These phases are congruent with the Transactional Model of Stress/Adaptation outlined in Chapter 1. The relationship between the two perspectives is presented in Figure 9.1. Similarly, Aguilera and Messick (1982) spoke of "balancing factors" that affect the way in which an individual perceives and responds to a precipitating stressor. A schematic of these balancing factors is illustrated in Figure 9.2.

As previously set forth, it is assumed that crises are acute, not chronic, situations and will be resolved in one way or another within a brief period. Barrell (1974) states, "Crises are by definition self-limiting and generally last from 4 to 6 weeks. During this brief period the person is psychologically vulnerable and is, consequently, *ready* for the learning and growth opportunity." Crises can become growth opportunities when individuals learn new methods of coping that can be preserved and used when similar stressors reoccur.

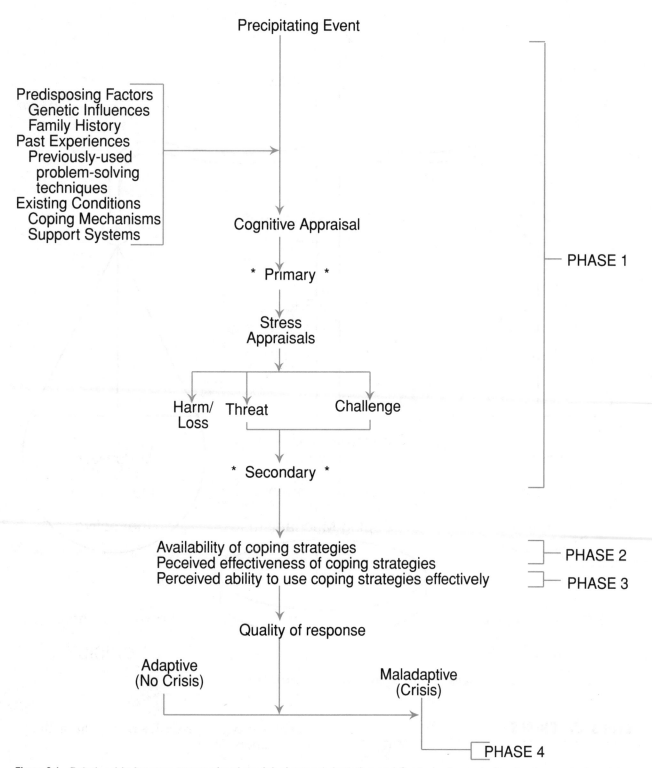

Figure 9.1   Relationship between transactional model of stress/adaptation and Caplan's phases in the development of a crisis.

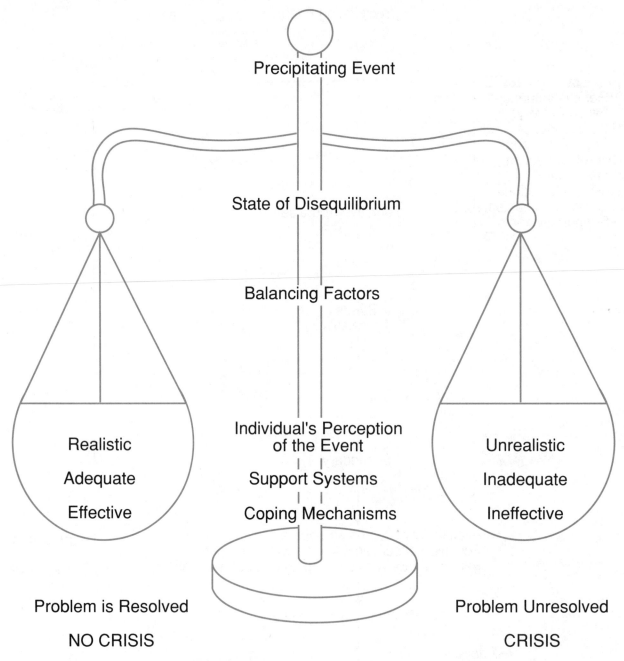

Precipitating Event

State of Disequilibrium

Balancing Factors

Realistic	Individual's Perception of the Event	Unrealistic
Adequate	Support Systems	Inadequate
Effective	Coping Mechanisms	Ineffective

Problem is Resolved   Problem Unresolved

NO CRISIS   CRISIS

Figure 9.2   The effects of balancing factors in a stressful event.

TYPES OF CRISES

Baldwin (1978) has identified six classes of emotional crisis, which progress by degree of severity. As the measure of psychopathology increases, the source of the stressor changes from external to internal. The type of crisis determines the method of intervention selected.

Class 1: Dispositional Crises

Definition: An acute response to an external situational stressor.

Example: Nancy and Ted have been married for 3 years. They have a 1-year-old daughter. Ted has been having difficulty with his boss at work. Twice during the past 6 months he has exploded in anger at home and become abusive with Nancy. Last night, he became angry that dinner was not ready when he expected. He grabbed the baby from Nancy and tossed her, screaming, into her crib. He hit and punched Nancy until she feared for her life. This morning when he left for work, she took the baby and went to the emergency department of the city hospital, not having anywhere else to go.

Intervention: Nancy's physical wounds were cared for in the emergency department. The mental health counselor provided support and guidance in terms of presenting alternatives to her. Needs and issues were clarified, and referrals for agency assistance were made.

Class 2: Crises of Anticipated Life Transitions

Definition: Normal life-cycle transitions that may be anticipated, but over which the individual may feel a lack of control.

Example: College student J.T. is placed on probationary status due to low grades this semester. His wife had a baby and had to quit her job. He increased his working hours from part time to full time to compensate, and therefore had little time for studies. He presents himself to the student-health nurse clinician complaining of numerous vague physical complaints.

Intervention: Perform physical examination (physical symptoms could be caused by depression). Encourage ventilation of feelings. Provide reassurance and support as needed. Suggest referrals to services that can provide financial and other types of needed assistance. Identify problematic areas and discuss approaches to change.

Class 3: Crises Resulting from Traumatic Stress

Definition: These crises are precipitated by unexpected, external stresses over which the individual has little or no control, and from which

he or she feels emotionally overwhelmed and defeated.

Example: Sally was a waitress whose shift ended at midnight. Two weeks ago, while walking to her car in the deserted parking lot, she was abducted by two men with guns, taken to an abandoned building, raped, and beaten. Since that time, her physical wounds have nearly healed. However, Sally cannot be alone, she is constantly fearful, she relives the experience in flashbacks and dreams, and is unable to eat, sleep, or work on her job at the restaurant. Her friend offers to accompany her to the mental health clinic.

Intervention: Encourage her to talk about the experience and to ventilate feelings associated with it. Offer reassurance and support. Discuss stages of grief and how rape causes a loss of self-worth, triggering the grief response. Identify support systems who can help her to resume her normal activities. Explore new methods of coping with emotions arising from a situation with which she has had no previous experience.

Class 4: Maturational/Developmental Crises

Definition: These types of crises occur in response to situations that trigger emotions related to unresolved conflicts in one's life. These crises are of internal origin and reflect underlying developmental issues that involve dependency, value conflicts, sexual identity, control, and capacity for emotional intimacy.

Example: Bob is 40 years old. He has just been passed over for job promotion for the third time. He has moved many times within the large company for which he works, usually after angering and alienating himself from the supervisor. His father was domineering and became abusive when Bob did not comply with his every command. Over the years, Bob's behavioral response became one of passive-aggressiveness, first with his father, then with his supervisors. This third rejection has created feelings of depression and intense anxiety in Bob. At his wife's insistence, he has sought help at the mental health clinic.

Intervention: The primary intervention is to assist the individual to identify the unresolved developmental issue that is creating the conflict. Support and guidance are offered during the initial crisis period, then assistance is given to help the individual work through the underlying conflict in an effort to change response patterns that are creating problems in his current life situation.

Class 5: Crises Reflecting Psychopathology

Definition: Emotional crises in which preexisting psychopathology has been instrumental in precipitating the crisis or in which psychopathology significantly impairs or complicates adaptive resolution. Examples of psychopathology that may precipitate crises include borderline personality, severe neuroses, characterological disorders, or schizophrenia. (Baldwin, 1978).

Example: Sonja, aged 29, was diagnosed with borderline personality at age 18. She has been in therapy on a weekly basis for 10 years, with several hospitalizations for suicide attempts during that time. She has had the same therapist for the past 6 years. This therapist told Sonja today that she is to be married in 1 month and will be moving across the country with her new husband. Sonja is distraught and experiencing intense feelings of abandonment. She is found wandering in and out of traffic on a busy expressway, oblivious to her surroundings. Police bring her to the emergency room of the hospital.

Intervention: The initial intervention is to help bring down the level of anxiety in Sonja that has created feelings of unreality in her. She requires that someone stay with her and reassure her of her safety and security. After the feelings of panic have subsided, encourage verbalizations related to feelings of abandonment. Discourage regressive behaviors. Give positive reinforcement for independent activities and accomplishments. The primary therapist will need to pursue this issue of termination with Sonja at length. Referral to a long-term care facility may be required.

Class 6: Psychiatric Emergencies

Definition: Crisis situations in which general functioning has been severely impaired and the individual rendered incompetent or unable to assume personal responsibility. Examples include acutely suicidal individuals, drug overdoses, reactions to hallucinogenic drugs, acute psychoses, uncontrollable anger, and alcohol intoxication (Baldwin, 1978).

Example: Jennifer, age 16, had been dating Joe, the star high school football player, for 6 months. After the game on Friday night, Jennifer and Joe went to Jackie's house, where a number of high school students had gathered for an after-game party. No adults were present. About midnight, Joe told Jennifer that he did not want to date her anymore. Jennifer became hysterical, and Jackie was frightened by her behavior. She took Jennifer to her parents' bedroom and gave her a Valium from a bottle in her mother's medicine cabinet. She left Jennifer lying on her parents' bed and returned to the party downstairs. About an hour later, she returned to her parents' bedroom and found that Jennifer had removed the bottle of Valium from the cabinet and swallowed all of them. Jennifer was unconscious and Jackie could not awaken her. An ambulance was called, and Jennifer was transported to the local hospital.

Intervention: The crisis team monitored vital signs, ensured maintenance of adequate airway, initiated gastric lavage, and administered activated charcoal to minimize absorption. Jennifer's parents were notified and rushed to the hospital. The situation was explained to them, and they were encouraged to stay by her side. When the physical crisis was resolved, Jennifer was transferred to the psychiatric unit. In therapy, she was encouraged to ventilate her feelings regarding the rejection and subsequent overdose. Family therapy sessions were conducted in an effort to clarify interpersonal issues and to identify areas for change. On an individual level, Jennifer's therapist worked with her to establish more adaptive methods of coping with stressful situations.

CRISIS INTERVENTION

Individuals experiencing crises have an urgent need for assistance. In crisis intervention, the therapist, or other intervener, becomes a part of the individual's life situation. Because of the individual's emotional state, he or she is unable to problem solve, so requires guidance and support from another to help mobilize the resources needed to resolve the crisis.

Lengthy psychologic interpretations are obviously not appropriate for crisis intervention. It is a time for doing what is needed to help the individual get relief. It is a time for calling into action all the people and other resources required to do so.

Aguilera and Messick (1982) state:

> The minimum therapeutic goal of crisis intervention is psychological resolution of the individual's immediate crisis and restoration to at least the level of functioning that existed before the crisis period. A maximum goal is improvement in functioning above the precrisis level.

Crisis intervention takes place in both inpatient and outpatient settings. The basic methodology relies heavily on orderly problem-solving techniques and structured activities that are focused on change. Through adaptive change, crises are resolved and growth occurs. Because of the time limitation of crisis intervention, the individual must experience some degree of relief almost from the first interaction. Crisis intervention, then, is not aimed at major personality change or reconstruction (as may be the case in long-term psychotherapy), but rather at using a given crisis situation to, at the very least, restore functioning and, optimistically, to also enhance personal growth.

PHASES OF CRISIS INTERVENTION: THE ROLE OF THE NURSE

Nurses respond to crisis situations on a daily basis. Crises can occur on every unit in the general hospital, in the home setting, in the community health-care setting, in schools, offices, and in private practice. Indeed, nurses may be called upon to function as crisis helpers in virtually any setting committed to the practice of nursing.

Aguilera and Messick (1982) have described four specific phases in the technique of crisis intervention. These phases are clearly comparable to the steps of the nursing process.

Phase 1. Assessment

In this phase, the crisis helper gathers information regarding the precipitating stressor and the resulting crisis that prompted the individual to seek professional help. A nurse in crisis intervention might perform some of the following assessments:

1. Ask the individual to describe the event that precipitated this crisis.
2. Determine when it occurred.
3. Assess the individual's physical and mental status.
4. Determine if the individual has experienced this stressor before. If so, what method of coping was used? Have these methods been tried this time?
5. If previous coping methods were tried, what was the result?
6. If new coping methods were tried, what was the result?
7. Assess suicide or homicide potential, plan, and means.
8. Assess adequacy of support systems.
9. Determine level of precrisis functioning. Assess usual coping methods, available support systems, and ability to problem solve.
10. Assess individual's perception of own strengths and limitations.
11. Assess individual's use of substances.

Information from the comprehensive assessment is then analyzed, and appropriate nursing diagnoses reflecting the immediacy of the crisis situation are identified. Some nursing diagnoses that may be relevant include:

1. Ineffective individual coping
2. Anxiety (severe to panic)
3. Altered thought processes
4. Potential for violence, self-directed or directed at others
5. Rape-trauma syndrome
6. Post-trauma response
7. Fear

Phase 2. Planning of Therapeutic Intervention

In the planning phase of the nursing process, the nurse selects the appropriate nursing actions for the identified nursing diagnoses. In planning the interventions, the type of crisis, as well as the individual's strengths and available resources for support, are taken into consideration. Goals are established for crisis resolution and a return to, or increase in, the precrisis level of functioning.

Phase 3. Intervention

During phase 3, the actions that were identified in phase 2 are implemented. Smith, Karasik, and Meyer (1984) have outlined the following interventions as the focus of nursing in crisis intervention:

1. Use a reality-oriented approach. The focus of the problem is on the here and now.
2. Remain with the individual who is experiencing panic anxiety.
3. Establish a rapid working relationship by showing unconditional acceptance, by active listening, and by attending to immediate needs.
4. Discourage lengthy explanations or rationalizations of the situation; promote an atmosphere for verbalization of true feelings.
5. Set firm limits on aggressive, destructive behaviors. At high levels of anxiety, behavior is likely to be impulsive and regressive. Establish at the outset what is acceptable and what is not and maintain consistency.
6. Clarify the problem that the individual is facing. The nurse does this by describing his or her perception of the problem and comparing it with the individual's perception of the problem.
7. Help the individual determine what he or she believes precipitated the crisis.
8. Acknowledge feelings of anger, guilt, helplessness, and powerlessness, while taking care not to provide positive feedback for these feelings.
9. Guide the individual through a problem-solving process by which he or she may move in the direction of positive life change:
   a. Help the individual confront the source of the problem that is creating the crisis response.
   b. Encourage the individual to discuss changes he or she would like to make. Jointly determine whether or not desired changes are realistic.
   c. Encourage exploration of feelings about aspects that cannot be changed, and explore alternative ways of coping more adaptively in these situations.
   d. Discuss alternative strategies for creating changes that are realistically possible.
   e. Weigh benefits and consequences of each alternative.
   f. Assist the individual to select alternative coping strategies that will help alleviate future crisis situations.
10. Identify external support systems and new social networks from whom the individual may seek assistance in times of stress.

Phase 4. Evaluation of Crisis Resolution and Anticipatory Planning

To evaluate the outcome of crisis intervention, a reassessment is made to determine if the stated objective was achieved. Have positive behavioral changes occurred? Has the individual developed more adaptive coping strategies? Have they been effective? Has the individual grown from the experience by gaining insight into his or her responses to crisis situations? Does the individual believe that he or she could respond with healthy adaptation in future stressful situations to prevent crisis development? Can the individual describe a plan of action for dealing with stressors similar to the one which precipitated this crisis?

During the evaluation period, the nurse and patient summarize what has occurred during the intervention. They review what the individual has learned and "anticipate" how he or she will respond in the future. A determination is made regarding follow-up therapy; if needed, the nurse provides referral information.

SUMMARY

A *crisis* is a situation that produces "psychological disequilibrium in a person who confronts a hazardous circumstance that for him constitutes an important problem, which he can for the time being neither escape nor solve with his customary problem-solving resources" (Caplan, 1964). All individuals experience crises at one time or another. This does not necessarily indicate psychopathology.

Crises are precipitated by specific identifiable events and are determined by an individual's personal perception of the situation. They are acute, not chronic, and generally last no more than 4 to 6 weeks.

Crises occur when an individual is exposed to a stressor and previous problem-solving techniques are ineffective. This causes the level of anxiety to rise. Panic may ensue when new techniques are employed and resolution fails to occur.

Baldwin (1978) identified six types of crises. They include dispositional crises, crises of anticipated life transitions, crises resulting from traumatic stress, maturational/developmental crises, crises reflecting psychopathology, and psychiatric emergencies. The type of crisis determines the method of intervention selected.

Crisis intervention is designed to provide rapid assistance for individuals who have an urgent need. Aguilera and Messick (1982) have identified the minimum therapeutic goal of crisis intervention as "psychological resolution of the individual's immediate crisis and restoration to at least the level of functioning that existed before the crisis period. A maximum goal is improvement in functioning above the precrisis level."

Nurses regularly respond to individuals in crisis in all types of settings. Nursing process is the vehicle by which nurses assist individuals in crisis with a short-term problem-solving approach to change. A four-phase technique was outlined: assessment/analysis, planning of therapeutic intervention, intervention, and evaluation of crisis resolution and anticipatory planning. Through this structured method of assistance, nurses assist individuals in crisis to develop more adaptive coping strategies for dealing with stressful situations in the future.

REVIEW QUESTIONS
Self-Examination/Learning Exercise

*Select the **best** response to each of the following questions.*

1. Which of the following is a correct assumption regarding the concept of crisis?
   a. Crises occur only in individuals with psychopathology.
   b. The stressful event that precipitates crisis is seldom identifiable.
   c. A crisis situation contains the potential for psychological growth or deterioration.
   d. Crises are chronic situations that reoccur many times during an individual's life.

2. Crises occur when an individual:
   a. Is exposed to a precipitating stressor.
   b. Perceives a stressor to be threatening.
   c. Has no support systems.
   d. Experiences a stressor and perceives coping strategies to be ineffective.

3. Amanda's mobile home was destroyed by a tornado. Amanda received only minor injuries, but is experiencing disabling anxiety in the aftermath of the event. This type of crisis is called:
   a. Crisis resulting from traumatic stress
   b. Maturational/developmental crisis
   c. Dispositional crisis
   d. Crisis of anticipated life transitions

4. The most appropriate crisis intervention with Amanda would be to:
   a. Encourage her to recognize how lucky she is to be alive.
   b. Discuss stages of grief and feelings associated with each.
   c. Identify community resources that can help Amanda.
   d. Suggest that she find a place to live that provides a storm shelter.

5. Jenny reported to the high school nurse that her mother drinks too much. She is drunk every afternoon when Jenny gets home from school. Jenny is afraid to invite friends over because of her mother's behavior. This type of crisis is called:
   a. Crisis resulting from traumatic stress
   b. Maturational/developmental crisis
   c. Dispositional crisis
   d. Crisis reflecting psychopathology

6. The most appropriate nursing intervention with Jenny would be to:
   a. Make arrangements for her to start attending Al-Ateen meetings.
   b. Help her identify the positive things in her life and recognize that her situation could be a lot worse than it is.
   c. Teach her about the effects of alcohol on the body and that it can be hereditary.
   d. Refer her to a psychiatrist for private therapy to learn to deal with her home situation.

7. Ginger, age 19 and an only child, left 3 months ago to attend a college of her choice 500 miles away from her parents. It is Ginger's first time away from home. She has difficulty making decisions and will not undertake anything new without first consulting her mother. They talk on the phone almost every day. Ginger has recently started having anxiety attacks. She consults the nurse clinician in the student health center. This type of crisis is called:
   a. Crisis resulting from traumatic stress
   b. Dispositional crisis
   c. Psychiatric emergency
   d. Maturational/developmental crisis

8. The most appropriate nursing intervention with Ginger would be to:
   a. Suggest she move to a college closer to home.
   b. Work with Ginger on unresolved dependency issues.
   c. Help her find someone in the college town from whom she could seek assistance rather than calling her mother regularly.
   d. Recommend that the college physician prescribe an antianxiety medication for Ginger.

9. Marie, age 56, is the mother of five children. Her youngest child, who had been living at home and attending the local college, recently graduated and accepted a job in another state. Marie has never worked outside the home and has devoted her life to satisfying the needs of her husband and children. Since the departure of her last child from home, Marie has become more and more despondent. Her husband has become very concerned, and takes her to the local mental health center. This type of crisis is called:
   a. Dispositional crisis
   b. Crisis of anticipated life transitions
   c. Psychiatric emergency
   d. Crisis resulting from traumatic stress

10. The most appropriate nursing intervention with Marie would be to:
    a. Refer her to her family physician for a complete physical examination.
    b. Suggest she seek outside employment now that her children have left home.

c. Identify convenient support systems for times when she is feeling particularly despondent.

d. Begin grief work and assist her to recognize areas of self-worth separate and apart from her children.

REFERENCES

Aguilera, D. C. & Messick, J. M. (1982). *Crisis intervention: Theory and methodology* (4th ed.). St. Louis: CV Mosby.

Baldwin, B. A. (1978, July). A paradigm for the classification of emotional crises: Implications for crisis intervention. *Am J Orthopsychiatry, 48*(3), pp. 538–551.

Barrell, L. M. (1974, March). Crisis intervention: Partnership in problem-solving. *Nurs Clin North Am, 9*(1), pp. 5–16.

Caplan, G. (1964). *Principles of preventive psychiatry.* New York: Basic Books.

France, K. (1982). *Crisis intervention: A handbook of immediate person-to-person help.* Springfield, IL: Charles C. Thomas Publisher.

Geissler, E. M. (1984, July). Crisis: What it is and is not. *Adv Nurs Sci, 6*(4), pp. 1–9.

Smith, S. F., Karasik, D. A., & Meyer, B. J. (1984). *Psychiatric and psychosocial nursing.* Los Altos, CA: National Nursing Review.

BIBLIOGRAPHY

Brownell, M. J. (1984, July). The concept of crisis: Its utility for nursing. *Adv Nurs Sci, 6*(4), pp. 10–21.

Duggan, H. A. (1984). *Crisis intervention: Helping individuals at risk.* Lexington, MA: Lexington Books.

Goldstein, D. (1978, December). Crisis intervention: A brief therapy model. *Nurs Clin North Am, 13*(4), pp. 657–663.

Hatch, C. & Schut, L. (1980, April). Description of a crisis-oriented psychiatric home visiting service. *J Psychosoc Nurs, 18*(4), pp. 31–35.

Hoff, L. A. (1989). *People in crisis: Understanding and helping* (3rd ed.). Redwood City, CA: Addison-Wesley Publishing Co.

Johnson, R. (1981). Applying crisis intervention techniques. In J. Robinson (Ed.), *Using crisis intervention wisely.* Nursing Skillbook Series. Horsham, PA: Intermed Communications, Inc.

10

RELAXATION THERAPY

OBJECTIVES

After reading this chapter, the student will be able to:
1. Identify conditions for which relaxation is appropriate therapy.
2. Describe physiological and behavioral manifestations of relaxation.
3. Discuss various methods of achieving relaxation.
4. Describe the role of the nurse in relaxation therapy.

THE STRESS EPIDEMIC

Individuals experience stress as a daily fact of life. It cannot be avoided. It is generated by both positive and negative experiences that require adjustment to various changes in one's current routine. Whether or not there is more stress today than in the past is unknown, but some experts have suggested that it has become more pervasive. Perhaps this is due to the many uncertainties and salient risks that challenge our most basic value systems on a day-to-day basis.

In Chapter 1, a lengthy discussion was presented regarding the "fight or flight" response of the human body to stressful situations. This response served our ancestors well. The extra burst of adrenaline primed their muscles and focused their attention on the danger at hand. Indeed, the response provided early Homo sapiens with the essentials to deal with life and death situations, such as an imminent attack by a saber-toothed tiger or grizzly bear.

Today, with stress rapidly permeating our society, large segments of the population experience the "fight or flight" response on a regular basis. However, the physical reinforcements are not used in a manner by which the individual is returned to the homeostatic condition within a short period. The "fight or flight" emergency response is inappropriate to today's psychosocial stresses that persist over long periods. In fact, in today's society, rather than assisting with life and death situations, the response may actually be a contributing factor in some life and death situations. Dr. Joel Elkes, director of the behavioral medicine program at the University of Louisville (Kentucky) has said, "Our mode of life itself, the way we live, is emerging as today's principal cause of illness." Stress is now known to be a major contributor, either directly or indirectly, to coronary heart disease, cancer, lung ailments, accidental injuries, cirrhosis of the liver, and suicide — six of the leading causes of death in the United States (Wallis, 1983).

Stress management has become a multimillion dollar business in this country. Corporation managers have realized increases in production by providing employees with stress reduction programs. Hospitals and clinics have responded to the need for services that offer stress management information to individuals and groups.

When, then, is relaxation therapy required? The answer to this question is largely dependent upon *predisposing factors*, the genetic influences, past experiences, and existing conditions that influence how an individual perceives and responds to stress. For example, temperament, that is, behavioral characteristics that are present at birth, often plays a determining role in the individual's manner of responding to stressful situations. Some individuals, by temperament, naturally respond with a greater degree of anxiety than others.

Past experiences are occurrences that result in learned patterns that can influence an individual's adaptation response. They include previous exposure to the stressor or other stressors, learned coping responses, and degree of adaptation to previous stressors.

Existing conditions are the individual vulnerabilities that can influence the adequacy of the physical, psychological, and social resources for dealing with stressful situations. Examples include current health status, motivation, developmental maturity, severity and duration of the stressor, financial and educational resources, age, existing coping strategies, and a support system of caring others.

All individuals react to stress with predictable physiological and psychosocial responses. These predisposing factors determine the degree of severity of the response. Undoubtedly, there are very few people who would not benefit from some form of relaxation therapy. Homes and Rahe (1967) developed the Social Readjustment Rating Scale, which correlated an individual's susceptibility to physical or psychological illness with his or her level of stress (see Chapter 1). The lay literature now provides various self-tests that individuals may perform to determine one's vulnerability to stress. Two of these are presented in Tables 10.1 and 10.2.

PHYSIOLOGICAL, COGNITIVE, AND BEHAVIORAL MANIFESTATIONS OF RELAXATION

The physiological and behavioral manifestations of stress are well documented (see Chapters 1 and 2). A review of these symptoms is presented in Table 10.3. The persistence of these symptoms over long periods can contribute to the development of numerous stress-related illnesses.

Table 10.1 HOW VULNERABLE ARE YOU TO STRESS?

Score each item from 1 (almost always) to 5 (never), according to how much of the time each statement applies to you.

_____ 1. I eat at least one hot, balanced meal a day.

_____ 2. I get 7 to 8 hours sleep at least four nights a week.

_____ 3. I give and receive affection regularly.

_____ 4. I have at least one relative within 50 miles on whom I can rely.

_____ 5. I exercise to the point of perspiration at least twice a week.

_____ 6. I smoke less than half a pack of cigarettes a day.

_____ 7. I take fewer than five alcoholic drinks a week.

_____ 8. I am the appropriate weight for my height.

_____ 9. I have an income adequate to meet basic expenses.

_____ 10. I get strength from my religious beliefs.

_____ 11. I regularly attend club or social activities.

_____ 12. I have a network of friends and acquaintances.

_____ 13. I have one or more friends to confide in about personal matters.

_____ 14. I am in good health (including eyesight, hearing, and teeth).

_____ 15. I am able to speak openly about my feelings when angry or worried.

_____ 16. I have regular conversations with the people I live with about domestic problems (e.g., chores, money, and daily living issues).

_____ 17. I do something for fun at least once a week.

_____ 18. I am able to organize my time effectively.

_____ 19. I drink fewer than three cups of coffee (or tea or colas) a day.

_____ 20. I take quiet time for myself during the day.

_____ TOTAL

To get your score, add up the figures and subtract 20. Any number over 30 indicates a vulnerability to stress. You are seriously vulnerable if your score is between 50 and 75, and extremely vulnerable if it is over 75.

Source: From Miller and Smith (1983), p. 54.

The achievement of relaxation can counteract many of these symptoms. In a state of deep relaxation, the respiration rate may slow to as few as 4 to 6 breaths per minute and the heart rate to as low as 24 beats per minute (Pelletier, 1977). Blood pressure decreases, and the metabolic rate slows down. Muscle tension diminishes, pupils constrict, and blood vessels in the periphery dilate, leading to increased temperature and a feeling of warmth in the extremities.

One's level of consciousness moves from beta activity, which occurs when one is mentally alert and actively thinking, to alpha activity, a state that falls between full consciousness and unconsciousness (DiMotto, 1984). Benefits associated with achievement of alpha consciousness include an increase in creativity, memory, and the ability to concentrate. Ultimately, an improvement in adaptive functioning may be realized.

When deeply relaxed, individuals are less attentive to distracting stimuli in the external environment. They will respond to questions directed at them but do not initiate verbal interaction. Physical demeanor is very composed. Virtually no muscle activity is observed. Eyes are closed, jaws may be slightly parted, palms are open with fingers curled but not clenched. Head may be slightly tilted to the side.

A summary of the physiological, cognitive, and behavioral manifestations of relaxation is presented in Table 10.4.

METHODS OF ACHIEVING RELAXATION

Deep-Breathing Exercises

Deep breathing is a simple technique that is basic to most other relaxation skills. Tension is released when the lungs are allowed to breathe in as much oxygen as possible (Krames Communications, 1985). Breathing exercises have been found to be effective in reducing anxiety, depression, irritability, muscular tension, and fatigue (Davis, Eshelman, & McKay, 1982). An advantage of this exercise is that it may be accomplished anywhere and at any time. A good guideline is to practice deep breathing for a few minutes three or four times a day or whenever a feeling of tenseness occurs.

TECHNIQUE

1. Sit, stand, or lie in a comfortable position, ensuring that spine is straight.
2. Place one hand on your abdomen and the other on your chest.
3. Inhale slowly and deeply through the nose.

Table 10.2　ARE YOU "STRESSED OUT?"

Check yes or no for each of the following questions.

	Yes	No
1. Do you have recurrent headaches, neck tension, or back pain?	___	___
2. Do you often have indigestion, nausea, or diarrhea?	___	___
3. Have you unintentionally gained or lost 5–10 lb in the last month?	___	___
4. Do you have difficulty falling or staying asleep?	___	___
5. Do you often feel restless?	___	___
6. Do you have difficulty concentrating?	___	___
7. Do you drink alcohol, smoke, or take drugs to relax?	___	___
8. Have you had a major illness, surgery, or an accident in the past year?	___	___
9. Have you lost 5 or more days of work due to illness in the past 6 months?	___	___
10. Have you had a change in job status in the past 6 months? (been fired, laid off, promoted, demoted, etc.)	___	___
11. Do you work more than 48 hours a week?	___	___
12. Do you have serious financial problems?	___	___
13. Have you recently experienced family or marital problems?	___	___
14. Has a person of significance in your life died in the past year?	___	___
15. Have you been divorced or separated in the past year?	___	___
16. Do you find you've lost interest in hobbies, physical activity, and leisure time?	___	___
17. Have you lost interest in your relationship with your spouse, relative, or friend?	___	___
18. Do you find yourself watching more TV than you should?	___	___
19. Are you emotional or easily irritated lately?	___	___
20. Do you seem to experience more distress and discomfort than most people?	___	___

Scoring:

Each yes is worth 1 point; each no is worth 0.

Total your points: _____

0–3 = mildly stressed

4–6 = moderately stressed

7 or more = extremely vulnerable. You may be at risk for stress-related illness.

Source: From the Department of Psychiatry, St. Joseph Medical Center, Wichita, KS. Printed in *The Wichita Eagle*, November 10, 1990.

Table 10.3　PHYSIOLOGICAL, COGNITIVE, AND BEHAVIORAL MANIFESTATIONS OF STRESS

Physiological	Cognitive	Behavioral
Epinephrine and norepinephrine are released into the bloodstream	Anxiety increases	Restlessness
Pupil dilates	Confusion and disorientation may be evident	Irritability
Respiration rate increases	Inability to problem solve	Use or misuse of defense mechanisms
Heart rate increases	Unable to concentrate	Routine functioning may be disorganized
Blood pressure increases	Cognitive processes focus on achieving relief from anxiety	Insomnia and anorexia
Digestion subsides	Learning is inhibited	Compulsive or bizarre behaviors (depending on level of anxiety being experienced)
Blood sugar increases	Thoughts may reflect obsessions and ruminations	
Metabolism increases		
Serum-free fatty acids, cholesterol, and triglycerides increase		

Table 10.4 PHYSIOLOGICAL, COGNITIVE, AND BEHAVIORAL MANIFESTATIONS OF RELAXATION

Physiological	Cognitive	Behavioral
Lower levels of epinephrine and norepinephrine in the blood	Change from beta consciousness to alpha consciousness	Distractability to environmental stimuli is decreased
Respiration rate decreases (sometimes as low as 4–6 breaths per minute)	Creativity and memory are enhanced	Will respond to questions but does not initiate verbal interaction
Heart rate decreases (sometimes as low as 24 beats per minute)	Increased ability to concentrate	Calm, tranquil demeaner. No evidence of restlessness.
Blood pressure decreases		Common mannerisms include eyes closed, jaws parted, palms open, fingers curled, and head slightly tilted to the side.
Metabolic rate slows down		
Muscle tension diminishes		
Pupils constrict		
Vasodilation and increased temperature in the extremities		

The abdomen should be expanding and pushing up on your hand. The chest should be moving only slightly.

4. When you have breathed in as much as possible, hold your breath for a few seconds before exhaling.
5. Begin exhaling slowly through the mouth, pursing your lips as if you were going to whistle. Pursing the lips helps to control how fast you exhale and keeps airways open as long as possible.
6. Feel the abdomen deflate as the lungs are emptied of air.
7. Begin the inhale-exhale cycle again. Focus on the sound and feeling of your breathing as you become more and more relaxed.
8. Continue the deep-breathing exercises for 5 to 10 minutes at a time. Once mastery has been achieved, the technique may be employed as often as is required to relieve tension.

Progressive Relaxation

This method of deep-muscle relaxation was developed in 1929 by Chicago physician Edmond Jacobson. His technique is based on the premise that the body responds to anxiety-provoking thoughts and events with muscle tension. Excellent results have been observed with this method in the treatment of muscular tension, anxiety, insomnia, depression, fatigue, irritable bowel, muscle spasms,

neck and back pain, high blood pressure, mild phobias, and stuttering (Davis et al., 1982).

TECHNIQUE

Each muscle group is tensed for 5 to 7 seconds and then relaxed for 20 to 30 seconds, during which time the individual concentrates on the difference in sensations between the two conditions. Soft, slow background music may facilitate relaxation.

1. Sit in a comfortable chair with hands in lap and feet flat on floor, eyes closed.
2. Begin by taking three deep, slow breaths, inhaling through the nose and releasing the air slowly through the mouth.
3. Now starting with the feet, pull the toes forward toward the knees, stiffen your calves, and hold for a count of 5.
4. Now release the hold. Let go of the tension. Feel the sensation of relaxation and warmth as the tension flows out of the muscles.
5. Next, tense the muscles of the thighs and buttocks. Hold for a count of 5.
6. Now release the hold. Feel the tension drain away, and be aware of the difference in sensation—perhaps a heaviness or feeling of warmth that you did not feel when the muscles were tensed. Concentrate on this feeling for a few seconds.
7. Next, tense the abdominal muscles. Hold for a count of 5.

8. Now release the hold. Concentrate on the feeling of relaxation in the muscles. You may feel a warming sensation. Hold on to the feeling for 15 or 20 seconds.

9. Next, tense the muscles in the back. Hold for a count of 5.

10. Now release the hold. Feel the sensation of relaxation and warmth as the tension flows out of the muscles.

11. Next, tense the muscles of the hands, biceps, and forearms. Clench the hands into a tight fist. Hold for a count of 5.

12. Now release the hold. Notice the sensations. You may feel tingling, warmth, or a light, airy feeling. Recognize these sensations as tension leaves the muscles.

13. Next, tense the muscles of the shoulders and neck. Shrug the shoulders tightly and hold for a count of 5.

14. Now release the hold. Sense the tension as it leaves the muscles and experience the feeling of relaxation.

15. Next, tense the muscles of the face. Wrinkle the forehead. Frown, squint the eyes, and purse the lips. Hold for a count of 5.

16. Now release the hold. Recognize a light, warm feeling flowing into the muscles.

17. Now feel the relaxation in your whole body. Feel the tenseness leave your entire being, and you feel completely relaxed.

18. Open your eyes and enjoy renewed energy.

Modified (or Passive) Progressive Relaxation

TECHNIQUE

In this version of total-body relaxation, the muscles are not tensed. The individual learns to relax muscles by concentrating on the feeling of relaxation within the muscle. These instructions may be presented by one person for another or they may be self-administered. Relaxation may be facilitated by playing soft, slow background music during the activity.

1. Assume a comfortable position. Some suggestions include:
   a. Sitting straight up in a chair with hands in lap or at sides and feet flat on floor
   b. Sitting in a reclining chair with hands in lap or at sides and legs up on elevated foot of chair
   c. Lying flat with head slightly elevated on pillow, arms at sides

2. Close your eyes and take three deep breaths through your nose, slowly releasing the air through your mouth.

3. Allow a feeling of peacefulness to descend over you — a pleasant, enjoyable sensation of being comfortable and at ease.

4. Remain in this state for several minutes.

5. It is now time to turn your attention to various parts of your body.

6. We will begin with the muscles of the head, face, throat, and shoulders. Concentrate on these muscles. Pay particular attention to those in the forehead and jaws. Feel the tension leave the area. The muscles start to feel relaxed, heavy, and warm. Concentrate on this feeling for a few minutes.

7. Now let the feeling of relaxation continue to spread downward to the muscles of your biceps, forearms, and hands. Concentrate on these muscles. Feel the tension dissolve away. The muscles start to feel relaxed and heavy. A feeling of warmth spreads through these muscles all the way to the fingertips. They are feeling very warm and very heavy. Concentrate on this feeling for a few minutes.

8. The tension is continuing to dissolve now, and you are feeling very relaxed. Turn your attention to the muscles in your chest, abdomen, and lower back. Feel the tension leave these areas. Allow these muscles to become very relaxed. They start to feel very warm, very heavy. Concentrate on this feeling for a few minutes.

9. The feeling of relaxation continues to move downward now as we move to the muscles of the thighs, buttocks, calves, and feet. Feel the tension moving down and out of the body. These muscles feel very relaxed now. The legs are feeling very heavy, very limp. A feeling of warmth spreads over the area, all the way to the toes. You can feel that all the tension has been released.

10. Your whole body feels relaxed and warm. Listen to the music for a few moments and concentrate on this relaxed, warm feeling. Take several deep, slow breaths through your nose, releasing the air through your mouth. Continue

to concentrate on how relaxed and warm you feel.

11. It is now time to refocus your concentration back to the present and wake up your body to resume activity. Open your eyes and stretch or massage your muscles. Wiggle your fingers and toes. Take another deep breath, arise, and enjoy the feeling of renewed energy.

Meditation

Records and phenomenological accounts of meditative practices date back more than 2,000 years, but only recently have empirical studies revealed the psychophysiological benefits of regular use (Pelletier, 1977). The goal of meditation is to gain "mastery over attention." It brings on a special state of consciousness as attention is concentrated solely on one thought or object.

Historically, meditation has been associated with religious doctrines and disciplines by which individuals sought enlightenment with God or another higher power. However, meditation can be practiced independently from any religious philosophy and purely as a means of achieving inner harmony and increasing self-awareness.

During meditation, the respiration rate, heart rate, and blood pressure decrease. The overall metabolism declines, and the need for oxygen consumption is reduced. Alpha brain waves, those associated with brain activity during periods of deep relaxation, predominate (Pelletier, 1977).

Meditation has been used successfully in the prevention and treatment of various cardiovascular diseases. It has proved helpful in curtailing obsessive thinking, anxiety, depression, and hostility. Meditation improves concentration and attention (Davis et al., 1982).

TECHNIQUE

1. Select a quiet place and a comfortable position. Various sitting positions are appropriate for meditation. Examples include:
   a. In a chair with feet flat on floor approximately 6 inches apart, arms resting comfortably in lap.
   b. Cross-legged on the floor or on a cushion.
   c. In the Japanese fashion with knees on floor, great toes together, pointed backward, and buttocks resting comfortably on bottom of feet.
   d. In the yoga lotus position on the floor with legs flexed at knees. Ankles are crossed and each foot rests on the top of the opposite thigh.

2. Select an object, word, or thought on which to dwell. During meditation, the individual becomes preoccupied with the selected focus. This total preoccupation serves to prevent distractions from interrupting attention. Examples of foci include:
   a. Counting one's breaths. All attention is focused on breathing in and out.
   b. Mantras. A *mantra* is a syllable, word, or name that is repeated many times as you free your mind of thoughts. Any mantra is appropriate if it works to focus attention and prevent distracting thoughts.
   c. Objects for contemplation. Select an object, such as a rock, a marble, or anything that does not hold a symbolic meaning that might cause distraction. Contemplate the object both visually and tactiley. Focus total attention on the object.
   d. A thought that has special meaning to you. With eyes closed, focus total attention on a specific thought or idea.

3. Practice directing attention on your selected focus for 10 to 15 minutes a day for several weeks. It is essential that the individual does not become upset if intrusive thoughts find their way into the meditation practice. They should merely be dealt with and dismissed as the individual returns to the selected focus of attention. Worrying about one's progress in the ability to meditate is a self-inhibiting behavior.

Mental Imagery

This method of relaxation employs the imagination in an effort to reduce the body's response to stress. The frame of reference is very personal, based upon what each individual considers to be a relaxing environment. Some might select a scene at the seashore, some a mountain atmosphere, and some might choose floating through the air on a fluffy, white cloud. The choices are as limitless as one's imagination. Following is an example of how one individual uses imagery for relaxation. The information is most useful when taped and played back at a time when the individual wishes to achieve relaxation.

TECHNIQUE

Sit or lie down in a comfortable position. Close your eyes. Imagine that you and someone you love are walking along the seashore. Not one other person is in sight in any direction. The sun is shining; the sky is blue; and a gentle breeze is blowing. You select a spot to stop and rest. You lie on the sand and close your eyes. You hear the sound of the waves as they splash against the shore. The sun feels warm on your face and body. The sand feels soft and warm against your back. An occasional wave splashes you with a cool mist that dries rapidly in the warm sun. The coconut fragrance of your suntan lotion wafts gently and pleasantly in the air. You lie in this quiet place for what seems like a very long time, taking in the sounds of the waves, the warmth of the sun, and the cooling sensations of the mist and ocean breeze. It is very quiet. It is very warm. You feel very relaxed, very contented. This is your special place. You may come to this special place whenever you want to relax.

Biofeedback

Biofeedback is the use of instrumentation to become aware of processes in your body that you usually do not notice and to help bring them under voluntary control. Biofeedback machines give immediate information about an individual's own biological conditions, such as muscle tension, skin surface temperature, brain-wave activity, skin conductivity, blood pressure, and heart rate (Davis et al., 1982). Some conditions that can be treated successfully with biofeedback include spastic colon, hypertension, tension and migraine headaches, muscle spasms/pain, anxiety, phobias, stuttering, and teeth grinding.

TECHNIQUE

Biological conditions are monitored by the biofeedback equipment. Sensors relate muscle spasticity, body temperature, brain-wave activity, heart rate, and blood pressure. Each of these conditions will elicit a signal from the equipment, such as a blinking light, a measure on a meter, or an audible tone. The individual practices using relaxation and voluntary control to modify the signal, in turn indicating a modification of the autonomic function it represents.

Various types of biofeedback equipment have been developed in recent years for home use. However, they have not proved very effective, as they generally only measure one autonomic function when, in fact, modification of several functions may be required to achieve the benefits of total relaxation.

Biofeedback can provide assistance in monitoring the progress an individual is making toward learning to relax. It is often used together with other relaxation techniques, such as deep breathing, progressive relaxation, and mental imagery.

Special training is required to become a biofeedback practitioner. Nurses can offer support and encouragement to individuals learning to use this method of stress management. Nurses can also teach other techniques of relaxation that enhance the results of biofeedback training.

Physical Exercise

Regular exercise is viewed by many as one of the most effective methods for relieving stress. Physical exertion provides a natural outlet for the tension produced by the body in its state of arousal for "fight or flight." Following exercise, physiological equilibrium is restored, resulting in a feeling of relaxation and revitalization. A sedentary life-style and physical inactivity are thought to be major contributors to coronary heart disease, obesity, joint and spinal disk disease, fatigue, muscular tension, and depression (Davis et al., 1982).

Aerobic exercises strengthen the cardiovascular system and increase the body's ability to use oxygen more efficiently. Aerobic exercises include brisk walking, jogging, running, cycling, swimming, and dancing, among other activities. To achieve the benefits of aerobic exercises, they must be performed on a regular basis — for at least 30 minutes, three times per week.

Individuals can also benefit from low-intensity physical exercise. Although there is little benefit to the cardiovascular system, low-intensity exercise can help prevent obesity, relieve muscular tension, prevent muscle spasms, and increase flexibility.

Examples of low-intensity exercise include slow walking, house cleaning, shopping, light gardening, calisthenics, and weight lifting.

Studies indicate that physical exercise can be effective in reducing general anxiety and depression. Fifteen to twenty minutes of vigorous exercise has been shown to stimulate the secretion of both norepinephrine and serotonin into the brain and the release of endorphins into the blood (Davis et al., 1982). Depressed people are often deficient in norepinephrine and serotonin. Endorphins act as natural narcotics and mood elevators.

THE ROLE OF THE NURSE IN RELAXATION THERAPY

Nurses work with anxious patients in all departments of the hospital and in community and home health services. Individuals experience stress on a daily basis. It cannot be eliminated. Management of stress must be considered a lifelong function. Nurses can help individuals recognize the sources of stress in their lives and identify methods of adaptive coping.

Assessment

Stress management requires a holistic approach. Physical and psychosocial dimensions are considered in determining the individual's adaptation to stress. Following are some examples of assessment data for collection. Other assessments may need to be made, depending on the specific circumstances of each individual.

1. *Genetic Influences*
   a. Identify medical/psychiatric history of patient and biological family members.
2. *Past Experiences*
   a. Describe your living/working conditions.
   b. When did you last have a physical examination?
   c. Do you have a spiritual or religious position from which you derive support?
   d. Do you have a job? Have you experienced any recent employment changes or other difficulties on your job?
   e. What significant changes have occurred in your life in the last year?

f. What is your usual way of coping with stress?
   g. Do you have someone to whom you can go for support when you feel stressed?
3. *Patient's Perception of the Stressor*
   a. What do you feel is the major source of stress in your life right now?
4. *Adaptation Responses*
   a. Do you ever feel anxious? Confused? Unable to concentrate? Fearful?
   b. Do you have tremors? Stutter or stammer? Sweat profusely?
   c. Do you often feel angry? Irritable? Moody?
   d. Do you ever feel depressed? Do you ever feel like harming yourself or others?
   e. Do you have difficulty communicating with others?
   f. Do you experience pain? What part of your body? When do you experience it? When does it worsen?
   g. Do you ever experience stomach upset? Constipation? Diarrhea? Nausea and vomiting?
   h. Do you ever feel your heart pounding in your chest?
   i. Do you take any drugs (either prescription or street)?
   j. Do you drink alcohol? Smoke cigarettes? How much?
   k. Are you eating (more) (less) than usual?
   l. Do you have difficulty sleeping?
   m. Do you have a significant other? Describe the relationship.
   n. Describe your relationship with other family members.
   o. Do you perceive any problems in your sexual life-style or behavior?

Analysis

Possible nursing diagnoses for individuals requiring assistance with stress management are listed here. Others may be appropriate for individuals with other particular problems.

1. Adjustment, impaired
2. Anxiety (specify level)
3. Body image disturbance
4. Coping, defensive
5. Coping, ineffective, individual
6. Decisional conflict (specify)
7. Denial, ineffective

8. Fear
9. Grieving, anticipatory
10. Hopelessness
11. Knowledge deficit (specify)
12. Pain (acute or chronic)
13. Parental role conflict
14. Post-trauma response
15. Powerlessness
16. Rape-trauma syndrome
17. Role performance, altered
18. Self-esteem, disturbance
19. Sexual dysfunction
20. Sexuality patterns, altered
21. Grieving, dysfunctional
22. Sleep pattern disturbance
23. Social isolation
24. Social interaction, impaired
25. Spiritual distress
26. Violence, high risk for, directed at self/others

Implementation/Evaluation

The immediate goal for nurses working with individuals needing assistance with stress management is to help minimize current maladaptive symptoms. The long-term goal is to assist individuals toward achievement of their highest potential for wellness. Implementation of nursing actions has a strong focus on the role of patient teacher. Relaxation therapy, as described in this chapter, is one method for assisting individuals in the management of stress. These techniques are well within the scope of nursing practice.

Evaluation requires that the nurse and patient assess whether or not these techniques are achieving the desired outcomes. Various alternatives may be attempted. Life-style changes may be required. Examples of outcome criteria may include:

1. Patient will verbalize a reduction in pain following progressive relaxation techniques.
2. Patient will be able to voluntarily control a decrease in blood pressure following 3 weeks of biofeedback training.
3. Patient will be able to maintain stress at a manageable level by performing deep-breathing exercises when feeling anxious.

Relaxation therapy provides alternatives to old, maladaptive methods of coping with stress. Change does not come easily. Nurses must help individuals analyze the usefulness of these techniques in the management of stress in their daily lives.

SUMMARY

Stress is a part of our everyday lives. It can be positive or negative, but it cannot be eliminated. Keeping stress at a manageable level is a lifelong process.

Individuals under stress respond with a physiological arousal that can be dangerous over long periods. Indeed, the stress response has been shown to be a major contributor, either directly or indirectly, to coronary heart disease, cancer, lung ailments, accidental injuries, cirrhosis of the liver, and suicide — six of the leading causes of death in the United States.

Relaxation therapy is an effective means of reducing the stress response in some individuals. The degree of anxiety that an individual experiences in response to stress is related to certain predisposing factors, such as characteristics of temperament with which he or she was born, past experiences resulting in learned patterns of responding, and existing conditions, such as health status, coping strategies, and adequate support systems.

Deep relaxation can counteract the physiological and behavioral manifestations of stress. Various methods of relaxation therapy were presented: deep-breathing exercises, progressive relaxation, passive progressive relaxation, meditation, mental imagery, biofeedback, and physical exercise.

Nurses use the nursing process in assisting individuals in the management of stress. Assessment data are collected, from which nursing diagnoses are derived. Goals are established to help individuals reduce current maladaptive symptoms and to ultimately achieve their highest potential for wellness. Implementation includes instructing patients and their families in the various techniques for achieving relaxation. Behavioral changes provide outcome criteria for evaluation.

REVIEW QUESTIONS
Self-Examination/Learning Exercise

1. **Learning exercise:**

   Practice some of the relaxation exercises presented in this chapter. It may be helpful to tape some of the exercises with soft music in the background. These tapes may be used with anxious patients or during times when you are feeling anxious yourself.

2. **Clinical activity:**

   Teach a relaxation exercise to a patient. Practice it together. Evaluate the patient's ability to achieve relaxation by performing the exercise.

3. **Case study:**

   Linda has just been admitted to the psychiatric unit. She was experiencing attacks of severe anxiety. Linda has worked in the typing pool of a large corporation for 10 years. She was recently promoted to private secretary for one of the executives. Some of her new duties include attending the board meetings and taking minutes, screening all calls and visitors for her boss, keeping track of his schedule, reminding him of important appointments, and making decisions for him in his absence. Linda felt comfortable in her old position but has become increasingly fearful of making errors and incorrect decisions in her new job. Even though she is proud to have been selected for this position, she is constantly "nervous," has lost 10 pounds in 3 weeks, is having difficulty sleeping, and is having a recurrance of the severe migraine headaches she experienced as a teenager. She is often irritable with her husband and children for no apparent reason.

   a. Identify some possible nursing diagnoses for Linda.
   b. Describe some relaxation techniques that may be helpful for her.
   c. Define outcome criteria for Linda.

REFERENCES

Davis M. D., Eshelman, E. R., & McKay, M. (1982). *The relaxation and stress reduction workbook* (2nd ed.). Oakland, CA: New Harbinger Publications.

DiMotto, J. W. (1984, June). Relaxation. *Am J Nurs*, pp. 754–758.

Homes and Rahe (1967). The social readjustment scale. J Psychosom Res 11:213–218.

Krames Communications. (1985). *A guide to managing stress.* Daly City, CA: Krames Communications.

Miller, L. H. & Smith, A. D. (1983, June 6). How vulnerable are you to stress? *Time*, p. 54.

Pelletier, K. R. (1977). *Mind as healer, mind as slayer.* New York: Dell Publishing Co.

Wallis, C. (1983, June 6). Stress: Can we cope? *Time*, pp. 48–54.

BIBLIOGRAPHY

Bakal, D. A. (1979). *Psychology and medicine.* New York: Springer Publishing Company.

Bernstein, D. A. & Borkovec, T. D. (1973). *Progressive relaxation training: A manual for the helping professions.* Champaign, IL: Research Press.

Everly, G. S., Jr. (1989). *A clinical guide to the treatment of the human stress response*. New York: Plenum Press.

Leepson, M. (1984). *The alive and well stress book*. New York: Bantam Books.

Maier, S. F. & Laudenslager, M. (1985 August). Stress and health: Exploring the links. *Psychology Today*, pp. 44–49.

McGuigan, F. J., Sime, W. E., & Wallace, J. M. (1989). *Stress and tension control*. New York: Plenum Press.

Rachman, S. J. & Philips, C. (1980). *Psychology and behavioral medicine*. Cambridge, England: Cambridge University Press.

Rosenbaum, L. (1989). *Biofeedback frontiers*. New York: AMS Press.

Selye, H. *Stress without distress*. (1974). New York: The New American Library, Inc.

Sethi, A. S. (1989). *Meditation as an intervention in stress reactivity*. New York: AMS Press.

Smith, J. C. (1990). *Cognitive-behavioral relaxation training*. New York: Springer Publishing.

Sutherland, V. J. & Cooper, C. L. (1990). *Understanding stress: A psychological perspective for health professionals*. London: Chapman and Hall.

11

ASSERTIVENESS TRAINING

KEY TERMS
nonassertiveness
assertiveness
aggressiveness
passive-aggressiveness
thought stopping

OBJECTIVES

After reading this chapter, the student will be able to:
1. Define *assertive behavior.*
2. Discuss basic human rights.
3. Differentiate between nonassertive, assertive, aggressive, and passive-aggressive behaviors.
4. Describe techniques that promote assertive behavior.
5. Demonstrate thought-stopping techniques.
6. Discuss the role of the nurse in assertiveness training.

ASSERTIVE COMMUNICATION

Alberti and Emmons (1990) have defined assertive behavior as "behavior that enables individuals to act in their own best interests, to stand up for themselves without undue anxiety, to express their honest feelings comfortably, or to exercise their own rights without denying the rights of others."

Assertive behavior helps us feel good about ourselves and increases our self-esteem. It helps us feel good about other people and increases our ability to develop satisfying relationships with others. This is accomplished out of honesty, directness, appropriateness, and respecting one's own basic rights as well as the rights of others (Jakubowski & Lange, 1978).

Honesty is basic to assertive behavior. Assertive honesty is not an outspoken declaration of everything that is on one's mind. It is instead an accurate representation of feelings, opinions, or preferences expressed in a manner that promotes self-respect and respect for others.

Directness implies stating what one wants to convey with clarity and candor. Hinting and "beating around the bush" are indirect forms of communication.

Communication must occur in an appropriate context to be considered assertive. The location and timing, as well as the manner (tone of voice, nonverbal gestures) in which the communication is presented, must be correct for the situation.

BASIC HUMAN RIGHTS

A number of authors have identified a variety of "assertive rights" (Baer, 1976; Bloom, Coburn, & Peralman, 1975; Davis, McKay, & Eshelman, 1982; Jakubowski & Lange, 1978; Kelly, 1979; Powell & Enright, 1990; Smith, 1975). Many of these rights have been identified by participants in assertiveness training groups. Following is a composite of ten basic assertive human rights adapted from the aggregation of sources.

1. The right to be treated with respect.
2. The right to express feelings, opinions, and beliefs.
3. The right to say "no" without feeling guilty.
4. The right to make mistakes and accept the responsibility for them.
5. The right to be listened to and taken seriously.
6. The right to change one's mind.
7. The right to ask for what you want.
8. The right to put yourself first, sometimes.
9. The right to set one's own priorities.
10. The right to refuse justification for one's feelings or behavior.

In accepting these rights, an individual also accepts the responsibilities that accompany them. Rights and responsibilities are reciprocal entities. To experience one without the other is inherently destructive to an individual. Some responsibilities associated with basic assertive human rights are presented in Table 11.1

RESPONSE PATTERNS

Kelly (1979) identified six ways in which individuals develop patterns of responding to others. They include:

1. By watching other people (role modeling).
2. By being positively reinforced or punished for a certain response.
3. By inventing a response.
4. By not thinking of a better way to respond.
5. By not developing the proper skills for a better response.
6. By consciously choosing a response style.

The nurse should be able to recognize his or her own pattern of responding as well as that of others. Four response patterns will be discussed here: nonassertive, assertive, aggressive, and passive-aggressive.

Nonassertive Behavior

Individuals who are nonassertive (sometimes called *passive*) seek to please others at the expense of denying their own basic human rights. They seldom let their true feelings show and often feel hurt and anxious since they allow others to choose for them. They seldom achieve their own desired goals (Alberti & Emmons, 1990). They come across as being very apologetic and tend to be self-deprecat-

Table 11.1 ASSERTIVE RIGHTS AND RESPONSIBILITIES

Rights	Responsibilities
1. To be treated with respect	To treat others in a way that recognizes their human dignity
2. To express feelings, opinions, and beliefs	To accept ownership of our feelings and show respect for those that differ from our own
3. To say "no"	To analyze each situation individually, recognizing all human rights as equal (others have the right to say "no," too)
4. To make mistakes	To accept responsibility for own mistakes and to try to correct them
5. To be listened to	To listen to others
6. To change one's mind	To accept the possible consequences that the change may incur; to accept the same flexibility in others
7. To ask for what you want	To accept others' right to refuse your request
8. To put yourself first, sometimes	To put others first, sometimes
9. To set one's own priorities	To consider one's limitations as well as strengths in directing independent activities; to be a dependable person
10. To refuse to justify feelings or behavior	To accept ownership of own feelings/behavior; to accept others without requiring justification for their feelings/behavior

ing. They use actions instead of words and hope someone will "guess" what they want. Their voices are hesitant, weak, and expressed in a monotone. Eyes are generally downcast. They feel uncomfortable in interpersonal interactions. All they want is to please and to be liked by others. Their behavior helps them avoid unpleasant situations and confrontations with others. However, they often harbor anger and resentment.

Assertive Behavior

Assertive individuals stand up for their own rights while protecting the rights of others. Feelings are expressed openly and honestly. They assume responsibility for their own choices and allow others to choose for themselves. They maintain self-respect and respect for others by treating everyone equally and with human dignity. They communicate tactfully, using lots of "I" statements. Their voices are warm and expressive, and eye contact is intermittent but direct. These individuals desire to communicate effectively with, and be respected by, others. They are self-confident and experience satisfactory and pleasurable relationships with others.

Aggressive Behavior

Individuals who are aggressive defend their own basic rights by violating the basic rights of others. Feelings are often expressed dishonestly and inappropriately. They say what is on their mind, often at the expense of others. Aggressive behavior commonly results in a *putdown* of the receiver. Rights denied, the receiver feels hurt, defensive, and humiliated (Alberti & Emmons, 1990). Aggressive individuals devalue the self-worth of others upon whom they impose their choices. They express an air of superiority, and their voices are often loud, demanding, angry, or cold, without emotion. Eye contact may be "to intimidate others by staring them down." They want to increase their feeling of power by dominating or humiliating others. Aggressive behavior hinders interpersonal relationships.

Passive-Aggressive Behavior

Passive-aggressive individuals defend their own rights by expressing resistance to social and occupational demands (American Psychiatric Association, 1987). Sometimes called *indirect aggression*, this behavior takes the form of passive, nonconfrontative action (Alberti & Emmons, 1990). These individuals are devious, manipulative, sly, and they undermine others with behavior that expresses the opposite of what they are feeling. They are highly critical and sarcastic. They allow others to make choices for them, then resist by using passive behaviors, such as procrastination, dawdling, stubbornness, and "forgetfulness." They use actions instead of words to convey their message, and the actions express covert aggression. They become sulky, irritable, or argumentative when asked to do something they do not want to do. They may protest to others about the demands but will not confront the person who is making the demands. Instead, they may deal with the demand by "forgetting" to do it. The goal is domination through retaliation. This behavior offers a feeling of control and power, although they actually feel resentment and as though they are being taken advantage of. They possess extremely low self-confidence.

A comparison of these four behavior patterns is presented in Table 11.2.

BEHAVIORAL COMPONENTS OF ASSERTIVE BEHAVIOR

Alberti & Emmons (1990) have identified several defining characteristics of assertive behavior. They include:

1. *Eye contact.* Eye contact is considered appro-

Table 11.2 COMPARISON OF BEHAVIORAL RESPONSE PATTERNS

	Nonassertive	Assertive	Aggressive	Passive-Aggressive
Behavioral characteristics	Passive, does not express true feelings, self-deprecating, denies own rights	Stands up for own rights, protects rights of others, honest, direct, appropriate	Violates rights of others, expresses feelings dishonestly and inappropriately	Defends own rights with passive resistance, is critical and sarcastic; often expresses opposite of true feelings
Examples	"Uh, well, uh, sure, I'll be glad to stay and work an extra shift."	"I don't want to stay and work an extra shift today. Perhaps I will next time someone is needed."	"You've got to be kidding!"	"Okay, I'll stay and work an extra shift." (Then to peer: "How dare she ask us to work over! Well, we'll just see how much work she gets out of me!)
Goals	To please others; to be liked by others	To communicate effectively; to be respected by others	To dominate or humiliate others	To dominate through retaliation
Feelings	Anxious, hurt, disappointed with self, angry, resentful	Confident, successful, proud, self-respecting	Self-righteous, controlling, superior	Anger, resentment, manipulated, controlled
Compensation	Is able to avoid unpleasant situations and confrontations with others	Increased self-confidence, self-respect, respect for others, satisfying interpersonal relationships	Anger is released, increasing feeling of power and superiority	Feels self-righteous and in control
Outcomes	Goals not met; others meet *their* goals at nonassertive person's expense; anger and resentment grow; feels violated and manipulated	Goals met; desires most often fulfilled while defending own rights as well as rights of others	Goals may be met but at the expense of others; they feel hurt and vengeful	Goals not met, nor are the goals of others met due to retaliatory nature of the interaction

Source: Adapted from Jakubowski and Lange (1978), pp. 42–43.

priate when it is intermittent, that is, looking directly at the person to whom one is speaking but looking away now and then. Individuals feel uncomfortable when someone stares at them continuously and intently. Intermittent eye contact conveys the message that one is interested in what is being said.

2. *Body posture*. Sitting and leaning slightly toward the other person in a conversation suggests an active interest in what is being said. Emphasis on an assertive stance can be achieved by standing with an erect posture, squarely facing the other person. A slumped posture conveys passivity or nonassertiveness.

3. *Distance/physical contact*. The distance between two individuals in an interaction or the physical contact between them has a strong cultural influence. For example, in the United States, intimate distance is considered approximately 18 inches from the body. We are very careful about whom we allow to enter this intimate space. Invasion of this space may be interpreted by some individuals as very aggressive.

4. *Gestures*. Nonverbal gestures may also be culturally related. Gesturing can add emphasis, warmth, depth, or power to the spoken word.

5. *Facial expression*. Various facial expressions convey different messages (e.g., frown, smile, surprise, anger, fear). It is difficult to "fake" these messages. In assertive communication, the facial expression is congruent with the verbal message.

6. *Voice*. The voice conveys a message by its loudness, softness, degree and placement of emphasis, and evidence of emotional tone.

7. *Fluency*. Being able to discuss a subject with ease and with obvious knowledge conveys assertiveness and self-confidence. This message is impeded by numerous pauses or filler words such as, "and, uh . . .," or "you know . . ."

8. *Timing*. Assertive responses are most effective when they are spontaneous and immediate. However, most people have experienced times when it was not appropriate to respond (e.g., in front of a group of people) or times when an appropriate response is generated only after the fact ("If only I had said . . ."). Alberti and Emmons state that ". . . it is never too late to be assertive!" It is correct and worthwhile to seek out the individual at a later time and express the assertive response.

9. *Listening*. Assertive listening means giving the other individual full attention, with eye contact, nodding to indicate acceptance of what is being said, and taking time to understand what is being said before giving a response.

10. *Thoughts*. Cognitive processes affect one's assertive behavior. Two of these include: (1) an individual's attitudes about the appropriateness of assertive behavior in general and (2) the appropriateness of assertive behavior for himself or herself specifically.

11. *Content*. Many times individuals do not respond to an unpleasant situation because ". . . I just didn't know what to say." Perhaps *what* is being said is not as important as *how* it is said. Emotions should be expressed when they are experienced. It is also important to accept ownership of those emotions and not devalue the worth of another individual to assert oneself. Examples:

Assertive: "I'm really angry about what you said!"

Aggressive: "You're a real jerk for saying that!"

TECHNIQUES THAT PROMOTE ASSERTIVE BEHAVIOR

Various guidelines have been established as beneficial in the process of becoming an assertive person (Bakdash, 1978; Davis et al., 1982; Smith, 1975). The following techniques have been shown to be effective in responding to criticism and avoiding manipulation by others.

1. **Standing up for one's basic human rights.**

   Example:
   "I have the right to express my opinion."

2. **Assuming responsibility for one's own statements.**

Example:
"I *won't* work the extra shift," instead of "I *can't* work the extra shift." The latter implies a lack of power or ability.

3. **Responding as a "broken record."** Persistently repeating in a calm voice what is wanted.

Example:

Telephone salesperson:	"I want to help you save money by changing long-distance services."
Assertive response:	"I don't want to change my long-distance service."
Telephone salesperson:	"I can't believe you don't want to save money!"
Assertive response:	"I don't want to change my long-distance service."

4. **Agreeing assertively.** Assertively accepting negative aspects about oneself. Admitting when an error has been made.

Example:

Ms. Jones:	"You sure let that meeting get out of hand. What a waste of time."
Ms. Smith:	"Yes, I didn't do a very good job of conducting the meeting today."

5. **Inquiring assertively.** Seeking additional information about critical statements.

Example

Male Board Member:	"You made a real fool of yourself at the board meeting last night."
Female Board Member:	"Of what about my behavior did you not approve?"
Male Board Member:	"You were so damned pushy!"
Female Board Member:	"What is it about my speaking out that bothers you?"

6. **Shifting from content to process.** Changing the focus of the communication from discussing the topic at hand to analyzing what is actually going on in the interaction.

Example:

Wife:	"Would you please call me if you will be late for dinner?"
Husband:	"I've always had to account for every minute of my time with you!"
Wife:	"It seems as though we need to take the time to discuss this anger you are feeling toward me."

7. **Clouding/fogging.** Concurring with the critic's argument without becoming defensive and without agreeing to change.

Example:

Nurse #1:	"You make so many mistakes. I don't know how you ever got this job!"
Nurse #2:	"You're right. I have made some mistakes since I started this job."

8. **Defusing.** Putting off further discussion with an angry individual until he or she is calmer.

Example:
"You are very angry right now. I don't want to discuss this matter with you while you are so upset. I will discuss it with you in my office at 3 o'clock this afternoon."

9. **Delaying assertively.** Putting off further discussion with another individual until one is calmer.

Example:
"That's a very challenging position you have taken, Mr. Brown. I'll need time to give it some thought. I'll call you later this afternoon."

10. **Responding assertively with irony.**

Example:

Man:	"I bet you're one of them so-called 'women's libbers,' aren't you?"
Woman:	"Yes, thank you for noticing."

THOUGHT-STOPPING TECHNIQUES

Assertive thinking is sometimes inhibited by repetitive, negative thoughts of which the mind refuses to let go. Individuals with low self-worth may be obsessed with thoughts such as, "I know he'd never want to go out with me. I'm too ugly (or plain, or fat, or dumb, etc.)," or "I just know I'll never be able to do this job well," or "I just can't seem to do anything right." This type of thinking fosters the belief that one's individual rights are not deserving of the same consideration as those of others and reflects nonassertive communication and behavioral response patterns.

Thought-stopping techniques, as described below, were developed by psychiatrist Joseph Wolpe (1973) and are intended to eliminate intrusive, unwanted thoughts.

Method:

In a practice setting, with eyes closed, concentrate on an unwanted thought that continues to recur. Once the thought is clearly established in the mind, shout aloud: "STOP!" This action will interrupt the thought, and it is actually removed from one's awareness. The individual then immediately shifts his or her thoughts to one that is considered pleasant and desirable.

It is possible that the unwanted thought may soon recur, but with practice, the length of time for recurrence will increase until the unwanted thought is no longer intrusive.

Obviously, one cannot go about his or her daily life shouting "STOP!" in public places. After a number of practice sessions, the technique is equally as effective if the word "stop!" is employed silently in the mind.

THE ROLE OF THE NURSE

It is important for nurses to become aware of and recognize their own behavioral responses. Are they mostly nonassertive? Assertive? Aggressive? Passive-aggressive? Do they consider their behavioral responses effective? Do they wish to change? Remember, all individuals have the right to choose whether or not they want to be assertive.

The ability to respond assertively is especially important to those nurses who are committed to further development of the profession. Assertive skills facilitate the implementation of change—change that is required if the image of nursing is to be upgraded to the level of professionalism that most nurses desire. Assertive communication is useful in the political arena for nurses who choose to become involved at both state and national levels in striving to influence legislation and, ultimately, to improve the system of health care in our country.

Nurses who understand and use assertiveness skills themselves can in turn assist patients who wish to effect behavioral change in an effort to increase self-esteem and improve interpersonal relationships. The nursing process is a useful tool for nurses who are involved in helping patients increase their assertiveness.

Assessment

Nurses can assist patients to become more aware of their behavioral responses. Many tools for assessing level of assertiveness have been attempted over the years. None have been terribly effective. Perhaps this is because it is so difficult to *generalize* when attempting to measure assertive behaviors. Table 11.3 and Figure 11.1 represent examples of assertiveness inventories that could be personalized to describe life situations of individual patients more specifically. Obviously, "everyday situations that may require assertiveness" are not the same for all individuals.

Analysis

Possible nursing diagnoses for individuals needing assistance with assertiveness include:

1. Coping, defensive
2. Coping, ineffective, individual
3. Decisional conflict (specify)
4. Denial, ineffective
5. Personal identity disturbance
6. Powerlessness
7. Rape-trauma syndrome
8. Self-esteem, disturbance
9. Social interaction, impaired
10. Social isolation

Table 11.3 EVERYDAY SITUATIONS THAT MAY REQUIRE ASSERTIVENESS

At Work

How do you respond when:

1. You receive a compliment on your appearance or someone praises your work?
2. You are criticized unfairly?
3. You are criticized legitimately by a superior?
4. You have to confront a subordinate for continual lateness or sloppy work?
5. Your boss makes a sexual innuendo or makes a pass at you?

In Public

How do you respond when:

1. In a restaurant, the food you ordered arrives cold or overcooked?
2. A fellow passenger in a no-smoking compartment lights a cigarette?
3. You are faced with an unhelpful shop assistant?
4. Somebody barges in front of you in a waiting line?
5. You take an inferior article back to a shop?

Among Friends

How do you respond when:

1. You feel angry with the way a friend has treated you?
2. A friend makes what you consider to be an unreasonable request?
3. You want to ask a friend for a favor?
4. You ask a friend for repayment of a loan of money?
5. You have to negotiate with a friend on which film to see or where to meet?

At Home

How do you respond when:

1. One of your parents criticizes you?
2. You are irritated by a persistant habit in someone you love?
3. Everybody leaves the cleaning-up chores to you?
4. You want to say "no" to a proposed visit to a relative?
5. Your partner feels amorous but you are not in the mood?

Source: From Powell and Enright (1990), with permission.

Planning/Implementation

The goal for nurses working with individuals needing assistance with assertiveness is to help them recognize that they are worthwhile and to help increase self-esteem. Individuals who do not feel good about themselves either allow others to violate their rights or cover up their low self-esteem by being overtly or covertly aggressive.

Individuals should be given information regarding their individual human rights. They must know what these rights are before they can stand up for them.

Nurses can teach patients the techniques to use to increase their assertive responses. This can be done on a one-to-one basis or in group situations. Once these techniques have been discussed, nurses can assist patients to practice them through role play. Each patient should compose a list of specific personal examples of situations that create difficulties for him or her. These situations will then be simulated in the therapy setting so that the patient may practice assertive responses in a nonthreatening environment. In a group situation, feedback from peers can provide valuable insight about the effectiveness of the response.

Evaluation

Evaluation requires that the nurse and patient assess whether or not these techniques are achieving the desired outcomes. Examples of outcome criteria may include:

1. Patient will be able to accept criticism without becoming defensive.
2. Patient will be able to express true feelings to (spouse, friend, boss, etc.) when his or her individual rights are violated.
3. Patient will be able to decline a request without feeling guilty.

Assertiveness training serves to extend and create more flexibility in an individual's communication style so that he or she has a greater choice of responses in various situations. Although change does not come easily, assertiveness training can be an effective way of changing behavior. Nurses can assist individuals to become more assertive, thereby encouraging them to become what they want to be, promoting an improvement in self-esteem, and fostering a respect for their own rights as well as the rights of others.

SUMMARY

Assertive behavior helps individuals feel better about themselves by encouraging them to stand up for their own basic human rights. These rights have equal representation for all individuals. But along

DIRECTIONS: Fill in each block with a rating of your assertiveness on a 5-point scale. A rating of 0 means you have no difficulty asserting yourself. A rating of 5 means that you are completely unable to assert yourself. Evaluation can be made by analyzing the scores:

1. totally by activity, including all of the different people categories
2. totally by people, including all of the different activity categories
3. on an individual basis, considering specific people and specific activities

PEOPLE / ACTIVITY	Friends of the same sex	Friends of the opposite sex	Intimate relations or spouse	Authority figures	Relatives/ family members	Colleagues and sub-ordinates	Strangers	Service workers; waiters; shop assistants, etc.
Giving and receiving compliments								
Asking for favors/help								
Initiating and maintaining conversation								
Refusing requests								
Expressing personal opinions								
Expressing anger/dis-pleasure								
Expressing liking, love, affection								
Stating your rights and needs								

Figure 11.1 Rating your assertiveness.

with rights comes an equal number of responsibilities. Part of being assertive includes living up to these responsibilities.

Assertive behavior increases self-esteem and the ability to develop satisfying interpersonal relationships. This is accomplished through honesty, directness, appropriateness, and respecting one's own rights, as well as the rights of others.

Individuals develop patterns of responding in various ways, such as role modeling, by receiving positive or negative reinforcement, or by conscious choice. These patterns can take the form of nonassertiveness, assertiveness, aggressiveness, or passive-aggressiveness.

Nonassertive individuals seek to please others at the expense of denying their own basic human rights. *Assertive* individuals stand up for their own rights while protecting the rights of others. Those who respond *aggressively* defend their own rights by violating the basic rights of others. Individuals who respond in a *passive-aggressive* manner defend their own rights by expressing resistance to social and occupational demands.

Some important behavioral considerations of assertive behavior include eye contact, body posture, distance/physical contact, gestures, facial expression, voice, fluency, timing, listening, thoughts, and content. Various techniques have been developed to assist individuals in the process of becoming more assertive.

Negative thinking can sometimes interfere with one's ability to respond assertively. Thought-stopping techniques help individuals remove negative, unwanted thoughts from awareness and promote the development of a more assertive attitude.

Nurses can assist individuals to learn and practice assertiveness techniques. The nursing process is an effective vehicle for providing the information and support to patients as they strive to create positive change in their lives.

REVIEW QUESTIONS
Self-Examination/Learning Exercise

Beside each response identify if it is nonassertive (NA), assertive (AS), aggressive (AG), or passive-aggressive (PA).

1. Your husband says, "You're crazy to think about going to college! You're not smart enough to handle the studies and the housework, too." You respond:

    _____ a. "I will do what I can, and the best that I can."

    _____ b. (Thinking to yourself): "We'll see how HE likes cooking dinner for a change.")

    _____ c. "You're probably right. Maybe I should reconsider."

    _____ d. "I'm going to do what I want to do, when I want to do it, and you can't stop me!"

2. You are having company for dinner and they are due to arrive in 20 minutes. You are about to finish cooking and still have to shower and dress. The doorbell rings and it is a man selling a new product for cleaning windows. You respond:

    _____ a. "I don't do windows!" and slam the door in his face.

    _____ b. "I'll take a case," and write him a check.

    _____ c. "Sure, I'll take three bottles." Then to yourself you think: 'I'm calling this company tomorrow and complaining to the manager about their salespeople coming around at dinnertime!'

    _____ d. "I'm very busy at the moment. I don't wish to purchase any of your product. Thank you."

3. You are in a movie theater that prohibits smoking. The person in the seat next to you just lit a cigarette and the smoke is very irritating. Your response is:

_____ a. You say nothing.

_____ b. "Please put your cigarette out. Smoking is prohibited."

_____ c. You say nothing, but begin to frantically fan the air in front of you and cough loudly and convulsively.

_____ d. "Put your cigarette out, you slob! Can't you read the 'no smoking' sign?"

4. You have been studying for a nursing examination all afternoon and lost track of time. Your husband expects dinner on the table when he gets home from work. You have not started cooking yet when he walks in the door and shouts, "Why the heck isn't dinner ready?" You respond:

_____ a. "I'm sorry. I'll have it done in no time, honey." But then you move very slowly and take a long time to cook the meal.

_____ b. "I'm tired from studying all afternoon. Make your own dinner, you bum! I'm tired of being your slave!"

_____ c. "I haven't started dinner yet. I'd like some help from you."

_____ d. "I'm so sorry. I know you're tired and hungry. It's all my fault. I'm such a terrible wife!"

5. You and your best friend, Jill, have had plans for 6 months to go on vacation together to Hawaii. You have saved your money and have plane tickets to leave in 3 weeks. She has just called you and reported that she is not going. She has a new boyfriend, they are moving in together, and she doesn't want to leave him. You respond:

_____ a. "I'm very disappointed and very angry. I'd like to talk to you about this later. I'll call you."

_____ b. "I'm very happy for you, Jill, I think it's wonderful that you and Jack are moving in together."

_____ c. You tell Jill that you are very happy for her, but then say to another friend, "Well, that's the end of my friendship with Jill!"

_____ d. "What!? You can't do that to me! We've had plans! You're acting like a real slut!"

6. A typewritten report for your psychiatric nursing class is due tomorrow at 8:00 A.M. The assignment was made 4 weeks ago and you have yours ready to turn in. Your roommate says, "I finally finished writing my report, but now I have to go to work and I don't have time to type it. Please be a dear and type it for me, otherwise I'll fail!" You have a date with your boyfriend. You respond:

_____ a. "Okay, I'll call Ken and cancel our date."

_____ b. "I don't want to stay here and type your report. I'm going out with Ken."

_____ c. "You've got to be kidding! What kind of a fool do you take me for, anyway?"

_____ d. "Okay, I'll do it." However, when your roommate returns from work at midnight, you are asleep and the report has not been typed.

7. You are asked to serve on a committee on which you do not wish to serve. You respond:

_____ a. "Thank you, but I don't wish to be a member of that committee."

_____ b. "I'll be happy to serve." But then you don't show up for any of the meetings."

_____ c. "I'd rather have my teeth pulled!"

_____ d. "Okay, if I'm really needed, I'll serve."

8. You're on your way to the laundry room when you encounter a fellow dorm tenant who often asks you to "throw a few of my things in with yours." You view this as an imposition. He asks you where you're going. You respond:

_____ a. "I'm on my way to the Celtics game. Where do you think I'm going?"

_____ b. "I'm on my way to do some laundry. Do you have anything you want me to wash with mine?"

_____ c. "It's none of your damn business!"

_____ d. "I'm going to the laundry room. Please don't ask me to do some of yours. I resent being taken advantage of in that way."

9. At a hospital committee meeting, a fellow nurse who is the chairperson has interrupted you each time you have tried to make a statement. The next time it happens, you respond:

_____ a. "You make a lousy leader! You won't even let me finish what I'm trying to say!"

_____ b. You say nothing.

_____ c. "Excuse me. I would like to finish my statement."

_____ d. You say nothing, but fail to complete your assignment and do not show up for the next meeting.

10. A fellow worker often borrows small amounts of money from you with the promise that she will pay you back "tomorrow." She currently owes you $15.00 and has not yet paid back any that she has borrowed. She asks if she can borrow a couple of dollars for lunch. You respond:

_____ a. "I've decided not to loan you any more money until you pay me for that which you have already borrowed."

_____ b. "I'm so sorry. I only have enough to pay for my own lunch today."

_____ c. "Get a life, will you? I'm tired of you sponging off me all the time!"

_____ d. "Sure, here's two dollars." Then to the other workers in the office: "Be sure you never lend Cindy any money. She never pays her debts. I'd be sure never to go to lunch with HER if I were you!"

REFERENCES

Alberti, R. E. & Emmons, M. L. (1990). *Your perfect right — A guide to assertive living* (6th ed.). San Luis Obispo, CA: Impact Publishers.

American Psychiatric Association. (1987). *Diagnostic and statistical manual of mental disorders* (3rd ed., rev). Washington, DC: American Psychiatric Association.

Bakdash, D. P. (1978, October). Becoming an assertive nurse. *Am J Nurs*, pp. 1710–1712.

Baer, J. (1976). *How to be an assertive (not aggressive) woman in life, love, and on the job.* New York: New American Library, Inc.

Bloom, L., Coburn, K., & Peralman, J. (1976). *The new assertive woman.* New York: Dell.

Davis, M., McKay, M., & Eshelman, E. R. (1982). *The relaxation and stress reduction workbook.* Oakland, CA: New Harbinger Publications.

Jakubowski, P. & Lange, A. J. (1978). *The assertive option — Your rights and responsibilities.* Champaign, IL: Research Press Co.

Kelly, C. (1979). *Assertion training: A facilitator's guide.* LaJolla, CA: University Associates, Inc.

Powell, T. J. & Enright, S. J. (1990). *Anxiety and stress management.* London: Routledge.

Smith, M. J. (1975). *When I say no, I feel guilty.* New York: The Dial Press.

Wolpe, J. (1973). *The practice of behavior therapy* (2nd ed.). Elmsford, NY: Pergamon Press.

BIBLIOGRAPHY

Alberti, R. E. (1977). *Assertiveness: Innovations, applications, issues.* San Luis Obispo, CA: Impact Publishers.

Alberti, R. E. & Emmons, M. L. (1975). *Stand up, speak out, talk back!* New York: Pocket Books.

Angel, G. & Petronko, D. K. (1983). *Developing the new assertive nurse.* New York: Springer Publishing.

Chenevert, M. (1978). *Special techniques in assertiveness training for women in the health professions.* St. Louis: CV Mosby.

Clark, C. C. (1978). *Assertive skills for nurses.* Wakefield, MA: Contemporary Publishing, Inc.

Dawley, H. H. & Wenrich, W. W. (1976). *Achieving assertive behavior.* Monterey, CA: Brooks/Cole Publishing Co.

Hauck, P. A. (1979). *How to stand up for yourself.* Philadelphia: The Westminster Press.

Herman, S. (1978). *Becoming assertive: A guide for nurses.* New York: D. Van Nostrand.

Moniz, D. (1978, October). Putting assertiveness techniques into practice. *Am J Nurs*, p. 1713.

Zappe, C. & Epstein, D. (1987). Assertive training. *J Psychosoc Nurs*, *25*(8), pp. 23–25.

12

PSYCHOPHARMACOLOGY

KEY TERMS
hypertensive crisis
priapism
retrograde ejaculation
gynecomastia
amenorrhea
agranulocytosis
extrapyramidal symptoms
akinesia
akathisia
dystonia
oculogyric crisis
tardive dyskinesia
neuroleptic malignant syndrome

OBJECTIVES

After reading this chapter, the student will be able to:

1. Discuss historical perspectives related to psychopharmacology.
2. Describe indications, actions, contraindications, and precautions of the following classifications of drugs:
   a. antianxiety agents
   b. antidepressants
   c. antimanics
   d. antipsychotics
   e. antiparkinsonian agents
   f. anticonvulsants
   g. sedative-hypnotics
3. Discuss common side effects and nursing implications for each classification, including patient/family education.

HISTORICAL PERSPECTIVES*

Historically, reaction to and treatment of the mentally ill ranged from benign involvement to intervention some would consider inhumane. Mentally ill individuals were feared because of common beliefs associating them with demons or the supernatural. They were looked upon as loathsome and were often mistreated.

Beginning in the late 18th century, a type of "moral reform" in the treatment of the mentally ill began to occur. This resulted in the establishment of community and state hospitals concerned with the needs of the mentally ill. Considered a breakthrough in the humanization of care, these institutions, however well-intentioned, fostered the concept of custodial care. Patients were assured the provision of food and shelter but with little or no hope of change for the future. As they became increasingly dependent on the institution to fill their needs, the likelihood of their return to the family or community diminished.

The early part of the 20th century saw the advent of the somatic therapies in psychiatry. Mentally ill individuals were treated with insulin shock therapy, wet sheet packs, ice baths, electroconvulsive therapy, and psychosurgery. Before 1950, no important chemical agents existed in psychiatric practice except sedatives and amphetamines, which had limited use due to their toxicity and addicting effects (Burgess, 1985). Since the 1950s, the development of psychopharmacology has expanded to include widespread use of antipsychotic, antidepressant, and antianxiety medications. Research into how these drugs work has provided an understanding of the etiology of many psychiatric disorders.

Psychotropic medications are not intended to "cure" the mental illness. Most physicians who prescribe these medications for their patients use them as an adjunct to individual or group psychotherapy. Although their contribution to psychiatric care cannot be minimized, it must be emphasized that psychotropic medications relieve physical/behavioral symptoms. They do not resolve emotional problems.

Nurses must understand the legal implications associated with administration of psychotropic medications. Laws differ from state to state, but most adhere to the patient's right to refuse treatment. Exceptions exist in emergency situations when it has been determined that patients are likely to harm themselves or others.

ANTIANXIETY AGENTS

Indications

Antianxiety drugs are also called *anxiolytics* and *minor tranquilizers.* They are used in the treatment of anxiety disorders, anxiety symptoms, acute alcohol withdrawal, skeletal muscle spasms, convulsive disorders, status epilepticus, preoperative sedation, and relief of anxiety. Their use and efficacy for periods greater than 4 months have not been evaluated.

Action

Antianxiety drugs depress subcortical levels of the central nervous system (CNS), particularly the limbic system and reticular formation. They may potentiate the effects of the powerful inhibitory neurotransmitter gamma-aminobutyric acid in the brain, thereby producing a calmative effect. All levels of CNS depression can be effected, from mild sedation to hypnosis to coma.

> EXCEPTION: Buspirone (BuSpar) does not depress the CNS. Its action is unknown, but the drug is believed to produce the desired effects through interactions with serotonin, dopamine, and other neurotransmitter receptors.

Contraindications/Precautions

Antianxiety drugs are contraindicated in individuals with hypersensitivity to any of the drugs within the classification (i.e., anxiolytics) or group (e.g., benzodiazepines). They should not be taken in combination with other CNS depressants and are contraindicated in pregnancy and lactation, narrow-angle glaucoma, shock, and coma.

Caution should be taken in administering these drugs to elderly or debilitated patients and patients with hepatic or renal dysfunction. (The dosage will generally have to be decreased.) Caution is also required with individuals who have a history of drug

---

*From Townsend, M. C. (1990), pp 1–2.

abuse/addiction and with individuals who are depressed or suicidal. In depressed patients, CNS depressants can exacerbate symptoms.

Examples of Commonly Used Antianxiety Agents (by Chemical Group) and the Daily Adult Dosage Range

Chemical Group	Generic (Trade) Name	Daily Dosage Range
Antihistamines	hydroxyzine (Vistaril, Atarax)	100–400 mg
Benzodiazepines	alprazolam (Xanax)	0.75–4 mg
	chlordiazepoxide (Librium)	15–100 mg
	clorazepate (Tranxene)	15–60 mg
	diazepam (Valium)	5–40 mg
	halazepam (Paxipam)	60–160 mg
	lorazepam (Ativan)	2–9 mg
	oxazepam (Serax)	30–120 mg
	prazepam (Centrax)	10–60 mg
Metathiazanones	chlormezanone (Trancopal)	100–800 mg
Propanediols	meprobamate (Equanil, Miltown)	200–2400 mg
Miscellaneous	buspirone (BuSpar)	15–60 mg

Side Effects and Nursing Implications

Nursing implications are designated by an asterisk [*].

1. **Drowsiness, confusion, lethargy** (most common side effects)
   * Instruct patient not to drive or operate dangerous machinery while taking medication.

2. **Tolerance; physical and psychological dependence** (does not apply to buspirone)
   * Instruct patient on long-term therapy not to quit taking the drug abruptly. Abrupt withdrawal can be life threatening. Symptoms include depression, insomnia, increased anxiety, abdominal and muscle cramps, tremors, vomiting, sweating, convulsions, and delirium.

3. **Potentiates the effects of other CNS depressants**
   * Instruct patient not to drink alcohol or take other medications that depress the CNS while taking this medication.

4. **May aggravate symptoms in depressed persons**
   * Assess mood daily.
   * Take necessary precautions for potential suicide.

5. **Orthostatic hypotension**
   * Monitor vital signs.
   * Instruct patient to arise slowly from a lying or sitting position.

6. **Paradoxical excitement**
   * Withhold drug and notify physician.

7. **Dry mouth**
   * Have patient take frequent sips of water, suck on ice chips or hard candy, or chew sugarless gum.

8. **Nausea and vomiting**
   * May take drug with food or milk.

9. **Blood dyscrasias**
   * Symptoms of sore throat, fever, malaise, easy bruising, or unusual bleeding should be reported to the physician immediately.

10. **Delayed onset** (buspirone only)
    * Ensure that patient understands there is a lag time of 7 to 10 days between onset of therapy with buspirone and subsiding of anxiety symptoms. Patient should continue to take medication during this time.

    NOTE: This medication is not recommended for p.r.n. administration because of this delayed therapeutic onset. There is no evidence that buspirone creates tolerance or physical dependence as do the CNS depressant anxiolytics.

Patient/Family Education

Patient should:

* Not drive or operate dangerous machinery. Drowsiness and dizziness can occur.
* Not stop taking the drug abruptly. Can produce serious withdrawal symptoms, such as depres-

sion, insomnia, anxiety, abdominal and muscle cramps, tremors, vomiting, sweating, convulsions, and delirium.

* (With *buspirone* only): Be aware of lag time between start of therapy and subsiding of symptoms. Relief is usually evident within 7 to 10 days. Be sure to take medication regularly, as ordered, so that it has sufficient time to take effect.
* Not consume other CNS depressants, including alcohol.
* Not take nonprescription medication without approval from physician.
* Rise slowly from sitting or lying position to prevent sudden drop in blood pressure.
* Report symptoms of sore throat, fever, malaise, easy bruising, unusual bleeding, or motor restlessness to physician immediately.
* Be aware of risks of taking this drug during pregnancy. (Congenital malformations have been associated with use during first trimester.) Notify physician of desirability to discontinue drug if pregnancy is suspected or planned.
* Be aware of possible side effects. Refer to written materials furnished by health-care providers regarding correct method of self-administration.
* Carry card or piece of paper at all times stating names of medications being taken.

ANTIDEPRESSANTS

Indications

Antidepressant medications are used in the treatment of dysthymic disorder; major depression with melancholia or psychotic symptoms; depression associated with organic disease, alcoholism, schizophrenia, or mental retardation; depressive phase of bipolar disorder; and depression accompanied by anxiety. These drugs elevate mood and alleviate other symptoms associated with moderate-to-severe depression.

Action

These drugs ultimately work to increase the concentration of norepinephrine and serotonin in the body. This is accomplished in the brain by blocking the reuptake of these chemicals by the neurons (unicyclics, bicyclics, tricyclics, tetracyclics, and others). It also occurs when an enzyme, monoamine oxidase (MAO), that is known to inactivate norepinephrine and serotonin is inhibited at various sites in the body (MAO inhibitors).

Contraindications/Precautions

Antidepressant drugs are contraindicated in individuals with hypersensitivity. They are also contraindicated in the acute recovery phase following myocardial infarction and in individuals with angle-closure glaucoma.

Caution should be taken in administering these drugs to elderly or debilitated patients and patients with hepatic, renal, or cardiac insufficiency. (The dosage will generally have to be decreased.) Caution is also required with psychotic patients, with patients who have benign prostatic hypertrophy, and with individuals who have a history of seizures (may decrease seizure threshold).

> NOTE: As these drugs take effect, and mood begins to lift, the individual may have increased energy with which to implement a suicide plan. Suicide potential often increases as level of depression decreases. The nurse should be particularly alert to *sudden* lifts in mood.

Examples of Commonly Used Antidepressant Medications (by Chemical Group) and the Daily Adult Dosage Range

> NOTE: Dosage requires slow titration; onset of therapeutic response may be 1 to 4 weeks.

Chemical Group	Generic (Trade) Name	Daily Dosage Range
Unicyclic	bupropion (Wellbutrin)	200–450 mg
Bicyclic	fluoxetine (Prozac)	20–80 mg
Tricyclics	amitriptyline (Elavil)	75–300 mg
	amoxapine (Asendin)	100–600 mg
	clomipramine (Anafranil)	75–150 mg
	desipramine (Norpramin)	75–300 mg
	doxepin (Sinequan; Adapin)	30–300 mg
	imipramine (Tofranil)	75–300 mg
		(*continued*)

Chemical Group	Generic (Trade) Name	Daily Dosage Range
	nortriptyline (Aventyl; Pamelor)	75–150 mg
	protriptyline (Triptil; Vivactil)	15–60 mg
	trimipramine (Surmontil)	75–300 mg
Tetracyclics	maprotiline (Ludiomil)	75–225 mg
Monoamine oxidase inhibitors	phenelzine (Nardil)	45–90 mg
	isocarboxazid (Marplan)	10–30 mg
	tranylcypromine (Parnate)	10–60 mg
Other	trazodone (Desyrel)	150–600 mg
	sertraline (Zoloft)	50–200 mg

Side Effects and Nursing Implications

Nursing implications are designated by an asterisk [*].

1. **Anticholinergic effects**
   a. **Dry mouth**
      * Offer patient sugarless candy, ice, frequent sips of water.
      * Strict oral hygiene is very important.
   b. **Blurred vision**
      * Offer reassurance that symptom will subside after a few weeks.
      * Instruct patient not to drive until vision is clear.
      * Clear small items from routine pathway to prevent falls.
   c. **Constipation**
      * Order foods high in fiber; increase fluid intake if not contraindicated; encourage patient to increase physical exercise, if possible.
   d. **Urinary retention**
      * Instruct patient to report hesitancy or inability to urinate.
      * Monitor intake and output.
      * Various methods to stimulate urination may be tried, such as running water in the bathroom or pouring water over the perineal area.

2. **Sedation**
   * Request an order from the physician for drug to be given at bedtime.
   * Request that physician decrease the dosage or perhaps order a less sedating drug.
   * Instruct patient not to drive or use dangerous equipment while experiencing sedation.

3. **Orthostatic hypotension**
   * Instruct patient to rise slowly from a lying or sitting position.
   * Monitor blood pressure (lying and standing) frequently; document and report significant changes.
   * Avoid long hot showers or tub baths.

4. **Reduction of seizure threshold**
   * Patients with history of seizures should be observed closely.
   * Institute seizure precautions as specified in hospital procedure manual.
   * Bupropion (Wellbutrin) should be administered in doses of no more than 150 mg and should be given at least 4 hours apart. Bupropion has been associated with a relatively high incidence of seizure activity in anorexic and cachectic patients.

5. **Tachycardia; arrhythmias**
   * Carefully monitor blood pressure and pulse rate/rhythm; report significant change to physician.

6. **Photosensitivity** (with tricyclics and tetracyclics)
   * Ensure that patient wears protective sunscreens, clothing, and sunglasses while spending time outdoors.

7. **Hypertensive crisis** (with MAO inhibitors)
   * Occurs if individual consumes foods containing tyramine while receiving MAO inhibitor therapy.
   * Products containing tyramine include aged cheeses; other aged, overripe, and fermented foods; broad beans; pickled herring; beef/chicken livers; preserved sausages; beer; wine (especially Chianti); yeast products; chocolate; caffeinated drinks; canned figs; sour cream; yogurt; soy sauce; over-the-counter cold medications; and diet pills.
   * Symptoms of hypertensive crisis include se-

vere occipital headache, palpitations, nausea/vomiting, nuchal rigidity, fever, sweating, marked increase in blood pressure, chest pain, and coma.

* Treatment of hypertensive crisis: discontinue drug immediately; monitor vital signs; administer short-acting antihypertensive medication, as ordered by physician; use external cooling measures to control hyperpyrexia.

8. **Priapism** (with trazodone)

* This is a rare side effect but has occurred in some men taking trazodone (Desyrel).
* If patient complains of prolonged or inappropriate penile erection, withhold medication dosage and notify physician immediately.
* Can become very problematic, requiring surgical intervention, and if not treated successfully, can result in impotence.

9. **Weight loss** (with fluoxetine and sertraline)

* A significant weight loss has been noted as a side effect with fluoxetine (Prozac) and sertraline (Zoloft), especially in underweight depressed patients.
* Caution should be taken in prescribing these drugs for anorectic patients.
* Patient should be weighed daily or every other day, at same time and on same scale, if possible.

Patient/Family Education

Patient should:

* Continue to take medication even though symptoms have not subsided. Therapeutic effect may not be seen for as long as 4 weeks. If after this length of time no improvement is noted, physician may prescribe a different medication.
* Use caution when driving or operating dangerous machinery. Drowsiness and dizziness can occur. If these side effects become persistent or interfere with activities of daily living, report to physician. Adjustment may be necessary.
* Not stop taking the drug abruptly. To do so might produce withdrawal symptoms, such as nausea, vertigo, insomnia, headache, malaise, and nightmares.
* Use sunscreens and wear protective clothing

when spending time outdoors. Skin may be sensitive to sunburn.

* Report occurrence of any of the following symptoms to physician immediately: sore throat, fever, malaise, unusual bleeding, easy bruising, persistent nausea/vomiting, severe headache, rapid heart rate, difficulty urinating, anorexia/weight loss, seizure activity, stiff or sore neck, and chest pain.
* Rise slowly from a sitting or lying position to prevent a sudden drop in blood pressure.
* Take frequent sips of water, chew sugarless gum, or suck on hard candy if dry mouth is a problem. Good oral care (frequent brushing, flossing) is very important.
* Not consume the following foods/medications while taking MAO inhibitors: aged cheese, wine (especially Chianti), beer, chocolate, colas, coffee, tea, sour cream, beef/chicken livers, canned figs, soy sauce, overripe and fermented foods, pickeled herring, preserved sausages, yogurt, yeast products, broad beans, cold remedies, and diet pills. To do so could cause a life-threatening hypertensive crisis.
* Avoid smoking while on tricyclic therapy. Smoking increases metabolism of tricyclics, requiring adjustment in dosage to achieve therapeutic effect.
* Not drink alcohol while on antidepressant therapy. These drugs potentiate the effects of each other.
* Not consume other medications, including over-the-counter medications, without physician's approval while on antidepressant therapy. Many medications contain substances that, in combination with antidepressant medication, could precipitate a life-threatening hypertensive crisis.
* Notify physician immediately if inappropriate or prolonged penile erections occur while taking trazodone (Desyrel). If the erection persists longer than 1 hour, seek emergency room treatment. This condition is rare but has occurred in some men who have taken trazodone. If measures are not instituted immediately, impotence can result.
* Not "double up" on medication if a dose of bupropion (Wellbutrin) is missed, unless advised to do so by physician. Taking bupropion in divided doses will decrease risk of seizures and other adverse effects.

* Be aware of possible risks of taking antidepressants during pregnancy. Safe use during pregnancy and lactation has not been fully established. These drugs are believed to readily cross the placental barrier; if so, the fetus could experience adverse effects of the drug. Inform physician immediately if pregnancy occurs, is suspected, or is planned.
* Be aware of side effects of antidepressants. Refer to written materials furnished by healthcare providers for safe self-administration.
* Carry card or other identification at all times describing medications being taken.

ANTIMANIC AGENTS

Drug of Choice

Lithium Carbonate

Indications

Lithium is used in the prevention and treatment of manic episodes associated with bipolar disorder. It may also be effective for depression associated with bipolar disorder.

Following initiation of lithium therapy, there is a lag period of 1 to 3 weeks before the symptoms of mania are alleviated. During this time, an antipsychotic, such as chlorpromazine (Thorazine), may be administered to decrease the level of hyperactivity.

Action

Lithium alters sodium metabolism within nerve and muscle cells and enhances the reuptake of biogenic amines (norepinephrine and serotonin) in the brain, lowering levels in the body and resulting in decreased hyperactivity. It may block development of sensitive dopamine receptors in the CNS of manic patients. Lithium has both antimanic and antidepressant properties.

Contraindications/Precautions

Lithium is contraindicated in individuals with hypersensitivity to the drug. It is also contraindicated in individuals with severe cardiovascular or renal disease, severe dehydration, sodium deple-

tion, brain damage, and during pregnancy and lactation.

Caution should be taken in administering these drugs to elderly patients and to patients with thyroid disorders, diabetes mellitus, urinary retention, or a history of seizure disorders.

Common Trade Names

Eskalith, Lithane, Lithobid, Lithonate, Lithotabs, Carbolith, Duralith, Lithizine

Daily Dosage

Acute mania: 1800 to 2400 mg
Maintenance: 300 to 1200 mg

Side Effects and Nursing Implications

Nursing implications are designated by an asterisk [*].

1. **Drowsiness, dizziness, headache**
   * Ensure that the patient does not participate in activities that require alertness until this response has stabilized.

2. **Dry mouth; thirst**
   * Provide patient with sugarless candy, ice, frequent sips of water.
   * Strict oral hygiene is very important.

3. **Gastrointestinal (GI) upset; nausea/vomiting**
   * Schedule medication dosages with meals to minimize GI upset.

4. **Fine hand tremors**
   * Report to physician, who may decrease dose of medication.
   * Some physicians prescribe a small dose of the beta blocker propranolol (Inderal) to counteract this side effect.

5. **Hypotension; pulse irregularities; arrhythmias**
   * Monitor vital signs on a regular basis (bid or tid).
   * Physician may decrease dose of medication.

6. **Polyuria; dehydration**
   * May subside after initial week or two.
   * Monitor daily intake and output and weight.
   * Monitor skin turgor daily.

* Report changes (e.g., altered ratio of intake and output, sudden weight gain or loss) to physician immediately.

7. **Weight gain**
   * Instruct patient regarding reduced calorie diet.
   * Emphasize importance of maintaining adequate intake of sodium.

TOXICITY

There is a narrow margin between the therapeutic and toxic levels of lithium carbonate. The usual ranges of therapeutic serum concentrations are:

* For acute mania: 1.0 to 1.5 mEq/L
* For maintenance: 0.6 to 1.2 mEq/L

Serum lithium levels should be monitored once or twice a week after initial treatment until dosage and serum levels are stable, then monthly during maintenance therapy. Blood samples should be drawn 12 hours after the last dose.

Symptoms of lithium toxicity begin to appear at blood levels greater than 1.5 mEq/L and are dosage determinate. Symptoms include:

* **At serum levels of 1.5 to 2.0 mEq/L:** blurred vision, ataxia, tinnitis, persistent nausea and vomiting, and severe diarrhea
* **At serum levels of 2.0 to 3.5 mEq/L:** excessive output of dilute urine, increasing tremors, muscular irritability, psychomotor retardation, mental confusion, and giddiness
* **At serum levels greater than 3.5 mEq/L:** impaired consciousness, nystagmus, seizures, coma, oliguria/anuria, arrhythmias, myocardial infarction, and cardiovascular collapse

Lithium levels should be monitored prior to medication administration. Dosage should be withheld and physician notified if level reaches 1.5 mEq/L or at the earliest observation or report by the patient of even the mildest symptom. If left untreated, lithium toxicity can be life threatening.

Lithium is similar in chemical structure to sodium, behaving in the body in much the same manner and competing at various sites in the body with sodium. If sodium intake is reduced or the body is depleted of its normal sodium (e.g., due to excessive sweating, fever, diuresis), lithium is reabsorbed by the kidneys, increasing the possibility of toxicity. Therefore, the patient must consume a diet adequate in sodium as well as 2500 to 3000 ml of fluid per day. Accurate records of intake, output, and the patient's weight should be kept on a daily basis.

Patient/Family Education

Patient should:

* Take medication on a regular basis, even when feeling well. Discontinuation can result in return of symptoms.
* Not drive or operate dangerous machinery until lithium levels are stabilized. Drowsiness and dizziness can occur.
* Not skimp on dietary sodium intake. Choose foods from the four food groups. Avoid "junk" foods. Drink six to eight large glasses of water each day. Avoid excessive use of beverages containing caffeine (coffee, tea, colas), which promote increased urine output.
* Notify physician if vomiting or diarrhea occurs. These symptoms can result in sodium loss and an increased risk of toxicity.
* Carry card or other identification noting patient is taking lithium.
* Be aware of appropriate diet should weight gain become a problem. Include adequate sodium and other nutrients while decreasing number of calories.
* Be aware of risks of becoming pregnant while on lithium therapy. Use information furnished by health-care providers regarding methods of contraception. Notify physician as soon as possible if pregnancy is suspected or planned.
* Be aware of side effects and symptoms associated with toxicity. Notify physician if any of the following symptoms occur: persistent nausea and vomiting, severe diarrhea, ataxia, blurred vision, tinnitis, excessive output of urine, increasing tremors, and mental confusion.
* Refer to written materials furnished by health-care providers while on self-administered maintenance therapy. Keep appointments for outpatient follow up; have serum lithium level

checked every 1 to 2 months or as advised by physician.

ANTIPSYCHOTICS

Indications

Antipsychotic drugs are also called *major tranquilizers* and *neuroleptics*. They are used in the treatment of acute and chronic psychoses, particularly when accompanied by increased psychomotor activity. Selected agents are used as antiemetics (chlorpromazine, perphenazine, prochlorperazine), in the treatment of intractable hiccoughs (chlorpromazine, perphenazine), and for the control of tics and vocal utterances in Tourette's disorder (haloperidol, pimozide).

Action

The exact mechanism of action is not known. These drugs are believed to work by blocking postsynaptic dopamine receptors in the basal ganglia, hypothalamus, limbic system, brainstem, and medulla. Antipsychotic effects may also be related to inhibition of dopamine-mediated transmission of neural impulses at the synapses.

Contraindications/Precautions

These drugs are contraindicated in patients with hypersensitivity (cross sensitivity may exist among phenothiazines). They should not be used when CNS depression is evident, when blood dyscrasias exist, in patients with Parkinson's disease, or those with liver, renal, or cardiac insufficiency.

Caution should be taken in administering these drugs to patients who are elderly, severely ill, or debilitated and to diabetic patients or patients with respiratory insufficiency, prostatic hypertrophy, or intestinal obstruction. Antipsychotics may lower seizure threshold. Individuals should avoid exposure to extremes in temperature while taking antipsychotic medication. Safety in pregnancy and lactation has not been established.

Examples of Commonly Used Antipsychotic Agents (by Chemical Group) and the Daily Adult Dosage Range

Chemical Group	Generic (Trade) Name	Daily Dosage Range
Phenothiazines	acetophenazine (Tindal)	60–120 mg
	chlorpromazine (Thorazine)	30–800 mg
	fluphenazine (Prolixin)	1–40 mg
	mesoridazine (Serentil)	30–400 mg
	perphenazine (Trilafon)	12–64 mg
	prochlorperazine (Compazine)	15–150 mg
	promazine (Sparine)	40–1200 mg
	thioridazine (Mellaril)	150–800 mg
	trifluoperazine (Stelazine)	2–40 mg
	triflupromazine (Vesprin)	60–150 mg
Thioxanthenes	chlorprothixene (Taractan)	75–600 mg
	thiothixene (Navane)	8–30 mg
Butyrophenone	haloperidol (Haldol)	1–100 mg
Dibenzoxazepine	loxapine (Loxitane)	20–250 mg
Dihydroindolone	molindone (Moban)	15–225 mg
Dibenzodiazepine	clozapine (Clozaril)	300–900 mg

Side Effects and Nursing Implications

Nursing implications are designated by an asterisk [*].

1. **Anticholinergic effects**
   a. **Dry mouth**
      * Provide patient with sugarless candy, ice, and frequent sips of water.
      * Ensure that patient practices strict oral hygiene.
   b. **Blurred vision**
      * Explain that symptom will most likely subside after a few weeks.

* Advise patient not to drive a car until vision clears.
* Clear small items from pathway to prevent falls.

c. **Constipation**

* Order foods high in fiber; encourage increase in physical activity and fluid intake if not contraindicated.

d. **Urinary retention**

* Instruct patient to report any difficulty urinating; monitor intake and output.

2. **Nausea; gastrointestinal (GI) upset**

* Tablets or capsules may be administered with food to minimize GI upset.
* Concentrate forms may be diluted and administered with fruit juice or other liquid; they should be mixed immediately prior to administration.

3. **Skin rash**

* Report appearance of any rash on skin to physician.
* Avoid spilling any of the liquid concentrate on skin; contact dermatitis can occur.

4. **Sedation**

* Discuss with physician possibility of administering drug at bedtime.
* Discuss with physician possible decrease in dosage or order for less sedating drug; instruct patient not to drive or use dangerous equipment while experiencing sedation.

5. **Orthostatic hypotension**

* Instruct patient to rise slowly from a lying or sitting position; monitor blood pressure (lying and standing) each shift; document and report significant changes.

6. **Photosensitivity**

* Ensure that patient wears protective sunscreens, clothing, and sunglasses while spending time outdoors.

7. **Hormonal effects**

a. **Decreased libido; retrograde ejaculation; gynecomastia (men)**

* Provide explanation of the effects and reassurance of reversibility; may discuss with physician possibility of ordering alternate medication.

b. **Amenorrhea (women)**

* Offer reassurance of reversibility; instruct patient to continue use of contraception, as amenorrhea does not indicate cessation of ovulation.

c. **Weight gain**

* Weigh patient every other day; order calorie-controlled diet; provide opportunity for physical exercise; provide diet/exercise instruction.

8. **Reduction of seizure threshold**

* Closely observe patients with history of seizures.
* NOTE: This is particularly important with patients taking clozapine (Clozaril). Reportedly, seizures affect 1% to 5% of individuals who take this drug, depending on the dosage (Pokalo, 1991).

9. **Agranulocytosis**

* Relatively rare with most of the antipsychotic drugs. Usually occurs within the first 3 months of treatment. Observe for symptoms of sore throat, fever, and malaise; complete blood count should be monitored if these symptoms appear
* EXCEPTION: With clozapine (Clozaril), agranulocytosis occurs in 1% to 2% of all patients taking the drug (Pokalo, 1991). It is a potentially fatal blood disorder in which the patient's white blood cell (WBC) count can drop to extremely low levels. Individuals on clozapine therapy are required to have blood levels drawn weekly to continue therapy. They are administered a 1-week supply of medication at a time. If the WBC count falls below 3000 mm^3 or the granulocyte count falls below 1500 mm^3, clozapine therapy is discontinued. The disorder is reversible if discovered in the early stages. However, this additional required technology of weekly blood tests has made this drug cost prohibitive for many people.

10. **Extrapyramidal symptoms**

* Observe for symptoms and report; administer antiparkinsonian drugs, as ordered.

a. **Pseudoparkinsonism** (tremor, shuffling gait, drooling, rigidity)

* Symptoms may appear 1 to 5 days following initiation of antipsychotic medication; occurs most often in women, the elderly, and dehydrated patients.

b. **Akinesia** (muscular weakness)

* Same as above.

c. **Akathisia** (continuous restlessness and fidgeting)

* Occurs most frequently in women; symptoms may occur 50 to 60 days following initiation of therapy.

d. **Dystonia** (involuntary muscular movements [spasms] of face, arms, legs, and neck)

* Occurs most often in men and patients younger than 25 years of age.

e. **Oculogyric crisis** (uncontrolled rolling back of the eyes)

* May appear as part of syndrome described as dystonia; may be mistaken for seizure activity; dystonia and oculogyric crisis should be treated as an emergency situation; contact physician; intravenous benztropine mesylate (Cogentin) is commonly administered; stay with the patient and offer reassurance and support during this frightening time.

11. **Tardive dyskinesia** (bizarre facial and tongue movements, stiff neck, and difficulty swallowing)

* All patients on long-term (months or years) antipsychotic therapy are at risk.
* Symptoms are potentially irreversible.
* Drug should be withdrawn at first sign, which is usually vermiform movements of the tongue; prompt action may prevent irreversibility.

12. **Neuroleptic malignant syndrome**

* A rare, but potentially fatal, complication of treatment with neuroleptic drugs. Routine assessments should include temperature and observation for parkinsonian symptoms.
* Onset can occur within hours or even years after drug initiation, and progression is rapid during the following 24 to 72 hours.

* Symptoms include severe parkinsonian muscle rigidity, hyperpyrexia up to 107°F, tachycardia, tachypnea, fluctuations in blood pressure, diaphoresis, and rapid deterioration of mental status to stupor and coma.
* Discontinue neuroleptic medication immediately.
* Monitor vital signs, degree of muscle rigidity, intake and output, and level of consciousness.
* Physician may order bromocriptine (Parlodel) or dantrolene (Dantrium) to counteract the effects of neuroleptic malignant syndrome.

Patient/Family Education

Patient should:

* Use caution when driving or operating dangerous machinery. Drowsiness and dizziness can occur.
* Not stop taking the drug abruptly after long-term use. To do so might produce withdrawal symptoms, such as nausea, vomiting, gastritis, headache, tachycardia, insomnia, and tremulousness.
* Use sunscreens and wear protective clothing when spending time outdoors. Skin is more susceptible to sunburn. Can happen in as little as 30 minutes.
* Report weekly (if on clozapine therapy) to have blood levels drawn and to obtain weekly supply of the drug.
* Report occurrence of any of the following symptoms to physician immediately: sore throat, fever, malaise, unusual bleeding, easy bruising, persistent nausea/vomiting, severe headache, rapid heart rate, difficulty urinating, muscle twitching, tremors, darkly colored urine, pale stools, yellow skin or eyes, muscular incoordination, skin rash, or seizures.
* Rise slowly from a sitting or lying position to prevent a sudden drop in blood pressure.
* Take frequent sips of water, chew sugarless gum, or suck on hard candy if dry mouth is a problem. Good oral care (frequent brushing, flossing) is very important.
* Consult physician regarding smoking while on neuroleptic therapy. Smoking increases me-

tabolism of neuroleptics, requiring adjustment in dosage to achieve therapeutic effect.

* Dress warmly in cold weather and avoid extended exposure to very high or low temperatures. Body temperature is harder to maintain with this medication.
* Not drink alcohol while on neuroleptic therapy. These drugs potentiate each other's effects.
* Not consume other medications, including over-the-counter medications, without physician's approval. Many medications contain substances that interact with neuroleptics in a way that may be harmful.
* Be aware of possible risks of taking neuroleptics during pregnancy. Safe use during pregnancy and lactation has not been established. Neuroleptics are believed to readily cross the placental barrier; if so, a fetus could experience adverse effects of the drug. Inform physician immediately if pregnancy occurs, is suspected, or is planned.
* Be aware of side effects of neuroleptic drugs. Refer to written materials furnished by healthcare providers for safe self-administration.
* Continue to take medication, even if feeling well and as though it is not needed. Symptoms may return if medication is discontinued.
* Carry card or other identification at all times describing medications being taken.

ANTIPARKINSONIAN AGENTS

Indications

These drugs are used in the treatment of parkinsonism of various causes, including degenerative, toxic, infective, neoplastic, or drug induced.

Action

Drugs used in the treatment of the parkinsonian syndrome and other dyskinesias are aimed at restoring the natural balance of two major neurotransmitters in the CNS: acetylcholine and dopamine. The imbalance is a deficiency in dopamine that results in excessive cholinergic activity. Drugs used are either anticholinergics (e.g., benztropine,

trihexyphenidyl), antihistamine (e.g., diphenhydramine), or dopaminergic agonists (e.g., amantadine, bromocriptine, levodopa).

Contraindications/Precautions

Antiparkinsonian agents are contraindicated in individuals with hypersensitivity. Anticholinergics should be avoided by individuals with angle-closure glaucoma; pyloric, duodenal, or bladder neck obstructions; prostatic hypertrophy; or myasthenia gravis.

Caution should be taken in administering these drugs to patients with hepatic, renal, or cardiac insufficiency; elderly and debilitated patients; those with a tendency toward urinary retention; or those exposed to high environmental temperatures.

Examples of Commonly Used Antiparkinsonian Agents (by Chemical Group) and the Daily Adult Dosage Range

Chemical Class	Generic (Trade) Name	Daily Dosage Range
Anticholinergics	benztropine (Cogentin)	0.5–6 mg
	biperiden (Akineton)	2–8 mg
	ethopropazine (Parsidol)	50–600 mg
	orphenadrine (Disipal)	150–250 mg
	procyclidine (Kemadrin)	6–20 mg
	trihexyphenidyl (Artane)	1–15 mg
Antihistamines	diphenhydramine (Benadryl)	10–400 mg
Dopaminergic agonists	amantadine (Symmetrel)	100–300 mg
	bromocriptine (Parlodel)	2.5–100 mg
	carbidopa/ levodopa (Sinemet)	10/100–200/2000 mg
	levodopa (Dopar, Larodopa)	500–8000 mg

Side Effects and Nursing Implications

Nursing implications are designated by an asterisk [*].

1. **Anticholinergic effects**
These side effects are identical to those produced by antipsychotic drugs. Taking both medications compounds these effects. Because of this, the physician may elect to prescribe anticholinergics only at the onset of extrapyramidal symptoms rather than as routine adjunctive therapy.
   a. **Dry mouth**
      * Offer patient sugarless candy, ice, frequent sips of water.
      * Ensure that patient practices strict oral hygiene.
   b. **Blurred vision**
      * Explain that symptom will most likely subside after a few weeks.
      * Advise patient not to drive until vision clears.
      * Clear small items from routine pathway to prevent falls.
   c. **Constipation**
      * Order foods high in fiber; encourage increase in physical activity and fluid intake, if not contraindicated.
   d. **Paralytic ileus**
      * A rare, but a potentially very serious side effect of anticholinergic drugs. Monitor for abdominal distention, absent bowel sounds, nausea, vomiting, and epigastric pain.
      * Report any of these symptoms to physician immediately.
   e. **Urinary retention**
      * Instruct patient to report any difficulty urinating; monitor intake and output.
   f. **Tachycardia, decreased sweating, elevated temperature**
      * Assess vital signs each shift; document and report significant changes to physician.
      * Ensure that patient remains in cool environment, as the body is not able to cool itself naturally with this medication.

2. **Nausea; GI upset**
   * Tablets or capsules may be administered with food to minimize GI upset.

3. **Sedation, drowsiness, dizziness**
   * Discuss with physician possibility of administering drug at bedtime.
   * Discuss with physician possible decrease in dosage or order for less sedating drug; instruct patient not to drive or use dangerous equipment while experiencing sedation or dizziness.

4. **Exacerbation of psychoses**
   * Assess for signs of loss of contact with reality.
   * Intervene during a hallucination; talk about real people and real events; reorient patient to reality.
   * Stay with patient during period of agitation and delirium; remain calm and reassure patient of his or her safety.
   * Discuss with physician possible decrease in dosage or change in medication.

5. **Orthostatic hypotension**
   * Instruct patient to rise slowly from a lying or sitting position; monitor blood pressure (lying and standing) each shift; document and report significant changes.

Patient/Family Education

Patient should:

* Take medication with food if GI upset occurs.
* Use caution when driving or operating dangerous machinery. Drowsiness and dizziness can occur.
* Not stop taking the drug abruptly. To do so might produce unpleasant withdrawal symptoms.
* Report occurrence of any of the following symptoms to physician immediately: pain or tenderness in area in front of ear; extreme dryness of mouth; difficulty urinating; abdominal pain; constipation; fast, pounding heart beat; rash; visual disturbances; or mental changes.
* Rise slowly from a sitting or lying position to prevent a sudden drop in blood pressure.
* Stay inside in air-conditioned room when

weather is very hot. Perspiration is decreased with antiparkinsonian agents, and the body cannot cool itself as well. There is greater susceptibility to heatstroke. Inform physician if air-conditioned housing is not available.

* Take frequent sips of water, chew sugarless gum, or suck on hard candy if dry mouth is a problem. Good oral care (frequent brushing, flossing) is very important.
* Not drink alcohol while on antiparkinsonian therapy.
* Not consume other medications, including over-the-counter medications, without physician's approval. Many medications contain substances that interact with antiparkinsonian agents in a way that may be harmful.
* Be aware of possible risks of taking antiparkinsonian agents during pregnancy. Safe use during pregnancy and lactation has not been fully established. Antiparkinsonian agents are believed to readily cross the placental barrier; if so, the fetus could experience adverse effects of the drug. Inform physician immediately if pregnancy occurs, is suspected, or is planned.
* Be aware of side effects of antiparkinsonian agents. Refer to written materials furnished by health-care providers for safe self-administration.
* Continue to take medication, even if feeling well and as though it is not needed. Symptoms may return if medication is discontinued.
* Carry card or other identification at all times describing medications being taken.

ANTICONVULSANTS

A seizure is a transient, paroxysmal, pathophysiological disturbance of cerebral function caused by a spontaneous, excessive discharge of cortical neurons (Kaplan & Sadock, 1985). Seizures are treated with a variety of anticonvulsant drugs, depending on the site of origin and the pattern of spread of the discharge. Nurses should be familiar with the use of anticonvulsant medications because personality problems and psychiatric symptoms are not uncommon in patients with seizure disorders. Some anticonvulsant medications are now being used investigationally to treat various psychiatric disorders. Long-acting barbiturates, ben-

zodiazepines, hydantoins, and carbamazepine will be discussed in this section.

Long-Acting Barbiturates

INDICATIONS

These drugs are used in the long-term management of tonic-clonic, absence, and complex partial seizures. They are also used for control in moderate states of anxiety.

ACTION

Barbiturates depress the CNS. These drugs are believed to reduce monosynaptic and polysynaptic transmission, resulting in decreased excitability of the entire nerve cell. Barbiturates also increase the threshold for electrical stimulation of the motor cortex.

Chemical Class	Generic (Trade) Name	Daily Dosage Range
Barbiturates	mephobarbital (Mebaral)	400–600 mg
	metharbital (Gemonil)	300–800 mg
	phenobarbital (Luminal)	100–300 mg
	primidone (Mysoline)	750–1500 mg

Hydantoins

INDICATIONS

Hydantoins are used in the management of tonic-clonic seizures and partial seizures with complex symptomatology. Mephenytoin is also used in the management of focal and Jacksonian seizures. Phenytoin is also used intravenously in the treatment of status epilepticus (second-choice drug when intravenous diazepam is not effective).

ACTION

Hydantoins act by increasing the seizure threshold in the cerebral cortex. By promoting sodium efflux from neurons in the motor cortex, they encourage stabilization of the threshold against hyperexcitability. Maximal activity of the brainstem centers responsible for the tonic phase of grand mal seizures is also reduced.

Chemical Group	Generic (Trade) Name	Daily Dosage Range
Hydantoins	ethotoin (Peganone)	2000–3000 mg
	mephenytoin (Mesantoin)	200–600 mg
	phenytoin (Dilantin)	300–600 mg

Benzodiazepines

INDICATIONS

Clonazepam is used in the management of absence, akinetic, and myoclonic seizures. Clorazepate is indicated as adjunctive therapy for partial seizures. Intravenous diazepam is the drug of choice for treatment of status epilepticus.

ACTION

Benzodiazepines cause depression of the CNS. They may potentiate the effects of the powerful inhibitory neurotransmitter gamma-aminobutyric acid in the brain.

Chemical Class	Generic (Trade) Name	Daily Dosage Range
Benzodiazepines	clonazepam (Klonopin)	1.5–20 mg
	clorazepate (Tranxene)	22.5–90 mg
	diazepam (Valium)	IV push for status epilepticus (adults) 5–10 mg initially; repeat every 10–15 min; maximum dose 30 mg

Carbamazepine

INDICATIONS

Carbamazepine is used in the management of tonic-clonic, complex partial, and mixed-type seizures. Investigational uses include bipolar affective disorder, schizoaffective disorder, resistant schizophrenia, rage reactions, and alcohol withdrawal.

ACTION

Action is unknown. May reduce polysynapatic responses and block post-tetanic potentiation of synaptic transmission.

Chemical Group	Generic (Trade) Name	Daily Dosage Range
Iminostilbene derivative	carbamazepine (Tegretol)	600–1200 mg

See Table 12.1 for a list of therapeutic serum levels and symptoms of toxicity for anticonvulsant medications.

Contraindications/Precautions

Anticonvulsants are contraindicated in individuals with hypersensitivity to the drug or any drug within the same chemical class. Most are contraindicated in lactating mothers.

Caution should be taken in administering these drugs to elderly or debilitated patients; patients with hepatic, cardiac, or renal disease; and patients who are pregnant. Anticonvulsants should not be discontinued abruptly.

Side Effects and Nursing Implications for Anticonvulsants

Nursing implications are designated by an asterisk [*].

1. **Drowsiness, dizziness, unsteadiness**
   * Ensure that patient is protected from injury. Supervise and assist with ambulation if required.
   * Pad siderails and headboard for patient who experiences seizures during the night.

2. **Decreased mental alertness**
   * Avoid or monitor activities that require mental alertness (including smoking).

3. **Nausea and vomiting**
   * Administer medication with food or milk if nausea and vomiting are a problem.

4. **Agranulocytosis, thrombocytopenia**
   * Report the presence of sore throat, fever,

Table 12.1 THERAPEUTIC SERUM LEVELS OF ANTICONVULSANTS AND SYMPTOMS OF TOXICITY		
Drug	**Therapeutic Serum Level**	**Symptoms of Toxicity**
Phenobarbital	10–30 mcg/ml	Confusion, drowsiness, dyspnea, slurred speech, staggering
Phenytoin	10–20 mcg/ml	At serum levels of 25–30 mcg/ml: nystagmus, ataxia, diplopia. At serum levels of 30–50 mcg/ml: confusion, nausea, slurred speech, drowsiness, dizziness, lethargy. Levels above 50 mcg/ml are marked by comatose states. Death may result from respiratory and circulatory depression.
Ethotoin	15–50 mcg/ml	Dermatitis, skin rash, pigmentation changes, ataxia, confusion, nausea, vomiting, slurred speech, dizziness
Clonazepam	20–80 ng/ml	Euphoria, relaxation, drowsiness, slurred speech, disorientation, mood lability, incoordination, unsteady gait, disinhibition of sexual and aggressive impulses, judgment or memory impairment
Primidone	5–12 mcg/ml (is metabolized to phenobarbital, 10–30 mcg/ml)	Lethargy, vision changes, confusion, dyspnea, hypoventilation, hypotension, coma
Carbamazepine	4–12 mcg/ml	Restlessness, twitching, tremor, ataxia, drowsiness, dizziness, nystagmus, stupor, agitation, involuntary movements, mydriasis, flushing, cyanosis, urinary retention, tachycardia, hypotension or hypertension, nausea and vomiting, convulsions, oliguria, shock, respiratory depression, coma

Source: From Townsend, M. C. (1990) and *Facts and Comparisons* (1990).

malaise, unusual bleeding, or easy bruising to physician immediately.

* Ensure that patient receives routine blood studies to determine onset of myelosuppression.

5. **Liver damage**

* Report evidence of yellowish skin or eyes to physician immediately.
* Ensure that patient has routine liver function tests.

6. **Gingival hyperplasia (hydantoins)**

* Ensure that patient practices good oral care by brushing after eating with a soft toothbrush. Flossing daily to remove plaque and massaging the gums may also be helpful.

Patient/Family Education for Anticonvulsants

Patient should:

* Not drive or operate dangerous machinery until individual response has been determined. Drowsiness and dizziness can occur.
* Not stop taking the drug abruptly. Doing so can result in status epilepticus.

* Avoid alcohol intake or nonprescription medication without approval from physician.
* Be aware of risks of taking anticonvulsants during pregnancy. There is an association between use of these drugs by women with epilepsy and the incidence of birth defects in offspring of these women. A patient who requires the medication to prevent seizures may be maintained on it; however, she must be fully aware of potential risks to her unborn child. If pregnancy occurs, or is suspected or planned, notify physician immediately.
* Use an alternate method of birth control during therapy because of decreased effectiveness of oral contraceptives with some anticonvulsants.
* Report any of the following symptoms to physician promptly: sore throat, fever, malaise, unusual bleeding, easy bruising, yellow skin or eyes, decrease in urine output, fluid retention, or pale stools.
* Be protected during a seizure: In the case of tonic-clonic (grand mal) seizure, do not restrain. Padding may be used (towels, blankets, pillows) to prevent bumping against hard objects. When convulsion has subsided, turn patient on side to allow secretions to drain and

prevent aspiration. Keep records of occurrence, characteristics, and duration of seizures, so that accurate reports may be given to physician for providing assistance in stabilization and control of seizures. If patient has difficulty breathing or continues to experience subsequent seizures, family should immediately call for emergency assistance.

* Be aware of potential side effects. Refer to written materials furnished by health-care providers regarding correct method of self-administration.
* Carry card or other identification at all times stating condition and names of medications being taken. Include name of physician and medical facility to which patient should be transported in event of an emergency.

SEDATIVE-HYPNOTICS

Indications

Sedative-hypnotics are used in the short-term management of various anxiety states and to treat insomnia. Selected agents are used as anticonvulsants and preoperative sedatives (phenobarbital, pentobarbital, secobarbital) and to reduce anxiety associated with drug withdrawal (chloral hydrate).

Action

Sedative-hypnotics cause generalized CNS depression. They may produce tolerance with chronic use and have the potential for psychological or physical dependence.

Contraindications/Precautions

Sedative-hypnotics are contraindicated in individuals with hypersensitivity to the drug or to any drug within the chemical class.

Caution should be taken in administering these drugs to patients with hepatic dysfunction or severe renal impairment. Use with caution in patients who may be suicidal or who may have been addicted to drugs previously. Hypnotic use should be short term. Elderly patients may be more sensitive to CNS depressant effects, and dosage reduction may be required.

Chemical Group	Generic (Trade) Name	Daily Dosage Range
Barbiturates	amobarbital (Amytal)	30–200 mg
	aprobarbital (Alurate)	40–160 mg
	butabarbital (Butisol)	45–120 mg
	pentobarbital (Nembutal)	40–200 mg
	phenobarbital (Luminal)	30–320 mg
	secobarbital (Seconal)	90–200 mg
	talbutal (Lotusate)	60–180 mg
Benzodiazepines	flurazepam (Dalmane)	15–30 mg
	temazepam (Restoril)	15–30 mg
	triazolam (Halcion)	0.25–0.5 mg
Miscellaneous	chloral hydrate (Noctec)	500–1000 mg
	ethchlorvynol (Placidyl)	500–1000 mg
	ethinamate (Valmid)	500–1000 mg
	glutethimide (Doriden)	250–500 mg
	methyprylon (Noludar)	200–400 mg

Side Effects, Nursing Implications, and Patient/Family Education

Refer to this section in the discussion of antianxiety medications.

SUMMARY

Psychotropic medications are intended to be used as adjunctive therapy to individual or group psychotherapy. *Antianxiety agents* are used in the treatment of anxiety disorders and to alleviate acute anxiety symptoms. The benzodiazepines are the most commonly used group. They are CNS depressants and have a potential for physical and psychological dependence. They should not be discontinued abruptly following long-term use as they can produce a life-threatening withdrawal syndrome. The most common side effects are drowsiness, confusion, and lethargy.

Antidepressants elevate mood and alleviate other symptoms associated with moderate-to-severe depression. These drugs work to increase the concentration of norepinephrine and serotonin in the body. The tricyclics and related drugs accomplish this by blocking the reuptake of these chemicals by the neurons. Another group of antidepressants inhibit MAO, an enzyme that is known to inactivate norepinephrine and serotonin. They are called MAO inhibitors. Some antidepressant medications take 1 to 4 weeks to produce the desired effect. The most common side effects are anticholinergic effects, sedation, and orthostatic hypotension. They also reduce the seizure threshold. MAO inhibitors can cause hypertensive crisis if products containing tyramine are consumed while taking these medications.

The *antimanic agent* of choice is lithium carbonate. It enhances the reuptake of norepinephrine and serotonin in the brain, thereby lowering the levels in the body, resulting in decreased hyperactivity. The most common side effects are dry mouth, GI upset, polyuria, and weight gain. There is a very narrow margin between the therapeutic and toxic levels of lithium. Serum levels must be drawn regularly to monitor for toxicity. Symptoms of lithium toxicity begin to appear at serum levels of approximately 1.5 mEq/L. If left untreated, lithium toxicity can be life threatening.

Antipsychotic drugs are used in the treatment of acute and chronic psychoses. Their action is unknown but is thought to decrease the activity of dopamine in the brain. The phenothiazines are the most commonly used group. Their most common side effects include anticholinergic effects, sedation, weight gain, reduction in seizure threshold, photosensitivity, and extrapyramidal symptoms.

Antiparkinsonian agents are used to counteract the extrapyramidal symptoms associated with antipsychotic medications. Antiparkinsonian drugs work to restore the natural balance of acetylcholine and dopamine in the brain. The most common side effects of these drugs are the anticholinergic effects. They may also cause sedation and orthostatic hypotension.

Anticonvulsant medications are used in the management of a variety of seizure disorders. Commonly used groups include barbiturates, hydantoins, benzodiazepines, and carbamazepine, an iminostilbene derivative. Side effects include drowsiness, dizziness, unsteadiness, and decreased mental alertness. Blood dyscrasias and liver damage can also occur. These drugs should not be discontinued abruptly. To do so could result in status epilepticus.

Sedative-hypnotics are used in the management of anxiety states and to treat insomnia. They are CNS depressants and have the potential for physical and psychological dependence. They are indicated for short-term use only. Side effects and nursing implications are similar to those described for antianxiety medications.

REVIEW QUESTIONS
Self-Examination/Learning Exercise

*Select the answer that is **most** appropriate for each of the following questions.*

1. Antianxiety medications produce a calming effect by:
   a. Depressing the CNS
   b. Decreasing levels of norepinephrine and serotonin in the brain
   c. Decreasing levels of dopamine in the brain
   d. Inhibiting production of the enzyme MAO

2. Nancy has a new diagnosis of panic disorder. Dr. S. has written a prn order for alprazolam (Xanax) for when Nancy is feeling anxious. She says to the nurse, "Dr. S. prescribed BuSpar for my friend's anxiety. Why did he order something different for me?" The nurse's answer is based on which of the following?
   a. BuSpar is not an antianxiety medication.

b. Xanax and BuSpar are essentially the same medication, so either one is appropriate.

c. BuSpar has delayed onset of action and cannot be used on a prn basis.

d. Xanax is the only medication that really works for panic disorder.

3. Patient education for the person who is taking MAO inhibitors should include which of the following?

a. Fluid and sodium replacement when appropriate, frequent drug blood levels, signs and symptoms of toxicity

b. Lifetime of continuous use, possible tardive dyskinesia, advantages of an injection every 2 to 4 weeks

c. Short-term use, possible tolerance to beneficial effects, careful taper at end of treatment

d. Tyramine-restricted diet, prohibited concurrent use of over-the-counter medications without physician notification

4. There is a very narrow margin between the therapeutic and toxic levels of lithium carbonate. Symptoms of toxicity are most likely to appear if the serum levels exceed:

a. 0.15 mEq/L

b. 1.5 mEq/L

c. 15.0 mEq/L

d. 150 mEq/L

5. Initial symptoms of lithium toxicity include:

a. Constipation, dry mouth, drowsiness, oliguria

b. Dizziness, thirst, dysuria, arrhythmias

c. Ataxia, tinnitus, blurred vision, diarrhea

d. Fatigue, vertigo, anuria, weakness

6. Antipsychotic medications are thought to decrease psychotic symptoms by:

a. Blocking reuptake of norepinephrine and serotonin

b. Blocking the action of dopamine in the brain

c. Inhibiting production of the enzyme MAO

d. Depressing the CNS

7. Part of the nurse's continual assessment of the patient taking antipsychotic medications is to observe for extrapyramidal symptoms. Examples include:

a. Muscular weakness, rigidity, tremors, facial spasms

b. Dry mouth, blurred vision, urinary retention, orthostatic hypotension

c. Amenorrhea, gynecomastia, retrograde ejaculation

d. Elevated blood pressure, severe occipital headache, stiff neck

8. If the above extrapyramidal symptoms should occur, which of the following would be a priority nursing intervention?

a. Notify the physician immediately.

b. Administer prn trihexyphenidyl (Artane).

c. Withhold the next dose of antipsychotic medication.

d. Explain to the patient that these symptoms are only temporary and will disappear shortly.

9. Anticonvulsants should not be discontinued abruptly because:

a. The patient may experience hypertensive crisis.

b. The patient may develop neuroleptic malignant syndrome.

c. The patient may experience status epilepticus.

d. The patient may develop tardive dyskinesia.

10. Should the above condition occur, the drug of choice for treatment is:

a. Intravenous phenytoin (Dilantin)

b. Intravenous diazepam (Valium)

c. Intravenous benztropine (Cogentin)

d. Intravenous phenobarbital (Luminal)

REFERENCES

Burgess, A. W. (1985). *Psychiatric nursing in the hospital and the community* (4th ed.). Englewood Cliffs, NJ: Prentice-Hall.

Facts and comparisons. (1990). St. Louis: JB Lippincott.

Kaplan, H. I. & Sadock, B. J. (1985). *Modern synopsis of comprehensive textbook of psychiatry* (4th ed.). Baltimore: Williams & Wilkins.

Pokalo, C. L. (1991). Clozapine: Benefits and controversies. *J Psychosoc Nurs, 29*(2), pp. 33–36.

Townsend, M. C. (1990). *Drug guide for psychiatric nursing.* Philadelphia: FA Davis.

BIBLIOGRAPHY

Baer, C. L. & Williams, B. R. (1992). *Clinical pharmacology and nursing.* Springhouse, PA: Springhouse.

Baldessarini, R. J. (1985). *Chemotherapy in psychiatry: Principles and practice* (rev. ed.). Cambridge, MA: Harvard University Press.

Deglin, J. H., Vallerand, A. H. and Russin, M. M. (1992). *Davis's drug guide for nurses* (3rd ed.). Philadelphia: FA Davis.

Gahart, B. L. (1992). *Intravenous medications: A handbook for nurses and allied health personnel* (8th ed.). St. Louis: CV Mosby.

Kuhn, M. M. (1991). *Pharmacotherapeutics: A nursing process approach* (2nd ed.). Philadelphia: FA Davis.

Lickey, M. E. & Gordon, B. (1983). *Drugs for mental illness: A revolution in psychiatry.* New York: WH Freeman.

Schatzberg, A. F. & Cole, J. O. (1986). *Manual of clinical psychopharmacology.* Washington: American Psychiatric Press.

Townsend, M. C. (1991). *Nursing diagnoses in psychiatric nursing: A pocket guide for care plan construction.* Philadelphia: FA Davis.

ELECTROCONVULSIVE THERAPY

KEY TERMS
electronconvulsive therapy
insulin coma therapy
pharmacoconvulsive therapy

OBJECTIVES

After reading this chapter, the student will be able to:
1. Define electroconvulsive therapy (ECT).
2. Discuss historical perspectives related to ECT.
3. Discuss indications, contraindications, mechanism of action, and side effects of ECT.
4. Identify risks associated with ECT.
5. Describe the role of the nurse in the administration of ECT.

ELECTROCONVULSIVE THERAPY, DEFINED

Electroconvulsive therapy is the induction of a grand mal (generalized) seizure through the application of electrical current to the brain. The stimulus is applied through electrodes that are placed either bilaterally in the frontotemporal region or unilaterally on the same side as the dominant hand (American Psychiatric Association [APA], 1978). Controversy exists over optimal placement of the electrodes in terms of possible greater efficacy, with bilateral placement versus the potential in some patients for less confusion and acute amnesia with unilateral placement.

The amount of electrical stimulus applied is administered in accordance with the directions for the machine being employed (APA, 1978). The patient's physical condition is also a consideration. A typical range of application might be 70 to 125 volts of electrical current for 0.7 to 1.5 seconds. The duration of the resulting seizure is 25 to 90 seconds (Endler & Persad, 1988). Movements are very minimal due to the administration of a muscle relaxant prior to the treatment. The tonic phase of the seizure usually lasts 10 to 15 seconds and may be identified by a rigid plantar flexion of the feet. The clonic phase, which lasts for approximately 30 to 60 seconds, follows and is usually characterized by rhythmic movements of the muscles. Because of the muscle relaxant, movements may be observed merely as a rhythmic twitching of the toes. Weiner (1979) has suggested that a seizure duration of 25 to 60 seconds per treatment is appropriate for a therapeutic response.

Most patients require an average of 6 to 10 treatments, but some may not reach a maximal response until after 20 to 25 treatments (Kaplan & Sadock, 1985). Treatments are usually administered every other day, three times per week. Treatments are performed on an inpatient basis for those who require close observation and care (e.g., patients who are suicidal, agitated, delusional, catatonic, or acutely manic). Those at less risk may have the option of receiving therapy at an outpatient treatment facility.

HISTORICAL PERSPECTIVES

The first ECT treatment was performed in April 1938 by Italian psychiatrists Ugo Cerletti and Lucio Bini in Rome. Other somatic therapies had been tried prior to that time, in particular insulin coma therapy and pharmaconconvulsive therapy.

Insulin coma therapy was introduced by the German psychiatrist Manfred Sakel in 1933. His therapy was used for patients with schizophrenia. The insulin injection treatments would induce a hypoglycemic coma, which Sakel claimed was effective in alleviating schizophrenic symptoms. This therapy required vigorous medical and nursing intervention through the stages of induced coma. Some fatalities occurred when patients failed to respond to efforts directed at termination of the coma. The efficacy of insulin coma therapy has been questioned, and it is very rarely used in the United States today (Kaplan & Sadock, 1985).

Pharmacoconvulsive therapy was introduced in Budapest in 1934 by Ladislas Meduna (Endler & Persad, 1988). He induced convulsions with intramuscular injections of camphor in oil in patients with schizophrenia. He based his treatment on clinical observation and on his theory that there was a biological antagonism between schizophrenia and epilepsy. Thus, by inducing seizures, he hoped to reduce schizophrenic symptoms. Because he discovered that camphor was unreliable for inducing seizures, he began using pentylenetetrazol (Cardiazol/Metrazol). Some successes were reported in terms of reduction of psychotic symptoms, and until the advent of ECT in 1938, Metrazol was the most frequently used procedure for producing seizures in psychotic patients. There was a brief resurgence of pharmacoconvulsive therapy in the late 1950s, when flurothyl (Indoklon), a potent inhalant convulsant, was introduced as an alternative for individuals who were unwilling to consent to ECT for the treatment of depression and schizophrenia (Cherkin, 1974). Pharmacoconvulsive therapy is no longer used in psychiatry.

Periodic recognition of the important contribution of ECT in the treatment of mental illness has been evident in the United States. An initial acceptance was observed from 1940 to 1955, followed by a 20-year period in which ECT was considered objectionable by both the psychiatric profession and the lay public. A second wave of acceptance began around 1975 and has been increasing to the present. The period of nonacceptability coincided with the introduction of tricyclic and monoamine oxidase inhibitor antidepressant drugs and ended with the realization among many psychiatrists that the widely heralded replacement of ECT with these chemical agents had failed to materialize (Abrams,

1988). Some individuals showed improvement with ECT after failing to respond to other forms of therapy.

Undoubtedly, the disapproval that ECT has encountered within the lay community has been fueled by unfavorable media presentations, such as movies like *One Flew Over the Cuckoo's Nest*, in which the treatment is exposed as physically and emotionally brutal, imposed as a punitive measure on patients who are noncompliant with institutional regulations.

Approximately 60,000 to 100,000 people per year receive ECT treatments in the United States (Sackeim, 1985). The typical patient is white, female, middle-aged, and from a middle- to upper-income background, receiving treatment in a private or university hospital for major depression, usually after drug therapy has proved ineffective. Due largely to the expense involved, including a team of highly skilled medical specialists, most public hospitals are not able to offer this service to their patients.

INDICATIONS

Major Depression

Electroconvulsive therapy has been shown to be effective in the treatment of severe depression. It appears to be particularly effective in depressed patients who are also experiencing psychotic symptoms and those with psychomotor retardation and neurovegetative changes, such as disturbances in sleep, appetite, and energy (Endler & Persad, 1988). Electroconvulsive therapy is not often used as the treatment of choice for depressive disorders, but is considered only after a trial of therapy with antidepressant medication has proved ineffective.

Mania

Electroconvulsive therapy is also indicated in the treatment of manic episodes of bipolar affective disorder (Endler & Persad, 1988). At present, it is rarely used for this purpose, having been superseded by the widespread use of antipsychotic drugs and/or lithium. However, it has been shown to be effective in the treatment of manic patients who do not tolerate or fail to respond to lithium or other drug treatment, or when life is threatened by dangerous behavior or exhaustion.

Schizophrenia

Electroconvulsive therapy can induce a remission in some patients who present with acute schizophrenia, particularly if it is accompanied by catatonic or affective (depression or mania) symptomatology (Kaplan & Sadock, 1985). It does not appear to be of value to individuals with chronic schizophrenic illness (Endler & Persad, 1988).

Other Conditions

Electroconvulsive therapy has also been tried with patients experiencing a variety of neuroses, obsessive-compulsive disorders, and personality disorders (Kendell, 1981). Little evidence exists to support the efficacy of ECT in the treatment of these conditions.

CONTRAINDICATIONS

The only absolute contraindication for ECT is increased intracranial pressure (from brain tumor, recent cardiovascular accident, or other cerebrovascular lesion). Electroconvulsive therapy is associated with a physiologic rise in cerebrospinal fluid pressure during the treatment, resulting in increased intracranial pressure that could lead to herniation (Crowe, 1984).

Various other conditions, not considered absolute contraindications but rendering patients at high risk for the treatment, have been identified (Endler & Persad, 1988; Kaplan & Sadock, 1985; Abrams, 1988). They are largely cardiovascular in nature and include myocardial infarction or cerebrovascular accident within the preceding 3 months, aortic or cerebral aneurysm, severe underlying hypertension, and congestive heart failure. Patients with cardiovascular problems are placed at risk due to the response of the body to the seizure itself. The initial vagal response results in a sinus bradycardia and drop in blood pressure. This is followed immediately by tachycardia and a hypertensive response. These changes can be life threatening to an individual with an already compromised cardiovascular system. Other factors that place patients at high risk for ECT include severe osteoporosis, acute and chronic pulmonary disorders, and pregnancy.

MECHANISM OF ACTION

The exact mechanism by which ECT effects a therapeutic response is unknown. Several theories exist, but the one to which the most credibility has been given is the biochemical theory. A number of researchers have demonstrated that electric stimulation results in significant increases in the circulating levels of several neurotransmitters (Endler & Persad, 1988). These neurotransmitters include serotonin, norepinephrine, and dopamine, the same biogenic amines that are affected by antidepressant drugs.

SIDE EFFECTS

The most common side effects of ECT are temporary memory loss and confusion. Critics of the therapy argue that these changes represent irreversible brain damage. Proponents insist they are temporary and reversible. In a review of a number of studies dealing with this question, Kendell (1981) could find no evidence of memory deficits persisting beyond 3 months. Other researchers have suggested that varying degrees of memory loss may be evident in some patients up to 6 to 9 months following ECT (Squire, 1977; Weiner et al., 1986).

The controversy continues regarding the choice of unilateral versus bilateral ECT. Studies have shown that unilateral placement of the electrodes decreases the amount of memory disturbance. However, unilateral ECT is not as effective in the relief of depression, and a greater number of treatments may be required than with bilateral ECT (Endler & Persad, 1988).

RISKS ASSOCIATED WITH ELECTROCONVULSIVE THERAPY

Mortality

Recent studies indicate that the mortality rate from ECT falls somewhere in the range between 0.01% and 0.04% (Abrams, 1988). Although the occurrence is rare, the major cause of death with ECT is cardiovascular complications, such as acute myocardial infarction, acute coronary insuffi-

ciency, ventricular fibrillation, myocardial rupture, cardiac arrest, cardiovascular collapse, stroke, and ruptured cerebral or aortic aneurysm. Assessment and management of cardiovascular disease *prior* to treatment is vital in the reduction of morbidity and mortality rates associated with ECT.

Permanent Memory Loss

Freeman and associates (1980) conducted a study of cognitive dysfunction in a group of individuals who had received a course of ECT treatments an average of 10 years previously. These patients were given a battery of cognitive memory tasks, on several of which they were found to be significantly impaired; a few even scored in the organic impairment range. The authors concluded that a small subgroup of patients receiving ECT might suffer permanent memory impairment.

Brain Damage

Brain damage from ECT remains a concern for those who continue to believe in its usefulness and efficacy as a treatment for depression. Critics of the procedure remain adamant in their beliefs that ECT always results in some degree of immediate brain damage (Endler & Persad, 1988). However, evidence is based largely on animal studies in which the subjects received excessive electrical dosages, and the seizures were unmodified by muscle paralysis and oxygenation (Abrams, 1988). Although this is an area for continuing study, there are no current data to substantiate that ECT produces any permanent changes in brain structure or functioning.

THE ROLE OF THE NURSE IN ELECTROCONVULSIVE THERAPY

Nurses routinely assist with ECT, providing support before, during, and after the treatment to the patient, family, and medical professionals who are conducting the therapy. The nursing process provides a systematic approach to the provision of care for the patient receiving ECT.

Assessment

A complete physical examination must be completed by the appropriate medical professional prior to the initiation of ECT. This evaluation should include a thorough assessment of cardiovascular and pulmonary status as well as laboratory blood and urine studies. A skeletal history and x-ray assessment should also be considered.

The nurse may be responsible for ensuring that informed consent has been obtained from the patient. If the depression is severe and the patient is clearly unable to consent to the procedure, permission may be obtained from family or other legally responsible individual. Consent is secured only after the patient or responsible individual acknowledges understanding of the procedure, including possible side effects and potential risks involved.

Nurses may also be required to assess:

- Patient's mood and level of interaction with others
- Evidence of suicidal ideation, plan, and means
- Level of anxiety and fears associated with receiving ECT
- Thought and communication patterns
- Baseline memory for short- and long-term events
- Patient and family knowledge of indications for, side effects of, and potential risks involved with ECT
- Current and past use of medications
- Baseline vital signs and history of allergies
- Patient's ability to carry out activities of daily living

Analysis

Selection of appropriate nursing diagnoses for the patient undergoing ECT is based on continual assessment before, during, and after treatment. Following are selected potential nursing diagnoses with projected outcomes for evaluation.

Nursing Diagnoses	Projected Outcomes
Anxiety (moderate to severe) related to impending therapy	Patient will verbalize a decrease in anxiety following explanation of procedure and expression of fears.

Nursing Diagnoses	Projected Outcomes
Knowledge deficit related to necessity for and side effects or risks of ECT	Patient will verbalize understanding of need for and side effects/risks of ECT following explanation.
High risk for injury related to risks involved with ECT	Patient will undergo treatment without sustaining injury.
High risk for aspiration related to altered level of consciousness immediately following treatment	Patient will experience no aspiration during ECT.
Decreased cardiac output related to vagal stimulation occurring during ECT	Patient will demonstrate adequate tissue perfusion during and after treatment (absence of cyanosis or severe change in mental status).
Altered thought processes related to side effects of temporary memory loss and confusion	Patient will maintain reality orientation following ECT treatment.
Self-care deficit related to incapacitation during postictal stage	Patient's self-care needs will be fulfilled at all times.
High risk for activity intolerance related to post-ECT confusion and memory loss	Patient will gradually increase level of participation in therapeutic activities to the highest level of personal capability.

Intervention

Electroconvulsive therapy treatments are usually performed in the morning. The patient is NPO at least 4 hours prior to the treatment. Some institutional policies require that the patient be placed on NPO status at midnight. The treatment team routinely consists of the psychiatrist, anesthesiologist, and two or more nurses.

Nursing interventions prior to the treatment include:

- Ensure that the physician has obtained informed consent and that a signed permission form is on the chart.
- Ensure that the most recent laboratory reports (complete blood count, urinalysis) and results of ECG and x-ray are available.

- Approximately 1 hour before treatment is scheduled, take vital signs and record. Have patient void, remove dentures, eyeglasses or contact lenses, jewelry, and hairpins. Following institutional requirements, patient should change into hospital gown, or if permitted, into own loose clothing or pajamas. Patient should remain in bed with bedrails up.
- Approximately 30 minutes before treatment, administer the pretreatment medication as prescribed by the physician. The usual order is for atropine sulfate or glycopyrrolate (Robinul) given intramuscularly. Either of these medications may be ordered to decrease secretions and counteract the effects of vagal stimulation induced by ECT.
- Stay with the patient to help allay fears and anxiety. Maintain a positive attitude about the procedure, and encourage the patient to verbalize feelings.

In the treatment room, the patient is placed on the treatment table in a supine position. The anesthesiologist intravenously administers a short-acting anesthetic, such as thiopental sodium (Pentothal) or methohexital sodium (Brevital). A muscle relaxant, usually succinylcholine (Anectine), is given intravenously to prevent severe muscle contractions during the seizure, thereby reducing the possibility of fractured or dislocated bones. Because succinylcholine paralyzes respiratory muscles as well, the patient is oxygenated with pure oxygen prior to the treatment.

An airway/bite block is placed in the patient's mouth, and he or she is positioned to facilitate airway patency. Electrodes are placed (either bilaterally or unilaterally) on the temples to deliver the electrical stimulation.

Nursing interventions during the treatment include:

- Ensure patency of airway. Provide suctioning if needed.
- Assist anesthesiologist with oxygenation as required.
- Observe readouts on machines monitoring vital signs and cardiac functioning.
- Provide support to patient's arms and legs during the seizure.
- Observe and record type and amount of movement induced by the seizure.

Following the treatment, the anesthesiologist continues to oxygenate the patient with pure oxygen until spontaneous respirations return. Most patients awaken within 10 or 15 minutes of the treatment and are confused and disoriented. Some patients will sleep for 1 to 2 hours following the treatment. All patients require close observation in this immediate posttreatment period.

Nursing interventions in the posttreatment period include:

- Monitor pulse, respirations, and blood pressure every 15 minutes for the first hour, during which time the patient should remain in bed.
- Position patient on side to prevent aspiration.
- Orient patient to time and place.
- Describe what has occurred.
- Provide reassurance that memory loss the patient may be experiencing is only temporary.
- Allow patient to verbalize fears and anxieties related to receiving ECT.
- Stay with the patient until he or she is fully awake, oriented, and able to perform self-care activities without assistance.
- Provide patient with a highly structured schedule of routine activities to minimize confusion.

Evaluation

Evaluation of the effectiveness of nursing interventions is based on the achievement of the projected outcomes.

Example

- Was the patient's anxiety maintained at a manageable level?
- Was the patient/family teaching completed satisfactorily?
- Did patient/family verbalize understanding of the procedure, its side effects, and risks involved?
- Did patient undergo treatment without experiencing injury or aspiration?
- Has patient maintained adequate tissue perfusion during and following treatment? Have vital signs remained stable?
- With consideration to individual patient condition and response to treatment, is patient reoriented to time, place, and situation?
- Have all of patient's self-care needs been fulfilled?

- Is patient participating in therapeutic activities to his or her maximum potential? What is the patient's level of social interaction?

Careful documentation is an important part of the evaluation process. Some routine observations may be evaluated on flow sheets specifically identified for ECT. However, progress notes with detailed descriptions of patient behavioral changes are essential to evaluate improvement and provide assistance in determining the number of treatments that will be administered. Continual reassessment, planning, and evaluation provide assurance that the patient will receive adequate and appropriate nursing care throughout the course of therapy.

SUMMARY

Electroconvulsive therapy is the induction of a grand mal seizure through the application of electrical current to the brain. It is a safe and effective treatment alternative for individuals with depression, mania, or schizoaffective disorder who do not respond to other forms of therapy.

Electroconvulsive therapy is contraindicated for individuals with increased intracranial pressure. Individuals with cardiovascular problems are at high risk for ECT. Other factors that place patients at high risk include severe osteoporosis, acute and chronic pulmonary disorders, and pregnancy.

The exact mechanism of action of ECT is unknown, but it is thought that the electrical stimulation results in significant increases in the circulating levels of the neurotransmitters serotonin, norepinephrine, and dopamine.

The most common side effects with ECT are temporary memory loss and confusion. Although it is rare, death must be considered a risk associated with ECT. When it does occur, the most common cause is cardiovascular complications. Other possible risks include permanent memory loss and brain damage, for which there is little substantiating evidence.

The nurse assists with ECT using the steps of the nursing process before, during, and following treatment. Important nursing interventions include ensuring patient safety, managing patient anxiety, and providing adequate patient education. Nursing input into the ongoing evaluation of patient behavior is an important factor in determining the therapeutic effectiveness of ECT.

REVIEW QUESTIONS
Self-Examination/Learning Exercise

*Select the answer that is **most** appropriate for each of the following questions.*

1. Electroconvulsive therapy is most commonly prescribed for:
   a. Bipolar disorder, manic
   b. Paranoid schizophrenia
   c. Major depression
   d. Obsessive-compulsive disorder

2. Which of the following best describes the *average* number of ECT treatments given and the timing of administration?
   a. 1 treatment per month for 6 months
   b. 1 treatment every other day for a total of 6 to 10
   c. 1 treatment three times per week for a total of 20 to 30
   d. 1 treatment every day for a total of 10 to 15

3. Which of the following conditions is considered to be the only *absolute* contraindication for ECT?
   a. Increased intracranial pressure
   b. Recent myocardial infarction
   c. Severe underlying hypertension
   d. Congestive heart failure

4. Electroconvulsive therapy is believed to effect a therapeutic response by:
   a. Stimulation of the CNS
   b. Decreasing the levels of acetylcholine and monoamine oxidase
   c. Increasing the levels of serotonin, norepinephrine, and dopamine
   d. Altering sodium metabolism within nerve and muscle cells

5. The most common side effects of ECT are:
   a. Permanent memory loss and brain damage
   b. Fractured and dislocated bones
   c. Myocardial infarction and cardiac arrest
   d. Temporary memory loss and confusion

Sam has just been admitted to the inpatient psychiatric unit with a diagnosis of major depression. Sam has been treated with antidepressant medication for 6 months without improvement. His psychiatrist has suggested a series of ECT treatments. Sam says to the nurse on admission, "I don't want to end up like McMurphy in *One Flew Over the Cuckoo's Nest!* I'm scared!" The following questions pertain to Sam.

6. Sam's priority nursing diagnosis at this time would be:
   a. Anxiety related to knowledge deficit about ECT
   b. High risk for injury related to risks associated with ECT
   c. Knowledge deficit related to negative media presentation of ECT·
   d. Altered thought processes related to side effects of ECT

7. The priority nursing intervention prior to initiation of Sam's therapy is to:
   a. Take vital signs and record
   b. Have the patient void
   c. Administer succinylcholine (Anectine)
   d. Ensure that consent form has been signed

8. Atropine sulfate is administered to Sam for what purpose?
   a. To alleviate anxiety
   b. To decrease secretions
   c. To relax muscles
   d. As a short-acting anesthetic

9. Succinylcholine (Anectine) is administered to Sam for what purpose?
   a. To alleviate anxiety
   b. To decrease secretions
   c. To relax muscles
   d. As a short-acting anesthetic

REFERENCES

Abrams, R. (1988). *Electroconvulsive therapy.* New York: Oxford University Press.

American Psychiatric Association. (1978). *Electroconvulsive therapy — Report of the task force on ECT.* Washington, DC: American Psychiatric Association.

Cherkin, A. (1974). Effects of flurothyl (Indoklon) upon memory in the chick. In M. Fink, Kety, S. and McGaugh, J. (Eds.), *Psychobiology of convulsive therapy.* New York: John Wiley & Sons.

Crowe, R. R. (1984, July 19). Electroconvulsive therapy — A current perspective. *N Engl J Med,* pp. 163–166.

Endler, N. S. & Persad, E. (1988). *Electroconvulsive therapy — The myths and the realities.* Toronto: Hans Huber Publishers.

Freeman, C. P. et al. (1980). ECT: Patients who complain. *Br J Psychiatry, 137,* pp. 17–25.

Kaplan, H. I. & Sadock, B. J. (1985). *Modern synopsis of comprehensive textbook of psychiatry* (4th ed.). Baltimore: Williams & Wilkins.

Kendell, R. E. (1981). The present status of electroconvulsive therapy. *Br J Psychiatry, 139*, pp. 265–283.

Sackeim, H. A. (1985, June). The case for ECT. *Psychology Today*, pp. 36–40.

Squire, L. R. (1977, September). ECT and memory loss. *Am J Psychiatry, 134*:9, pp. 997–1001.

Weiner, R. D. (1979). The psychiatric use of electrically induced seizures. *Am J Psychiatry, 136*, pp. 1507–1517.

Weiner, R. D., Rogers, H. J., Davidson, J. R., and Squire, L. R. (1986). Effects of stimulus parameters on cognitive side effects. *Ann NY Acad Sci, 462*, pp. 315–325.

BIBLIOGRAPHY

Culver, C. M. et al. (1980, May). ECT and special problems of informed consent. *Am J Psychiatry, 137*:5, pp. 586–591.

Fink, M. (1977, September). Myths of shock therapy. *Am J Psychiatry, 134*:9, pp. 991–996.

Fink, M. (1979). *Convulsive therapy: Theory and practice.* New York: Raven Press.

Fine, M. & Jenike, M. A. (1985, September). Electroshock—Exploding the myths. *RN*, pp. 58–66.

Fink, M., Kety, S. and McGaugh, J. (1974). *Psychobiology of convulsive therapy.* New York: John Wiley & Sons.

Frankel, F. H. (1977, September). Current perspectives on ECT: A discussion. *Am J Psychiatry, 134*:9, pp. 1014–1019.

Friedberg, J. (1977, September). Shock treatment, brain damage, and memory loss: A neurological perspective. *Am J Psychiatry, 134*:9, pp. 1010–1014.

Greenblatt, M. (1977, September). Efficacy of ECT in affective and schizophrenic illness. *Am J Psychiatry, 134*:9, pp. 1001–1005.

Mulaik, J. S. (1979, February). Nurses' questions about electroconvulsive therapy. *J Psychosoc Nurs*, pp. 15–19.

Rosenfeld, A. H. (1985, June). Depression: Dispelling despair. *Psychology Today*, pp. 29–34.

Salzman, C. (1977, September). ECT and ethical psychiatry. *Am J Psychiatry, 134*:9, pp. 1006–1009.

Yudofsky, S. C. (1982, July). Electroconvulsive therapy in the eighties: Technique and technologies. *Am J Psychotherapy, 36*:3, pp. 391–397.

BEHAVIOR THERAPY

KEY TERMS
classical conditioning
unconditioned response
conditioned response
unconditioned stimulus
conditioned stimulus
stimulus generalization
operant conditioning
positive reinforcement
negative reinforcement
aversive stimulus
discriminative stimulus
shaping
modeling
Premack principle
extinction
contingency contracting
token economy
time out
reciprocal inhibition
overt sensitization
covert sensitization
systematic desensitization
flooding

OBJECTIVES

After reading this chapter, the student will be able to:
1. Discuss the principles of classical and operant conditioning as foundations for behavior therapy.
2. Identify various techniques used in the modification of patient behavior.
3. Implement the principles of behavior therapy using the steps of the nursing process.

INTRODUCTION

A behavior is considered to be maladaptive when it is age-inappropriate, when it interferes with adaptive functioning, or when it is misunderstood by others in terms of cultural inappropriateness. The behavioral approach to therapy is that people have become what they are through learning processes, or more correctly, through the interaction of the environment with their genetic endowment (Chambless & Goldstein, 1979). The basic assumption is that problematic behaviors occur when there has been inadequate learning and therefore can be corrected through the provision of appropriate learning experiences. The principles of behavior therapy as we know it today are based upon the early studies of *classical conditioning* by Pavlov (1927) and *operant conditioning* by Skinner (1938).

CLASSICAL CONDITIONING

Classical conditioning is a process of learning that was introduced by the Russian physiologist Pavlov. In his experiments with dogs, during which he hoped to learn more about the digestive process, he inadvertently discovered that organisms can learn to respond in specific ways if they are conditioned to do so.

In his trials, he found that, as expected, the dogs salivated when they began to eat the food that was offered to them. This was a reflexive response that Pavlov called an *unconditioned response*. However, he also noticed that with time, the dogs began to salivate when the food came into their range of view, before it was even presented to them for consumption. Pavlov, concluding that this response was not reflexive but had been learned, called it a *conditioned response*. He carried the experiments even further by introducing an unrelated stimulus, one that had had no previous connection to the animal's food. He simultaneously presented the food with the sound of a bell. The animal responded with the expected reflexive salivation to the food. After a number of trials with the combined stimuli (food and bell), Pavlov found that the reflexive salivation began to occur when the dog was presented with the sound of the bell in the absence of food.

This was an important discovery in terms of how learning can occur. Pavlov found that unconditioned responses (salivation) occur in response to unconditioned stimuli (eating food). He also found that, over time, an unrelated stimulus (sound of the bell) introduced with the *unconditioned stimulus* can elicit the same response alone, that is, the conditioned response. The unrelated stimulus is called the *conditioned stimulus*. A graphic of Pavlov's classical conditioning model is presented in Figure 14.1. An example of the application of Pavlov's classical conditioning model to humans is shown in Figure 14.2. The process by which the fear response is elicited from similar stimuli (all individuals in white uniforms) is called *stimulus generalization*.

OPERANT CONDITIONING

The focus of operant conditioning differs from that of classical conditioning. With classical conditioning, the focus is on behavioral responses that are elicited by specific objects or events. With operant conditioning, additional attention is given to the consequences of the behavioral response.

Operant conditioning was introduced by Skinner (1938), an American psychologist whose work was largely influenced by Thorndike's (1911) law of effect, that is, that the connection between a stimulus and a response is strengthened or weakened by the consequences of the response. There are a number of terms that must be defined to understand the concept of operant conditioning.

Stimuli are environmental events that interact with and influence an individual's behavior. Stimuli may precede or follow a behavior. A stimulus that follows a behavior (or response) is called a reinforcing stimulus or *reinforcer*. The function is called *reinforcement*. When the reinforcing stimulus increases the probability that the behavior will recur, it is called a *positive reinforcer*. *Negative reinforcement* is increasing the probability that a behavior will recur by *removal* of an undesirable reinforcing stimulus. A stimulus that follows a behavioral response and decreases the probability that the behavior will recur is called an *aversive stimulus* or *punisher*. Examples of these reinforcing stimuli are presented in Table 14.1.

Sequences of Conditioning Operations:

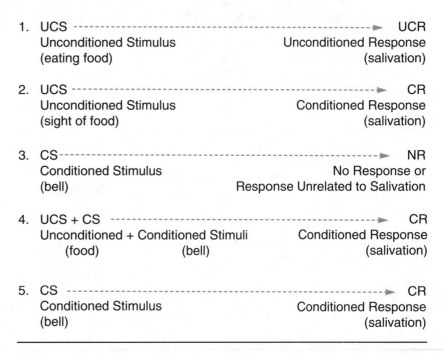

1. UCS --➤ UCR
   Unconditioned Stimulus   Unconditioned Response
   (eating food)   (salivation)

2. UCS --➤ CR
   Unconditioned Stimulus   Conditioned Response
   (sight of food)   (salivation)

3. CS --➤ NR
   Conditioned Stimulus   No Response or
   (bell)   Response Unrelated to Salivation

4. UCS + CS --➤ CR
   Unconditioned + Conditioned Stimuli   Conditioned Response
   (food)   (bell)   (salivation)

5. CS --➤ CR
   Conditioned Stimulus   Conditioned Response
   (bell)   (salivation)

Figure 14.1 Pavlov's model of classical conditioning.

Classic Conditioning and Stimulus Generalization

Subject: 6-month-old baby
Sequence of Conditioning Operations:

1. CS --➤ NR
   Conditioned Stimulus   No Response
   (Nurse A in white uniform walks into room)

2. UCS --➤ UCR
   Unconditioned Stimulus   Unconditioned Response
   (Nurse A in white uniform gives shot)   (Cries; clings to Mom)

3. CS --➤ CS
   Conditioned Stimulus   Conditioned Response
   (Nurse A in white uniform walks into room)   (Cries; clings to Mom)

4. CS --➤ CS
   Conditioned Stimulus   Conditioned Response
     (Nurse B in white uniform walks into room)   (Cries; clings to Mom)
     or:
   (Family friend comes to visit wearing white dress)

Figure 14.2 Example: classical conditioning and stimulus generalization.

Table 14.1 EXAMPLES OF REINFORCING STIMULI

Type	Stimulus	Behavioral Response	Reinforcing Stimulus
Positive	Messy Room	Child cleans her messy room	Child gets allowance for cleaning room
Negative	Messy Room	Child cleans her messy room	Child does not receive scolding from Mom
Aversive	Messy Room	Child does not clean her messy room	Child receives scolding from Mom

Stimuli that precede a behavioral response and predict that a particular reinforcement will occur are called *discriminative stimuli*. Discriminative stimuli are under the control of the individual. The individual is said to be able to *discriminate* between stimuli and to *choose* according to the type of reinforcement he or she has come to associate with a specific stimulus. Following is an example of the concept of discrimination.

Example

Mrs. M. was admitted to the hospital from a nursing home 2 weeks ago. She has no family, and no one visits her. She is very lonely. Nurse A and Nurse B have taken care of Mrs. M. on a regular basis during her hospital stay. When she is feeling particularly lonely, Mrs. M. calls Nurse A to her room, for she has learned that Nurse A will stay and talk to her for a while, but Nurse B only takes care of her physical needs and leaves. She no longer seeks out Nurse B for emotional support and comfort.

After several attempts, Mrs. M. is able to discriminate between stimuli. She can predict with assurance that calling Nurse A (and not Nurse B) will result in the reinforcement she desires.

TECHNIQUES FOR MODIFYING PATIENT BEHAVIOR

Shaping

In shaping the behavior of another, reinforcements are given for increasingly closer approximations to the desired response. For example, in training a mute child to talk, the teacher may first reward the child for (a) watching the teacher's lips, then (b) for making any sound in imitation of the teacher, then (c) for forming sounds similar to the word uttered by the teacher, and so on, until only correct imitations are rewarded (Chambless & Goldstein, 1979).

Modeling

Modeling refers to the learning of new behaviors by imitating the behavior in others. Models are more likely to be imitated when they are perceived as prestigious, influential, or physically attractive, and when the behavior is followed by positive reinforcement (Bandura, 1969). Modeling occurs in various ways. Children imitate the behavior patterns of their parents, teachers, friends, and others. Adults and children alike model many of their behaviors after individuals whom they observe on television and in movies. Unfortunately, modeling can result in maladaptive, as well as adaptive, behaviors.

In the practice setting, patients may imitate the behaviors of those practitioners who are charged with their care. This can occur naturally in the therapeutic community environment. It can also occur in a therapy session where the patient observes a model demonstrate appropriate behaviors in a role play of the patient's problem. The patient is then instructed to imitate the model's behaviors in a similar role play and is positively reinforced for appropriate imitation (Sundel & Sundel, 1982).

Premack Principle

This technique, named for its originator, states that a frequently occurring response (R_1) can serve as a positive reinforcement for a response (R_2) that occurs less frequently (Premack, 1959). This is accomplished by allowing R_1 to occur only after R_2 has been performed. For example, 13-year-old Jennie has been neglecting her homework for the past few weeks. She spends a lot of time on the tele-

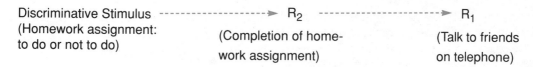

Figure 14.3 Example: premack principle.

phone talking to her friends. Applying the *Premack principle*, being allowed to talk on the telephone to her friends could serve as a positive reinforcement for completing her homework. A schematic of the Premack principle for this situation is presented in Figure 14.3.

Extinction

Extinction is the gradual decrease in frequency or disappearance of a response when the positive reinforcement is withheld. A classic example of this technique is its use with children who have temper tantrums. The tantrum behaviors continue as long as the parent gives attention to them but decrease and often disappear when the parent simply leaves the child alone in the room.

Contingency Contracting

With this technique, a contract is drawn up between all parties involved. The behavior change that is desired is stated, explicitly, in writing. The contract specifies the behavior change desired and the reinforcers to be given for performing the desired behaviors. The negative consequences or punishers that will be rendered for not fulfilling the terms of the contract are also delineated (Sundel & Sundel, 1982). The contract is specific about how reinforcers and punishment will be presented. However, flexibility is important so that renegotiations can occur if necessary.

Token Economy

Token economy is a type of contingency contracting (although there may or may not be a written and signed contract involved) in which the reinforcers for desired behaviors are presented in the form of *tokens*. Essential to this type of technique is the prior determination of items and situations of significance to the patient that can be em-

ployed as reinforcements. With this therapy, tokens are awarded when desired behaviors are performed and may be exchanged for designated privileges. For example, a patient may be able to "buy" a snack or cigarettes for 2 tokens, a trip to the coffee shop or library for 5 tokens, or even a trip outside the hospital (if that is a realistic possibility) for a designated number of tokens. The tokens themselves provide immediate positive feedback, and patients should be allowed to make the decision of whether to "spend" the token as soon as it is presented or to accumulate tokens that may be exchanged later for a more desirable reward.

Time Out

Time out is an aversive stimulus or punishment during which the patient is removed from the environment where the unacceptable behavior is being exhibited. The patient is usually isolated so that reinforcement from the attention of others is absent.

Reciprocal Inhibition

Also called counterconditioning, this technique serves to decrease or eliminate a behavior by introducing a more adaptive behavior, but one that is incompatible with the unacceptable behavior (Wolpe, 1958). An example is the introduction of relaxation exercises to an individual who is phobic. Relaxation is practiced in the presence of anxiety so that in time, the individual is able to manage the anxiety in the presence of the phobic stimulus by engaging in relaxation exercises. Relaxation and anxiety are incompatible behaviors.

Overt Sensitization

Overt sensitization is a type of aversion therapy that produces unpleasant consequences for undesirable behavior. For example, disulfiram (Antabuse) is a drug that is given to individuals who wish to stop drinking alcohol. If an individual consumes alcohol while on Antabuse therapy, symptoms of severe nausea and vomiting, dyspnea, palpitations, and headache will occur. Instead of the euphoric feeling normally experienced from the alcohol (the positive reinforcement for drinking), the individual receives a severe punishment that is intended to extinguish the unacceptable behavior (drinking alcohol).

Covert Sensitization

This aversion technique relies on the individual's imagination to produce unpleasant symptoms, rather than on medication. The technique is under the patient's control and can be used whenever and wherever it is required. The individual learns, through mental imagery, to visualize nauseating scenes and even to induce a mild feeling of nausea. This mental image is visualized when the individual is about to succumb to an attractive but undesirable behavior. It is most effective when paired with relaxation exercises that are performed instead of the undesirable behavior. The primary advantage of covert sensitization is that the individual does not have to perform the undesired behaviors but simply imagines them (Sundel & Sundel, 1982).

Systematic Desensitization

Systematic desensitization is a technique to assist individuals to overcome their fear of a phobic stimulus. It is "systematic" in that there is a hierarchy of anxiety-producing events through which the individual progresses during therapy. An example of a hierarchy of events associated with a fear of elevators may be as follows:

1. Discuss riding an elevator with the therapist.
2. Look at a picture of an elevator.
3. Walk into the lobby of a building and see the elevators.
4. Push the button for the elevator.
5. Walk into an elevator with a trusted person; disembark before doors close.
6. Walk into an elevator with a trusted person; allow doors to close; then open the doors and walk out.
7. Ride one floor with a trusted person, then walk back down the stairs.
8. Ride one floor with a trusted person and ride the elevator back down.
9. Ride elevator alone.

As each of these steps is attempted, it is paired with relaxation exercises as an antagonistic behavior to anxiety. Generally, the desensitization procedures occur in the therapy setting by instructing the patient to engage in relaxation exercises. When relaxation has been achieved, the patient uses mental imagery to visualize the step in the hierarchy being described by the therapist. If the patient becomes anxious, the therapist suggests relaxation exercises again and presents a scene that is lower in the hierarchy. Therapy continues until the individual is able to progress through the entire hierarchy with manageable anxiety. The effects of relaxation in the presence of imagined anxiety-producing stimuli have been found to transfer to the real situation, once the patient has achieved relaxation capable of suppressing or inhibiting anxiety responses (Sundel & Sundel, 1982). However, some patients are not successful in extinguishing phobic reactions through imagery. For these patients, *real-life desensitization* may be required. In these instances, the therapist arranges for the patient to be exposed to the hierarchy of steps in the desensitization process, but in real-life situations. Relaxation exercises may or may not be a part of real-life desensitization (Sherman, 1973).

Flooding

This technique, sometimes called *implosive therapy*, is also used to desensitize individuals to phobic stimuli. It differs from systematic desensitization in that, instead of working up a hierarchy of anxiety-producing stimuli, the individual is "flooded" with a continuous presentation (through mental imagery) of the phobic stimulus until it no longer elicits anxiety (Sundel & Sundel, 1982). Flooding is believed to produce results faster than systematic desensitization. However, some therapists report that patients are more likely to revert to previous phobic behaviors with flooding than with systematic desensitization (Mikulas, 1972). Some questions have also been raised in terms of the psychological discomfort that this therapy produces for the patient as well as the possibility of increased anxiety when faced with the phobic stimulus in real-life situations (Sundel & Sundel, 1982).

THE ROLE OF THE NURSE IN BEHAVIOR THERAPY

The nursing process is the vehicle for delivery of nursing care with the patient requiring assistance with behavior modification. The steps of the nursing process are illustrated in the following example case study.*

CASE STUDY

Assessment

Jordan, age 6, has been admitted to the child psychiatric unit following evaluation by a child psychiatrist. The parents' already shaky marriage was being severely tested by conflict over their son's behavior at home and at school. The mother complained bitterly that the father, frequently away from home on business, "overindulged" their son. In point of fact, the son would argue and throw temper tantrums and insist on continuing games, books, and so forth, whenever his father put him to bed, so that a 7:30 PM bedtime was delayed until 10:30, 11:00, or even 11:30 at night. Similarly, the father had been known to cook four or five different meals for his son's dinner if Jordan stubbornly insisted that he would not eat what had been prepared. At school, several teachers had complained that the child was stubborn and spiteful, often spoke out of turn, and refused to comply with classroom rules.

On questioning by the psychiatric nurse, the parents denied that their son had ever been destructive of property, lied excessively, or stolen. When interviewed, the child was observed to be cheerful and able to sit quietly in his chair, listening attentively to the questions that were asked of him. His answers, however, were brief, and he tended to minimize the extent of the problems he was having with his parents and teachers.

During his first 3 days on the unit, the following assessments were made:

1. Jordan loses his temper when he cannot have his way. He screams, stomps his feet, and sometimes kicks the furniture.
2. Jordan refuses to follow directions given by staff. He merely responds, "No, I won't."
3. Jordan likes to engage in behaviors that annoy the staff and other children: belching loudly, scraping his fingernails across the blackboard, making loud noises when the other children are trying to watch television, opening his mouth when it is full of food.
4. Jordan blames others when he makes a mistake. He spilled his milk at lunchtime while racing to get to a spe-

cific seat he knew Tony wanted. He blamed the accident on Tony saying, "He made me do it! He tripped me!"

Upon completion of the initial assessments, the psychiatrist diagnosed Jordan with oppositional defiant disorder.

Analysis

Nursing diagnoses and goals for Jordan include:

Nursing Diagnoses	Goals
Noncompliance with therapy	Patient will participate in and cooperate during therapeutic activities.
Defensive coping	Patient will accept responsibility for own behaviors and interact with others without becoming defensive.
Impaired social interaction	Patient will be able to interact with staff and peers using age-appropriate, acceptable behaviors.

Planning/Intervention

A contract for Jordan's care was drawn up by the admitting nurse and others on the treatment team. Jordan's contact was based on a system of token economies. He discussed with the nurse the kinds of privileges he would like to earn. They included:

Getting to wear his own clothes (5 tokens)
Having a can of pop for a snack (2 tokens)
Getting to watch 30 minutes of TV (5 tokens)
Getting to stay up later on Friday nights with the other patients (7 tokens)
Getting to play with the video games (3 tokens)
Getting to walk with the nurse to the gift shop to spend some of his money (8 tokens)
Getting to talk to his parents/grandparents on the phone (5 tokens)
Getting to go on the outside therapeutic recreation activities, for example, movies, zoo, picnics (10 tokens)

Tokens were awarded for appropriate behaviors:

Gets out of bed when the nurse calls him (1 token)
Gets dressed for breakfast (1 token)
Presents himself for *all* meals in an appropriate manner, that is, no screaming, no belching, no opening his mouth when it is full of food, no throwing of food, staying in his chair during the meal, putting his tray away in the appropriate place when he is finished (2 tokens × 3 meals = 6 tokens)

---

*Adapted from Spitzer, R. L. et al. (1989).

Completes hygiene activities (1 token)

Accepts blame for own mistakes (1 token)

Does not fight; uses no obscene language; does not "sass" staff (1 token)

Remains quiet while others are watching TV (1 token)

Participates and is not disruptive in unit meetings and group therapy sessions (2 tokens)

Displays no temper tantrums (1 token)

Follows unit rules (1 token)

Goes to bed at designated hour without opposition (1 token)

Tokens are awarded at bedtime for absence of inappropriate behaviors during the day. For example, if Jordan has no temper tantrums during the day, he is awarded 1 token. Likewise, if Jordan *has* a temper tantrum (or exhibits other inappropriate behavior), he must pay back the token amount designated for that behavior. No other attention is given to inappropriate behaviors other than withholding and payback of tokens.

EXCEPTION: If Jordan is receiving reinforcement from peers for inappropriate behaviors, staff has the option of imposing time out or isolation until the behavior is extinguished.

The contract may be renegotiated at any time between Jordan and staff. Additional privileges or responsibilities may be added as they develop and are deemed appropriate.

All staff are consistent with the terms of the contract and do not allow Jordan to manipulate. There are no exceptions without renegotiation of the contract.

NOTE: Parents meet with the social worker from the treatment team on a regular basis. Effective parenting techniques are discussed as well as other problems identified within the marriage relationship. Parenting instruction coordinates with the pattern of behavior modification Jordan is receiving on the psychiatric unit. The importance of follow-through is stressed, along with strong encouragement that the parents manifest a united front in the disciplining of Jordan. Oppositional behaviors are nurtured by divided management.

Evaluation

In this step of the nursing process, a determination must be made if the goals of Jordan's care have been achieved. Outcome criteria might include that the patient:

- Participates in and cooperates during therapeutic activities
- Follows the rules of the unit (including mealtimes, hygiene, bedtimes) without opposition
- Accepts responsibility for own mistakes
- Does not become defensive when asked to complete a task
- Does not interrupt when others are talking or make noise in situations where quiet is in order
- Does not try to manipulate the staff

- Expresses anger appropriately without tantrum behaviors
- Expresses desire to form social relationships and demonstrates acceptable behavior in interactions with peers

SUMMARY

The basic assumption of behavior therapy is that problematic behaviors occur when there has been inadequate learning and, therefore, can be corrected through the provision of appropriate learning experiences. The antecedents of today's principles of behavior therapy are largely the products of laboratory efforts by Pavlov and Skinner.

Pavlov introduced a process that came to be known as classical conditioning. He demonstrated in his trials with laboratory animals that a neutral stimulus could acquire the ability to elicit a conditioned response through pairing with an unconditioned stimulus. Previous responses had been reflexive in nature. Pavlov considered the conditioned response to be a new, learned response.

Skinner, in his model of operant conditioning, gave additional attention to the consequences of the response as an approach to learning new behaviors. His work was largely influenced by Thorndike's law of effect, that is, that the connection between a stimulus and a response is strengthened or weakened by the consequences of the response.

Various techniques for modifying patient behavior have been applied. Those most widely used include shaping, modeling, the Premack principle, extinction, contingency contracting, token economy, time out, reciprocal inhibition, overt and covert sensitization, systematic desensitization, and flooding.

Nurses are important members of the treatment team in the implementation of behavior therapy. Because nurses are the only members of the team who manage patient behavior on a 24-hour basis, it is essential that they have input into the treatment plan. The nursing process provides a systematic method of directing care for patients who need assistance with modification of maladaptive behaviors. It is a dynamic process that allows each plan of care to be individualized for the personal requirements of each patient.

REVIEW QUESTIONS
Self-Examination/Learning Exercise

Select the correct answer for each of the following questions:

1. A positive reinforcer:
   a. Increases the probability that a behavior will recur
   b. Decreases the probability that a behavior will recur
   c. Has nothing to do with modifying behavior
   d. Always results in positive behavior

2. A negative reinforcer:
   a. Increases the probability that a behavior will recur
   b. Decreases the probability that a behavior will recur
   c. Has nothing to do with modifying behavior
   d. Always results in unacceptable behavior

3. An aversive stimulus or punisher:
   a. Increases the probability that a behavior will recur
   b. Decreases the probability that a behavior will recur
   c. Has nothing to do with modifying behavior
   d. Always results in unacceptable behavior

Situation: B.J. has been out with his friends. He is late getting home. He knows his wife will be angry and will yell at him for being late. He stops at the florist's and buys a dozen red roses for her. The following three questions are related to this situation.

4. Which of the following behaviors represents positive reinforcement on the part of the wife?
   a. She meets him at the door, accepts the roses, and says nothing further about his being late.
   b. She meets him at the door, yelling that he is late, and makes him spend the night on the couch.
   c. She meets him at the door, expresses delight with the roses, and kisses him on the cheek.
   d. She meets him at the door and says, "How could you? You know I'm allergic to roses!"

5. Which of the following behaviors represents negative reinforcement on the part of the wife?
   a. She meets him at the door, accepts the roses, and says nothing further about his being late.
   b. She meets him at the door, yelling that he is late, and makes him spend the night on the couch.
   c. She meets him at the door, expresses delight with the roses, and kisses him on the cheek.
   d. She meets him at the door and says, "How could you? You know I'm allergic to roses!"

6. Which of the following behaviors represents an aversive stimulus on the part of the wife?
   a. She meets him at the door, accepts the roses, and says nothing further about his being late.
   b. She meets him at the door, yelling that he is late, and makes him spend the night on the couch.

    c. She meets him at the door, expresses delight with the roses, and kisses him on the cheek.

    d. She meets him at the door and says, "How could you? You know I'm allergic to roses!"

7. Fourteen-year-old Sally has been spending many hours after school watching TV. She has virtually stopped practicing her piano lessons. Her parents have told her that she may watch TV only after she has practiced the piano for 1 hour. This is an example of which behavior modification technique?
   a. Shaping
   b. Extinction
   c. Contingency contracting
   d. The Premack principle

8. Nancy has a fear of dogs. In helping her overcome this fear, the therapist is using systematic desensitization. List the following steps in the hierarchial order that the therapist would proceed.
   a. Look at a real dog.
   b. Look at a stuffed toy dog.
   c. Pet a real dog.
   d. Pet the stuffed toy dog.
   e. Walk past a real dog.
   f. Look at a picture of a dog.

REFERENCES

Bandura, A. (1969). *Principles of behavior modification.* New York: Holt, Rinehart & Winston.

Chambless, D. L. & Goldstein, A. J. (1979). Behavioral psychotherapy. In *Current psychotherapies* (2nd ed.). Itasca, IL: FE Peacock Publishers, Inc.

Mikulas, W. L. (1972). *Behavior modification: An overview.* New York: Harper & Row.

Pavlov, I. P. (1927). *Conditioned reflexes.* London: Oxford University Press.

Premack, D. (1959). Toward empirical behavior laws: I. Positive reinforcement. *Psychol Rev 66*, 219–233.

Sherman, R. A. (1973). *Behavior modification: Theory and practice.* Monterey, CA: Brooks/Cole Publishing Co.

Skinner, B. F. (1938). *The behavior of organisms.* New York: Appleton-Century-Crofts.

Spitzer, R. L., Gibbon, M., Skodol, A. E., Williams, J. B. W., and First, M. B. (1989). *DSM-III-R casebook.* Washington, DC: American Psychiatric Press, Inc.

Sundel, M. & Sundel, S. S. (1982). *Behavior modification in the human services: A systematic introduction to concepts and applications* (2nd ed.). Englewood Cliffs, NJ: Prentice-Hall.

Thorndike, E. L. (1911). *Animal intelligence.* New York: Macmillan.

Wolpe, J. (1958). *Psychotherapy by reciprocal inhibition.* Stanford, CA: Stanford University Press.

BIBLIOGRAPHY

Berni, R. & Fordyce, W. E. (1973). *Behavior modification and the nursing process.* St. Louis: CV Mosby.

Hersen, M. & Last, C. G. (1985). *Behavior therapy casebook.* New York: Springer.

Kaplan, H. I. & Sadock, B. J. (1988). *Modern synopsis of comprehensive textbook of psychiatry* (4th ed.). Baltimore: Williams & Wilkins.

Lebow, M. D. (1973). *Behavior modification: A significant method in nursing practice.* Englewood Cliffs, NJ: Prentice-Hall.

Loomis, M. E. & Horsley, J. A. (1974). *Interpersonal change: A behavioral approach to nursing practice.* New York: McGraw-Hill.

Skinner, B. F. (1953). *Science and human behavior.* New York: The Macmillan Company.

Wenrich, W. W. (1970). *A primer of behavior modification.* Belmont, CA: Wadsworth Publishing.

Yates, A. J. (1970). *Behavior therapy.* New York: John Wiley & Sons.

NURSING CARE OF PATIENTS WITH ALTERATIONS IN PSYCHOSOCIAL ADAPTATION

15

DISORDERS USUALLY FIRST EVIDENT IN INFANCY, CHILDHOOD, OR ADOLESCENCE

OBJECTIVES
After reading this chapter, the student will be able to:
1. Identify psychiatric disorders usually first evident in infancy, childhood, or adolescence.
2. Discuss predisposing factors implicated in the etiology of mental

retardation, autistic disorder, behavior disorders, anxiety disorders of childhood/adolescence, eating disorders, and gender identity disorders.
3. Identify symptomatology and use the information in the assessment of patients with the above disorders.
4. Identify nursing diagnoses common to patients with these disorders and select appropriate nursing interventions for each.
5. Discuss relevant criteria for evaluating nursing care of patients with selected infant, childhood, and adolescent psychiatric disorders.
6. Describe various treatment modalities relevant to care of patients with these disorders.

INTRODUCTION

This chapter deals with various disorders in which the symptoms usually first become evident during infancy, childhood, or adolescence. That is not to say that some of the disorders discussed in this chapter do not appear later in life or that symptoms associated with other disorders, such as major depression or schizophrenia, do not appear in childhood or adolescence. The basic concepts of care are applied to treatment in those instances, with consideration for the variances in age and developmental level.

Developmental theories were discussed at length in Chapter 3. Any nurse working with children or adolescents should be knowledgeable regarding "normal" stages of growth and development. In any case, the developmental process is one that is fraught with frustrations and difficulties at best. Behavioral responses are individual and idiosyncratic. They are, indeed, *human* responses.

Whether or not a child's behavior is indicative of emotional problems is often difficult to determine. The *Diagnostic and Statistical Manual of Mental Disorders (DSM-III-R)* (American Psychiatric Association [APA], 1987) includes the following criteria among many of its diagnostic categories. An emotional problem exists if the behavioral manifestations:

1. Are not age appropriate
2. Deviate from cultural norms
3. Create deficits or impairments in adaptive functioning

This chapter will focus on the nursing process in care of patients with developmental disorders, disruptive behavior disorders, anxiety disorders of childhood/adolescence, eating disorders, and gender identity disorders.

DEVELOPMENTAL DISORDERS

Mental Retardation

Mental retardation is defined by deficits in general intellectual functioning and adaptive functioning (APA, 1987). General intellectual functioning is measured by an individual's performance on intelligence quotient (IQ) tests. Adaptive functioning refers to the person's ability to adapt to the requirements of daily living and the expectations of his or her age and cultural group. The *DSM-III-R* diagnostic criteria for mental retardation are presented in Table 15.1.

Table 15.1 DIAGNOSTIC CRITERIA FOR MENTAL RETARDATION
A. Significantly subaverage general intellectual functioning: an IQ of 70 or less on an individually administered IQ test (for infants, a clinical judgment of significantly subaverage intellectual functioning, since available intelligence tests do not yield numerical IQ values).
B. Concurrent deficits or impairments in adaptive functioning, that is, the person's effectiveness in meeting the standards expected for his or her age by his or her cultural group in areas such as social skills and responsibility, communication, daily living skills, personal independence, and self-sufficiency.
C. Onset before the age of 18.

Source: From APA, (1987) with permission.

PREDISPOSING FACTORS

The *DSM-III-R* (APA, 1987) states that the etiology of mental retardation may be primarily biologic, psychosocial, or a combination of both. In approximately 30% of cases seen clinically, the etiology cannot be determined. Five major causes have been implicated as etiological factors in the remaining 70% of cases of mental retardation.

Heredity Factors Heredity factors are implicated as the cause in approximately 5% of the cases. These include inborn errors of metabolism, such as Tay-Sachs disease, phenylketonuria, and hyperglycinemia. Also included are chromosomal disorders, such as Down's syndrome and Klinefelter's syndrome, and single-gene abnormalities, such as tuberous sclerosis and neurofibromatosis.

Prenatal Factors Prenatal factors that result in early alterations in embryonic development account for 30% of mental retardation cases. Damages may occur in response to toxicity associated with maternal ingestion of alcohol or other drugs. Maternal illnesses and infections during pregnancy (e.g., rubella and cytomegalovirus) can also result in congenital mental retardation, as can complications of pregnancy, such as toxemia and uncontrolled diabetes (Kaplan & Sadock, 1985).

Perinatal Factors Approximately 10% of cases of mental retardation are the result of trauma or complications of the birth process that deprive the infant of oxygen, causing damage to the brain. Examples include trauma to the head incurred during the process of birth, placenta previa or premature separation of the placenta, and prolapse of the cord. Prematurity has also been associated with higher risk for mental retardation.

Postnatal Factors These conditions encountered in childhood account for approximately 5% of cases of mental retardation. They include infections, such as meningitis and encephalitis; poisonings, such as from insecticides, medications, and lead; and physical traumas, such as head injuries, asphyxiation, and hyperpyrexia (Scipien et al, 1975).

Social, Cultural, and Environmental Factors Approximately 20% of cases of mental retardation are attributed to deprivation of nurturance and social stimulation (APA, 1987). Nutritional deficiencies have also been implicated (Scipien et al, 1975).

Recognition of the cause and period of inception provides information regarding what to expect in terms of behavior and potential. However, each child is different, and consideration must be given on an individual basis in every case.

APPLICATION OF THE NURSING PROCESS

Background Assessment Data (Symptomatology) Degree of severity of mental retardation is identified by IQ level. Four levels have been delineated: mild, moderate, severe, and profound. Various behavioral manifestations and abilities are associated with each of these levels of retardation. They are outlined in Table 15.2.

Nurses should assess and focus upon each patient's strengths and individual abilities. Knowledge regarding level of independence in the performance of self-care activities is essential to the development of an adequate plan for the provision of nursing care.

Nursing Diagnoses Selection of appropriate nursing diagnoses for the patient with mental retardation will be largely dependent on the degree of severity of the condition and the capabilities of the patient. Possible nursing diagnoses include:

High risk for injury related to altered physical mobility or aggressive behavior
Self-care deficit related to altered physical mobility or lack of maturity
Impaired verbal communication related to developmental alteration
Impaired social interaction related to speech deficiencies or difficulty adhering to conventional social behavior
Altered growth and development related to isolation from significant others; inadequate environmental stimulation; hereditary factors
Anxiety (moderate to severe) related to hospitalization and absence of familiar surroundings
Defensive coping related to feelings of powerlessness and threat to self-esteem
Ineffective individual coping related to inadequate coping skills secondary to developmental delay

Nursing diagnoses for the patient with mental retardation are by no means limited to those listed here. Each individual must be assessed and the data analyzed on an individual basis. There are, however, some commonalities that are identifiable and useful in the planning of nursing care.

Table 15.2 DEVELOPMENTAL CHARACTERISTICS OF MENTAL RETARDATION BY DEGREE OF SEVERITY

Level (IQ)	Ability to Perform Self-Care Activities	Cognitive/Educational Capabilities	Social/Communication Capabilities	Psychomotor Capabilities
Mild (50–70)	Capable of independent living, with assistance during times of stress.	Capable of academic skills to 6th grade level. As adult can achieve vocational skills for minimum self support.	Capable of developing social skills. Functions well in a structured, sheltered setting.	Psychomotor skills usually not affected, although may have some slight problems with coordination.
Moderate (35–49)	Can perform some activities independently. Requires supervision.	Capable of academic skill to 2nd grade level. As adult may be able to contribute to own support in sheltered workshop.	May experience some limitation in speech communication. Difficulty adhering to social convention may interfere with peer relationships.	Motor development is fair. Vocational capabilities may be limited to unskilled gross motor activities.
Severe (20–34)	May be trained in elementary hygiene skills. Requires complete supervision.	Unable to benefit from academic or vocational training. Profits from systematic habit training.	Minimal verbal skills. Wants and needs often communicated by acting-out behaviors.	Poor psychomotor development. Only able to perform simple tasks under close supervision.
Profound (Below 20)	No capacity for independent functioning. Requires constant aid and supervision.	Unable to profit from academic or vocational training. May respond to minimal training in self-help if presented in the close context of a one-to-one relationship.	Little, if any, speech development. No capacity for socialization skills.	Lack of ability for both fine and gross motor movements. Requires constant supervision and care. May be associated with other physical disorders.

Sources: Adapted from APA (1987); Kaplan and Sadock (1985).

Planning/Implementation   Table 15.3 provides a plan of care for the mentally retarded child using selected nursing diagnoses, goals of care, and appropriate nursing interventions for each. Rationale is provided in italics.

Although this plan of care is directed toward the individual patient, it is essential that family members or primary caregivers participate in the ongoing care of the mentally retarded patient. They need to receive information regarding the scope of the condition, realistic expectations and patient potentials, methods for modifying behavior as required, and community resources from which they may seek assistance and support.

Evaluation   Evaluation of care given to the mentally retarded patient should reflect positive behavioral changes. Evaluation is accomplished by determining if the goals of care have been met through implementation of the nursing actions selected. The nurse reassesses the plan and makes changes where required. Reassessment data may include information gathered by asking the following questions:

Have nursing actions providing for patient safety been sufficient to prevent injury? Have all of the patient's self-care needs been fulfilled? Can he or she fulfill some of these needs independently? Has the patient been able to communicate needs and desires so that he or she can be understood? Has the patient learned to interact with others in an appropriate manner? When regressive behaviors surface, can the patient accept constructive feedback and discontinue the inappropriate behavior? Has anxiety been maintained at a manageable level? Has patient learned new coping skills through behavior modification? Does patient demonstrate evidence

Table 15.3 CARE PLAN FOR MENTALLY RETARDED CHILD

Nursing Diagnoses	Objectives	Nursing Interventions
High risk for injury related to altered physical mobility of aggressive behavior	Patient will not experience injury.	Create a safe environment for the patient. Ensure that small items are removed from area where patient will be ambulating and that sharp items are out of reach. Store items that patient uses frequently within easy reach. Pad siderails and headboard of patient with history of seizures. Prevent physical aggression and acting out behaviors by learning to recognize signs that patient is becoming agitated. *Patient safety is a nursing priority.*
Self-care deficit related to altered physical mobility or lack of maturity	Patient will be able to participate in aspects of self-care.	Identify aspects of self-care that may be within the patient's capabilities. Work on one aspect of self-care at a time. Provide simple, concrete explanations. Offer positive feedback for efforts. *Positive reinforcement enhances self-esteem and encourages repetition of desirable behaviors.* When one aspect of self-care has been mastered to the best of the patient's ability, move on to another. Encourage independence but intervene when patient is unable to perform. *Patient comfort and safety are nursing priorities.*
Impaired verbal communication related to developmental alteration	Patient will be able to communicate needs and desires to staff.	Maintain consistency of staff assignment over time. *This facilitates trust and the ability to understand patient's actions and communication.* Anticipate and fulfill patient's needs until satisfactory communication patterns are established. Learn (from family, if possible) special words patient uses that are different from the norm. Identify nonverbal gestures or signals that patient may use to convey needs if verbal communication is absent. Practice these communication skills over and over. *Some mentally retarded children, particularly at the severe level, can only learn by systematic habit training.*
Impaired social interaction related to speech deficiencies or difficulty adhering to conventional social behavior	Patient will be able to interact with others using behaviors that are socially acceptable and appropriate to developmental level.	Remain with patient during initial interactions with others on the unit. *Presence of a trusted individual provides a feeling of security.* Explain to other patients the meaning behind some of patient's nonverbal gestures and signals. Use simple language to explain to patient which behaviors are acceptable and which are not. Establish a procedure for behavior modification that offers rewards for appropriate behaviors and renders punishment in response to the use of inappropriate behaviors. *Positive, negative and aversive reinforcements can contribute to desired changes in behavior.* Those privileges and penalties are individually determined as staff learns the likes and dislikes of the patient.

of increased self-esteem due to the accomplishment of these new skills and adaptive behaviors? Have primary caregivers been taught realistic expectations of patient's behavior and methods for attempting to modify unacceptable behaviors? Have primary caregivers been given information regarding various resources from which they can seek assistance and support within the community?

Autistic Disorder

Autistic disorder is characterized by a withdrawal of the child into the self and into a fantasy world of his or her own creation. The child has marked impairments in the ability to interact with others, in interpersonal communication, and in imaginative play. Activities and interests are restricted and may be considered somewhat bizarre.

The disorder is relatively rare and occurs three to five times more often in the male than in the female population. In most cases, the disorder runs a chronic course, with symptoms persisting into adulthood. The *DSM-III-R* further categorizes the disorder by age of the child at the onset of symptoms:

1. Infantile onset (before 36 months of age)
2. Childhood onset (after 36 months of age)

PREDISPOSING FACTORS

Although the exact underlying pathology associated with autistic disorder is unknown, several theories have evolved that speculate about etiology. Attention has been focused on the relationship between autistic children and their social environment and basic biological factors (Schreibman & Charlop, 1989).

Social Environment The proponents of this theory suggest that autistic disorder is caused by the parents and the social environment they provide. Some of the specific causative factors proposed in these theories are parental rejection, child responses to deviant parental personality characteristics, family breakup, family stress, insufficient stimulation, and faulty communication patterns (Schreibman & Charlop, 1989).

One of the first theorists to espouse this view was Kanner (1973). In his studies, he described the parents of autistic children as well-educated upper-class individuals, involved in careers and intellectual pursuits, who were aloof, obsessive, and emotionally cold. The term *refrigerator parents* was coined to describe their lack of warmth and affectionate behavior. However, because Kanner's studies also showed that many parents of autistic children also have children without the disorder, and other parents who could be described as cold and aloof produce no autistic children, he came to believe that autistic disorder has no single cause. He believed that children must have a predisposing biologic condition that combines with the unfavorable social environment and gives rise to the autistic behavior.

Mahler and associates (1975) suggested that the autistic child is fixed in the presymbiotic phase of development. In this phase, the child creates a barrier between self and others. The normal symbiotic relationship between mother and child, followed by the progression to separation/individuation, does not occur. Ego development is inhibited, and the child fails to achieve a sense of self.

Biological Factors

Genetics Recent research has revealed strong evidence that genetic factors may play a significant role in the etiology of autism (Schreibman & Charlop, 1989). Some studies have shown that siblings of autistic children have a 50 times greater chance of being autistic than the general population. Studies with both monozygotic and dizygotic twins have provided strong evidence of a genetic involvement. The understanding of how genetic factors influence the development of autistic disorder has only just begun. Future research is indicated to delineate these factors more clearly.

Neurological Factors The *DSM-III-R* (APA, 1987) identifies various conditions that cause brain dysfunction as possible contributors in the predisposition to autistic disorder. They include maternal rubella, untreated phenylketonuria, tuberous sclerosis, anoxia during birth, encephalitis, infantile spasms, and fragile X syndrome. Schreibman and Charlop (1989) describe various other diseases and syndromes that affect the central nervous system and may be implicated in the etiology of autistic disorder. These include mental retardation, retrolental fibroplasia, congenital syphilis, neurolipidosis, epilepsy, congenital rubella, Down's syndrome, hydrocephaly, and microencephaly. A number of studies are currently being investigated that relate autistic disorder to structural or functional abnormalities of the brain.

APPLICATION OF THE NURSING PROCESS

Background Assessment Data (Symptomatology)

Impairment in Social Interaction Autistic children do not form interpersonal relationships with others. They do not respond to, or show interest in, people. As infants, they may have an aversion to affection and physical contact. As toddlers, the attachment to a significant adult may be either absent or manifested as exaggerated adherence behaviors. In childhood, there is failure to develop cooperative play, imaginative play, and friendships. Those children with minimal handicaps may eventually progress to the point of recognizing other children as part of their environment, if only in a passive manner (APA, 1987).

Impairment in Communication and Imaginative Activity Both verbal and nonverbal skills are affected. Language may be totally absent, or characterized by immature structure or idiosyncratic utterances whose meaning is clear only to those who are familiar with the child's past experiences. Nonverbal communication, for example, facial expression and gesture, is absent or minimal or, if present, is socially inappropriate in form (APA, 1987). The child does not participate in imaginative activities or fantasy ("pretend") play.

Restricted Activities and Interests Even minor changes in the environment are often met with resistance or sometimes with hysterical responses. Attachment to, or extreme fascination with, objects that move or spin (e.g., fans) is common. Routine may become an obsession, with minor alterations in routine leading to marked distress. Stereotyped body movements (hand clapping, rocking, whole-body swaying) and verbalizations (repetition of words or phrases) are typical. Diet abnormalities may include eating only a few specific foods or consuming an excessive amount of fluids. Behaviors that are self-injurious, such as head banging or biting the hands or arms, may be evident.

The *DSM-III-R* (APA, 1987) diagnostic criteria for autistic disorder are presented in Table 15.4.

Nursing Diagnoses Based upon data collected during the nursing assessment, possible nursing diagnoses for the patient with autistic disorder include:

> High risk for self-mutilation related to lack of nurturing; neurological alterations
>
> Impaired social interaction related to lack of nurturing; inability to trust; neurological alterations
>
> Impaired verbal communication related to withdrawal into the self; inadequate sensory stimulation; neurological alterations
>
> Personal identity disturbance related to fixation in presymbiotic phase of development; lack of nurturing; inadequate sensory stimulation

Planning/Implementation Table 15.5 provides a plan of care for the child with autistic disorder using selected nursing diagnoses, goals of care, and appropriate nursing interventions for each. Rationale is provided in italics.

Evaluation Evaluation of care for the autistic child reflects whether or not the nursing actions have been effective in achieving the established goals. The nursing process calls for reassessment of the plan. Questions for gathering reassessment data may include:

Has the child been able to establish trust with at least *one* caregiver? Have the nursing actions directed toward preventing mutilative behaviors been effective in protecting the patient from self-harm? Has the child attempted to interact with others? Has he or she received positive reinforcement for these efforts? Has eye contact improved? Has the child established a means of communicating his or her needs/desires to others? Have all self-care needs been met? Does the child demonstrate an awareness of self as separate from others? Can he or she name own body parts and body parts of caregiver? Can he or she accept touch from others? Does he or she willingly and appropriately touch others?

DISRUPTIVE BEHAVIOR DISORDERS

These disorders are characterized by behavior that is socially disruptive and inappropriate. They generally create more distress for others than they do for the individuals manifesting the maladaptive behaviors. The disorders in this category include attention-deficit hyperactivity disorder (ADHD),

Table 15.4 DIAGNOSTIC CRITERIA FOR AUTISTIC DISORDER

At least 8 of the following 16 items are present, these to include at least 2 items from A, 1 from B, and 1 from C.

A. Qualitative impairment in reciprocal social interaction as manifested by the following:
 1. Marked lack of awareness of the existence or feelings of others (e.g., treats a person as if he or she were a piece of furniture; does not notice another person's distress; apparently has no concept of the need of others for privacy)
 2. No or abnormal seeking of comfort at times of distress (e.g., does not come for comfort even when ill, hurt, or tired; seeks comfort in a stereotyped way, for example, says "cheese, cheese, cheese" whenever hurt)
 3. No or impaired imitation (e.g., does not wave bye-bye; does not copy mother's domestic activities; mechanical imitation of others' actions out of context)
 4. No or abnormal social play (e.g., does not actively participate in simple games; prefers solitary play activities; involves other children in play only as "mechanical aids")
 5. Gross impairment in ability to make peer friendships (e.g., no interest in making peer friendships; despite interest in making friends, demonstrates lack of understanding of conventions of social interaction (e.g., reads phone book to uninterested peer)

B. Qualitative impairment in verbal and nonverbal communication, and in imaginative activity as manifested by the following:
 1. No mode of communication, such as communicative babbling, facial expression, gesture, mime, or spoken language
 2. Markedly abnormal nonverbal communication, as in the use of eye-to-eye gaze, facial expression, body posture, or gestures to initiate or modulate social interaction (e.g., does not anticipate being held, stiffens when held, does not look at the person or smile when making a social approach, does not greet parents or visitors, has a fixed stare in social situations)
 3. Absence of imaginative activity, such as playacting of adult roles, fantasy characters, or animals; lack of interest in stories about imaginary events
 4. Marked abnormalities in the production of speech, including volume, pitch, stress, rate, rhythm, and intonation (e.g., monotonous tone, questionlike melody, or high pitch)
 5. Marked abnormalities in the form or content of speech, including stereotyped and repetitive use of speech (e.g., immediate echolalia or mechanical repetition of television commercial); use of "you" when "I" is meant (e.g., using "You want cookie?" to mean "I want a cookie"); idiosyncratic use of words or phrases (e.g., "Go on green riding" to mean "I want to go on the swing"); or frequent irrelevant remarks (e.g., starts talking about train schedules during a conversation about sports)
 6. Marked impairment in the ability to initiate or sustain a conversation with others, despite adequate speech (e.g., indulging in lengthy monologues on one subject regardless of interjections from others)

C. Markedly restricted repertoire of activities and interests as manifested by the following:
 1. Stereotyped body movements (e.g., hand flicking or hand twisting, spinning, head banging, or complex whole-body movements)
 2. Persistent preoccupation with parts of objects (e.g., sniffing or smelling objects, repetitive feeling of texture of materials, spinning wheels of toy cars) or attachment to unusual objects (e.g., insists on carrying around a piece of string)
 3. Marked distress over changes in trivial aspects of environment (e.g., when a vase is moved from usual position)
 4. Unreasonable insistence on following routines in precise detail (e.g., insisting that exactly the same route always be followed when shopping)
 5. Markedly restricted range of interests and a preoccupation with one narrow interest (e.g., interested only in lining up objects, in amassing facts about meteorology, or in pretending to be a fantasy character)

D. Onset during infancy or childhood

Source: From APA (1987) with permission.

oppositional defiant disorder, and conduct disorder.

Attention-Deficit Hyperactivity Disorder

The essential features of this disorder are developmentally inappropriate degrees of inattention, impulsiveness, and hyperactivity (APA, 1987).

These children are highly distractible and unable to contain stimuli. Motor activity is excessive and movements are random and impulsive. In approximately half of the cases, onset of the disorder is before age 4, but frequently the disorder is not recognized until the child enters school. It is six to nine times more common in the male than in the female population, and may occur in as many as 3% of children.

Table 15.5   CARE PLAN FOR CHILD WITH AUTISTIC DISORDER

Nursing Diagnoses	Objectives	Nursing Interventions
High risk for self-mutilation related to lack of nurturing; neurological alterations	Patient will not harm self.	Work with the child on a one-to-one basis to *establish trust.* Try to determine if the self-mutilative behavior occurs in response to increasing anxiety, and if so, to what the anxiety may be attributed. *Mutilative behaviors may be averted if the cause can be determined.* Try to intervene with diversion or replacement activities and offer self to the child as anxiety level starts to rise. *These activities may provide needed feelings of security and substitute for self-mutilative behaviors.* Protect the child when self-mutilative behaviors occur. Devices such as a helmet, padded hand mitts, or arm covers may *provide protection when the potential for self-harm exists.*
Impaired social interaction related to lack of nurturing; inability to trust; neurological alterations	Patient will initiate social interactions with caregiver.	Assign a limited number of caregivers to the child. Ensure that warmth, acceptance, and availability are conveyed. *These characteristics, along with consistency of assignment, enhance the establishment and maintenance of a trusting relationship.* Provide child with familiar objects, such as familiar toys or a blanket. Support child's attempts to interact with others. *Familiar objects and presence of trusted individual provides security during times of distress.* Give positive reinforcement for eye contact with something acceptable to the child (e.g., food, familiar object). Gradually replace with social reinforcement (e.g., touch, smelling, hugging). *Being able to establish eye contact is essential to the child's ability to form satisfactory interpersonal relationships.*
Impaired verbal communication related to withdrawal into the self; inadequate sensory stimulation; neurological alterations	Patient will establish a means of communicating needs and desires to others.	Maintain consistency in assignment of caregivers. *Consistency facilitates trust and enhances the caregiver's ability to understand child's attempts to communicate.* Anticipate and fulfill the child's needs until communication can be established. *Minimizes frustration while the child is learning communication skills.* Seek clarification and validation *to ensure that intended message has been conveyed.* Give positive reinforcement when eye contact is used to convey nonverbal expressions.
Personal identity disturbance related to fixation in presymbiotic phase of development; lack of nurturing; inadequate sensory stimulation	Patient will name own body parts as separate and individual from those of others.	Assist child to recognize separateness during self-care activities, such as dressing and feeding. *These activities increase the child's awareness of self as separate from others.* Assist the child in learning to name own body parts. This can be facilitated with the use of mirrors, drawings, and pictures of the child. Encourage appropriate touching of, and being touched by, others. *All of these activities may help increase the child's awareness of self as separate from others.*

PREDISPOSING FACTORS

Biological Influences

Genetics A number of studies have revealed supportive evidence of genetic influences in the etiology of ADHD. Results have indicated that a large number of parents of hyperactive children showed signs of hyperactivity during their own childhood; that hyperactive children are more likely than normal children to have siblings who are also hyperactive; and that full siblings of hyperactive children are more likely than half siblings to show hyperactive behavior patterns (Whalen, 1989).

Biochemical Theory Shaywitz and associates (1983) have implicated a deficit of the catecholamines dopamine and norepinephrine in the overactivity attributed to ADHD. This deficit of neurotransmitters is believed to lower the threshold for stimuli input. The controversy surrounding this theory relates to cause and effect. Does the deficit of neurotransmitters result in hyperactive behavior, or does the stress associated with these problem behaviors result in altered neurotransmitter metabolism? Obviously, more investigation is required for validation of this theory.

Pre-, Peri-, and Postnatal Factors A recent study is consistent with an earlier finding that links maternal smoking during pregnancy and hyperkinetic-impulsive behavior in offspring (Nichols & Chen, 1981). This is one variable that must be examined carefully in future studies.

Perinatal influences that may contribute to ADHD are prematurity, signs of fetal distress, precipitated or prolonged labor, and perinatal asphyxia and low Apgar scores (Clunn, 1991). Postnatal factors that have been implicated include cerebral palsy, epilepsy, and other central nervous system abnormalities resulting from trauma, infections, or other neurologic disorders (APA, 1987; Clunn, 1991).

Environmental Influences

Environmental Lead Studies continue to provide evidence of the adverse effects on cognitive and behavioral development in children with elevated body levels of lead. Lead is pervasive in our environment, even though the government has placed tighter restrictions on the substance in recent years. Even though gasoline lead additives have been reduced, auto exhausts still spew more than 50,000 tons of lead into the air each year (Needleman & Bellinger, 1984). A possible causal link between elevated lead levels and behavior associated with ADHD is still being investigated.

Diet Factors The possible link between food dyes and additives was introduced in the mid-1970s by a San Francisco pediatrician (Feingold, 1976). Striking improvement in behavior is often reported by parents and teachers when hyperactive children are placed on this diet. However, results are inconsistent.

Another diet factor that has been receiving much attention in its possible link to ADHD is sugar. A number of studies have been conducted in an effort to determine the effect of sugar on hyperactive behavior. The results have been less than revealing.

What has been clear is that the etiological roles of both food additives and sugar have been greatly exaggerated. There are no reliable indications to date that either of these diet components plays a significant role in the development or exacerbation of hyperactivity (Whalen, 1989).

Psychosocial Influences
The *DSM-III-R* (APA, 1987) suggests that disorganized or chaotic environments and child abuse or neglect may be predisposing factors in some cases of ADHD. Other psychosocial influences that have been implicated include family history of alcoholism, hysterical and sociopathic behaviors, and parental history of hyperactivity. Developmental learning disorders may also predispose to ADHD (Clunn, 1991).

APPLICATION OF THE NURSING PROCESS

Background Assessment Data (Symptomatology) A major portion of the hyperactive child's problems relate to difficulties in performing age-appropriate tasks. They are highly distractible and have extremely limited attention spans. They often shift from one uncompleted activity to another. Impulsivity, or deficit in inhibitory control, is also common.

Hyperactive children have difficulty forming satisfactory interpersonal relationships. They demonstrate behaviors that inhibit acceptable social interaction. They are disruptive and intrusive in group endeavors. They have difficulty complying with social norms. Some ADHD children are very aggressive or oppositional, while others exhibit more regressive and immature behaviors. Low frustration tolerance and outbursts of temper are not uncommon.

Children with ADHD have boundless energy, exhibiting excessive levels of activity, restlessness, and fidgeting. They have been described as "perpetual motion machines," continuously running, jumping, wiggling, or squirming. They experience a greater than average number of accidents, from minor mishaps to more serious incidents that may lead to physical injury or the destruction of property.

The *DSM-III-R* diagnostic criteria for ADHD are presented in Table 15.6.

Nursing Diagnoses Based upon the data collected during the nursing assessment, possible nursing diagnoses for the child with ADHD include:

Table 15.6 DIAGNOSTIC CRITERIA FOR ATTENTION-DEFICIT HYPERACTIVITY DISORDER

A. A disturbance of at least 6 months during which at least eight of the following are present:

1. Often fidgets with hands or feet or squirms in seat (in adolescents, may be limited to subjective feelings of restlessness)
2. Has difficulty remaining seated when required to do so
3. Is easily distracted by extraneous stimuli
4. Has difficulty awaiting turn in games or group situations
5. Often blurts out answers to questions before they have been completed
6. Has difficulty following through on instructions from others (not due to oppositional behavior or failure of comprehension), for example, fails to finish chores
7. Has difficulty sustaining attention in tasks or play activities
8. Often shifts from one uncompleted activity to another
9. Has difficulty playing quietly
10. Often talks excessively
11. Often interrupts or intrudes on others (e.g., butts into other children's games)
12. Often does not seem to listen to what is being said to him or her
13. Often loses things necessary for tasks or activities at school or at home (e.g., toys, pencils, books, assignments)
14. Often engages in physically dangerous activities without considering possible consequences (not for the purpose of thrill seeking), for example, runs into street without looking

B. Onset before the age of 7

Source: From APA (1987) with permission.

High risk for injury related to impulsive and accident-prone behavior and the inability to perceive self-harm

Impaired social interaction related to intrusive and immature behavior

Self-esteem disturbance related to dysfunctional family system and possible child abuse or neglect

Noncompliance with task expectations related to low frustration tolerance and short attention span

Planning/Implementation Table 15.7 provides a plan of care for the child with ADHD using nursing diagnoses common to the disorder, goals of care, and appropriate nursing interventions for each. Rationale is provided in italics.

Evaluation Evaluation of the care of a patient with ADHD involves examining patient behaviors following implementation of the nursing actions to determine if the goals of therapy have been achieved. Collecting data by using the following types of questions may provide appropriate information for evaluation.

Have the nursing actions directed toward patient safety been effective in protecting the child from injury? Has the child been able to establish a trusting relationship with the primary caregiver? Is the patient responding to limits set on unacceptable behaviors? Is the patient able to interact appropriately with others? Is the patient able to verbalize positive statements about self? Is the patient able to complete tasks independently or with a minimum of assistance? Can he or she follow through after listening to simple instructions? Is the patient able to apply self-control to decrease motor activity?

PSYCHOPHARMACOLOGICAL INTERVENTION*

Central nervous system stimulants are sometimes given to children with ADHD. Those most commonly used include dextroamphetamine (Dexedrine), methylphenidate (Ritalin), and pemoline (Cylert). The actual mechanism by which these medications improve behavior associated with ADHD is not known. In most individuals, they pro-

---

*From Townsend, M. (1990). *Drug guide for psychiatric nursing.* Philadelphia: FA Davis.

Table 15.7 CARE PLAN FOR CHILD WITH ATTENTION-DEFICIT HYPERACTIVITY DISORDER

Nursing Diagnoses	Objectives	Nursing Interventions
High risk for injury related to impulsive and accident-prone behavior and the inability to perceive self-harm	Patient will be free of injury.	Ensure that patient has a safe environment. Remove objects from immediate area on which patient could injure self due to random, hyperactive movements. *Objects that are appropriate to the normal living situation can be hazardous to the child whose motor activities are out of control.* Identify deliberate behaviors that put the child at risk for injury. Institute consequences for repetition of this behavior. *Behavior can be modified with negative reinforcement.* If there is risk of injury associated with specific therapeutic activities, provide adequate supervision and assistance, or limit patient's participation if adequate supervision is not possible. *Patient safety is a nursing priority.*
Impaired social interaction related to intrusive and immature behavior	Patient will observe limits set on intrusive behavior and will demonstrate ability to interact appropriately with others.	Develop a trusting relationship with the child. Convey acceptance of the child separate from the unacceptable behavior. *Unconditional acceptance increases feelings of self-worth.* Discuss with patient which behaviors are and are not acceptable. Describe in a matter-of-fact manner the consequences of unacceptable behavior. Follow through. *Aversive reinforcement can alter undesirable behaviors.* Provide group situations for patient. *Appropriate social behavior is often learned from the positive and negative feedback of peers.*
Self-esteem disturbance related to dysfunctional family system and possible child abuse or neglect	Patient will demonstrate increased feelings of self-worth by verbalizing positive statements about self and exhibiting fewer demanding behaviors.	Ensure that goals are realistic. *Unrealistic goals set patient up for failure, which diminishes self-esteem.* Plan activities that provide opportunities for success. *Success enhances self-esteem.* Convey unconditional acceptance and positive regard. *Communication of patient as worthwhile human being may increase self-esteem.* Offer recognition of successful endeavors and positive reinforcement for attempts made. Give immediate positive feedback for acceptable behavior. *Positive reinforcement enhances self-esteem and may increase the desired behaviors.*
Noncompliance with task expectations related to low frustration tolerance and short attention span	Patient will be able to complete assigned tasks independently or with a minimum of assistance.	Provide an environment for task efforts that is as free of distractions as possible. *Patient is highly distractible and is unable to perform in the presence of even minimal stimulation.* Provide assistance on a one-to-one basis, beginning with simple, concrete instructions. *Patient lacks the ability to assimilate information that is complicated or has abstract meaning.* Ask patient to repeat instructions to you to *determine level of comprehension.* Establish goals that allow patient to complete a part of the task, rewarding each step-completion with a break for physical activity. *Short-term goals are not so overwhelming to one with such a short attention span. The positive reinforcement (physical activity) increases self-esteem and provides incentive for patient to pursue the task to completion.* Gradually decrease the amount of assistance given to task performance, while assuring the patient that assistance is still available if deemed necessary. *This encourages the patient to perform independently while providing a feeling of security with the presence of a trusted individual.*

duce stimulation, excitability, and restlessness. In children with ADHD, the effects include an increased attention span, the control of hyperactive behavior, and improvement in learning ability.

Side effects include insomnia, anorexia, weight loss, tachycardia, and temporary decrease in rate of growth and development. Physical tolerance can occur (less with pemoline than with dextroamphetamine or methylphenidate).

Route and Dosage Information

Dextroamphetamine (Dexadrine)

- PO (Children 3 to 5 years): Initial dosage: 2.5 mg/day. May be increased in increments of 2.5 mg/day at weekly intervals until desired response is achieved.
- PO (Children 6 years and older): Initial dosage: 5 mg daily or bid. May be increased in increments of 5 mg/day at weekly intervals until desired response is achieved. Dosage will rarely exceed 40 mg/day. Give first dose of tablets or elixir forms on awakening; additional doses at intervals of 4 to 6 hours. Sustained-release forms may be used for once-a-day dosage, given in the morning.

Methylphenidate (Ritalin)

- PO (Children 6 and older): Initial dosage: 5 mg before breakfast and lunch. Dosage may be increased gradually in increments of 5 to 10 mg/day at weekly intervals. Maximum daily dosage: 60 mg. Sustained-release form may be used for once-a-day dosage, given in the morning.

Pemoline (Cylert)

- PO (Children 6 and older): Initial dosage: 37.5 mg/day, administered as single dose each morning. Dosage may be gradually increased at 1-week intervals in increments of 18.75 mg/day until desired effect is achieved. Effective dosage usually ranges from 56.25 to 75 mg/day. Maximum recommended dose: 112.5 mg/day.

Nursing Implications

- Assess mental status for changes in mood, level of activity, degree of stimulation, and aggressiveness.
- Ensure that patient is protected from injury.

Keep stimuli low and environment as quiet as possible to discourage overstimulation.

- To reduce anorexia, the medication may be administered immediately after meals. The patient should be weighed regularly (at least weekly) during hospitalization and at home while on therapy with central nervous system stimulants due to the potential for anorexia/weight loss and temporary interruption of growth and development.
- To prevent insomnia, administer last dose at least 6 hours before bedtime. Administer sustained-release forms in the morning.
- In children with behavior disorders, a drug "holiday" should be attempted periodically under direction of the physician to determine effectiveness of the medication and need for continuation.
- Ensure that parents are aware of the delayed effects of pemoline. Therapeutic response may not be seen for 2 to 4 weeks. Drug should not be discontinued for lack of immediate results.
- Inform parents that over-the-counter (OTC) medications should be avoided while child is on stimulant medication. Some OTC medications, particularly cold and hay fever preparations, contain sympathomimetic agents that could compound the effects of the stimulant and create a drug interaction that may be toxic to the child.
- Ensure that parents are aware that drug should not be withdrawn abruptly. Withdrawal should be gradual and under the direction of the physician.

Conduct Disorder

With this disorder, there is a persistent pattern of conduct in which the basic rights of others and major age-appropriate societal norms or rules are violated (APA, 1987). Physical aggression is common. The *DSM-III-R* further delineates this disorder into subgroups:

1. *Group type.* With this subgroup, the predominance of conduct problems occur mainly as a group activity with peers. Aggressive physical behavior may or may not be present.
2. *Solitary aggressive type.* The essential feature is the predominance of aggressive physical behavior, usually toward both adults and

peers, initiated by the person (not as a group activity).

3. *Undifferentiated type.* These individuals have been diagnosed with conduct disorder but exhibit a mixture of clinical features that cannot be classified as either solitary aggressive type or group type. Approximately 9% of boys and 2% of girls younger than age 18 have the disorder. Onset is usually prepubertal. Onset of the disorder beyond puberty is more common among females than males.

PREDISPOSING FACTORS

Biological Influences

Genetics Studies with monozygotic and dizygotic twins as well as with nontwin siblings have revealed a significantly higher number of conduct disorders among those who have family members with the disorder (Baum, 1989). Although genetic factors appear to be involved in the etiology of conduct disorders, little is yet known about the actual mechanisms involved in genetic transmission. A reasonable assumption is that environmental factors play an important role in the manifestation of the disorder in those who are genetically susceptible.

Temperament The term *temperament* refers to personality traits that become evident very early in life and may be present at birth. Evidence suggests a genetic component in temperament and an association between temperament and behavioral problems later in life (Plomin, 1983). In a study of children who had been identified as temperamentally difficult in early childhood, Rutter (1987) found a significantly higher degree of aggressive behavior at age 6 than in children who had not been described as difficult.

Biochemical Various studies have reported a possible correlation between elevated plasma levels of testosterone and aggressive behavior (Baum, 1989). There is, however, insufficient data available at this time to identify a positive relationship. Olweus and colleagues (1980) suggest that testosterone may increase in response to aversive, stressful, or physically strenuous events. Thus, although these hormonal differences are not sufficient to account for aggressive and antisocial behavior, they may serve a mediating role in individual responses to particular environmental circumstances (Baum, 1989).

Psychosocial Influences

Impaired Social-Cognition Studies indicate that children rejected by their peers (i.e., actively disliked as opposed to neglected) have been observed to behave more aggressively, to engage in lower rates of task-appropriate behaviors, and higher rates of task-inappropriate behaviors (Dodge et al, 1982). These children may suffer from cognitive deficits that result in behavior that is aggressive and inappropriate. These inappropriate responses are in turn causally related to peer rejection, which contributes to a cycle of maladaptive behavior.

Family Influences The *DSM-III-R* (APA, 1987) has identified the following factors related to family dynamics as contributors in the predisposition to this disorder:

- Parental rejection
- Inconsistent management with harsh discipline
- Early institutional living
- Frequent shifting of parental figures
- Large family size
- Absent father
- Parents with antisocial personality disorder or alcohol dependence
- Association with a delinquent subgroup

In addition to those aspects of family dynamics described above, Baum (1989) reports on various studies that implicate additional family influences in the predisposition to conduct disorder. They include:

- Marital conflict and divorce
- Inadequate communication patterns
- Parental permissiveness

APPLICATION OF THE NURSING PROCESS

Background Assessment Data (Symptomatology) The classic characteristic of conduct disorder is the use of physical aggression in the violation of the rights of others. The behavior pattern manifests itself in virtually all areas of the child's life (at home, at school, with peers, and in the community). Stealing, lying, and truancy are common problems. The child lacks feelings of guilt or remorse.

The use of tobacco, liquor, or nonprescribed drugs, as well as the participation in sexual activities, occurs earlier than the peer group's expected age. Projection is a common defense mechanism.

Low self-esteem is manifested by a "tough guy" image. Characteristics include poor frustration tolerance, irritability, and frequent temper outbursts. Symptoms of anxiety and depression are not uncommon.

Level of academic achievement may be low in relation to age and IQ. Manifestations associated with ADHD (e.g., attention difficulties, impulsiveness, and hyperactivity) are very common in children with conduct disorder.

The *DSM-III-R* diagnostic criteria for conduct disorder are presented in Table 15.8.

Nursing Diagnoses Based upon the data collected during the nursing assessment, possible nursing diagnoses for the patient with conduct disorder include:

Table 15.8 DIAGNOSTIC CRITERIA FOR CONDUCT DISORDER

A. A disturbance of conduct lasting at least 6 months, during which at least three of the following have been present:

1. Has stolen without confrontation of a victim on more than one occasion (including forgery)
2. Has run away from home overnight at least twice while living in parental or parental surrogate home (or once without returning)
3. Often lies (other than to avoid physical or sexual abuse)
4. Has deliberately engaged in fire setting
5. Is often truant from school (for older person, absent from work)
6. Has broken into someone else's house, building, or car
7. Has deliberately destroyed others' property (other than by fire setting)
8. Has been physically cruel to animals
9. Has forced someone into sexual activity with him or her
10. Has used a weapon in more than one fight
11. Often initiates physical fights
12. Has stolen with confrontation of a victim (e.g., mugging, purse snatching, extortion, armed robbery)
13. Has been physically cruel to people

B. If 18 years of age or older, does not meet criteria for antisocial personality disorder.

Source: From APA (1987) with permission.

High risk for violence directed toward others related to characteristics of temperament, peer rejection, negative parental role models, dysfunctional family dynamics

Impaired social interaction related to negative parental role models, impaired social cognition leading to inappropriate social behaviors

Defensive coping related to low self-esteem and dysfunctional family system

Self-esteem disturbance related to lack of positive feedback and unsatisfactory parent/child relationship

Planning/Implementation Table 15.9 provides a plan of care for the child with conduct disorder using nursing diagnoses common to the disorder, goals of care, and appropriate nursing interventions of each. Rationale is provided in italics.

Evaluation Following the planning and implementation of care, evaluation is made of the behavioral changes in the child with conduct disorder. This is accomplished by determining if the goals of therapy have been achieved. Reassessment is the next step in the nursing process and may be initiated by gathering information using the following questions.

Have the nursing actions directed toward managing the patient's aggressive behavior been effective? Have interventions prevented harm to others or others' property? Is the patient able to express anger in an appropriate manner? Has the patient developed more adaptive coping strategies to deal with anger and feelings of aggression? Does the patient demonstrate the ability to trust others? Is he or she able to interact with staff and peers in an appropriate manner? Is patient able to accept responsibility for own behavior? Is there less blaming of others? Is patient able to accept feedback from others without becoming defensive? Is patient able to verbalize positive statements about self? Is patient able to interact with others without engaging in manipulation?

Oppositional Defiant Disorder

This disorder is characterized by a pattern of negativistic, hostile, and defiant behavior without the more serious violations of the basic rights of others that are seen in conduct disorder (APA, 1987). The diagnosis is made only if the oppositional and defiant behavior is much more common than that

Table 15.9 CARE PLAN FOR CHILD/ADOLESCENT WITH CONDUCT DISORDER

Nursing Diagnoses	Objectives	Nursing Interventions
High risk for violence directed toward others related to characteristics of temperament, peer rejection, negative parental role models, dysfunctional family dynamics	Patient will not harm others or others' property.	Observe patient's behavior frequently through routine activities and interactions. Become aware of behaviors that indicate a rise in agitation. *Recognition of behaviors that precede the onset of aggression may provide the opportunity to intervene before violence occurs.* Redirect violent behavior with physical outlets for suppressed anger and frustration. *Excess energy is released through physical activities, and a feeling of relaxation is induced.* Encourage patient to express anger and act as a role model for appropriate expression of anger. *Discussion of situations that create anger may lead to more effective ways of dealing with them.* Ensure that a sufficient number of staff is available to indicate a show of strength if necessary. *This conveys an evidence of control over the situation and provides physical security for staff.* Administer tranquilizing medication, if ordered, or use mechanical restraints or isolation room only if situation cannot be controlled with less restrictive means. *It is the patient's right to expect the use of techniques that ensure safety of the patient and others by the least restrictive means.*
Impaired social interaction related to negative parental role models, impaired social cognition leading to inappropriate social behavior	Patient will be able to interact with staff and peers using age-appropriate, acceptable behaviors.	Develop a trusting relationship with the patient. Convey acceptance of the person separate from the unacceptable behavior. *Unconditional acceptance increases feelings of self-worth.* Discuss with patient which behaviors are and are not acceptable. Describe in matter-of-fact manner the consequence of unacceptable behavior. Follow through. *Aversive reinforcement can alter undesirable behaviors.* Provide group situations for patient. *Appropriate social behavior is often learned from the positive and negative feedback of peers.*
Defensive coping related to low self-esteem and dysfunctional family system	Patient will accept responsibility for own behaviors and interact with others without becoming defensive.	Explain to patient the correlation between feelings of inadequacy and the need for acceptance from others, and how these feelings provoke defensive behaviors, such as blaming others for own behaviors. *Recognition of the problem is the first step in the change process toward resolution.* Provide immediate, matter-of-fact, nonthreatening feedback for unacceptable behaviors. *Patient may not realize how these behaviors are being perceived by others.* Help identify situations that provoke defensiveness and practice more appropriate responses through role-play. *Role-playing provides confidence to deal with difficult situations when they actually occur.* Provide immediate positive feedback for acceptable behaviors. *Positive feedback encourages repetition, and immediacy is significant for these children who respond to immediate gratification.*

(continued)

Table 15.9 CONTINUED		
Nursing Diagnoses	**Objectives**	**Nursing Interventions**
Self-esteem disturbance related to lack of positive feedback and unsatisfactory parent/child relationship	Patient will demonstrate increased feelings of self-worth by verbalizing positive statements about self and exhibiting fewer manipulative behaviors.	Ensure that goals are realistic. *Unrealistic goals set patient up for failure, which diminishes self-esteem.* Plan activities that provide opportunities for success. *Success enhances self-esteem.* Convey unconditional acceptance and positive regard. *Communication of patient as worthwhile human being may increase self-esteem.* Set limits on manipulative behavior. Take caution not to reinforce manipulative behaviors by providing desired attention. Identify the consequences of manipulation. Administer consequences matter-of-factly when manipulation occurs. *Aversive consequences may work to decrease unacceptable behaviors.* Help patient understand that he or she uses this behavior to try to increase own self-esteem. Interventions should reflect other actions to accomplish this goal. *When patient feels better about self, the need to manipulate others will diminish.*

seen in other people of the same mental age. The disorder typically begins by 8 years of age and usually not later than early adolescence.

PREDISPOSING FACTORS

Biological Influences Because the behaviors associated with oppositional defiant disorder are very similar to those of conduct disorder, with the exception of violation of the rights of others, it is reasonable to speculate that they may share at least *some* of the same biological influences. What role, if any, genetics, temperament, or biochemical alterations plays in the etiology of oppositional defiant disorder has not been determined.

Family Influences Opposition during various developmental stages is both normal and healthy. Children first exhibit oppositional behaviors at around 10 or 11 months of age, again as a toddler between 18 and 36 months of age, and finally during adolescence. Pathology is only considered when the developmental phase is prolonged, or when there is overreaction in the child's environment to his or her behavior.

About 10% of children exhibit these behaviors in a more intense form than others (Kaplan & Sadock, 1985). Some parents interpret average or increased level of developmental oppositionalism as hostility and a deliberate effort on the part of the child to be

in control. If power and control are issues for parents, or if they exercise authority for their own needs, a power struggle can be established between the parents and the child that sets the stage for the development of oppositional defiant disorder.

APPLICATION OF THE NURSING PROCESS

Background Assessment Data (Symptomatology) The focal issue of oppositional defiant disorder is passive-aggression, and is exhibited by obstinacy, procrastination, disobedience, carelessness, negativism, dawdling, provocation, resistance to change, violation of minor rules, blocking out communications from others, and resistance to authority (Kaplan & Sadock, 1985). Other symptoms that may be evident are enuresis, encopresis, elective mutism, running away, school avoidance, school underachievement, eating and sleeping problems, temper tantrums, fighting, and argumentativeness.

The oppositional attitude is directed toward adults, most particularly the parents. Symptoms of the disorder may or may not be evident in school or elsewhere outside the home (APA, 1987).

Usually these children do not see themselves as being oppositional but view the problem as arising from others whom they believe are making unreasonable demands on them. Interpersonal relationships are fraught with difficulty, including those with peers. They are often friendless, perceiving human relationships as negative and unsatisfactory. School performance is poor due to their refusal to participate and resistance to external demands (Kaplan & Sadock, 1985).

The *DSM-III-R* (APA, 1987) diagnostic criteria for oppositional defiant disorder are presented in Table 15.10.

Nursing Diagnoses Based upon the data collected during the nursing assessment, possible nursing diagnoses for the patient with oppositional defiant disorder include:

Noncompliance with therapy related to negative temperament, denial of problems, underlying hostility

Defensive coping related to retarded ego development, low self-esteem, unsatisfactory parent/child relationship

Self-esteem disturbance related to lack of positive feedback, retarded ego development

Impaired social interaction related to negative temperament, underlying hostility, manipulation of others

Planning/Implementation Table 15.11 provides a plan of care for the child with oppositional defiant disorder using nursing diagnoses common to the disorder, goals of care, and appropriate nursing interventions for each. Rationale is provided in italics.

Table 15.10 DIAGNOSTIC CRITERIA FOR OPPOSITIONAL DEFIANT DISORDER

A. A disturbance of at least 6 months during which at least five of the following are present:
  1. Often loses temper
  2. Often argues with adults
  3. Often actively defies or refuses adult requests or rules (e.g., refuses to do chores at home)
  4. Often deliberately does things that annoy other people (e.g., grabs other children's hats)
  5. Often blames others for his or her own mistakes
  6. Is often touchy or easily annoyed by others
  7. Is often angry and resentful
  8. Is often spiteful or vindictive
  9. Often swears or uses obscene language

Source: From APA (1987) with permission.

Evaluation The evaluation step of the nursing process calls for reassessment of the plan of care to determine if the nursing actions have been effective in achieving the goals of therapy. The following questions can be used with the child/adolescent with oppositional defiant disorder to gather information for the evaluation.

Is the patient cooperating with schedule of therapeutic activities? Is level of participation adequate? Is attitude toward therapy less negative? Is patient accepting responsibility for problem behavior? Is patient verbalizing the unacceptableness of his or her passive-aggressive behavior? Is he or she able to identify which behaviors are unacceptable and substitute more adaptive behaviors? Is patient able to interact with staff and peers without defending behavior in an angry manner? Is patient able to verbalize positive statements about self? Is increased self-worth evident with fewer manifestations of manipulation? Is patient able to make compromises with others when issues of control emerge? Is anger and hostility expressed in an appropriate manner? Can patient verbalize ways of releasing anger adaptively? Is he or she able to verbalize true feelings instead of allowing them to emerge through use of passive-aggressive behaviors?

ANXIETY DISORDERS OF CHILDHOOD OR ADOLESCENCE

In this disorder, anxiety is the predominant clinical feature. The three subcategories include separation anxiety disorder, avoidant disorder of childhood or adolescence, and overanxious disorder. In separation anxiety disorder and avoidant disorder, the anxiety is focused on specific situations, while in overanxious disorder, the anxiety is generalized to a variety of situations (APA, 1987).

Predisposing Factors

BIOLOGICAL INFLUENCES

Genetics Studies have been conducted in which the children of adult patients diagnosed as having an anxiety disorder were studied. A second method, in which parents and other relatives of children diagnosed as having anxiety disorders,

Table 15.11 CARE PLAN FOR THE CHILD/ADOLESCENT WITH OPPOSITIONAL DEFIANT DISORDER

Nursing Diagnoses	Objectives	Nursing Interventions
Noncompliance with therapy related to negative temperament, denial of problems, underlying hostility	Patient will participate in and cooperate during therapeutic activities.	Set forth a structured plan of therapeutic activities. Start with minimum expectations and increase as patient begins to manifest evidence of compliance. *Structure provides security, and one or two activities may not seem as overwhelming as the whole schedule of activities presented at one time.* Establish a system of rewards for compliance with therapy and consequences for noncompliance. Ensure that the rewards and consequences are concepts of value to the patient. *Positive, negative, and aversive reinforcements can contribute to desired changes in behavior.* Convey acceptance of the patient separate from the undesirable behaviors being exhibited. ("It is not *you*, but your *behavior*, that is unacceptable.") *Unconditional acceptance enhances self-worth and may contribute to a decrease in the need for passive-aggression toward others.*
Defensive coping related to retarded ego development, low self-esteem, unsatisfactory parent/child relationship	Patient will accept responsibility for own behaviors and interact with others without becoming defensive.	Help patient recognize that feelings of inadequacy that provoke defensive behaviors, such as blaming others for problems and the need to "get even." *Recognition of the problem is the first step toward initiating change.* Provide immediate, nonthreatening feedback for passive-aggressive behaviors. *Since patient denies responsibility for problems, he or she is denying the inappropriateness of behavior.* Help identify situations that provoke defensiveness and practice through role play more appropriate responses. *Role playing provides confidence to deal with difficult situations when they actually occur.* Provide immediate positive feedback for acceptable behaviors. *Positive feedback encourages repetition, and immediacy is significant for these children who respond to immediate gratification.*
Self-esteem disturbance related to lack of positive feedback, retarded ego development	Patient will demonstrate increased feelings of self-worth by verbalizing positive statements about self and exhibiting fewer manipulative behaviors.	Ensure that goals are realistic. *Unrealistic goals set patient up for failure, which diminishes self-esteem.* Plan activities that provide opportunities for success. *Success enhances self-esteem.* Convey unconditional acceptance and positive regard. *Communication of patient as worthwhile human being may increase self-esteem.* Set limits on manipulative behavior. Take caution not to reinforce manipulative behaviors by providing desired attention. Identify the consequences of manipulation. Administer consequences matter-of-factly when manipulation occurs. *Aversive reinforcement may work to decrease unacceptable behaviors.* Help patient understand that he or she uses this behavior to try to increase own self-esteem. Interventions should reflect other actions to accomplish this goal. *When patient feels better about self, the need to manipulate others will diminish.*

(continued)

Table 15.11 CONTINUED

Nursing Diagnoses	Objectives	Nursing Interventions
Impaired social interaction related to negative temperament, underlying hostility, manipulation of others	Patient will be able to interact with staff and peers using age-appropriate, acceptable behaviors.	Develop a trusting relationship with the patient. Convey acceptance of the person separate from the unacceptable behavior. *Unconditional acceptance increases feelings of self-worth and may serve to diminish feelings of rejection that have accumulated over a long period.* Explain to the patient about passive-aggressive behavior. Explain how these behaviors are perceived by others. Describe which behaviors are not acceptable and role play more adaptive responses. Give positive feedback for acceptable behaviors. *Role playing is a way to practice behaviors that do not come easy for the patient, making it easier when the situation actually occurs. Positive feedback enhances repetition of desirable behaviors.* Provide peer group situations for the patient. *Appropriate social behavior is often learned from the positive and negative feedback of peers. Groups also provide an atmosphere for using the behaviors rehearsed in role play.*

has also been used (Klein & Last, 1989). The results of these studies have shown that a greater number of children with relatives who manifest anxiety problems develop anxiety disorders themselves than do children with no such family patterns. The results are significant enough to speculate that there is a hereditary influence in the development of anxiety disorders, but the mode of genetic transmission has not been determined.

Temperament It is well established that children differ from birth or shortly thereafter on a number of temperamental characteristics (Rutter et al., 1964; Berger, 1985). These studies indicate that from a hereditary perspective, individual differences in temperament may be related to the acquisition of fear and anxiety disorders in childhood. This may be referred to as *anxiety proneness* or *vulnerability* and may denote an inherited "disposition" toward developing anxiety disorders.

ENVIRONMENTAL INFLUENCES

Stressful Life Events Studies have shown a relationship between life events and the development of anxiety disorders (Klein & Last, 1989). Children who already are vulnerable or predisposed to developing anxiety disorders may be affected significantly by stressful life events. More research is needed before firm conculsions can be drawn.

FAMILY INFLUENCES

Various theories expound on the idea that anxiety disorders in children are related to an overattachment to the mother (Last, 1989). Kaplan and Sadock (1985) attribute the major determinants of anxiety disorders to transactions relating to separation conflicts between parent and child. The *DSM-III-R* (APA, 1987) suggests that children with separation anxiety disorders come from families that are close-knit and caring. Overanxious disorder seems to be more common in eldest children, in small families, in upper socioeconomic groups, and in families in which there is a concern about achievement.

Some parents may instill anxiety in their children by overprotecting them from expectable dangers or by exaggerating the dangers of the present and the future (Kaplan & Sadock, 1985). Some parents may also transfer their fears and anxieties to their children through role modeling. For example, a parent who becomes fearful in the presence of a small, harmless dog and retreats with dread and apprehension teaches the young child by example that this is an appropriate response.

Application of the Nursing Process

BACKGROUND ASSESSMENT DATA (SYMPTOMATOLOGY)

Separation Anxiety Disorder   Age at onset of this disorder may be as early as preschool age; rarely as late as adolescence. In most cases, the child has difficulty separating from the mother. Occasionally, the separation reluctance is directed toward the father, siblings, or other significant individual to whom the child is attached. Anticipation of separation may result in tantrums, crying, screaming, complaints of physical problems, and "clinging" behaviors.

Reluctance or refusal to attend school is especially common in adolescence. Younger children may "shadow" or follow around the person from whom they are afraid to be separated. During middle childhood or adolescence, they may refuse to sleep away from home (e.g., at a friend's house or at camp). Interpersonal peer relationships are usually not a problem with these children. They are generally well liked by their peers and are reasonably socially skilled (Last, 1989).

Worrying is common, and relates to the possibility of harm coming to self or to the attachment figure. Younger children may even have nightmares to this effect.

Specific phobias are not uncommon (e.g., fear of the dark, ghosts, animals). Depressed mood is frequently present and often precedes the onset of the anxiety symptoms, which commonly occur following a major stressor. The *DSM-III-R* diagnostic criteria for separation anxiety disorder are presented in Table 15.12.

Avoidant Disorder of Childhood or Adolescence   The essential feature of this disorder is an excessive and irrational fear of being around unfamiliar people. The child is extremely reluctant to enter situations in which there is someone with whom he or she is unacquainted. These children are generally warm and loving with family and other people whom they know well.

Children with avoidant disorder are very nonassertive and lack self-confidence. They typically have few or no friends, as their ability to interact with new acquaintances is severely limited (Last, 1989). The impairment of social functioning is often severe. In adolescence, inhibition of normal psychosexual activity is common (APA, 1987). Characteristic sequelae include social isolation and depression.

The *DSM-III-R* diagnostic criteria for avoidant disorder are presented in Table 15.13.

Overanxious Disorder   The essential feature of overanxious disorder includes unrealistic worrying about future events and about the appropriateness of one's behavior in the past. Excessive or unrealistic concern about competence is characteristic of overanxious children (Last, 1989). They are perfectionistic and desire to excel in all aspects of their life.

Somatic complaints are common in overanxious disorder. Common ones include headaches, stom-

---

Table 15.12 DIAGNOSTIC CRITERIA FOR SEPARATION ANXIETY DISORDER

A. Excessive anxiety concerning separation from those to whom the child is attached, as evidenced by at least three of the following:
   1. Unrealistic and persistent worry about possible harm befalling major attachment figures or fear that they will leave and not return
   2. Unrealistic and persistent worry that an untoward calamitous event will separate the child from a major attachment figure (e.g., the child will be lost, kidnapped, killed, or be the victim of an accident)
   3. Persistent reluctance or refusal to go to school in order to stay with major attachment figures or at home
   4. Persistent reluctance or refusal to go to sleep without being near a major attachment figure or to go to sleep away from home
   5. Persistent avoidance of being alone, including "clinging" to and "shadowing" major attachment figures
   6. Repeated nightmares involving the theme of separation
   7. Complaints of physical symptoms (e.g., headaches, stomachaches, nausea, or vomiting) on many school days or on other occasions when anticipating separation from major attachment figures
   8. Recurrent signs or complaints of excessive distress in anticipation of separation from home or major attachment figures (e.g., temper tantrums or crying, pleading with parents not to leave)
   9. Recurrent signs of complaints of excessive distress when separated from home or major attachment figures (e.g., wants to return home, needs to call parents when they are absent or when child is away from home)

B. Duration of disturbance of at least 2 weeks

C. Onset before the age of 18

Source: From APA (1987) with permission.

Table 15.13 DIAGNOSTIC CRITERIA FOR AVOIDANT DISORDER OF CHILDHOOD OR ADOLESCENCE

A. Excessive shrinking from contact with unfamiliar people, for a period of 6 months or longer, sufficiently severe to interfere with social functioning in peer relationships.

B. Desire for social involvement with familiar people (family members and peers the person knows well), and generally warm and satisfying relations with family members and other familiar figures.

C. Age at least 2½ years.

Source: From APA (1987) with permission.

Table 15.14 DIAGNOSTIC CRITERIA FOR OVERANXIOUS DISORDER

A. Excessive or unrealistic anxiety or worry, for a period of 6 months or longer, as indicated by the frequent occurrence of at least four of the following:
1. Excessive or unrealistic worry about future events
2. Excessive or unrealistic concern about the appropriateness of past behavior
3. Excessive or unrealistic concern about competence in one or more areas (e.g., athletic, academic, social)
4. Somatic complaints, such as headaches or stomachaches, for which no physical basis can be established
5. Marked self-consciousness
6. Excessive need for reassurance about a variety of concerns
7. Marked feelings of tension or inability to relax

Source: From APA (1987) with permission.

---

achaches, back pains, or a general feeling of malaise. Generalized tension, manifested by "nervous habits," such as nail biting, foot tapping, hair pulling, and fidgeting, is common.

These patients lack self-confidence and require repeated reassurance from significant others. They are markedly self-conscious and have difficulty being in the limelight on any occasion.

Unlike separation anxiety disorder, which is often precipitated by a stressful event and may remit spontaneously with resolution of the stress, overanxious disorder appears to be more chronic in nature. Many children who enter the mental health system with the disorder have a symptom history of several years without remission. The symptoms may persist into adulthood or may predispose the individual to developing generalized anxiety disorder as an adult (Last, 1989).

The *DSM-III-R* diagnostic criteria for overanxious disorder are presented in Table 15.14.

NURSING DIAGNOSIS

Based upon the data collected during the nursing assessment, possible nursing diagnoses for the patient with anxiety disorders of childhood or adolescence include:

Anxiety (severe) related to family history, temperament, overattachment to parent, negative role modeling

Ineffective individual coping related to unresolved separation conflicts and inadequate coping skills evidenced by numerous somatic complaints

Impaired social interaction related to excessive self-consciousness and inability to interact with unfamiliar people

PLANNING/IMPLEMENTATION

Table 15.15 provides a plan of care for the child/adolescent with an anxiety disorder using nursing diagnoses common to these disorders, goals of care, and appropriate nursing interventions for each. Rationale is provided in italics.

EVALUATION

Evaluation of the child/adolescent with an anxiety disorder requires reassessment of the behaviors for which the family sought treatment. Behavioral change will be required on the part of both the patient and family members. The following types of questions may provide assistance in gathering data required for evaluating whether the nursing interventions have been effective in achieving the goals of therapy.

Is the patient able to maintain anxiety at a manageable level, that is, without temper tantrums, screaming, "clinging"? Have complaints of physical symptoms diminished? Has patient demonstrated the ability to cope in more adaptive ways in the face of escalating anxiety? Have parents identified their role in the separation conflict? Are they able to discuss more adaptive coping strategies?

Does the child verbalize intention to return to school? Have nightmares and fears of the dark subsided? Is the child able to interact in a group situation without excessive self-consciousness? Has the child established a satisfactory relationship with one person? Has the perfectionistic child accepted more realistic self-expectations? Is the child with avoidant disorder now able to enter situations in which there are people with whom he or she is not acquainted? In the case of separation anxiety, has

Table 15.15	CARE PLAN FOR PATIENT WITH ANXIETY DISORDER OF CHILDHOOD OR ADOLESCENCE SEPARATION ANXIETY DISORDER, AVOIDANT DISORDER, OVERANXIOUS DISORDER	
Nursing Diagnoses	**Objectives**	**Nursing Interventions**
Anxiety (severe) related to family history, temperament, overattachment to parent, negative role modeling	Patient will maintain anxiety at no higher than moderate level in the face of events that formerly have precipitated panic.	**Establish an atmosphere of calmness, trust, and genuine positive regard.** *Trust and unconditional acceptance are necessary for satisfactory nurse/patient relationship. Calmness is important because anxiety is easily transmitted from one person to another.* **Ensure patient of his or her safety and security.** *Symptoms of panic anxiety are very frightening.* **Explore the child/adolescent's fears of separating from the parents. Explore with the parents possible fears they may have of separation from the child.** *Some parents may have an underlying fear of separation from the child of which they are unaware and which they are unconsciously transferring to the child.* **Help parents and child initiate realistic goals (e.g., child to stay with sitter for 2 hours with minimal anxiety, or child to stay at friend's house without parents until 9 PM without experiencing panic anxiety).** *Parents may be so frustrated with child's clinging and demanding behaviors that assistance with problem solving may be required.* **Give, and encourage parents to give, positive reinforcement for desired behaviors.** *Positive reinforcement encourages repetition of desirable behaviors.*
Ineffective individual coping related to unresolved separation conflicts and inadequate coping skills evidenced by numerous somatic complaints	Patient will demonstrate use of more adaptive coping strategies (than physical symptoms) in response to stressful situations.	**Encourage child/adolescent to discuss specific situations in life that produce the most distress and describe his or her response to these situations. Include parents in the discussion.** *Patient and family may be unaware of the correlation between stressful situations and the exacerbation of physical symptoms.* **Help the child/adolescent who is perfectionistic to recognize that self-expectations may be unrealistic. Connect times of unmet self-expectations to the exacerbation of physical symptoms.** *Recognition of maladaptive patterns is the first step in the change process.* **Encourage parents and child to identify more adaptive coping strategies that the child could use in the face of anxiety that feels overwhelming. Practice through role play.** *Practice facilitates the use of the desired behavior when the individual is actually faced with the stressful situation.*

(continued)

Table 15.15 CONTINUED

Nursing Diagnoses	Objectives	Nursing Interventions
Impaired social interaction related to excessive self-consciousness and inability to interact with unfamiliar people	Patient will be able to interact within the hospital peer group and will verbalize intention of returning to school upon discharge.	Develop a trusting relationship with patient. *This is the first step in helping the patient learn to interact with others.* Attend groups with the child and support efforts to interact with others. Give positive feedback. *Presence of a trusted individual provides security during times of distress. Positive feedback encourages repetition.* Convey to the child the acceptability of his or her not participating in group in the beginning. Gradually encourage small contributions until patient is able to participate more fully. *Small successes will gradually increase self-confidence and decrease self-consciousness, so that patient will feel less anxious in the group situation.* Help patient set small personal goals (e.g., "Today I will speak to one person I don't know."). *Simple, realistic goals provide opportunities for success that increase self-confidence and may encourage the patient to attempt more difficult objectives in the future.*

the precipitating stressor been identified? Have strategies for coping more adaptively to similar stressors in the future been established?

EATING DISORDERS

This classification of disorders is characterized by gross disturbances in eating behavior. Anorexia nervosa and bulimia nervosa are examples of eating disorders that will be discussed in this chapter. The onset of these disorders usually occurs in adolescence or early adulthood and is most prevalent among white women of middle- to upper-class socioeconomic status.

Predisposing Factors

BIOLOGICAL INFLUENCES

Genetics A hereditary predisposition to eating disorders has been hypothesized on the basis of family histories and an apparent association with other disorders for which the likelihood of genetic influences exists. Anorexia nervosa is more common among sisters and mothers of those with the disorder than among the general population. Several studies have reported a higher than expected frequency of major depression and bipolar dis-

order among first-degree biologic relatives of people with the disorder (APA, 1987).

Neuroendocrine Abnormalities There has been some speculation about a primary hypothalamic dysfunction in anorexia nervosa. Other studies, consistent with this theory of hypothalamic dysfunction, have revealed elevated cerebral spinal fluid cortisol levels and a possible impairment of dopaminergic regulation in anorexics (Leon & Dinklage, 1989). Additional evidence in the etiologic implication of hypothalmic dysfunction is the fact that in many anorexics, amenorrhea occurs prior to the onset of starvation and significant weight loss.

PSYCHODYNAMIC INFLUENCES

Bruch (1970) theorizes that eating disorders are the result of very early and profound disturbances in mother-infant interactions. The result is retarded ego development in the child and an unfulfilled sense of separation-individuation. This problem is compounded when the mother responds to the child's physical and emotional needs with food. Manifestations include a disturbance in body identity and a distortion in body image. When events occur that threaten the vulnerable ego, the feelings of lack of control over one's body (self) emerge. Behaviors associated with food and eating serve to provide feelings of control over one's life.

FAMILY INFLUENCES

Conflict Avoidance Minuchin and associates (1978) have suggested that families promote and maintain psychosomatic symptoms, including anorexia nervosa, in an effort to avoid spousal conflict. Parents are able to deny marital conflict by defining the sick child as the family problem. In these families, there is an unhealthy involvement between the members (enmeshment); the members strive at all costs to maintain "appearances"; and the parents endeavor to retain the child in the dependent position. Conflict avoidance may be a strong factor in the interpersonal dynamics of some anorexic families.

Elements of Power and Control The issue of control may become the overriding factor in the family of the patient with an eating disorder. These families often consist of a passive father, a domineering mother, and an overly dependent child. There is a high value placed on perfectionism in this family, and the child feels he or she must satisfy these standards (Bruch, 1983). Parental criticism promotes an increase in obsessive and perfectionistic behavior on the part of the child, who continues to seek love, approval, and recognition. Feelings of helplessness and ambivalence toward the parents eventually develop. In adolescence, these distorted eating patterns may be a rebellion against the parents, viewed by the child as a means of gaining, and remaining in, control. The symptoms are often triggered by a stressor that the adolescent perceives as a loss of control in some aspect of his or her life.

Application of the Nursing Process

BACKGROUND ASSESSMENT DATA (SYMPTOMATOLOGY)

Anorexia Nervosa This disorder is characterized by a morbid fear of obesity. Symptoms include gross distortion of body image, preoccupation with food, and refusal to eat. The term *anorexia* is actually a misnomer. It was initially believed that anorexics did not experience sensations of hunger. However, research indicates that they do indeed suffer from pangs of hunger, and it is only with food intake of less than 200 calories per day that hunger sensations actually cease (Leon & Dinklage, 1989).

The distortion in body image is manifested by the individual's perception of being "fat" when he or she is obviously underweight or even emaciated. Weight loss is usually accomplished by reduction in food intake and often extensive exercising. Self-induced vomiting may also occur, along with the abuse of laxatives or diuretics.

Weight loss is marked. For example, the child may present for health-care services weighing less than 85% of expected weight. Other symptoms include hypothermia, bradycardia, hypotension, edema, lanugo, and a variety of metabolic changes. Amenorrhea usually follows weight loss but, in some instances, may appear before significant weight loss has occurred (APA, 1987).

There may be an obsession with food. For example, they may hoard or conceal food, talk about food and recipes at great length, or prepare elaborate meals for others, only to restrict themselves to a limited amount of low-calorie food intake. Compulsive behaviors, such as hand washing, may also be present.

Age at onset is usually early to late adolescence. This disorder occurs predominantly in the female population (95%). Psychosexual development is generally delayed.

Feelings of depression and anxiety often accompany this disorder. In fact, several studies have suggested a possible interrelationship between eating disorders and affective disorders (Leon & Dinklage, 1989). Table 15.16 outlines the *DSM-III-R*

Table 15.16 DIAGNOSTIC CRITERIA FOR ANOREXIA NERVOSA

A. Refusal to maintain body weight over a minimal normal weight for age and height (e.g., weight loss leading to maintenance of body weight 15% below that expected; or failure to make expected weight gain during period of growth, leading to body weight 15% below that expected).

B. Intense fear of gaining weight or becoming fat, even though underweight.

C. Disturbance in the way in which one's body weight, size, or shape is experienced (e.g., the person claims to "feel fat" even when emaciated, believes that one area of the body is "too fat" even when obviously underweight).

D. In female patients, absence of at least three consecutive menstrual cycles when otherwise expected to occur (primary or secondary amenorrhea).

Source: From APA (1987) with permission.

diagnostic criteria for anorexia nervosa. The dynamics of the disorder using the Transactional Model of Stress/Adaptation is presented in Figure 15.1.

Bulimia Nervosa Bulimia is an episodic, uncontrolled, compulsive, rapid ingestion of large quantities of food over a short period (binging), followed by episodes of self-induced vomiting (purging). The food consumed during a binge often has a high caloric content, a sweet taste, and a texture that facilitates rapid eating (APA, 1987). These episodes often occur in secret and are usually only terminated by abdominal discomfort, sleep, social interruption, or self-induced vomiting. Although the eating binges may bring pleasure while they are occurring, self-degradation and depressed mood commonly follow.

Other symptoms include abuse of laxatives or diuretics, strict dieting or fasting, or vigorous exercise to prevent weight gain. There is a persistent overconcern with personal appearance, particularly regarding how they believe others perceive them. Weight fluctuations are common due to the alternating binges and fasts. However, most bulimics are within a normal weight range, some slightly underweight, some slightly overweight.

Excessive vomiting and laxative/diuretic abuse may lead to problems with dehydration and electrolyte imbalance. Gastric acid in the vomitus also contributes to the erosion of tooth enamel.

Some people with this disorder are subject to psychoactive substance abuse or dependence, most frequently involving sedatives, amphetamines, cocaine, or alcohol (APA, 1987). Diagnostic criteria for bulimia nervosa are presented in Table 15.17.

NURSING DIAGNOSES

Based upon the data collected during the nursing assessment, possible nursing diagnoses for the patient with anorexia nervosa or bulimia nervosa include:

Altered nutrition: Less than body requirements related to refusal to eat

Fluid volume deficit (high risk for or actual) related to decreased fluid intake; self-induced vomiting; laxative and or diuretic abuse

Ineffective denial related to retarded ego development and fear of losing the only aspect of life over which he or she perceives some control (eating)

Body image/Self-esteem disturbance related to retarded ego development and dysfunctional family system

Anxiety (moderate to severe) related to feelings of helplessness and lack of control over life events

PLANNING/IMPLEMENTATION

Table 15.18 provides a plan of care for the patient with the eating disorders of anorexia nervosa and bulimia nervosa. Included are nursing diagnoses common to these disorders, goals of care, and appropriate nursing interventions for each. Rationale is provided in italics.

Some institutions are using a case management model to coordinate care (see Chapter 6 for a more detailed explanation). In case management models, the plan of care may take the form of a critical pathway. Table 15.18A depicts an example of a critical pathway of care for a patient with anorexia nervosa.

EVALUATION

Evaluation of the patient with anorexia nervosa or bulimia nervosa requires a reassessment of the behaviors for which the patient sought treatment. Behavioral change will be required on the part of both the patient and family members. The following types of questions may provide assistance in gathering data required for evaluating whether the nursing interventions have been effective in achieving the goals of therapy.

Has the patient steadily gained 2 to 3 lb/wk to at least 80% of body weight for age and size? Is patient free from signs and symptoms of malnutrition/dehydration? Does patient consume adequate calories as determined by dietitian? Have there been any attempts to stash food from tray to discard later? Have there been any attempts to self-induce vomiting? Has patient admitted that a problem exists and that eating behaviors are maladaptive? Have behaviors aimed at manipulating the environment been discontinued? Is patient willing to discuss the *real* issues concerning family roles, sexual-

Precipitating Event
(Some aspect in life over
which he or she feels
a lack of control)

Predisposing Factors
  Genetic Influences: Higher incidence among family members
                     Possible hypothalmic dysfunction
  Past Experiences: Disturbance in mother/infant relationship
                     Retarded ego development
  Existing conditions: Parents' marital conflict
                     Family issues related to control

Cognitive Appraisal

* Primary *

(Self-concept is threatened)

* Secondary *

Because of weak ego strength, patient is unable to use coping mechanisms effectively.
Defense mechanisms utilized: denial, regression, rationalization

Quality of response

Adaptive   Maladaptive

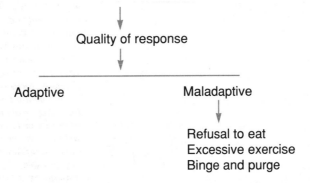

                                    Refusal to eat
                                      Excessive exercise
                                      Binge and purge

Figure 15.1 The dynamics of anorexia nervosa using the transactional model of stress/adaptation.

Table 15.17 DIAGNOSTIC CRITERIA FOR BULIMIA NERVOSA

A. Recurrent episodes of binge eating (rapid consumption of a large amount of food in a discrete period).

B. A feeling of lack of control over eating behavior during the eating binges.

C. The person regularly engages in either self-induced vomiting, use of laxatives or diuretics, strict dieting or fasting, or vigorous exercise to prevent weight gain.

D. A minimum average of two binge eating episodes a week for at least 3 months.

E. Persistent overconcern with body shape and weight.

Source: From APA (1987) with permission.

ity, dependence/independence, and the need for achievement? Does patient understand how he or she has used maladaptive eating behaviors in an effort to achieve a feeling of some control over life events? Has patient acknowledged that perception of body image as "fat" is incorrect? Has patient been able to develop a more realistic perception of body image? Has patient verbalized positive statements about self? Has patient acknowledged that past self-expectations may have been unrealistic? Does patient accept self as less than perfect? Has patient developed adaptive coping strategies to deal with stress without resorting to maladaptive eating behaviors?

Table 15.18 CARE PLAN FOR PATIENT WITH EATING DISORDERS
Anorexia Nervosa and Bulimia Nervosa

Nursing Diagnoses	Objectives	Nursing Interventions
Altered nutrition: Less than body requirements Fluid volume deficit (high risk for or actual) related to refusal to eat/drink; self-induced vomiting; abuse of laxatives/diuretics	Patient will achieve 80%–85% of body weight and be free of signs and symptoms of malnutrition/dehydration.	Dietitian will determine number of calories required to provide adequate nutrition and realistic weight gain. *Adequate calories are required to allow a weight gain of 2–3 lb per week.* Explain to the patient that privileges and restrictions will be based on compliance with treatment and direct weight gain. Do not focus on food and eating. *The real issues have little to do with food or eating patterns. Focus on the control issues that have precipitated these behaviors.* Weigh patient daily, immediately upon arising and following first voiding. Always use same scale, if possible. Keep strict record of intake and output. Assess skin turgor and integrity regularly. Assess moistness and color of oral mucous membranes. *These assessments are important measurements of nutritional status and provide guidelines for treatment.* Stay with patient during established time for meals (usually 30 minutes) and for at least 1 hour following meals. *Lengthy mealtimes put excessive focus on food and eating and provide the patient with attention and reinforcement. The hour following meals may be used to discard food stashed from tray or to engage in self-induced vomiting.* If weight loss occurs, employ restrictions. Patient must understand that if nutritional status deteriorates, tube feedings will be initiated. This is implemented in a matter-of-fact, nonpunitive way. *Restrictions and limits must be established and carried out consistently to avoid power struggles, to encourage patient compliance with therapy, and to ensure patient safety.*

(continued)

Table 15.18 CONTINUED

Nursing Diagnoses	Objectives	Nursing Interventions
Ineffective denial related to retarded ego development and fear of losing the only aspect of life over which patient perceives some control (eating)	Patient will verbalize understanding that eating behaviors are maladaptive and demonstrate the ability to cope with issues of control in a more adaptive manner.	Develop a trusting relationship. Convey positive regard. *Trust and unconditional acceptance promote dignity and self-worth and provide a strong foundation for a therapeutic relationship.* Avoid arguing or bargaining with the patient who is resistant to treatment. State matter-of-factly which behaviors are unacceptable and how privileges will be restricted for noncompliance. *The person who is denying a problem and who also has a weak ego will use manipulation to achieve control. Consistency and firmness by staff will decrease use of these behaviors.* Encourage patient to verbalize feelings regarding role within the family and issues related to dependence/independence, the intense need for achievement, and sexuality. Help patient recognize ways in which he or she can gain control over these problematic areas of life. *When patient feels control over major life issues, the need to gain control through maladaptive eating behaviors will diminish.*
Body image/self-esteem disturbance related to retarded ego development and dysfunctional family system	Patient will acknowledge misperception of body image as "fat" and verbalize positive self-attributes.	Help patient to develop a realistic perception of body image and relationship with food. Compare specific measurements of the patient's body with the patient's perceived calculations. *There may be a large discrepancy between the actual body size and the patient's perception of his or her body size. Patient needs to recognize that the misperception of body image is unhealthy and that maintaining control through maladaptive eating behaviors is dangerous — even life threatening.* Promote feelings of control within the environment through participation and independent decision making. Through positive feedback, help patient learn to accept self as is, including weaknesses as well as strengths. *Patient must come to understand that he or she is a capable, autonomous individual who can perform outside the family unit and who is not expected to be perfect. Control of his or her life must be achieved in other ways besides dieting and weight loss.* Help patient realize that perfection is unrealistic, and explore this need with him or her. *As patient begins to feel better about self and identifies positive self-attributes, as well as develops the ability to accept certain personal inadequacies, the need for unrealistic achievement should diminish.*

Treatment Modalities

The immediate aim of treatment in eating disorders is to restore the patient's nutritional status. Complications of emaciation, dehydration, and electrolyte imbalance can lead to death. Once the physical condition is no longer life threatening, other treatment modalities may be initiated.

BEHAVIOR MODIFICATION

Efforts to change the maladaptive eating behaviors of anorexics and bulimics have become the widely accepted treatment. The importance of instituting a behavior modification program with these patients is to ensure that the program does not "control" them. Issues of control are central to

Table 15.18A CRITICAL PATHWAY OF CARE FOR PATIENT WITH ANOREXIA NERVOSA

Estimated Length of Stay: 28 days—Variations from Designated Pathway Should Be Documented in Progress Notes

Nursing Diagnoses and Categories of Care	Time Dimension	Goals and/or Actions	Time Dimension	Goals and/or Actions	Time Dimension	Discharge Outcome
Altered nutrition: Less than body requires Fluid volume deficit, high risk for	Ongoing	Patient will gain 3 lb/wk and maintain adequate state of hydration			Day 28	Patient will exhibit no signs/symptoms of malnutrition or dehydration.
Referrals	Day 1 and ongoing	Consult dietitian	Day 2–28	Fulfill nutritional needs. Patient consumes 75% of food provided and at least 1000 ml fluid/day.		
Diagnostic studies	Day 1	Electrolytes Electrocardiogram Blood urea nitrogen/creatinine Urinalysis Complete blood count Thyroid function	Day 14	Repeat of selected diagnostic studies.	Day 28	All laboratory values are within normal limits.
Additional assessments	Daily; q shift Daily; q shift Day 1 Day 1	Vital signs Input and output Weight Monitor for purging following meals.	Day 7–28 Day 7–28 Day 2–28 Day 1–21	Vital signs within normal limits Appropriate balance is achieved. Patient gains approximately ½ lb/day. Patient bathroom is locked for 1 hr following meals.	Day 22–28	Patient is able to refrain from self-induced vomiting.
Patient education	Day 1	Unit orientation; behavior modification plan	Day 7–14	Principles of nutrition; foods for maintenance of wellness	Day 15–18	Patient demonstrates ability to select appropriate foods for healthy diet.

(continued)

Table 15.18A   CONTINUED

Estimated Length of Stay: 28 days—Variations from Designated Pathway Should Be Documented in Progress Notes

Nursing Diagnoses and Categories of Care	Time Dimension	Goals and/or Actions	Time Dimension	Goals and/or Actions	Time Dimension	Discharge Outcome
Ineffective denial	Day 1	Patient will cooperate with orientation to unit and explanation of behavior modification plan.	Day 2–28	Patient cooperates with therapy to restore nutritional status.	Day 18–28	Patient accepts that eating behaviors are maladaptive and demonstrates ability to cope more adaptively.
Referrals	Day 7 (or when physical condition is stable).	Psychologist; social worker; psychodramatist	Day 8–28	Patient attends group psychotherapies daily.	Day 28	Patient verbalizes ways to gain control in life situation.
Additional assessments	Day 1–17	Assess patient's ability to trust; use of manipulation to achieve control	Day 14	Patient has developed trusting relationship with at least one staff member on each shift.	Day 28	Patient no longer manipulates others to achieve control.
Patient education	Day 1 and ongoing as required	Describe privileges and responsibilities of behavior modification program. Explain consequences of noncompliance.	Day 21	Discuss roll of support groups for individuals with eating disorders.	Day 28	Patient and family verbalize intention to attend community support group.
Body image/self-esteem disturbance	Day 7	Patient acknowledges that attention will not be given to the discussion of body image and food.	Day 21	Patient acknowledges misperception of body image as fat and verbalizes positive self-attributes.	Day 28	Patient perceives body image correctly, is not obsessed with food, and has given up the need for perfection.
Referrals	Day 1 (or when physical condition is stable).	Occupational therapy; recreational therapy; music therapy; art therapy	Day 2–28	Patient attends therapy sessions on a daily basis.	Day 28	Through self-expression, patient has gained self-awareness and verbalizes positive attributes of self.

(continued)

Table 15.18A CONTINUED

Estimated Length of Stay: 28 days — Variations from Designated Pathway Should Be Documented in Progress Notes

Nursing Diagnoses and Categories of Care	Time Dimension	Goals and/or Actions	Time Dimension	Goals and/or Actions	Time Dimension	Discharge Outcome
Additional assessments	Day 7	Compare specific measurements of patient's body with patient's perceived calculations. Clarify discrepancies.	Day 8–28	Discuss strengths and weaknesses. Patient should strive to achieve self-acceptance.	Day 28	Patient verbalizes acceptance of self, including "imperfections."
Patient education	Day 14–28	Discuss alternative coping strategies for dealing with feelings. Have patient keep diary of feelings, particularly when thinking about food.			Day 28	Patient demonstrates adaptive coping strategies unrelated to eating behaviors for dealing with feelings.

the etiology of these disorders, and in order for the program to be successful, the patient must perceive that he or she is in control of the treatment.

Successes have been observed when the patient is allowed to contract for privileges based on weight gain (Sanger & Cassino, 1984). The patient has input into the care plan and can clearly see what the treatment choices are. The patient has control over eating, over the amount of exercise pursued, and even over whether or not to induce vomiting. Goals of therapy are agreed upon by patient and staff, along with the responsibilities of each for goal achievement.

Staff and patient also agree upon a system of rewards and privileges that can be earned by the patient. Ultimate control is given to the patient. He or she has a choice of whether or not to abide by the contract — a choice of whether or not to gain weight — a choice of whether or not to earn the desired privilege.

FAMILY THERAPY

The usefulness of family therapy in conjunction with behavior therapy has been observed (Kaplan & Sadock, 1985). In many instances, eating disorders may be considered *family* disorders, and resolution cannot be achieved until dynamics within the family have improved.

Family therapy deals with education of the members about the disorder's manifestations, possible etiology, and prescribed treatment. Support is given to family members as they deal with feelings of guilt associated with the perception that they may have contributed to the onset of the disorder. Support is also given as they deal with the social stigma of having a family member with emotional problems.

In some instances where the dysfunctional family dynamics are related to conflict avoidance, the family may be noncompliant with therapy, as they attempt to maintain equilibrium by keeping a member in the sick role. When this occurs, it is essential to focus on the functional operations within the family and to provide assistance with managing conflict and creating change.

Referrals are made to local support groups for families of individuals with eating disorders. Resolution and growth can sometimes be achieved through interaction with others who are experiencing, or have experienced, the numerous problems of living with an anorexic or bulimic family member.

PSYCHOPHARMACOLOGY

There are no medications specifically indicated for eating disorders. Various medications have been prescribed for associated symptoms, such as anxiety and depression. Kaplan and Sadock (1985) report on the use of chlorpromazine (Thorazine) and amitriptyline (Elavil) in patients with anorexia nervosa. Cyproheptadine (Periactin), in its unlabeled use as an appetite stimulant, has also been used to treat this disorder.

Therapy for anorexia nervosa with other antidepressants, such as desipramine (Norpramin), doxepin (Sinequan), or trazodone (Desyrel), has been reported (Sanger & Cassino, 1984). Several investigators have indicated good results with imipramine (Tofranil) in the treatment of bulimia nervosa (Kaplan & Sadock, 1985).

Psychopharmacology in the treatment of eating disorders is in its infancy. A great deal of further study is required before efficacy can be established.

GENDER IDENTITY DISORDERS

Gender identity is the sense of knowing to which sex one belongs, that is, the awareness of one's masculinity or femininity. Gender identity disorders occur when there is an incongruence between anatomic sex and gender identity. The *DSM-III-R* describes three gender identity disorders: gender identity disorder of childhood, transsexualism, and gender identity disorder of adolescence or adulthood. Although individuals with these disorders may seek clinical assistance at almost any age, in the majority of cases the onset of the disorder can be traced back to childhood (APA, 1987). For this reason, they are categorized together. For purposes of this text, each of these disorders will be defined, but only gender identity disorder of childhood will be discussed at length. Treatment aimed at reversal in behavior is considered cautiously optimistic if initiated in childhood. After one has established a clear cut core gender identity, it is difficult later in life to instill attributes of an opposite identity (Kaplan & Sadock, 1985).

Predisposing Factors

BIOLOGICAL INFLUENCES

Little, if any, convincing biological evidence exists to explain the etiology of gender disorders (Zucker, 1985). There are currently a number of studies being conducted relating to the influence of prenatal gonadal hormones on postnatal psychosexual behavior.

Hoenig (1985) reported on several studies of familial incidence in the case of transsexualism. The disorder is relatively rare, so case collection is difficult. However, various studies with siblings, twins, and other biological relatives suggest that familial factors may indeed play a role in the etiology of the disorder. However, the biological marker remains elusive.

FAMILY INFLUENCES

It appears that family dynamics plays the most influential role in the etiology of gender disorders. In Green's (1974) study with feminine boys, he concluded that the requisite variable was that, as any feminine behavior began to emerge, there was no discouragement of that behavior by the child's principal caretaker. He found this to be the case in nearly every family.

This pattern coincides with the family dynamics described as predisposing factors to gender identity disorders in the *DSM-III-R*. These include strong interests in opposite-gender activities and weak reinforcement of normative gender-role behavior by the parents. In boys, there may also be an absence or unavailability of a father and encouragement of extreme physical and psychological closeness with her son by the mother.

Application of the Nursing Process

BACKGROUND ASSESSMENT DATA (SYMPTOMATOLOGY)

Gender Identity Disorder of Childhood   In this disorder, the prepubescent child manifests a profound disturbance in his or her sense of masculinity or femininity. There is intense distress about the anatomic sex assignment and insistence that he or she is, or desires to be, of the opposite sex (APA, 1987). There is aversion to the physical characteristics of the anatomic sex and a preoccupation with opposite sex stereotypic activities or dress. They may insist that they will grow up to be a member of the opposite sex.

They are subjected to teasing and rejection by their peers and disapproval from most family members. This occurs early in childhood for male patients, but rarely occurs before adolescence in female patients. Because of this rejection, interpersonal relationships are hampered.

The disorder is not common, but it occurs more frequently in boys than in girls. The *DSM-III-R* diagnostic criteria for gender identity disorder of childhood are presented in Table 15.19.

Transsexualism   This disorder occurs in a person who has reached puberty and who experiences persistent discomfort and a sense of inappropriateness about his or her anatomic sex. The diagnosis is made only if there has been persistent preoccupation, for at least 2 years, with getting rid of one's primary and secondary sex characteristics and acquiring the sex characteristics of the opposite gender (APA, 1987). These individuals desire to live as a member of the opposite sex, dress in clothes of the opposite sex, and often engage in activities that are culturally associated with the opposite sex. They may be repelled by the characteristics that define their anatomic sex and persist in their requests for hormonal therapy or surgery to generate a sex reassignment. Almost without exception, these individuals report having had a gender identity problem in childhood (APA, 1987).

Gender Identity Disorder of Adolescence or Adulthood, Nontranssexual Type   The *DSM-III-R* describes this disorder as one in which there is persistent or recurrent discomfort and sense of inappropriateness about one's assigned sex, and persistent or recurrent cross-dressing in the role of the other sex, either in fantasy or in actuality, in a

Table 15.19   DIAGNOSTIC CRITERIA FOR GENDER IDENTITY DISORDER OF CHILDHOOD

For Females:

A. Persistent and intense distress about being a girl and a stated desire to be a boy (not merely a desire for any perceived cultural advantages from being a boy), or insistence that she is a boy.

B. Either of the following:
1. Persistent marked aversion to normative feminine clothing and insistence on wearing stereotypical masculine clothing, e.g., boys' underwear and other accessories
2. Persistent repudiation of female anatomic structures, as evidenced by at least one of the following:
   a. an assertion that she has, or will grow, a penis
   b. rejection of urinating in a sitting position
   c. assertion that she does not want to grow breasts or menstruate

C. The girl has not yet reached puberty.

For males:

A. Persistent and intense distress about being a boy and an intense desire to be a girl, or more rarely, insistence that he is a girl.

B. Either of the following:
1. Preoccupation with female stereotypical activities, as shown by a preference for either cross-dressing or simulating female attire, or by an intense desire to participate in the games and pastimes of girls and rejection of male stereotypical toys, games, and activities
2. Persistent repudiation of male anatomic structures, as indicated by at least one of the following repeated assertions:
   a. That he will grow up to become a woman (not merely in role)
   b. That his penis or testes are disgusting or will disappear
   c. That it would be better not to have a penis or testes

C. The boy has not yet reached puberty.

Source: APA (1987) with permission.

person who has reached puberty. The cross-dressing is not for the purpose of sexual excitement, as in the case of transvestism, and there is no preoccupation with sex reassignment, as in transsexualism. Psychosocial history reveals evidence of gender identity problems in childhood, and the disorder may evolve into transsexualism.

NURSING DIAGNOSES

Based upon the data collected during the nursing assessment, possible nursing diagnoses for the patient with gender identity disorder of childhood include:

Personal identity disturbance related to parenting patterns that encourage culturally unacceptable behaviors for assigned sex
Impaired social interaction related to socially and culturally unacceptable behaviors
Self-esteem disturbance related to rejection by peers.

PLANNING/IMPLEMENTATION

Table 15.20 provides a plan of care for the patient with gender identity disorder of childhood using nursing diagnoses common to this disorder, goals of care, and appropriate nursing interventions for each. Rationale is provided in italics.

NOTE: Most of the treatment conducted with children with this disorder have been in outpatient clinics. Nurses working in these settings may encounter these patients from time to time, although the disorder is relatively rare. One-to-one nursing intervention may be provided by a nurse specialist with a master's-degree.

EVALUATION

The final step of the nursing process is to determine if the nursing interventions have been effective in achieving the intended goals of care. This evaluation process requires that the nurse reassess the patient's behaviors and determine if the changes at which the interventions had been directed have occurred. For the child with gender identity disorder, this may be accomplished by using the following types of questions:

Does patient demonstrate use of behaviors that are culturally accepted for his or her assigned sex? Does the patient perceive that a problem existed, and that a change in behavior is the solution to the problem? Is the patient able to use these culturally accepted behaviors in interactions with others? Is the patient accepted by peers when same-sex behaviors are used? If the patient is refusing to change behaviors, what is peer reaction? What is the patient's response to negative peer reaction? Is the patient able to verbalize positive statements about self? Can the patient discuss past accomplishments without dwelling on the perceived failures? Has the patient shown progress toward accepting self as a worthwhile person regardless of others' responses to his or her behavior?

Table 15.20 CARE PLAN FOR PATIENT WITH GENDER IDENTITY DISORDER OF CHILDHOOD		
Nursing Diagnoses	**Objective**	**Nursing Interventions**
Personal identity disturbance related to parenting patterns that encourage culturally unacceptable behaviors for assigned sex.	Patient will verbalize knowledge of and demonstrate behaviors that are appropriate and culturally acceptable for assigned sex.	Spend time with patient and show positive regard. *Trust and unconditional acceptance are essential to the establishment of a therapeutic nurse/patient relationship.* Be aware of own feelings and attitudes toward this patient and his or her behavior. *Attitudes influence behavior. The nurse must not allow negative attitudes to interfere with the effectiveness of interventions.* Allow patient to describe his or her perception of the problem. *It is important to know how the patient perceives the problem before attempting to correct misperceptions.* Discuss with patient the type of behaviors that are more culturally acceptable. Practice these behaviors through role playing or with play therapy strategies (i.e., male and female dolls). Positive reinforcement or social attention may be given for use of appropriate behaviors. No response is given for opposite-sex-stereotype behaviors. *The goal is to enhance culturally appropriate same-sex behaviors, but not necessarily to extinguish all coexisting opposite-sex behaviors (Rosen et al., 1982).*

(*continued*)

Table 15.20 CONTINUED

Nursing Diagnoses	Objective	Nursing Interventions
Impaired social interaction related to socially and culturally unacceptable behaviors.	Patient will interact with others using culturally acceptable behaviors.	Once patient feels comfortable with the new behaviors in role playing or one-to-one nurse/patient interactions, they may be tried in group situations. If possible, remain with patient during interactions with others. Observe patient behaviors and the responses he or she elicits from others. Give social attention (e.g., smile, nod) to desired behaviors. Follow up these "practice" sessions with one-to-one processing of the interaction. Give positive reinforcement for efforts. Offer support if patient is feeling hurt from peer ridicule. Matter-of-factly discuss the behaviors that elicited the ridicule. Offer no personal reaction to the behavior. *The goal is to create a trusting, nonthreatening atmosphere for the patient in an attempt to change behavior and improve social interactions. Long-term studies have not yet revealed the significance of therapy with these children on psychosexual relationship development in adolescence or adulthood. One variable that must be considered is the evidence of psychopathology within the families of many of these children (Zucker, 1985).*
Self-esteem disturbance related to rejection by peers.	Patient will verbalize positive statements about self, including past accomplishments and future prospects.	Encourage child to engage in activities in which he or she is likely to achieve success. Help the child to focus on aspects of his or her life for which positive feelings exist. Discourage rumination about situations that are perceived as failures or over which patient has no control. Give positive reinforcement for these behaviors. *Success and positive feedback enhance self-esteem.* Help patient identify behaviors or aspects of life he or she would like to change. If realistic, assist child in problem-solving ways to bring about the change. *Having some control over his or her life may decrease feelings of powerlessness and increase feelings of self-worth.* Offer to be available for support to the child when he or she is feeling rejected by peers. *Having an available support person who does not judge the child's behavior and who provides unconditional acceptance assists the child to progress toward acceptance of self as a worthwhile person.*

SUMMARY

Child and adolescent psychiatric nursing is a specialty that has been given very little attention. Most basic nursing curricula include little or no instruction in child psychiatric nursing, and the topic is generally ignored on state board examinations (Clunn, 1991). Even though nurses work in many areas that place them in ideal positions to identify emotionally disturbed children, many of them do not have sufficient knowledge of child psychopathology to recognize maladaptive behaviors.

This chapter has presented the most prevalent disorders identified by the *DSM-III-R* (APA, 1987) as first becoming evident in infancy, childhood, or adolescence. An explanation of various etiological factors was presented for each disorder in an effort to assist in the comprehension of underlying dynamics. These included biological, environmental, and family influences.

The nursing process was presented as the vehicle for delivery of care. Symptomatology for each of the disorders provided background assessment data. Nursing diagnoses identified specific behaviors that were targeted for change. Both the patient and family were considered in the planning and implementation. Behavior modification is the focus of nursing intervention with children and adoles-

cents. With families, attention is given to education and referrals to community resources from which they can derive support. Reassessment data provide information for evaluation of nursing interventions in achieving the desired outcomes.

Child psychiatry is an area where nursing can make a valuable contribution. Nurses who choose this field have an excellent opportunity to serve in the promotion of emotional wellness for children and adolescents.

REVIEW QUESTIONS
Self-Examination/Learning Exercise

*Select the answer that is **most** appropriate for each of the following questions.*

1. In an effort to help the mildly to moderately mentally retarded child develop satisfying relationships with others, which of the following nursing interventions is most appropriate?
   a. Interpret the child's behavior for others.
   b. Set limits on behavior that is socially inappropriate.
   c. Allow the child to behave spontaneously, for he or she has no concept of right or wrong.
   d. This child is not capable of forming social relationships.

2. The autistic child has difficulty with trust. With this in mind, which of the following nursing actions would be *most* appropriate?
   a. Encourage all staff to hold the child as often as possible, conveying trust through touch.
   b. Assign a different staff member each day so child will learn that everyone can be trusted.
   c. Assign same staff person as often as possible to promote feelings of security and trust.
   d. Avoid eye contact, as it is extremely uncomfortable for the child and may even discourage trust.

3. Which of the following nursing diagnoses would be considered the *priority* in planning care for the autistic child?
   a. High risk for self-mutilation evidenced by banging head against wall.
   b. Impaired social interaction evidenced by unresponsiveness to people.
   c. Impaired verbal communication evidenced by absence of verbal expression.
   d. Personal identity disturbance evidenced by inability to differentiate self from others.

4. Which of the following activities would be most appropriate for the child with ADHD?
   a. Monopoly
   b. Volleyball
   c. Pool
   d. Checkers

5. With regard to the literature (even though the results are inconclusive), which of the following foods might it be wise to omit when helping the hyperactive child select a snack?
   a. Peanut butter and crackers
   b. Popcorn and apple juice
   c. Peanuts and raisins
   d. Cookies and Koolaid

6. Drug management of the hyperactive child is most common with which of the following groups?
   a. Central nervous system depressants (e.g., Valium)
   b. Central nervous system stimulants (e.g., Ritalin)
   c. Anticonvulsants (e.g., Dilantin)
   d. Major tranquilizers (e.g., Haldol)

7. The nursing history and assessment of an adolescent with a conduct disorder might reveal all of the following behaviors *except:*
   a. Manipulation of others for fulfillment of own desires
   b. Chronic violation of rules
   c. Feelings of guilt associated with the exploitation of others
   d. Inability to form close peer relationships

8. Certain family dynamics often predispose adolescents to the development of conduct disorder. Which of the following patterns is thought to be a contributing factor?
   a. Parents who are overprotective
   b. Parents who have high expectations for their children
   c. Parents who consistently set limits on their children's behavior
   d. Parents who are alcohol dependent

9. The precipitating stressor that may trigger the symptoms characteristic of anorexia nervosa is:
   a. A preoccupation with beauty and appearance
   b. Any aspect of their life that produces feelings of lack of control
   c. Aggression as the dominant pattern of family dynamics
   d. Lack of satisfactory mother/infant relationship

10. The *primary* nursing consideration in working with the anorexic patient is to:
    a. Identify stressors
    b. Include family members
    c. Relieve depression
    d. Restore nutrition

11. With the above primary nursing consideration in mind, which corresponding nursing diagnosis becomes the *priority* on the care plan for the anorexic patient?
    a. Dysfunctional grieving
    b. Altered nutrition: Less than body requirements
    c. Alteration in family process
    d. Anxiety (severe)

12. In helping the child with a gender identity problem, which is the most appropriate nursing intervention?
    a. Give positive reinforcement when he or she engages in assigned sex behaviors

b. Give negative reinforcement when he or she engages in opposite sex behaviors
c. Do not allow the child to interact with others until he or she demonstrates only appropriate behaviors
d. Withdraw privileges if the child is noncompliant

REFERENCES

American Psychiatric Association. (1987). *Diagnostic and statistical manual of mental disorders* (3rd ed, rev.). Washington DC: American Psychiatric Association.

Baum, C. G. (1989). Conduct disorders. In T. H. Ollendick & M. Hersen (Eds.), *Handbook of child psychopathology* (2nd ed). New York: Plenum Press.

Berger, M. (1985). Temperament and individual differences. In M. Rutter & L. Hersov (Eds.), *Child and adolescent psychiatry: Modern approaches.* Oxford: Blackwell Scientific.

Bruch, H. (1970). Eating disorders in adolescence. *Proceedings of the American Psychopathology Association, 59,* pp. 181–202.

Bruch, H. (1983). Psychotherapy in anorexia nervosa and developmental obesity. In R. K. Goodstein (Ed.), *Eating and weight disorders,* New York: Springer.

Clunn, P. (Ed.). (1991). *Child psychiatric nursing.* St. Louis: Mosby-Year Book, Inc.

Dodge, KA, et al. (1982). Behavior patterns of socially rejected and neglected preadolescents: The roles of social approach and aggression. *J Abnorm Child Psychol, 10,* pp. 389–410.

Feingold, B. F. (1976). Hyperkinesis and learning disabilities linked to the ingestion of artificial food colors and flavors. *Journal of Learning Disabilities, 9,* pp. 551–559.

Green, R. (1974). *Sexual identity conflict in children and adults.* Baltimore: Penguin.

Hoenig, J. (1985). Etiology of transsexualism. In B. W. Steiner (Ed.), *Gender dysphoria: Development, research, management.* New York: Plenum Press.

Kanner, L. (1973). To what extent is early infantile autism determined by constitutional inadequacies? In *Childhood psychosis: Initial studies and new insights.* Washington, DC: VH Winston.

Kaplan, H. I. & Sadock B. J. (1985). *Modern synopsis of comprehensive textbook of psychiatry* (4th ed.). Baltimore: Williams & Wilkins.

Klein, R. G. & Last C. G. (1989). *Anxiety disorders in children.* Newbury Park: Sage Publications.

Last, C. (1989). Anxiety disorders. In T. H. Ollendick & M. Hersen (Eds.), *Handbook of child psychopathology* (2nd ed.). New York: Plenum Press.

Leon, G. R. & Dinklage, D. (1989). Obesity and anorexia nervosa. In T. H. Ollendick & M. Hersen (Eds.), *Handbook of child psychopathology* (2nd ed.). New York: Plenum Press.

Mahler, M., Pine, F. and Bergman, A. (1975). *Psychological birth of the human infant.* New York: Basic Books.

Minuchin, S., Rosman, B. and Baker, L. (1978). *Psychosomatic families.* Cambridge, MA: Harvard University Press.

Needleman, H. L. & Bellinger, D. (1984). The developmental consequences of childhood exposure to lead: Recent studies and methodological issues. In B. B. Lahey & A. E. Kazdin (Eds.), *Advances in clinical child psychology.* New York: Plenum Press.

Nichols, & Chen (1981). *Minimal brain dysfunction: A prospective study.* Hillsdale, N.J.: Lawrence Erlbaum.

Olweus, D., Mattsson, A., Shalling, D. and Low, H. (1980). Testosterone, aggression, physical, and personality dimensions in normal adolescent males. *Psychosom Med, 42,* pp. 253–269.

Plomin, R. (1983). Childhood temperament. In B. B. Lahey & A. E. Kazdin (Eds), *Advances in clinical child psychology* (Vol. 6). New York: Plenum Press.

Rutter, M. (1987). Temperament, personality, and personality disorder. *Br J Psychiatry, 100,* pp. 443–458.

Rutter, M. et al. (1964). Temperamental characteristics in infancy and the later development of behavioural disorders. *Br J Psychiatry, 110,* pp. 651–661.

Sanger, E. & Cassino, T. (1984, January). Eating disorders: Avoiding the power struggle. *AJN 84*(1):31–33.

Schreibman, L. & Charlop, M. H. (1989). Infantile autism. In T. H. Ollendick & M. Hersen (Eds.), *Handbook of child psychopathology* (2nd ed.). New York: Plenum Press.

Scipien, G. M., Barnard, M. U., Chard, M. A., Howe, J. and Phillips, P. J. (1975). *Comprehensive pediatric nursing.* New York: McGraw-Hill.

Shaywitz, S. E., Shaywitz, B. A., Cohen, D. J., and Young, J. G. (1983). Monoaminergic mechanisms in hyperactivity. In M. Rutter (Ed.), *Developmental neuropsychiatry*. New York: Guilford Press.

Whalen, C. K. (1989). Attention deficit and hyperactivity disorders. In T. H. Ollendick & M. Hersen (Eds.), *Handbook of child psychopathology*. New York: Plenum Press.

Zucker, K. J. (1985). Cross-gender-identified children. In B. W. Steiner (Ed), *Gender dysphoria: Development, research, management*. New York: Plenum Press.

BIBLIOGRAPHY

Achenbach, T. M. (1982). *Developmental psychopathology*. (2nd ed.) New York: The Ronald Press Co.

Bakwin, H. & Bakwin, R. M. (1972). *Behavior disorders in children* (4th ed.). Philadelphia: WB Saunders.

Devine, P. (1983, March). Mental retardation: An early subspecialty in psychiatric nursing. *J Psychosoc Nurs 21*(3):21–30.

Dizon, M. A. B. (1984, March). Secure attachment—Anxious attachment. *J Psychosoc Nurs 22*(3): 27–31.

Doenges, M, Townsend, M, & Moorhouse, M. (1989). *Psychiatric care plans: Guidelines for client care*. Philadelphia: FA Davis.

Gilliam, J. E. (1981). *Autism: Diagnosis, instruction, management, and research*. Springfield, IL: Charles C. Thomas.

Keltner, N. L. (1984, August). Bulimia: Controlling compulsive eating. *J Psychosoc Nurs, 22*(8):24–29.

Kiecolt-Glaser, J. & Dixon, K. (1984, January). Postadolescent onset male anorexia. *J Psychosoc Nurs, 22*(1):11–20.

Potts, N. L. (1984, January). Eating disorders: The secret pattern of binge/purge. *AJN 84*(1):33–35.

Reed, G. & Sech, E. P. (1985, May). Bulimia: A conceptual model for group treatment. *J Psychosoc Nurs, 23*(5):16–22.

Schopler, E. & Mesibon, G. B. (1988). *Diagnosis and assessment in Autism*. New York: Plenum Press.

Slade, R. (1984). *The anorexia nervosa reference book*. London: Harper and Row Publishers.

Stoller, R. J. (1985). *Presentations of gender*. New Haven, CT: Yale University Press.

Townsend, M. C. (1991). *Nursing Diagnoses in Psychiatric Nursing: A Pocket Guide for Care Plan Construction* (2nd ed.). Philadelphia: FA Davis.

Weiss, L., Katzman, M., & Wolchik, S. (1985). *Treating bulimia: A psychoeducational approach*. New York: Pergamon Press.

White, J. H. (1984, April). Bulimia—Utilizing individual and family therapy. *J Psychosoc Nurs, 22*(4):22–28.

16

ORGANIC MENTAL SYNDROMES AND DISORDERS

In Psychoactive Substance-
Induced Intoxication and/or
Withdrawal
SUMMARY

OBJECTIVES

After reading this chapter, the student will be able to:

1. Describe various organic mental syndromes and disorders.
2. Discuss predisposing factors implicated in the etiology of organic mental syndromes and disorders.
3. Identify symptomatology and use the information in the assessment of patients with organic mental syndromes and disorders.
4. Identify nursing diagnoses common to patients with organic mental syndromes and disorders and select appropriate nursing interventions for each.
5. Discuss relevant criteria for evaluating nursing care of patients with organic mental syndromes and disorders.
6. Describe various treatment modalities relevant to care of patients with organic mental syndromes and disorders.

INTRODUCTION

This chapter presents a discussion of disorders that represent the dysfunction, and in some instances the eventual loss, of mental functions in an otherwise alert and awake individual. These disorders constitute a large and growing public health problem that is expected to persist well into the next century. Today, an estimated 1.5 million Americans suffer from severe dementia—that is, they are so incapacitated that others must care for them continually (Cook-Deegan et al, 1988). An additional 1 million to 5 million Americans have mild or moderate dementia. Ten times as many people are affected now as were at the turn of the century, and the number of people with severe dementia is expected to increase 60 percent by 2000. Unless cures or means of prevention are found for the common causes of dementia, 7.4 million Americans will be affected by the year 2040—five times as many as today (Cook-Deegan et al, 1988). This proliferation is not the result of an "epidemic," but rather because more people now survive into the high-risk period for dementia, middle age and beyond.

This chapter presents predisposing factors, symptomatology, and nursing interventions for care of the patient with organic brain syndromes and disorders. The objective is to provide these individuals with the dignity and quality of life they deserve, while offering guidance and support to their families or primary caregivers.

SYNDROME *VS.* DISORDER

In the *Diagnostic and Statistical Manual of Mental Disorders, ed 3, Revised (DSM-III-R)* (American Psychiatric Association [APA], 1987) a distinction is made between organic mental *syndromes* (OMS) and organic mental *disorders* (OMD). Syndrome refers to a cluster of signs and symptoms for which no etiology is known (e.g., dementia or delirium). Disorders designate particular syndromes for which the etiology is known or presumed (e.g., multi-infarct dementia, or alcohol withdrawal delirium).

Organic mental syndromes and disorders may be categorized as chronic or acute, reversible or irreversible. The chronic conditions generally have a subtle and insidious onset. The progression of deterioration is slow and most often irreversible. This is particularly true in pathologic processes that cause structural damage to the brain, such as primary degenerative dementia of the Alzheimer type.

Acute conditions have a sudden onset of symptoms due to a disturbance in brain function (e.g., delirium associated with acute infection or dementia resulting from major head trauma). Impairment may be reversible with time and treatment, or may become permanent and progressive, depending on the extent and severity of the cause.

ORGANIC MENTAL SYNDROMES

As previously stated, OMS refers to clusters of signs and symptoms for which no etiology is known. An individual may be diagnosed with an OMS based solely on the behavioral evidence being exhibited. If the etiology is never established, the syndrome diagnosis is retained. Underlying organic pathology is assumed. If etiology is established, the diagnosis would change to OMD. For example, if an individual is diagnosed with the OMS of delirium, based on presenting symptomatology, and is later found to be withdrawing from alcohol,

the diagnosis would be changed to alcohol withdrawal delirium, an OMD. The *DSM-III-R* describes the symptomatology related to OMS within the following categories. Examples of etiological factors implicated in the development of these syndromes are presented in Table 16.1.

1. Delirium
2. Dementia
3. Amnestic syndrome
4. Organic hallucinosis
5. Organic delusional syndrome
6. Organic mood syndrome
7. Organic anxiety syndrome
8. Organic personality syndrome
9. Intoxication
10. Withdrawal

Delirium

Symptoms of delirium include difficulty sustaining and shifting attention. The person is extremely distractible and must be repeatedly reminded to focus attention. Disorganized thinking prevails and

Table 16.1   ETIOLOGICAL FACTORS IMPLICATED IN THE DEVELOPMENT OF ORGANIC MENTAL SYNDROMES

Biologic Factors	Exogenous Factors
Hypoxia: any condition leading to a deficiency of oxygen to the brain	Birth trauma: prolonged labor, damage from use of forceps, other obstetric complications
Nutritional deficiencies: vitamins (particularly the B vitamins and vitamin C); protein; fluid and electrolyte imbalances	Cranial trauma: concussion, contusions, hemorrhage, hematomas
Metabolic disturbances: porphyria; encephalopathies related to hepatic, renal, pancreatic, or pulmonary insufficiencies; hypoglycemia	Volatile inhalant compounds: gasoline, glue, paint, paint thinners, spray paints, cleaning fluids, typewriter correction fluid, varnishes and lacquers
Endocrine dysfunction: thyroid, parathyroid, adrenal, pancreas, pituitary	Heavy metals: lead, mercury, manganese
Cardiovascular disease: stroke, cardiac insufficiency, atherosclerosis	Other metallic elements: aluminum
Primary brain disorders: epilepsy, Alzheimer's disease, Pick's disease, Huntington's chorea, multiple sclerosis, Parkinson's disease	Organic phosphates: various insecticides
Infections: encephalitis, meningitis, pneumonia, septicemia, neurosyphilis (dementia paralytica), acquired immunodeficiency syndrome, acute rheumatic fever, Creutzfeldt-Jakob disease	Substance abuse/dependence: alcohol, amphetamines, caffeine, cannabis, cocaine, hallucinogens, inhalants, nicotine, opioids, phencyclidine, sedatives, hypnotics, anxiolytics
Intracranial neoplasms	Other medications: anticholinergics, antihistamines, antidepressants, antipsychotics, antiparkinsons, antihypertensives, steroids, digitalis
Congenital defects: prenatal infections, such as first-trimester maternal rubella	

is reflected by speech that is rambling, irrelevant, pressured, incoherent, and unpredictably switches from subject to subject. Reasoning ability and goal-directed behavior are impaired. Disorientation to time and place is common, and impairment of recent memory is invariably evident. Misperceptions of the environment, including illusions and hallucinations, prevail.

Level of consciousness is often affected, with a disturbance in the sleep-wake cycle. The state of awareness may range from that of hypervigilance to stupor or semicoma. Sleep may fluctuate between hypersomnolence and insomnia. Vivid dreams and nightmares are common.

Psychomotor activity may fluctuate between agitated, purposeless movements, such as restlessness, hyperactivity, and striking out at nonexistent objects, and a vegetative state resembling catatonic stupor. Various forms of tremor are frequently present.

Emotional instability may be manifested by fear, anxiety, depression, irritability, anger, euphoria, or apathy. These various emotions may be evidenced by crying, calls for help, cursing, muttering, moaning, acts of self-destruction, and fearful attempts to flee or attacks upon others who are falsely viewed as threatening.

Autonomic manifestations, such as tachycardia, sweating, flushed face, dilated pupils, and elevated blood pressure, are common.

The symptoms of delirium usually begin quite abruptly, such as following a head injury or seizure. At other times, it may be preceded by several hours or days of prodromal symptoms, such as restlessness, difficulty thinking clearly, insomnia or hypersomnolence, and nightmares. The slower onset is more common if the underlying etiology is systemic illness or metabolic imbalance.

The duration of delirium is usually brief (e.g., 1 week; rarely for more than 1 month) and subsides completely upon recovery from the underlying determinant. If the underlying determinant persists, the syndrome of delirium gradually shifts to a more stable syndrome (e.g., dementia) or may result in death (APA, 1987).

Dementia

Memory impairment is the most characteristic feature of dementia, with loss of memory for recent

events being most prominent. Memory disturbance is demonstrated by difficulty in learning new information (deficits in short-term memory) and in remembering past personal information or facts of common knowledge (deficits in long-term memory).

Impairment is also evident in abstract thinking, judgment, and impulse control. The conventional rules of social conduct are often disregarded. Behavior may be uninhibited and inappropriate. Personal appearance and hygiene are often neglected.

Language may or may not be affected. Some individuals may have difficulty naming objects, or the language may seem vague and imprecise. In severe forms of dementia, the individual may not speak at all (aphasia).

Personality change is common in dementia and may be manifested by either an alteration or accentuation of premorbid characteristics. For example, an individual who was normally very socially active may become apathetic and socially isolated. A previously neat person may become markedly untidy in his or her appearance. Conversely, an individual who may have had difficulty trusting others prior to the illness may exhibit extreme fear and paranoia as manifestations of the dementia.

The reversibility of a dementia is a function of the underlying pathology and of the availability and timely application of effective treatment (APA, 1987). Truly reversible dementia occurs in only 2 to 3 percent of cases (Cook-Deegan et al, 1988). In most patients, dementia runs a progressive, irreversible course.

As the disease progresses, apraxia, the inability to carry out motor activities despite intact motor function, may develop. The individual may be irritable, moody, or exhibit sudden outbursts over trivial issues. The ability to work or care for personal needs independently will no longer be possible. These individuals can no longer be left alone, as they do not comprehend their limitations and are therefore at serious risk for accidents. Wandering away from the home or care setting often becomes a problem.

Cook-Deegan et al (1988) describe the late stages of dementia in the following manner:

"The late stages of the disease often begin with the onset of incontinence. Gradually the apraxia progresses until these persons are unable to walk without help. Many are bedfast. They will need to be bathed, fed, dressed, and toileted. They will be essentially mute; language will consist only of one or two words or cries. Behavior problems disappear due to the severity of the overall impairment. Seizures are common. These people become feeble and emaciated. They may refuse to eat or be unable to swallow without choking, so that artificial feeding may be required. They are at risk of developing bedsores, infections, and pneumonia. Pneumonia is a common cause of death. There is significant variability in the symptoms from person to person and some symptoms never appear in some individuals."

Amnestic Syndrome

The primary characteristic of this syndrome is impairment in short- and long-term memory that is attributed to a specific organic factor (e.g., organic changes related to chronic use of alcohol). The individual with amnestic syndrome has both an ongoing inability to learn new material (short-term memory deficit) and an inability to recall material that was known in the past (long-term memory deficit). However, events from the very remote past are more easily recalled than recently occurring ones. The syndrome differs from dementia in that there is no impairment in abstract thinking or judgment, no other disturbances of higher cortical function, and no personality change.

The amnesia commonly results in disorientation. The individual may engage in confabulation, the creation of imaginary events to fill in memory gaps.

Some individuals will continue to deny that they have a problem, even with evidence to the contrary. Of those who do acknowledge that a problem exists, many appear unconcerned. Apathy, lack of initiative, and emotional blandness are common. The person may appear friendly and agreeable, but the emotionality is superficial.

The onset of symptoms is usually abrupt. Duration of the illness depends on the extent and severity of the cause. The course is usually chronic.

Organic Hallucinosis

The prominent feature of this organic syndrome is the presence of persistent or recurrent hallucinations that are attributed to a specific organic factor, such as cerebral changes related to chronic use of alcohol or recent hallucinogen use. Visual and auditory hallucinations are most common, although the individual may experience false perceptions through all of the five senses. Other symptoms, such as those that occur with delirium, are not present.

Most often, the content of the hallucinations is unpleasant and disturbing. The individual who has ingested a hallucinogenic drug may also experience physical symptoms, including pupillary dilation, tachycardia, sweating, palpitations, blurring of vision, tremors, and incoordination.

Duration of symptoms depends on the underlying etiology. With chronic use of alcohol, and particularly after an extended period of alcohol intoxication, symptoms develop soon after cessation of drinking and may last for several weeks or months.

After ingestion of a hallucinogen, onset of symptoms usually occurs within 1 hour and may last from a few hours to a few days. Symptoms may produce anxiety or depression in the individual.

Organic Delusional Syndrome

This syndrome is identified by prominent delusions that can be attributed to a specific organic factor, such as ingestion of amphetamines, cannabis, cocaine, hallucinogens, or phencyclidine. Other symptoms, such as those that occur with delirium, are not present. Delusions of persecution are the most common type.

Mild cognitive impairment may be evident, with disorientation and incoherent or rambling speech. Hyperactivity may be manifested by increased pacing or rocking; or the individual may sit apathetically immobile. Dysphoric mood is common.

Organic Mood Syndrome

The characteristic feature of this syndrome includes persistent depression or elevation of mood. Symptoms mimic episodes of major depression or mania and are attributed to a specific organic factor, such as use of hallucinogens, hyperthyroidism, or hypothyroidism.

When the syndrome mimics mania, symptoms include elation, hyperactivity, psychomotor agitation, inflated self-esteem, excessive talkativeness, flight of ideas, distractibility, delusions of grandeur or persecution, and decreased need for sleep.

When the syndrome mimics depression, symptoms include sad affect, diminished interest or pleasure in usual activities, psychomotor retardation, insomnia or hypersomnia, weight loss or gain, lack of energy, excessive somatic complaints, feelings of worthlessness, difficulty concentrating, and suicidal ideations.

Organic Anxiety Syndrome

This syndrome is characterized by prominent, recurrent, panic attacks or generalized anxiety attributed to a specific organic factor, such as stimulant intoxication, withdrawal from CNS depressants, or certain endocrine disorders (e.g., hypothyroidism or hyperthyroidism). Symptoms include excessive anxiety, fear, worry, restlessness, difficulty concentrating, irritability, shortness of breath, heart palpitations, sweating, dizziness, abdominal distress, hot flashes, or chills.

Duration of the syndrome depends on the extent and severity of the underlying cause. Recovery is generally expected when the etiologic factor is removed.

Organic Personality Syndrome

The characteristic feature of this syndrome is a persistent personality disturbance. The disturbance may represent a lifelong pattern of behavior or a change or accentuation of a previous personality trait. The symptoms are attributed to a specific organic factor, such as neoplasms of the brain, head trauma, cerebrovascular disease, or use of psychoactive substances.

Common symptoms include unstable mood, recurrent outbursts of aggression or rage, impaired social judgment, marked apathy and indifference, and suspiciousness. Changes in patterns of behavior are generally evident. For example, the individual who is usually mild-mannered by nature may respond with temper outbursts and belligerence that is grossly out of proportion to a situation. An individual who is normally very socially correct may exhibit socially inappropriate behaviors, such as sexual indiscretions.

Another pattern of behavior is seen in individuals who show sudden indifference and lack of interest in usual hobbies and other activities. Still another pattern of personality change may be the development of suspiciousness or paranoid ideation.

Duration of symptoms depends on the extent and severity of the etiology. The course may be of short duration if the syndrome was the result of a psychoactive substance that is no longer ingested or from a neoplasm that was successfully removed shortly after the symptoms appeared. However, if structural damage has occurred, or the etiology is a progressive disorder such as multiple sclerosis, the duration becomes chronic and is likely to eventually develop into a dementia.

NOTE: The final two categories, intoxication and withdrawal, are considered by the *DSM-III-R* as OMS. However, when they become substance specific, they are then categorized as OMD.

Intoxication

Symptoms of this syndrome are attributed to recent ingestion of a psychoactive substance that results in maladaptive behavioral changes. Symptoms of the substance-specific intoxication disorders include the following:

1. *Alcohol.* Disinhibition of sexual or aggressive impulses, mood lability, impaired judgment, impaired social or occupational functioning, slurred speech, incoordination, unsteady gait, nystagmus, and flushed face. Intoxication usually occurs at blood alcohol levels between 100 and 200 mg/dl. Death has been reported at levels ranging from 400 to 700 mg/dl.
2. *Amphetamines.* Fighting, grandiosity, hypervigilance, psychomotor agitation, impaired judgment, impaired social or occupational functioning, tachycardia, pupillary dilation, elevated blood pressure, perspiration or chills, and nausea or vomiting. The course of amphetamine intoxication is usually self-limited, with full recovery within 48 hours.
3. *Caffeine.* Restlessness, nervousness, excitement, insomnia, flushed face, diuresis, gastrointestinal disturbance, muscle twitching, rambling flow of thought and speech, tachycardia or cardiac arrhythmia, periods of inexhaustibility, and psychomotor agitation. Symptoms occur following recent consumption of caffeine in excess of 250 mg. (NOTE: one cup of coffee contains 100 to 150 mg of caffeine; one

cup of tea contains 50 to 75 mg; and one glass of cola contains 30 to 50 mg).

4. *Cannabis.* Euphoria, anxiety, suspiciousness or paranoid ideation, sensation of slowed time, impaired judgment, social withdrawal, conjunctival injection, increased appetite (often for "junk" food), dry mouth, and tachycardia. Intoxication from smoking marijuana occurs immediately and lasts about 3 hours. The substance is more slowly absorbed when orally ingested and has longer-lasting effects.

5. *Cocaine.* Euphoria, fighting, grandiosity, hypervigilance, psychomotor agitation, impaired judgment, impaired social or occupational functioning, tachycardia, pupillary dilation, elevated blood pressure, perspiration or chills, nausea or vomiting, and visual or tactile hallucinations. The course of cocaine intoxication is usually self-limited, with full recovery within 48 hours. Following large doses, seizures may occur. Death may result from cardiac arrhythmias or respiratory paralysis.

6. *Inhalants.* Belligerence, assaultiveness, apathy, impaired judgment, impaired social or occupational functioning, dizziness, nystagmus, incoordination, slurred speech, unsteady gait, lethargy, depressed reflexes, psychomotor retardation, tremor, generalized muscle weakness, blurred vision or diplopia, stupor or coma, and euphoria. Inhalant substances include gasoline, glue, paint, paint thinners, spray paints, and cleaning compounds. These inhalants are rapidly distributed through the lungs. Intoxication occurs within 5 minutes and lasts about 1 to 1½ hours.

7. *Opioids.* Initial euphoria followed by apathy, dysphoria, psychomotor retardation, impaired judgment, impaired social or occupational functioning, pupillary constriction, drowsiness, slurred speech, and impairment in attention or memory. Opioids include codeine, morphine, meperidine, methadone, oxycodone, and others. They are commonly prescribed as analgesics, anesthetics, or cough suppressants.

8. *Phencyclidine.* Belligerence, assaultiveness, impulsiveness, unpredictability, psychomotor agitation, impaired judgment, impaired social or occupational functioning, vertical or horizontal nystagmus, increased blood pressure or heart rate, numbness or diminished responsiveness to pain, ataxia, speech impairment, muscle rigidity, seizures, and hypersensitivity to sound. Intoxication lasts 4 to 6 hours. Effects can last for several days.

9. *CNS depressants.* Disinhibition of sexual or aggressive impulses, mood lability, impaired judgment, impaired social or occupational functioning, slurred speech, incoordination, unsteady gait, and impairment in attention and memory. Substances in this category include sedatives, hypnotics, and anxiolytics. Factors affecting onset and duration of intoxication include amount and rapidity of substance ingested and tolerance and body size of the individual.

Withdrawal

The essential feature of withdrawal is the development of a substance-specific syndrome that follows the cessation of, or reduction in, intake of a psychoactive substance that the person previously used regularly (APA, 1987). Symptoms of the substance-specific withdrawal disorders include the following:

1. *Alcohol.* Within several hours of cessation of or reduction in prolonged (several days or longer) heavy drinking, the following symptoms may appear: coarse tremor of hands, tongue, or eyelids, nausea or vomiting, malaise or weakness, tachycardia, sweating, elevated blood pressure, anxiety, depressed mood or irritability, transient hallucinations or illusions, headache, and insomnia. A complicated withdrawal syndrome may progress to *alcohol withdrawal delirium.* Onset of delirium is usually on the second or third day following cessation of or reduction in prolonged, heavy drinking. Symptoms include those described under the syndrome of delirium.

2. *Amphetamines and cocaine.* Symptoms occur following abrupt cessation of or reduction in prolonged (several days or longer) heavy use of amphetamines or cocaine. Symptoms include depression, irritability, anxiety, fatigue, insomnia or hypersomnia, and psychomotor agitation. Paranoia and suicidal ideation may be present. Symptoms peak in 2 to 4 days, al-

though depression and irritability may persist for months.

3. *Nicotine.* Symptoms occur within 24 hours of abrupt cessation of or reduction in use of nicotine (on a daily basis for at least several weeks). Symptoms include craving for nicotine, irritability, frustration, anger, anxiety, difficulty concentrating, restlessness, decreased heart rate, increased appetite, or weight gain.

4. *Opioids.* Symptoms occur following abrupt cessation of or reduction in prolonged, heavy use of opioids. In the case of morphine or heroin, symptoms usually appear within 6 to 8 hours of the last dose, reach a peak on the second or third day, and disappear in 7 to 10 days. The withdrawal process is quicker and shorter with meperidine, and slower and longer with methadone. Symptoms include craving for an opioid, nausea or vomiting, muscle aches, lacrimation or rhinorrhea, pupillary dilation, piloerection or sweating, diarrhea, yawning, fever, and insomnia.

5. *CNS depressants.* Symptoms occur following cessation of or reduction in prolonged (several weeks or more) moderate or heavy use of sedatives, hypnotics, or anxiolytics. Symptoms include nausea or vomiting; malaise or weakness; tachycardia; sweating; anxiety or irritability; orthostatic hypotension; coarse tremor of hands, tongue, and eyelids; marked insomnia; and grand mal seizures. The onset of benzodiazepine withdrawal is usually within 2 to 3 days after cessation of use; but with long-acting drugs, such as diazepam, there may be a latency period of 5 to 6 days before the withdrawal syndrome appears (APA, 1987). A complicated withdrawal syndrome may progress to *withdrawal delirium*, with onset within 1 week following cessation of or reduction in substance use. Symptoms include those described under the syndrome of delirium.

ORGANIC MENTAL DISORDERS

As previously stated, the difference between OMS and OMD is that in the latter the etiology is either known or presumed. The *DSM-III-R* identifies the following categories of organic mental disorders:

1. Dementias arising in the senium and presenium
   a. Primary degenerative dementia of the Alzheimer type
   b. Multi-infarct dementia
2. Psychoactive substance-induced organic mental disorders
3. Organic mental disorders associated with physical disorders or conditions, or whose etiology is unknown

Dementias Arising in the Senium and Presenium

PRIMARY DEGENERATIVE DEMENTIA OF THE ALZHEIMER TYPE

This disorder is characterized by the syndrome of dementia. The onset of symptoms is slow and insidious, and the course of the disorder is generally progressive and deteriorating. The *DSM-III-R* further categorizes this disorder as *senile onset* (first symptoms appear after age 65) and *presenile onset* (initial symptoms occur at age 65 or younger).

Although this disorder presents a distinct clinical picture, a definitive diagnosis requires biopsy or autopsy examination of brain tissue (Cook-Deegan et al, 1988). Gross examination reveals a degenerative pathology of the brain that includes atrophy, widened cortical sulci, and enlarged cerebral ventricles. Sometimes these changes can be viewed in life with a computerized axial tomography scan or pneumoencephalogram.

Microscopic examinations reveal numerous neurofibrillary tangles and senile plaques in the brains of patients with Alzheimer's disease. These changes apparently occur as a part of the normal aging process. However, in patients with Alzheimer's disease, they are found in dramatically increased numbers and their profusion is concentrated in the hippocampus and certain parts of the cerebral cortex. In aging patients who do not have dementia, the plaques and tangles are much less frequent and are more widely dispersed (Cook-Deegan et al, 1988).

Predisposing Factors The exact cause of Alzheimer's disease is unknown. Several hypotheses have been supported by varying amounts and quality of supporting data. These hypotheses include:

1. *Acetylcholine alterations.* Research has indi-

cated that in the brains of Alzheimer's patients, the enzyme required to produce acetylcholine is dramatically reduced. The reduction seems to be greatest in the areas of the brain where the senile plaques and neurofibrillary tangles occur in the greatest numbers (Cohen & Eisdorfer, 1986). This decrease in production of acetylcholine reduces the amount of the neurotransmitter that is released to cells in the cortex and hippocampus, resulting in a disruption of memory processes (Cook-Deegan et al, 1988).

2. *Accumulation of aluminum.* Several studies have reported higher concentrations of aluminum in the brains of Alzheimer's patients than in those of healthy older persons without dementia (Cohen & Eisdorfer, 1986). However, high concentrations of aluminum also have been reported in the brains of patients with other types of dementias. Therefore, aluminum as a contributing factor is probably not specific to Alzheimer's disease. More research is necessary to determine the role of aluminum in the etiology of all dementias.

3. *Alterations in the immune system.* Several studies have shown that antibodies are produced in the Alzheimer's brain. What the antibodies are produced in response to is unknown. The reactions are actually *auto*antibody production — a reaction against the self — suggesting a possible alteration in the body's immune system as an etiological factor in Alzheimer's disease.

4. *Head trauma.* The etiology of Alzheimer's disease has been associated with serious head trauma (Cook-Deegan et al, 1988). Studies have shown that a large number of individuals who had experienced head trauma had subsequently (after years) developed Alzheimer's disease. This hypothesis is currently being investigated as a possible cause.

5. *Genetic factors.* There is clearly a familial pattern with some forms of Alzheimer's disease. Some families exhibit a pattern of inheritance that suggests possible autosomal-dominant gene transmission (Cook-Deegan et al, 1988). Some studies indicate that early-onset cases (before age 65) are more likely to be familial than late-onset cases, and that from one-third to one-half of all cases may be of the genetic form. The *DSM-III-R* (APA, 1987) identifies

Down's syndrome as a predisposing factor to Alzheimer's disease.

MULTI-INFARCT DEMENTIA

In this disorder, the clinical syndrome of dementia is due to significant cerebrovascular disease. The blood vessels of the brain are affected, and progressive intellectual deterioration occurs. Multi-infarct dementia, believed to be the second most common cause of dementia, may be responsible for 15 to 25 percent of the cases (Cohen & Eisdorfer, 1986).

Multi-infarct dementia differs from Alzheimer's disease in that it has a relatively abrupt onset and runs a more variable course. Progression of the symptoms occurs in "steps" rather than gradual deterioration; that is, at times the dementia seems to clear up and the individual exhibits fairly lucid thinking. Memory may seem better, and the patient may become optimistic that improvement is occurring, only to experience further decline of functioning in a fluctuating pattern of progression. This irregular pattern of decline appears to be an intense source of anxiety for the patient with this disorder (Cohen & Eisdorfer, 1986).

In multi-infarct dementia, patients suffer the equivalent of small strokes that destroy many areas of the brain. The pattern of deficits is variable, depending on which regions of the brain have been destroyed (APA, 1987). Certain focal neurologic signs are commonly seen with multi-infarct dementia, including weakness of the limbs, small-stepped gait, and difficulty with speech.

Life expectancy is somewhat shorter for patients with multi-infarct dementia than for those with Alzheimer's disease (Cook-Deegan et al, 1988). The disorder is more common in men than in women (APA, 1987).

Predisposing Factors The cause of multi-infarct dementia is directly related to an interruption of blood flow to the brain. Symptoms result from death of nerve cells in regions nourished by diseased vessels. Various diseases and conditions that interfere with blood circulation have been implicated. These include:

1. *Arterial hypertension.* High blood pressure is the most significant factor in the etiology of multiple small strokes or cerebral infarcts (APA, 1987). Hypertension causes thickening

and degeneration of cerebral arterioles, making the small arteries vulnerable to rupture (Phipps et al, 1987).

2. ***Cerebral emboli.*** Dementia can result from infarcts related to occlusion of blood vessels by debris within the bloodstream. These emboli can arise from diseased heart valves, damage to cells lining the heart, the dislodging of clots in large vessels, the release of fat from large bones, or large sudden infusions of air or other gases (Cook-Deegan et al, 1988; APA, 1987).

3. ***Cerebral thrombosis.*** Multiple small thrombi may occur in persons whose blood pressure is normal or even below normal if atheromatous changes have occurred in the lining of cerebral arteries (Phipps et al, 1987). This condition causes frequent small and barely perceptible infarcts that can lead to personality changes and memory deficits.

Psychoactive Substance-Induced Organic Mental Disorders

These disorders are identified by various syndromes of symptoms caused by the direct effects of various psychoactive substances on the central nervous system (APA, 1987). These syndromes include all ten of those described under the section on OMS in the beginning of this chapter. In addition, substance-specific symptomatology was described for the syndromes of intoxication and withdrawal. The classes of substances that most commonly induce these organic syndromes include the following:

1. alcohol
2. amphetamines and related substances
3. caffeine
4. cannabis
5. cocaine
6. hallucinogens
7. inhalants
8. nicotine
9. opioids
10. phencyclidine and related substances
11. sedatives, hypnotics, or anxiolytics

Table 16.2 identifies the specific OMSs known to be caused by each class of psychoactive substance. These syndromes are classified as OMDs when they are identified with a specific substance. For example, organic delusional syndrome becomes cocaine delusional disorder when the symptoms are attributed to the substance cocaine.

PREDISPOSING FACTORS

The etiology of psychoactive substance-induced OMDs is the prolonged heavy use of substance(s) that are taken nonmedicinally to alter mood or behavior (APA, 1987). Substance dependence may be a factor. The dynamics of these disorders using the Transactional Model of Stress/Adaptation is presented in Figure 16.1.

Organic Mental Disorders Associated with Physical Disorders or Conditions, or Whose Etiology is Unknown

A number of physical disorders and conditions have been identified as etiological factors in the development of OMDs. Dementia is the most common syndrome of symptoms associated with these disorders, although in severe acute infections, such as pneumonia, the clinical picture is more likely to manifest symptoms of delirium.

PREDISPOSING FACTORS

Physical disorders and conditions that predispose to OMDs include, but are not limited to:

1. ***Parkinson's disease.*** Dementia occurs in about one-fifth of patients with Parkinson's disease (Fraser, 1987). In this disease, there is a loss of nerve cells located in the substantia nigra and dopamine activity is diminished, resulting in involuntary muscle movements, slowness, and rigidity. Tremor in the upper extremities is characteristic. In some instances, the cerebral changes that occur in dementia of Parkinson's disease closely resemble those of Alzheimer's disease.

2. ***Huntington's chorea.*** This disease is transmitted as a Mendelian dominant gene. Damage is seen in the basal ganglia and cerebral cortex. The onset of symptoms (i.e., involuntary twitching of the limbs or facial muscles) is usually between age 30 and 40. The patient usually declines into a profound state of de-

Table 16.2   ORGANIC MENTAL SYNDROMES ASSOCIATED WITH PSYCHOACTIVE SUBSTANCES

Psychoactive Substances	Delirium	Dementia	Amnestic Syndrome	Organic Halluci-nosis	Organic Delusional Syndrome	Organic Mood Syndrome	Organic Anxiety Syndrome	Organic Personality Syndrome	Intox-ication	With-drawal
Alcohol		X	X	X					X	X*
Amphetamine and related substances	X				X				X	X
Caffeine									X	
Cannabis					X				X	
Cocaine	X				X				X	X
Hallucinogens				X	X	X				
Inhalants									X	
Nicotine										X
Opioids									X	X
Phencyclidine and related substances	X				X	X			X	
Sedatives, hypnotics, or anxiolytics			X						X	X*

*May progress to withdrawal delirium.
Source: American Psychiatric Association (1987).

mentia and ataxia within 5 to 10 years of onset (Fraser, 1987).

3. *Pick's disease.* The cause of this disorder is unknown, but a genetic factor appears to be involved. The clinical picture is strikingly similar to Alzheimer's disease. In fact, diagnosis of Pick's disease is most often made on autopsy of a patient with clinically diagnosed Alzheimer's disease (Cook-Deegan et al, 1988). Onset of symptoms is usually in middle age, and women are affected more frequently than men (Fraser, 1987). Studies reveal that pathology results from atrophy in the frontal and temporal lobes of the brain.

4. *Multiple sclerosis.* This disease is characterized by a disseminating demyelination of nerve fibers within the central nervous system. Initial symptoms include weakness, numbness, vertigo, and visual changes. There may be periods of remission and exacerbation, or a steady progression of neurologic dysfunction. In the late stages of the disease, the individual may exhibit some symptoms of dementia, including memory deficits, confusion, and disorientation (Thompson et al, 1986).

5. *Epilepsy.* Uncontrolled epilepsy may lead to behavior and personality changes, and memory deficits (Patrick et al, 1991). This is especially true of uncontrolled temporal lobe epilepsy, but has also been reported in patients with generalized tonic-clonic seizures.

6. *Neurosyphilis.* This disorder causes cerebral atrophy that results in problems with a variety of higher cognitive functions and can lead to regressive, childlike behavior.

7. *Head trauma.* Symptoms of posttraumatic or postconcussion syndrome include headache, irritability, dizziness, diminished concentration, and hypersensitivity to certain stimuli. Intellectual function and memory may be minimally impaired (Patrick et al, 1991).

8. *Various medical conditions: diabetes, pulmonary disease, hepatic or renal failure, cardiopulmonary insufficiency, thyroid, parathyroid,*

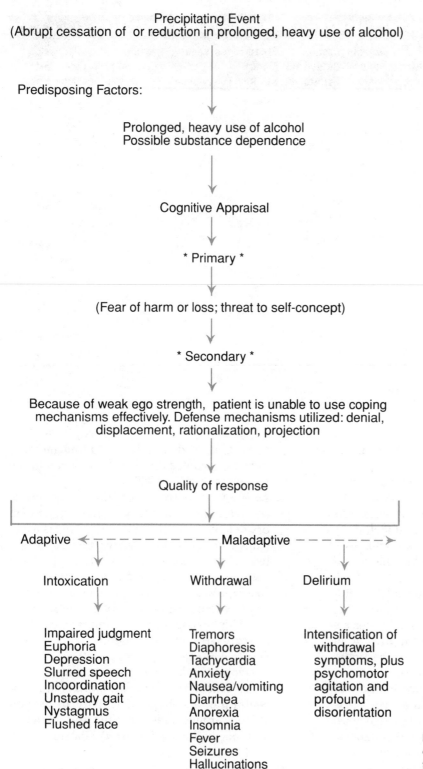

Figure 16.1 The dynamics of alcohol-induced organic mental disorders using the transactional model of stress/adaptation.

or adrenal dysfunction, fluid and electrolyte imbalances, and nutritional deficiencies. Any of these conditions may interfere with cognitive functions, such as attention, memory, language, perception, planning, judgment, insight, and problem solving (Patrick et al, 1991).

9. *Frontal or temporal lobe lesions.* Tumor (either benign or malignant) in these areas may result in personality changes, memory deficits, and other cognitive and behavioral changes.

10. *Central nervous system or systemic infections.* Various infectious processes (e.g., pneumonia, encephalitis, and meningitis) can interfere with thinking, attention, and memory.

11. *Acquired Immunodeficiency Syndrome (AIDS).* This disease is the most common cause of dementia due to infection (Cook-Deegan et al, 1988). The immune dysfunction of AIDS can lead to brain infections by other organisms, and the AIDS virus also appears to cause dementia directly. Neuropsychiatric symptoms may range from barely perceptible changes in a person's normal psychological presentation to acute delirium to profound dementia (Perkins, 1989).

APPLICATION OF THE NURSING PROCESS

Assessment

Nursing assessment of the patient with an OMS or OMD is based on knowledge of the symptomatology associated with the various OMSs described in the beginning of this chapter. Subjective and objective data are gathered by various members of the health-care team. Clinicians report use of a variety of methods for obtaining assessment information (Cook-Deegan et al, 1988; Cohen & Eisdorfer, 1986).

THE PATIENT HISTORY

Nurses play a significant role in acquiring the patient history, including the specific mental and physical changes that have occurred and the age at which the changes began. If the patient is unable to relate information adequately, the data should be obtained from family members or others who would be aware of the patient's physical and psy-

chosocial history. From the patient history, nurses should assess the following areas of concern: type, frequency, and severity of mood swings, personality and behavioral changes, and catastrophic emotional reactions; cognitive changes, such as problems with attention span, thinking process, problem solving, and memory (recent and remote); language difficulties; orientation to person, place, time, and situation; and appropriateness of social behavior.

The nurse also should obtain information regarding current and past medication usage, and history of other drug and alcohol use. Knowledge regarding the history of related symptoms or specific illnesses, such as Huntington's chorea, Alzheimer's disease, Pick's disease, or Parkinson's disease, in other family members may be useful.

PHYSICAL ASSESSMENT

Assessment of physical systems by both the nurse and physician has two main emphases: signs of damage to the nervous system and evidence of diseases of other organs that could affect mental function (Cook-Deegan et al, 1988). Diseases of various organ systems can induce confusion, loss of memory, and behavioral changes. These causes must be considered in diagnosing OMDs. In the neurological examination, the patient is asked to perform maneuvers or answer questions that are designed to elicit information about the condition of specific parts of the brain or peripheral nerves. Testing will assess mental status and alertness, muscle strength, reflexes, sensory perception, language skills, and coordination (Cohen & Eisdorfer, 1986). A battery of psychological tests may be ordered as part of the diagnostic examination. The results of these tests may be used to make a differential diagnosis between dementia and pseudodementia (depression). They can be very useful in establishing an effective treatment plan.

DIAGNOSTIC LABORATORY EVALUATIONS

The nurse also may be required to assist the patient in fulfilling the physician's orders for special diagnostic laboratory evaluations. Many of these tests are routinely included with the physical examination. They may include evaluation of blood and urine samples to test for various infections, hepatic and renal dysfunction, diabetes or hypoglycemia, electrolyte imbalances, metabolic and endocrine disorders, nutritional deficiencies, and presence of toxic substances, including alcohol and other drugs.

Other diagnostic evaluations may be made by electroencephalogram, which measures and records the brain's electrical activity. With computerized tomography scan, an image of the size and shape of the brain can be obtained. A new, and as yet experimental, technology called *positron emission tomography* reveals the metabolic activity of the brain, an evaluation some researchers believe will be important in the diagnosis of Alzheimer's disease. Magnetic resonance imaging is used to obtain a computerized image of soft tissue in the body. It provides a sharp and detailed picture of the tissues of the brain (Cohen & Eisdorfer, 1986). A lumbar puncture may be performed to examine the cerebrospinal fluid for evidence of central nervous system infection or hemorrhage.

Nursing Diagnoses

Using information collected during the assessment, the nurse completes the patient data base, from which the selection of appropriate nursing diagnoses is determined. Possible nursing diagnoses for patients with OMDs include:

High risk for trauma related to impairments in cognitive and psychomotor functioning

High risk for injury related to substance intoxication or withdrawal

High risk for self-directed violence related to depressed mood secondary to awareness in decline of mental and/or physical capability

High risk for violence directed toward others related to impairment of impulse control

Altered thought processes related to cerebral degeneration evidenced by disorientation, confusion, memory deficits, and inaccurate interpretation of the environment

Self-esteem disturbance related to loss of independent functioning evidenced by expressions of shame and self-degradation and progressive social isolation

Ineffective individual coping related to disorientation, confusion, and memory deficits evidenced by inability to fulfill activities of daily living.

Planning/Implementation

Table 16.3 provides a plan of care for the patient with dementia (irrespective of etiology). Selected nursing diagnoses are presented, along with goals of care and appropriate nursing interventions for each. Rationale is provided in italics.

Some institutions are using a case management

Table 16.3 CARE PLAN FOR PATIENT WITH DEMENTIA		
Nursing Diagnoses	**Objectives**	**Nursing Interventions**
High risk for trauma related to impairments in cognitive and psychomotor functioning	Patient will not experience injury.	The following measures may be instituted *to ensure patient safety:* a. Arrange furniture and other items in the room to accommodate patient's disabilities. b. Store frequently used items within easy access. c. Keep bed in unelevated position. Pad siderails and headboard if patient has history of seizures. Keep bedrails up when patient is in bed. d. Assign room near nurses' station; observe frequently. e. Assist patient with ambulation. f. Keep a dim light on at night. g. If patient is a smoker, cigarettes and lighter or matches should be kept at the nurses' station and dispensed only when someone is available to stay with patient while he or she is smoking. h. Frequently orient patient to place, time, and situation. i. Soft restraints may be required if patient is very disoriented and hyperactive.

(continued)

Table 16.3 CONTINUED

Nursing Diagnoses	Objectives	Nursing Interventions
Altered thought processes related to cerebral degeneration evidenced by disorientation, confusion, memory deficits, and inaccurate interpretation of the environment	Patient will interpret the environment accurately and maintain reality orientation to the best of his or her cognitive ability.	Frequently orient patient to reality. Use clocks and calendars with large numbers that are easy to read. Notes and large, bold signs may be useful as reminders. Allow patient to have personal belongings. *All of these items serve to help maintain orientation and aid in memory and recognition.* Keep explanations simple. Use face-to-face interaction. Speak slowly and do not shout. *These interventions facilitate comprehension. Shouting may create discomfort, and in some instances may provoke anger.* Discourage rumination of delusional thinking. Talk about real events and real people. *Rumination promotes disorientation. Reality orientation increases sense of self-worth and personal dignity.* Monitor for medication side effects. *Physiologic changes in the elderly can alter the body's response to certain medications. Toxic effects may intensify altered thought processes.*
Ineffective individual coping related to disorientation, confusion, and memory deficits evidenced by inability to fulfill activities of daily living	Patient will accomplish activities of daily living to the best of his or her ability. Unfulfilled needs will be met by caregivers.	Provide a simple, structured environment *to minimize confusion:* a. Identify self-care deficits and provide assistance as required. Promote independent actions as able. b. Allow plenty of time for patient to perform tasks. c. Provide guidance and support for independent actions by talking the patient through the task one step at a time. d. Provide a structured schedule of activities that does not change from day to day. e. Activities of daily living should follow home routine as closely as possible. f. Allow consistency in assignment of daily caregivers. *In planning for discharge:* a. Perform ongoing assessment of patient's ability to fulfill nutritional needs, ensure personal safety, follow medication regimen, and communicate need for assistance with those activities that he or she cannot accomplish independently. b. Assess prospective caregivers' ability to anticipate and fulfill patient's unmet needs. Provide information to assist caregivers with this responsibility. Ensure that caregivers are aware of available community support systems from which they can seek assistance when required. Examples include: adult day-care centers, housekeeping and homemaker services, respite care services, or perhaps a local chapter of the Alzheimer's Disease and Related Disorders Association. This organization sponsors a nationwide 24-hour hot line to provide information and link families who need assistance with nearby chapters and affiliates. The hot-line number is 1-800-621-0379.

model to coordinate care (see Chapter 6 for more detailed explanation). In case management models, the plan of care may take the form of a critical pathway.

Table 16.4 is an example of a critical pathway of care for a patient experiencing the syndrome associated with alcohol withdrawal.

Evaluation

In the final step of the nursing process, reassessment occurs to determine if the nursing interventions have been effective in achieving the intended goals of care. Evaluation of the patient with an OMS/OMD may be accomplished by using information gathered from the following reassessment questions.

FOR THE PATIENT WITH DEMENTIA

Evaluation of the patient with a progressive dementing disease is based on a series of short-term goals rather than long-term goals. Resolution of

Table 16.4   CRITICAL PATHWAY OF CARE FOR PATIENT IN ALCOHOL WITHDRAWAL

Estimated Length of Stay: 7 days — Variations from designated pathway should be documented in progress notes

Nursing Diagnoses and Categories of Care	Time Dimension	Goals and/or Actions	Time Dimension	Goals and/or Actions	Time Dimension	Discharge Outcome
Potential for injury related to central nervous system agitation					Day 7	Patient shows no evidence of injury obtained during ETOH withdrawal.
Referrals	Day 1	Psychiatrist Assess need for: Neurologist Cardiologist Internist			Day 7	Discharge with follow-up appointments as required
Diagnostic studies	Day 1	Blood alcohol level Drug screen SMAC 27 Urinalysis Chest x-ray ECG	Day 4	Repeat of selected diagnostic studies as necessary		
Additional assessments	Day 1 Day 1–5 ongoing ongoing	VS q4h I&O Restraints prn Assess withdrawal symptoms: tremors, nausea/vomiting, tachycardia, sweating, high blood pressure, seizures, insomnia, hallucinations	Day 2–3 Day 6 Day 4	VS q8h if stable DC I&O Marked decrease in objective symptoms	Day 4–7 Day 7	VS bid; remain stable Discharge; Absence of objective withdrawal symptoms

(continued)

Table 16.4 CONTINUED

Estimated Length of Stay: 7 days—Variations from designated pathway should be documented in progress notes

Nursing Diagnoses and Categories of Care	Time Dimension	Goals and/or Actions	Time Dimension	Goals and/or Actions	Time Dimension	Discharge Outcome
Medications	Day 1 Day 2 Day 1–6 Day 1–7	Librium 200 mg Librium 160 mg Librium prn Maalox ac and hs	Day 3 Day 4	Librium 120 mg Librium 80 mg	Day 5 Day 6 Day 7	Librium 40 mg DC Librium Discharge; no withdrawal symptoms
Patient education			Day 5	Discuss goals of Alcoholics Anonymous (AA) and need for outpatient therapy	Day 7	Discharge with information regarding AA attendance or outpatient treatment
Altered nutrition: Less than body requirements					Day 7	Nutritional condition has stabilized.
Referrals	Day 1	Consult Dietitian	Day 1–7	Fulfill nutritional needs		
Diet	Day 1	Bland as tolerated; fluids as tolerated	Day 2–3	Frequent, small, meals; easily digested foods; advance as tolerated	Day 4–7	High-protein, high-carbohydrate diet
Additional assessments	Day 1–7	Weight I&O Skin turgor Color of mucous membranes				
Medications	Day 1–4	Thiamine 100-mg injections	Day 2–7	Multiple vitamin tablet		
Patient education			Day 5	Principles of nutrition; foods for maintenance of wellness	Day 6–7	Patient demonstrates ability to select appropriate foods for healthy diet

identified problems is unrealistic for this patient. Instead, outcomes must be measured in terms of slowing down the process rather than stopping or curing the problem (Detwiler, 1989). Evaluation questions may include:

Has patient experienced injury?

Does patient maintain orientation to time, person, place, and situation most of the time?

Is patient able to fulfill basic needs?

Have those needs unmet by patient been fulfilled by caregivers?

Is confusion minimized by familiar objects and structured, routine schedule of activities?

Do prospective caregivers have information regarding the progression of patient's illness?

Do they have information regarding where to go for assistance and support in the care of their loved one?

Have prospective caregivers received instruction in how to promote patient safety, minimize confusion and disorientation, and cope with difficult patient behaviors (hostility, anger, depression, and agitation)?

FOR THE PATIENT WITH ALCOHOL WITHDRAWAL

Evaluation questions may include:

Has patient progressed through the withdrawal syndrome without injury?

Are vital signs stable?

Does patient exhibit any objective symptoms of alcohol withdrawal?

Have substitution medications been discontinued?

Has nutritional status stabilized?

Can patient verbalize principles of good nutrition?

Does he or she select appropriate foods from daily menu?

Does patient verbalize the need for aftercare?

Has patient made arrangements to begin outpatient treatment or attend Alcoholics Anonymous?

Does patient admit that alcohol is a problem in his or her life?

MEDICAL TREATMENT MODALITIES

Psychopharmacology In Progressive Degenerative Dementia

A number of pharmaceutical agents have been tried, with varying degrees of success, in the treatment of patients with dementia. The drugs that follow are described according to the symptomatology for which they are indicated (see Chapter 12), for side effects and nursing implications of the psychotrophics).

COGNITIVE IMPAIRMENT

The angiotensin-converting enzyme inhibitor physostigmine (Antilirium) has been shown to enhance the ability to assimilate new information into long-term memory (Fraser, 1987). Use of vasodilators, such as cyclandelate (Cyclan), has resulted in improvements in orientation, communication, and socialization in patients with multi-infarct dementia (Fraser, 1987). Probably the most extensively studied and widely prescribed drug for dementia is ergoloid mesylate (Hydergine). Its precise mode of action is unclear, but it is thought to enhance brain cell metabolism. The effects are exhibited by mild mental improvement, increased alertness, and relief of depression (Cook-Deegan, et al, 1988). Improvements have been observed with these drugs in the early stages of dementia only. They are of no benefit to patients with moderate or severe dementia.

AGITATION, AGGRESSION, HALLUCINATIONS, THOUGHT DISTURBANCES, AND WANDERING

Antipsychotic medications are used to control these behaviors in patients with dementia. Commonly used drugs include chlorpromazine (Thorazine), thioridazine (Mellaril), and haloperidol (Haldol). The usual adult dosage must be decreased in the elderly patient. Paradoxical effects are not uncommon. Haloperidol is extremely effective in calming a disturbed patient. However, it is generally not suitable for continual use as it tends to accumulate and produce heavy sedation. Extrapyramidal side effects are most common with haloperidol. Thioridazine is considered an excellent choice for tranquilization of the demented elderly both by day and by night (Fraser, 1987).

DEPRESSION

Depression has been observed in 15 to 20 percent of early dementia patients (Cohen & Eisdorfer, 1986). Recognizing the symptoms of depression in these individuals is often a challenge. Depression, which affects thinking, memory, sleep, appetite, and interferes with daily life, is sometimes difficult to distinguish from dementia. Clearly, the existence of depression in the patient with dementia complicates and worsens the individual's functioning. Antidepressant medication is sometimes used in the treatment of depression in dementia. The tricyclics are the most commonly used group. Examples of tricyclics are amitriptyline (Elavil), desipramine (Norpramin), doxepin (Adapin), and imipramine (Tofranil). The dosage for elderly individuals is usually one-fourth to one-half of the usual daily adult dose. Several newer antidepressants, including trazodone (Desyrel), bupropion (Wellbutrin), and fluoxetine (Prozac), are now on the market. Their long-term advantages and disadvantages have not yet been fully evaluated for use in older persons with dementia.

ANXIETY

The progressive loss of mental functioning is a significant source for anxiety in the early stages of dementia. Patients should be encouraged to verbalize their feelings and fears associated with this loss. These interventions may be useful in reducing the anxiety of patients with dementia. Antianxiety medications may be helpful but should not be used routinely or for prolonged periods. The least toxic and most effective of the antianxiety medications are the benzodiazepines. Examples include diazepam (Valium), chlordiazepoxide (Librium), alprazolam (Xanax), lorazepam (Ativan), and oxazepam (Serax). Barbiturates are not appropriate as antianxiety agents, as they frequently induce confusion and paradoxical excitement in elderly individuals.

SLEEP DISTURBANCES

Sleep problems are common in patients with dementia and often intensify as the disease progresses. Wakefulness and nighttime wandering create much distress and anguish in family members who are charged with protection of their loved one. Indeed, sleep disturbances are among the problems that most frequently cause families to place the patient in a long-term care facility (Cohen & Eisdorfer, 1986). Some physicians treat sleep problems with sedative-hypnotic medications. The benzodiazepines may be useful for some patients but are indicated for relatively brief periods only. Examples include flurazepam (Dalmane), temazepam (Restoril), and triazolam (Halcion). As stated above, barbiturates should not be used in elderly patients. Sleep problems are usually ongoing, and most clinicians prefer to use medications only to help an individual through a short-term stressful situation. Behavioral approaches to sleep problems, such as rising at the same time each morning, eliminating or minimizing afternoon naps, regular physical exercise, proper nutrition, stimulating activities, and retiring at the same time each night, may eliminate the need for sleep aids, particularly in the early stages of dementia (Cohen & Eisdorfer, 1986).

In Psychoactive Substance-Induced Intoxication and/or Withdrawal

Various medications have been used to decrease the intensity of symptoms in an individual who is withdrawing from, or who is experiencing the effects of excessive use of, alcohol and other drugs. Substitution therapy may be required to reduce the life-threatening effects of intoxication or withdrawal from some substances. The severity of the withdrawal syndrome depends on the particular drug used, how long it has been used, the dose used, and the rate at which the drug is eliminated from the body (Bennett & Woolf, 1991).

ALCOHOL

Benzodiazepines are the most widely used group of drugs for substitution therapy of alcohol withdrawal. Chlordiazepoxide (Librium) and diazepam

(Valium) are the most commonly used agents. The approach to treatment with benzodiazepines for alcohol withdrawal is to start with relatively high doses and reduce the dosage by 20 percent to 25 percent each day until withdrawal is complete. In patients with liver disease, accumulation of these longer-acting agents (Librium and Valium) may be problematic, and the use of shorter-acting benzodiazepines (e.g., oxazepam [Serax]) may be more appropriate.

Some physicians may order anticonvulsant medications (e.g., phenytoin, phenobarbital, or magnesium sulfate) for management of withdrawal seizures. This is not a universal intervention, and it is likely that most patients are adequately protected against seizures by the benzodiazepine used to stop the progression of withdrawal symptoms. If seizures do occur, diazepam (Valium) or lorazepam (Ativan) administered intravenously is probably indicated (Bennett & Woolf, 1991).

Multivitamin therapy, in combination with daily injections of thiamine, is common protocol. Thiamine is commonly deficient in chronic alcoholics. Replacement therapy is required to prevent neuropathy, confusion, and encephalopathy.

OPIOIDS

Examples of opioids include heroin, morphine, opium, meperidine, codeine, and methadone. Withdrawal symptoms generally begin within 8 to 12 hours after the last opioid dose and become most intense by 36 to 48 hours (Bennett & Woolf, 1991). The acute phase of withdrawal is over in approximately 10 days; however, symptoms of irritability and restlessness may persist for 2 to 3 months.

Opioid intoxication is treated with narcotic antagonists, such as naloxone (Narcan), nalorphine (Nalline), or levallorphan (Lorfan). Withdrawal therapy includes rest, adequate nutritional support, and methadone substitution. Methadone is given on the first day in a dose sufficient to suppress withdrawal symptoms. The dose is then gradually tapered so that methadone substitution is complete in 21 days. Propoxyphene (Darvon) has also been tried in opioid substitution therapy, usually with less than satisfactory results (Bennett & Woolf, 1991).

Clonidine (Catapres) has been used to suppress opiate withdrawal symptoms. Although it is not as effective as substitution with an opioid, it is nonaddicting and can serve as a bridge to enable the patient to stay opiate free long enough to initiate naltrexone (Trexan) therapy, which is used to facilitate termination of methadone maintenance (Bennett & Woolf, 1991).

DEPRESSANTS

Substitution therapy for central nervous system depressant withdrawal (particularly barbiturates) is most commonly with the long-acting barbiturate phenobarbital (Luminal). The dosage required to suppress withdrawal symptoms is given. When stabilization has been achieved, the dose is gradually decreased by 30 mg/day until withdrawal is complete. Long-acting benzodiazepines are commonly used for substitution therapy when the abused substance is a nonbarbiturate central nervous system depressant (Bennett & Woolf, 1991).

STIMULANTS

Treatment of stimulant intoxication usually begins with minor tranquilizers, such as chlordiazepoxide (Librium) and progresses to major tranquilizers, such as haloperidol (Haldol). Phenothiazines are avoided due to reduction in seizure threshold and anticholinergic side effects (Schuckit, 1979). Intravenous phentolamine (Regitine) may be administered for severe hypertension. Repeated seizures are treated with intravenous diazepam (Valium).

Withdrawal from central nervous system stimulants is not the medical emergency observed with central nervous system depressants. Treatment is usually aimed at reducing drug craving and managing severe depression. The patient is placed in a quiet atmosphere and allowed to sleep and eat as much as is needed or desired. Suicide precautions may need to be instituted. Therapy with tricyclic antidepressants (e.g., desipramine [Norpramin]) has been successful in treating the symptoms of cocaine withdrawal (Bennet & Woolf, 1991).

HALLUCINOGENS AND CANNABINOLS

Substitution therapy is not required with these drugs. When adverse reactions, such as anxiety or panic, occur, benzodiazepines (e.g., diazepam [Valium] or chlordiazepoxide [Librium]) may be prescribed to prevent harm to the patient or others. Should psychotic reactions occur, they may be treated with antipsychotics, such as the phenothiazines or haloperidol (Haldol).

SUMMARY

This chapter examined a group of disorders that constitute a large and growing public health concern. Organic mental syndromes refer to a cluster of signs and symptoms for which no etiology is known. Examples of OMSs include delirium, dementia, amnestic syndrome, organic hallucinosis, organic delusional syndrome, organic mood syndrome, organic anxiety syndrome, organic personality syndrome, intoxication, and withdrawal.

Organic mental disorders designate particular syndromes for which the etiology is known or presumed. Examples of OMDs include primary degenerative dementia of the Alzheimer type, multiinfarct dementia, psychoactive substance-induced OMDs, and OMDs associated with physical disorders or conditions, or with unknown etiology.

Organic mental syndromes and disorders may be categorized as acute or chronic, reversible or irreversible. Common behavioral changes include those that relate to thinking, memory, language, attention, sensory perception, and orientation. Various biologic, genetic, and exogenous factors have been implicated in the development of OMDs.

Nursing care of the patient with OMSs and OMDs is presented around the five steps of the nursing process. Objectives of care for the patient experiencing an acute syndrome are aimed at eliminating the etiology, promoting patient safety, and a return to highest possible functioning. Objectives of care for the patient experiencing a chronic, progressive disorder are aimed at preserving the dignity of the individual, promoting deceleration of the symptoms, and maximizing functional capabilities.

Nursing interventions are also directed toward assisting the family/primary caregivers of the patient with a chronic, progressive OMD. Education is provided about the disease process, expectations of patient behavioral changes, methods to facilitate care, and sources for assistance and support, as they struggle, both physically and emotionally, with the demands brought on by a disease process that is slowly taking their loved one away from them.

REVIEW QUESTIONS
Self-Examination/Learning Exercise

*Select the answer that is **most** appropriate for each of the following questions.*

Mrs. Gold is 67 years old. She is brought to the hospital by her husband. He explains that she has become increasingly confused and forgetful. Yesterday, she started a fire in the kitchen when she put some bacon on to fry and went off and forgot it on the stove. Her husband reports that sometimes she seems okay, and sometimes she is completely disoriented. The physician has made an admitting diagnosis of dementia, etiology unknown.

1. Because the etiology of Mrs. Gold's symptoms is unknown, the physician will attempt to rule out that the possibility of a reversible condition exists. An example of a treatable (reversible) form of dementia is one that is caused by:
   a. Multiple sclerosis
   b. Multiple small brain infarcts
   c. Electrolyte imbalances
   d. AIDS

2. The physician rules out all reversible etiological factors and diagnoses Mrs. Gold with primary degenerative dementia of the Alzheimer type, senile onset. The cause of this disorder is:
   a. Multiple small brain infarcts
   b. Chronic alcohol abuse
   c. Cerebral abscess
   d. Unknown

3. The *primary* nursing intervention in working with Mrs. Gold would be:
   a. Ensuring that she receives food she likes, to prevent hunger
   b. Ensuring that the environment is safe, to prevent injury
   c. Ensuring that she meets the other patients, to prevent social isolation
   d. Ensuring that she takes care of her own activities of daily living, to prevent dependence

4. Some medications have been indicated to decrease the agitation violence, and bizarre thoughts associated with dementia. A drug suggested for this use is:
   a. chlorpromazine (Thorazine)
   b. benztropine (Cogentin)
   c. ergoloid (Hydergine)
   d. diazepam (Valium)

5. Mrs. Gold says to the nurse, "I have a date tonight. I always have a date on Christmas." The most appropriate response is:
   a. "Don't by silly. It's not Christmas, Mrs. Gold."
   b. "Today is Tuesday, Oct. 21, Mrs. Gold. We will have supper soon, and then your daughter will come to visit."
   c. "Who is your date with, Mrs. Gold?"
   d. "I think you need some more medication, Mrs. Gold. I'll bring it to you now."

Mr. White is admitted to the hospital after an extended period of binge alcohol drinking. His wife reports that he has been a heavy drinker for a number of years. Lab reports reveal he has a blood alcohol level of 250 mg/dl. He is placed on the chemical dependency unit for detoxification.

6. When would the first signs of alcohol withdrawal symptoms be expected to occur?
   a. In several hours after the last drink
   b. In 2 to 3 days after the last drink
   c. In 4 to 5 days after the last drink
   d. In 6 to 7 days after the last drink

7. Symptoms of alcohol withdrawal include:
   a. Euphoria, hyperactivity, and hypersomnia
   b. Depression, suicidal ideation, and insomnia
   c. Diaphoresis, nausea and vomiting, and tremors
   d. Unsteady gait, nystagmus, and profound disorientation

8. Which of the following medications is the physician most likely to order for Mr. White during his withdrawal syndrome?
   a. haloperidol (Haldol)
   b. chlordiazepoxide (Librium)
   c. propranolol (Inderal)
   d. phenytoin (Dilantin)

9. If the above medication is not effective in controlling the withdrawal symptoms, a progression to which of the following may occur?
   a. Organic hallucinosis
   b. Amnestic syndrome
   c. Delirium
   d. Organic delusional syndrome

10. Characteristic manifestations of the above syndrome include:
    a. Stupor and respiratory depression
    b. Loss of memory and personality changes
    c. Psychomotor agitation and profound disorientation
    d. Ideas of reference and control

REFERENCES

American Psychiatric Association. (1987). *Diagnostic and statistical manual of mental disorders* (ed. 3, rev.). Washington, DC: American Psychiatric Association.

Bennett, G. & Woolf, D. S. (1991). *Substance abuse: Pharmacologic, developmental, and clinical perspectives* (ed 2.). Albany, NY: Delmar Publishers Inc.

Cohen, D. & Eisdorfer, C. (1986). *The loss of self.* New York: WW Norton & Company.

Cook-Deegan, R. M. et al. (1988). *Confronting Alzheimer's disease and other dementias.* Philadelphia: JB Lippincott.

Detwiler, C. S. (1989). Organic mental disorder. In B. S. Johnson (Ed.), *Psychiatric-mental health nursing: Adaptation and growth.* Philadelphia: JB Lippincott.

Fraser, M. (1987). *Dementia: Its nature and management.* Chichester, England: John Wiley & Sons.

Patrick, M. L., Woods, S. L., Craven, R. F., Rokosky, J. S. and Bruno, P. M. (1991). *Medical-surgical nursing: Pathophysiological concepts* (ed 2.). Philadelphia: JB Lippincott.

Perkins, K. R. (1989). Organic mental disorders and AIDS. In B. S. Johnson (Ed.), *Psychiatric-mental health nursing: Adaptation and growth.* Philadelphia: JB Lippincott.

Phipps, W. J., Long, B. C., & Woods, N. F. (1987). *Medical-surgical nursing: Concepts and clinical practice* (ed 3.). St. Louis: CV Mosby.

Schuckit, M. A. (1979). *Drug and alcohol abuse: A clinical guide to diagnosis and treatment.* New York: Plenum Medical Book Company.

Thompson, J. M., McFarland, G. K., Hirsch, J. E., Tucker, S. M. and Bowers, A. C. (1986). *Clinical nursing.* St. Louis: CV Mosby.

Wertheimer, J. & Marois, M. (1984). *Senile dementia: Outlook for the future.* New York: Alan R. Liss, Inc.

BIBLIOGRAPHY

Briley, M. et al. (1986). *New concepts in Alzheimer's disease.* London: The Macmillan Press LTD.

Brody, J. E. (1983, November 30). Guidance in the care of patients with Alzheimer's disease. *The New York Times.*

Clark, M. et al. (1984, December 3). A slow death of the mind. *Newsweek*, pp. 56–62.

Hendricks, J. & Hendricks, C. D. (1987). *Aging in mass society.* Cambridge, MA: Winthrop Publishers.

Mace, N. & Rabins, P. V. (1981). *The 36-hour day.* Baltimore: The Johns Hopkins University Press.

Mahendra, B. (1987). *Dementia: A survey of the syndrome of dementia* (2nd ed.). Boston: MTP Press.

Mayeux, R. et al. (1988). *Alzheimer's disease and related disorders.* Springfield, IL: Charles C. Thomas.

McNichol, R. W. (1970). *The treatment of delirium tremens and related states.* Springfield, IL: Charles C. Thomas.

Shamoian, C. A. (1984). *Biology and treatment of dementia in the elderly.* Washington, DC: American Psychiatric Press.

PSYCHOACTIVE SUBSTANCE USE DISORDERS

OBJECTIVES

After reading this chapter, the student will be able to:

1. Differentiate between *abuse* and *dependence.*
2. Discuss predisposing factors implicated in the etiology of substance use disorders.
3. Identify symptomatology and use the information in assessment of patients with various substance use disorders.
4. Identify nursing diagnoses common to patients with substance use disorders and select appropriate nursing interventions for each.
5. Describe relevant criteria for evaluating nursing care of patients with substance use disorders.
6. Discuss the issue of substance abuse and dependence within the profession of nursing.
7. Define *co-dependency* and identify behavioral characteristics associated with the disorder.
8. Discuss treatment of co-dependency.
9. Describe various modalities relevant to treatment of individuals with substance use disorders.

INTRODUCTION

This chapter explores the topics of substance abuse and dependency. To differentiate between the abuse and dependency described in this chapter and the substance-induced syndromes described in the previous chapter, the following explanation is offered from the *Diagnostic and Statistical Manual of Mental Disorders*, Third Edition, Revised (*DSM-III-R*) (American Psychiatric Association [APA], 1987):

"Psychoactive Substance Use Disorders refer to the maladaptive behavior associated with more or less regular use of the substances whereas Psychoactive Substance-Induced Organic Mental Disorders describe the direct acute [e.g., withdrawal, intoxication] or chronic [e.g., dementia] effects of such substances on the central nervous system.

Almost invariably, people who have a Psychoactive Substance Use Disorder will also have a Psychoactive Substance-Induced Organic Mental Disorder, such as intoxication or withdrawal."

Drugs are a pervasive part of our society. Certain mood-altering substances are quite socially acceptable and are used moderately by the majority of adult Americans. They include alcohol, caffeine, and nicotine. Society has even developed a relative indifference to an occasional abuse of these substances.

A wide variety of substances are produced for medicinal purposes. These include stimulants (e.g., amphetamines), central nervous system (CNS) depressants (e.g., sedatives, tranquilizers), as well as numerous over-the-counter preparations designed to relieve nearly every kind of human ailment, real or imagined.

Some illegal substances have achieved a degree of social acceptance by various subcultural groups within our society. These drugs, such as marijuana and hashish, are by no means harmless, and the long-term effects are still being studied. On the other hand, the dangerous effects of other illegal substances (e.g., LSD, phencyclidine, cocaine, and heroin) have been well documented.

This chapter discusses the physical and behavioral manifestations and personal and social consequences related to the abuse of or dependency on alcohol, other CNS depressants, CNS stimulants, opioids, hallucinogens, and cannabinols. The behavioral changes associated with abuse of these substances would be viewed as extremely undesirable in almost all cultures (APA, 1987).

The concept of co-dependency is described in this chapter, including aspects of treatment for the disorder. The issue of substance impairment within the profession of nursing is also explored. Nursing care for the person who abuses or is dependent on substances is presented in the context of the five steps of the nursing process.

PSYCHOACTIVE SUBSTANCE DEPENDENCE

Physical Dependence

This disorder is evidenced by a cluster of cognitive, behavioral, and physiologic symptoms that indicate a loss of control over use of the substance and a continual use of the substance despite adverse consequences (APA, 1987). As this condition develops, the repeated administration of the substance necessitates its continued use to prevent the appearance of unpleasant effects characteristic of the withdrawal syndrome associated with that particular drug (Bratter & Forrest, 1985). The development of physical dependence is promoted by the phenomenon of *tolerance*. Tolerance is indicated by the need for increasingly larger or more frequent doses of a substance to obtain the desired effects originally produced by a lower dose.

Psychological Dependence

An individual is considered to be psychologically dependent on a substance when its use is perceived by the user to be *necessary* to maintain an optimal state of personal well-being, interpersonal relations, or skill performance (Bratter & Forrest, 1985).

DSM-III-R Criteria for Psychoactive Substance Dependence

At least three of the following characteristics must be present for a diagnosis of psychoactive substance dependence:

1. The individual often consumes the substance in larger amounts or over a longer period than originally intended (e.g., decides to have one drink of alcohol but continues to drink until severely intoxicated).
2. Recognition that the substance use is excessive has led to unsuccessful attempts to reduce or control it (as long as the substance is available). This also includes evidence of the *desire* to reduce or control use of the substance without ever having attempted to do so.
3. A great deal of time is spent in activities necessary to procure the substance (including theft), using the substance, or recovering from its effects.
4. The individual is frequently intoxicated or recovering from withdrawal symptoms during times that interfere with fulfillment of major role obligations at work, school, or home, or during times in which substance use is physically hazardous (e.g., does not go to work because hung over; goes to school or work "high"; intoxicated while taking care of children; drives while intoxicated).
5. Important social, occupational, or recreational activities are discontinued or reduced because of substance use (e.g., may choose to spend time using substance alone or with substance-using friends rather than in activities with family).
6. The individual continues to use the substance despite knowledge of having a persistent or recurrent social, psychological, or physical problem that is caused or exacerbated by its use (e.g., continues to drink alcohol despite family arguments about it, depressed mood, or exacerbation of alcohol-induced gastritis).
7. Significant tolerance develops, evidenced by

the need for markedly increased amounts of the substance to achieve intoxication or the desired effect, or markedly diminished effect with continued use of the same amount.

NOTE: The following items may not apply to cannabis, hallucinogens, or phencyclidine.

8. Characteristic withdrawal symptoms develop when the person stops or reduces intake of the substance. (See Chapter 16 for detailed descriptions of substance-withdrawal syndromes. A summary of this information is presented in Table 17.1.)

9. The substance is often taken to relieve or avoid withdrawal symptoms.

PSYCHOACTIVE SUBSTANCE ABUSE

Bennett and Woolf (1991) define substance abuse as psychoactive drug use of any class or type, used alone or in combination, that poses significant hazards to health. The *DSM-III-R* (APA, 1987) identifies psychoactive substance abuse as a residual category for noting maladaptive patterns of psy-

Table 17.1   SUMMARY OF SYMPTOMS ASSOCIATED WITH THE ORGANIC MENTAL SYNDROMES OF INTOXICATION AND WITHDRAWAL

Class of Drugs	Intoxication	Withdrawal	Comments
Alcohol	Aggressiveness, impaired judgment, impaired attention, irritability, euphoria, depression, emotional lability, slurred speech, incoordination, unsteady gait, nystagmus, flushed face	Tremors, nausea/vomiting, malaise, weakness, tachycardia, sweating, elevated blood pressure, anxiety, depressed mood, irritability, hallucinations, headache, insomnia, seizures	Alcohol withdrawal begins within 4–6 hr after last drink. May progress to delirium tremens on 2nd or 3rd day. Use of Librium is common for substitution therapy.
Amphetamines and related substances	Fighting, grandiosity, hypervigilance, psychomotor agitation, impaired judgment, tachycardia, pupillary dilation, elevated blood pressure, perspiration or chills, nausea and vomiting	Anxiety, depressed mood, irritability, craving for the substance, fatigue, insomnia or hypersomnia, psychomotor agitation, paranoid and suicidal ideation	Withdrawal symptoms usually peak within 2–4 days, although depression and irritability may persist for months. Tricyclic antidepressants may be used.
Caffeine	Restlessness, nervousness, excitement, insomnia, flushed face, diuresis, gastrointestinal complaints, muscle twitching, rambling flow of thought and speech, cardiac arrhythmia, periods of inexhaustibility, psychomotor agitation	Headache	Caffeine is contained in coffee, tea, colas, cocoa, chocolate, some over-the-counter analgesics, "cold" preparations, and stimulants.
Cannabis	Euphoria, anxiety, suspiciousness, sensation of slowed time, impaired judgment, social withdrawal, tachycardia, conjunctival redness, increased appetite, hallucinations	Restlessness, irritability, insomnia, loss of appetite	Intoxication occurs immediately and lasts about 3 hours. Oral ingestion is more slowly absorbed and has longer-lasting effects.

(continued)

Table 17.1 CONTINUED

Class of Drugs	Intoxication	Withdrawal	Comments
Cocaine	Euphoria, fighting, grandiosity, hypervigilance, psychomotor agitation, impaired judgment, tachycardia, elevated blood pressure, pupillary dilation, perspiration or chills, nausea/vomiting, hallucinations, delirium	Depression, anxiety, irritability, fatigue, insomnia or hypersomnia, psychomotor agitation, paranoid or suicidal ideation, apathy, social withdrawal	Large doses of the drug can result in convulsions or death from cardiac arrhythmias or respiratory paralysis.
Inhalants	Belligerence, assaultiveness, apathy, impaired judgment, dizziness, nystagmus, slurred speech, unsteady gait, lethargy, depressed reflexes, tremor, blurred vision, stupor or coma, euphoria, irritation around eyes, throat, and nose		Intoxication occurs within 5 minutes of inhalation. Symptoms last 60–90 min. Large doses can result in death from CNS depression or cardiac arrhythmia.
Nicotine		Craving for the drug, irritability, anger, frustration, anxiety, difficulty concentrating, restlessness, decreased heart rate, increased appetite, weight gain, tremor, headaches, insomnia	Symptoms began within 24 hours of last drug use and decrease in intensity over days, weeks, or sometimes longer.
Opioids	Euphoria, lethargy, somnolence, apathy, dysphoria, impaired judgment, pupillary constriction, drowsiness, slurred speech, constipation, nausea, decreased respiratory rate and blood pressure	Craving for the drug, nausea/vomiting, muscle aches, lacrimation or rhinorrhea, pupillary dilation, piloerection or sweating, diarrhea, yawning, fever, insomnia	Withdrawal symptoms appear within 6–8 hours after last dose, reach a peak in the 2nd or 3rd day, and disappear in 7–10 days.
Phencyclidine and related substances	Belligerence, assaultiveness, impulsiveness, psychomotor agitation, impaired judgment, nystagmus, increased heart rate and blood pressure, diminished pain response, ataxia, dysarthria, muscle rigidity, seizures, hyperacusis, delirium		Delirium can occur within 24 hours after use of phencyclidine, or may occur up to a week following recovery from an overdose of the drug.
Sedatives, hypnotics, anxiolytics	Disinhibition of sexual or aggressive impulses, mood lability, impaired judgment, slurred speech, incoordination, unsteady gait, impairment in attention or memory, disorientation, confusion	Nausea/vomiting, malaise, weakness, tachycardia, sweating, anxiety, irritability, orthostatic hypotension, tremor, insomnia, seizures	Withdrawal may progress to delirium, usually within 1 week of last use. Long-acting barbiturates or benzodiazepines may be used in withdrawal substitution therapy.

choactive substance use that have never met the criteria for dependence for that particular class of substance.

DSM-III-R Criteria for Psychoactive Substance Abuse

A maladaptive pattern of psychoactive substance use is indicated by at least one of the following. Some symptoms of the disturbance have persisted for at least 1 month or have occurred repeatedly for a longer period.

1. Continued use despite knowledge of having a persistent or recurrent social, occupational, psychological, or physical problem that is caused or exacerbated by use of the psychoactive substance
2. Recurrent use in situations in which use is physically hazardous (e.g., driving while intoxicated)

CLASSES OF PSYCHOACTIVE SUBSTANCES

Ten classes of psychoactive substances are associated with abuse or dependence. They include:

1. Alcohol
2. Amphetamines and related substances
3. Cannabis
4. Cocaine
5. Hallucinogens
6. Inhalants
7. Nicotine
8. Opioids
9. Phencyclidine and related substances
10. Sedatives, hypnotics, or anxiolytics

PREDISPOSING FACTORS

A number of factors have been implicated in the predisposition to abuse of substances. At present, there is no single theory that can adequately explain the etiology of this problem. No doubt the interaction between various elements forms a complex collection of determinants that influence a person's susceptibility to abuse substances.

Biological Factors

GENETICS

An apparent hereditary factor is involved in the development of substance use disorders. This is especially evident with alcoholism, less so with other substances. Some studies have indicated that the development of alcoholism in first-degree relatives of alcoholics may be as high as 50 percent (Estes & Heinemann, 1986). Studies with monozygotic and dizygotic twins have also supported the genetic hypothesis. The monozygotic (one egg, identical genetically) twins reported a 54 percent concordance for alcoholism, while the dizygotic twins (two eggs, nonidentical genetically) showed only a 28 percent concordance (Kaij, 1960). Studies also have been conducted with children of alcoholics who were separated from their biologic parents shortly after birth and adopted by nonalcoholic parents (Goodwin et al, 1973). Results indicated that the number of these children who developed alcoholism as adults was significant to suggest a genetic link.

BIOCHEMICAL

A second biological hypothesis relates to the possibility that alcohol may produce morphinelike substances in the brain that are responsible for alcohol addiction. These substances are formed by the reaction of biologically active amines (e.g., dopamine, serotonin) with products of alcohol metabolism, such as acetaldehyde (Bennett & Woolf, 1991). Examples of these morphinelike substances include tetrahydropapaveroline and salsolinol. Some tests with animals have shown that injection of these compounds into the brain in small amounts results in patterns of alcohol addiction in animals who had previously avoided even the most dilute alcohol solutions (Estes & Heinemann, 1986).

Psychological Factors

DEVELOPMENTAL INFLUENCES

The psychodynamic approach to the etiology of substance abuse proposes that the predisposition relates to severe ego impairment and disturbances in the sense of self (Leigh, 1985). The person retains a highly dependent nature, with characteristics of poor impulse control, low frustration tolerance, and low self-esteem. Freud (1959) described this person as fixed in the oral stage of development and as one who seeks satisfaction through oral gratification (e.g., ingestion of substances). Having once experienced the gratification of a supportive, drug-induced pattern of ego functioning, users attempt to repeat this satisfying experience as a solution to their own conflicts (Milkman & Frosch, 1980).

PERSONALITY FACTORS

Research suggests that certain personality traits may play an important part in both the development and maintenance of alcohol dependence (Barnes, 1980). Characteristics that have been identified include impulsivity, negative self-concept, weak ego, low social conformity, neuroticism, and introversion. Substance abuse has also been associated with antisocial personality and depressive response styles (Leigh, 1985). This may be explained by the inability of the individual with antisocial personality to anticipate the aversive consequences of behavior. It is likely an effort on the part of the depressed person to treat the symptoms of discomfort associated with dysphoria. Achievement of relief then provides the positive reinforcement to continue abusing substances.

Sociocultural Factors

SOCIAL LEARNING

The effects of modeling, imitation, and identification on behavior can be observed from early childhood onward. In relation to drug consumption, the family appears to be an important influence. Various studies have shown that children and adolescents are more likely to use substances if they have parents who provide a model for substance use (Leigh, 1985). Peers often exert a great deal of influence in the life of the child or adolescent who is being encouraged to use substances for the first time. Modeling may continue to be a factor in the use of substances once the individual enters the work force. This is particularly true in the work setting that provides plenty of leisure time with coworkers and where drinking is valued and is used to express group cohesiveness (Cosper, 1979).

CONDITIONING

Another important learning factor is the effect of the substance itself. Many substances create a pleasurable experience that encourages the user to repeat it. Thus, it is the intrinsically reinforcing properties of addictive drugs that "condition" the individual to seek out their use again and again. The environment in which the substance is taken also contributes to the reinforcement. If the environment is pleasurable, substance use is usually increased. Aversive stimuli within an environment are thought to be associated with a decrease in substance use within that environment (Leigh, 1985).

CULTURAL AND ETHNIC INFLUENCES

Factors within an individual's culture help to establish patterns of substance use by molding attitudes, influencing patterns of consumption based on cultural acceptance, and determining the availability of the substance. For centuries, the French and Italians have considered wine an essential part of the family meal, even for the children. The incidence of alcohol dependency is low, and acute intoxication from alcohol is not common. However, the possibility of chronic physiologic effects associated with lifelong alcohol consumption cannot be ignored.

In the American Indian culture, there is a high incidence of alcohol dependency (Westermeyer & Baker, 1986). Drinking is the primary group activity, and failure to drink is considered a social offense. American Indian students in U.S. universities report personal conflict with the attempt to conform to the dominant white society while retaining their own cultural identity. This cognitive dissonance may be a predisposing factor to alcohol abuse among American Indians who have left their own culture (Baker, 1982).

The incidence of alcohol dependence is higher among northern Europeans than southern Europeans. The Finns and the Irish use excessive alcohol consumption for the release of aggression, and the English "pub" is known for its attraction as a social meeting place (Ahlstrom-Laakso, 1976).

Incidence of alcohol dependence among people of the Oriental culture is relatively low. This may be a result of a possible genetic intolerance of the substance. Some Orientals develop unpleasant symptoms, such as flushing, headaches, and palpitations, upon drinking of alcohol. Research indicates that this is due to an isoenzyme variant that quickly converts alcohol to acetaldehyde as well as the absence of an isoenzyme that is needed to oxidize acetaldehyde. This results in a rapid accumulation of acetaldehyde that produces the unpleasant symptoms (Madden, 1984).

THE DYNAMICS OF PSYCHOACTIVE SUBSTANCE USE DISORDERS

Alcohol Abuse and Dependence

A PROFILE OF THE SUBSTANCE

Alcohol is a natural substance formed by the reaction of fermenting sugar with yeast spores. Although there are many alcohols, the kind in alcoholic beverages is known scientifically as ethyl alcohol and chemically as C_2H_5OH. Its abbreviation, ETOH, is sometimes seen in medical records and in various other documents and publications.

By strict definition, alcohol is classified as a food because it contains calories. However, it has no nutritional value. Different alcoholic beverages are produced by using different sources of sugar for the fermentation process. For example, beer is made from malted barley, wine from grapes or berries, whiskey from malted grains, and rum from molasses. Distilled beverages (e.g., whiskey, scotch, gin, vodka, and other "hard" liquors) derive their name from further concentration of the alcohol through a process called distillation.

The alcohol content varies by type of beverage. For example, most American beers contain 3 percent to 6 percent alcohol, wines average 10 percent to 20 percent, and distilled beverages range from 40 percent to 50 percent alcohol. The average-sized drink, regardless of beverage, will contain a similar amount of alcohol. That is, 12 ounces of beer, 3 to 5 ounces of wine, and a cocktail with 1 ounce of whiskey would all contain approximately 0.5 ounce of alcohol, and if consumed at the same rate, would have an equal effect on the body.

Alcohol exerts a depressant effect on the CNS, resulting in behavioral changes and alterations in mood. The effects of alcohol on the CNS are proportional to the alcoholic concentration in the blood. Most states consider that an individual is legally intoxicated with a blood alcohol level of 0.10 g/dl (100 mg percent). The body burns alcohol at the rate of about one-half ounce per hour, so behavioral changes would not be expected to occur in an individual who slowly consumed only one average-sized drink per hour. Other factors do influence these effects, however, such as individual size and whether or not the stomach contains food at the time the alcohol is consumed. Alcohol is believed to have a more profound effect when an individual is emotionally stressed or fatigued (National Institute on Alcohol Abuse and Alcoholism [NIAAA], 1971).

HISTORICAL ASPECTS

The use of alcohol can be traced back to the Neolithic age (Blum, 1984). Beer and wine are known to have been used around 6400 B.C. Although alcohol has little therapeutic value, with the introduction of distillation by the Arabs in the Middle Ages, alchemists believed that alcohol was the answer to all of their ailments. The word "whiskey," meaning "water of life," became widely known.

In America, the Indians were drinking beer and wine at the time they met their first white visitors. Refinement of the distillation process made beverages with high alcohol content readily available. By the early 1800s, one renowned physician of the time, Benjamin Rush, had begun to identify the widespread excessive, chronic alcohol consumption as a disease and an addiction (Keller, 1979). The strong religious mores on which this country was founded soon led to a driving force aimed at prohibiting the sale of alcoholic beverages. By the middle of the nineteenth century, 13 states had passed prohibition laws. The most notable prohibition of major proportions was that in effect in the United States from 1920 until 1933. These mandatory restrictions on national social habits resulted in the creation of profitable underground markets that led to flourishing criminal enterprises. Furthermore, millions of dollars in federal, state, and local revenues from taxes and import duties on alcohol were lost. It is difficult to measure the value of this dollar loss compared to the human devastation and social costs that occur as a result of alcohol abuse in the United States today.

PATTERNS OF USE/ABUSE

Approximately 70 out of every 100 adults in the United States drink alcohol (Spence, 1987). Of these 70, about one-tenth (7 people) are alcoholics.

Why do people drink? Drinking patterns in the United States show that people use alcoholic beverages to enhance the flavor of food with meals; at social gatherings to encourage relaxation and conviviality among the guests; and to promote a feeling of celebration at special occasions, such as weddings, birthdays, and anniversaries. Alcoholic beverages (wine) are also used as part of the sacred ritual in some religious ceremonies. Therapeutically, alcohol is the major ingredient in many over-the-counter, as well as prescription, medicines that are prepared in concentrate form. Therefore, alcohol can be harmless and enjoyable, sometimes even beneficial, if it is used responsibly and in moderation. But, like any other mind-altering drug, alcohol has the potential for abuse. Indeed, it is the most widely abused drug in the United States today (Blum, 1984). Kaplan and Sadock (1985) have stated:

> "Alcoholism is usually referred to as the country's third most serious public health problem, following cardiovascular disease and cancer. However, in terms of total morbidity, as contrasted to mortality, it is the number one health problem in the United States."

Jellinek (1952) outlined four phases through which the alcoholic's pattern of drinking progresses. Some variability among individuals is to be expected within this model of progression.

Phase I. The Prealcoholic Phase   This phase is characterized by the use of alcohol to relieve the everyday stress and tensions of life. As a child, the individual may have observed parents or other adults drinking alcohol and enjoying the effects. The child learns that use of alcohol is an acceptable method of coping with stress. Tolerance develops, and the amount required to achieve the desired effect increases steadily.

Phase II. The Early Alcoholic Phase   This phase begins with blackouts—brief periods of amnesia that occur during or immediately after a period of drinking. Now the alcohol is no longer a source of pleasure or relief for the individual but rather a drug that is *required* by the individual. Common behaviors include sneaking drinks or secret drinking, preoccupation with drinking and maintaining the supply of alcohol, rapid gulping of drinks, and further blackouts. The individual feels enormous guilt and becomes very defensive about his or her drinking. Excessive use of denial and rationalization is evident.

Phase III. The Crucial Phase   In this phase, the individual has lost control, and physiologic dependence is clearly evident. This loss of control has been described as the inability to choose whether or not to drink. Binge drinking, lasting from a few hours to several weeks, is common. These episodes are characterized by sickness, loss of consciousness, squalor, and degradation. In this phase, the individual is extremely ill. Anger and aggression are common manifestations. Drinking is the total focus, and he or she is willing to risk losing everything that was once important in an effort to maintain the addiction. By this phase of the illness, it is not uncommon for the individual to have experienced the loss of job, marriage, family, friends, and most especially, self-respect.

Phase IV. The Chronic Phase   This phase is characterized by emotional and physical disintegration. The individual is usually intoxicated more than he or she is sober. Emotional disintegration is evidenced by profound helplessness and self-pity. An impairment in reality testing may result in psychosis. Life-threatening physical manifestations may be evident in virtually every system of the body. Abstention from alcohol results in a terrifying syndrome of symptoms that include hallucinations, tremors, convulsions, severe agitation, and panic. Depression and ideas of suicide are not uncommon.

EFFECTS ON THE BODY

Alcohol is capable of inducing a general, nonselective, reversible depression of the CNS. About 20 percent of a single dose of alcohol is absorbed directly and immediately into the bloodstream through the stomach wall. Unlike other "foods," it does not have to be digested. The blood carries it directly to the brain where the alcohol acts on the brain's central control areas, slowing down or depressing brain activity (NIAAA, 1971). The other 80 percent of the alcohol in one drink is processed only slightly slower through the upper intestinal tract and into the bloodstream. Only moments after alcohol is consumed, it can be found in all tissues, organs, and secretions of the body (NIAAA, 1971). Rapidity of absorption is influenced by various factors. For example, absorption is delayed when the drink is sipped, rather than gulped; when the stomach contains food, rather than being empty; and when the drink is wine or beer, rather than distilled beverages.

At low doses, alcohol produces relaxation, loss of inhibitions, lack of concentration, drowsiness, slurred speech, and sleep. Intoxication results in aggressiveness, impaired judgment, impaired attention, irritability, euphoria, depression, emotional lability, incoordination, and unsteady gait. At very high levels, alcohol can induce severe disorientation, stupor anesthesia, coma, and even death.

Chronic abuse results in multisystem physiological impairments. These complications include (but are not limited to) those outlined below.

Peripheral Neuropathy This disorder, characterized by peripheral nerve damage, results in pain, burning, tingling, or prickly sensations of the extremities. Researchers believe it is the direct result of deficiencies in the B vitamins, particularly thiamine. Nutritional deficiencies are common in chronic alcoholics because of insufficient intake of nutrients as well as the toxic effect of alcohol that results in malabsorption of nutrients. The process is reversible with abstinence from alcohol and restoration of nutritional deficiencies. Otherwise, permanent muscle wasting and paralysis can occur.

Alcoholic Myopathy This syndrome may occur as an acute or chronic condition. In the acute condition, the individual experiences pain, tenderness, and edema in the skeletal muscles of the extremities, pelvic and shoulder girdle, and the muscles of the thoracic cage following acute excesses of alcoholic ingestion (Estes & Heinemann, 1986). Laboratory studies show elevations of the enzymes CPK, LDH, aldolase, and AST (SGOT). The symptoms of chronic alcoholic myopathy include a gradual wasting and weakness in skeletal muscles. Neither the pain and tenderness nor the elevated muscle enzymes seen in acute myopathy are evident in the chronic condition.

Alcoholic myopathy is thought to be a result of the same B vitamin deficiency that contributes to peripheral neuropathy. Improvement is observed with abstinence from alcohol and the return to a nutritious diet with vitamin supplements.

Wernicke's Encephalopathy This disorder characterizes the most serious form of thiamine deficiency in alcoholics. Symptoms include paralysis of the ocular muscles, diplopia, ataxia, somnolence, and stupor. If thiamine replacement therapy is not undertaken quickly, death will ensue.

Korsakoff's Psychosis This disorder is identified by a syndrome of confusion, loss of recent memory, and confabulation in alcoholics. It is frequently encountered in patients recovering from Wernicke's encephalopathy. In the United States, the two disorders are usually considered together, and called *Wernicke-Korsakoff's syndrome*. Treatment is with parenteral or oral thiamine replacement.

Alcoholic Cardiomyopathy The effect of alcohol on the heart is an accumulation of lipids in the myocardial cells, resulting in enlargement and a weakened condition. The clinical findings of alcoholic cardiomyopathy generally relate to congestive heart failure or arrhythmia (Estes & Heinemann, 1986). Symptoms include decreased exercise tolerance, tachycardia, dyspnea, edema, palpitations, and nonproductive cough. Laboratory studies may show elevation of the enzymes CPK, AST (SGOT), ALT (SGPT), and LDH. Changes may be observed by electrocardiogram, and congestive failure may be evident on chest x-ray films.

Treatment includes total, permanent abstinence from alcohol. Treatment of the congestive failure may include rest, oxygen, digitalization, sodium restriction, and diuretics. Prognosis is encouraging if treated in the early stages. The death rate is high for individuals with advanced symptomatology.

Esophagitis This inflammation and pain in the esophagus occurs due to toxic effects of alcohol on the esophageal mucosa and also to frequent vomiting associated with alcohol abuse.

Gastritis The effects of alcohol on the stomach includes inflammation of the stomach lining characterized by epigastric distress, nausea, vomiting, and distention. Alcohol breaks down the stomach's protective mucosal barrier, allowing hydrochloric acid to erode the stomach wall. Damage to blood vessels may result in hemorrhage.

Pancreatitis This condition may be categorized

as *acute* or *chronic.* Acute pancreatitis usually occurs 1 or 2 days after a binge of excessive alcohol consumption. Symptoms include constant, severe epigastric pain, nausea and vomiting, and abdominal distention. The chronic condition leads to pancreatic insufficiency, resulting in steatorrhea, malnutrition, weight loss, and diabetes mellitus.

Alcoholic Hepatitis This disease often follows a severe, prolonged bout of drinking, and is usually superimposed on an already damaged alcoholic liver (Bratter & Forrest, 1985). It is characterized by a syndrome of inflammation and necrosis. Clinical manifestations include enlarged liver and spleen, abdominal pain, vomiting, weakness, low-grade fever, fatigability, loss of appetite, elevated white blood cell count, and jaundice. Ascites and weight loss may be evident in more severe cases. With treatment, which includes strict abstinence from alcohol, proper nutrition, and rest, the individual can experience complete recovery. Fatality or progression to cirrhosis occurs in the majority of the most severe cases.

Cirrhosis of the Liver Cirrhosis is the end stage of alcoholic liver disease and is believed to be caused by the direct toxic effect of alcohol on the liver (Bratter & Forrest, 1985). There is widespread destruction of liver cells, which are replaced by fibrous (scar) tissue. Clinical manifestations are similar to those described for alcoholic hepatitis. In more advanced stages, the liver may have shrunk to the point where it cannot be felt (Bratter & Forrest, 1985). Treatment includes abstention from alcohol, correction of malnutrition, and supportive care to prevent complications of the disease. Complications of cirrhosis include:

1. *Portal hypertension.* Elevation of blood pressure through the portal circulation results from defective blood flow through the cirrhotic liver.
2. *Ascites.* This condition, in which an excessive amount of serous fluid accumulates in the abdominal cavity, occurs in response to portal hypertension. The increased pressure results in the seepage of fluid from the surface of the liver into the abdominal cavity.
3. *Esophageal varices.* Veins in the esophagus may become distended due to excessive pressure from defective blood flow through the cirrhotic liver. As this pressure increases,

these varicosities can rupture, resulting in hemorrhage and sometimes death.

4. *Hepatic encephalopathy.* This serious complication occurs in response to the inability of the diseased liver to convert ammonia to urea for excretion. The continued rise in serum ammonia results in progressively impaired mental functioning, apathy, euphoria or depression, sleep disturbance, increasing confusion, and progression to coma and eventual death. Treatment requires complete abstention from alcohol, temporary elimination of protein from the diet, and reduction of intestinal ammonia using neomycin or lactulose (Bratter & Forrest, 1985).

Leukopenia The production, function, and movement of the white blood cells is impaired in chronic alcoholics. This places the individual at high risk for contracting infectious diseases as well as for complicated recovery.

Thrombocytopenia Platelet production and survival is impaired due to toxic effects of alcohol. This places the alcoholic at risk for hemorrhage. Abstinence from alcohol rapidly reverts this deficiency.

Sexual Dysfunction Alcohol has both short-term and long-term effects on sexual functioning. In the short-term, enhanced libido and failure of erection are common. Long-term effects include gynecomastia, sterility, impotence, and decreased libido (Blum, 1984).

Other CNS Depressant Abuse and Dependence

A PROFILE OF THE SUBSTANCE

The sedative-hypnotic compounds are drugs of diverse chemical structures that are all capable of inducing varying degrees of CNS depression, from tranquilizing relief of anxiety to anesthesia, coma, and even death. They are generally categorized as (1) barbiturates, (2) nonbarbiturate hypnotics, and (3) antianxiety agents. Effects produced by these substances depend on the size of the dose and the potency of the drug administered.

Following is a selected list of drugs included in these categories. Generic names are followed in parentheses by the trade names. Common street names for each category are also included.

Barbiturates

pentobarbital (Nembutal):	yellow jackets; yellow birds
secobarbital (Seconal):	
amobarbital (Amytal):	red birds; red devils
secobarbital/amobarbital (Tuinal):	blue birds; blue angels tooies

Nonbarbiturate Hypnotics

methaqualone (Quaalude):	ludes, sopers, love drug
ethchlorvynol (Placidyl):	dyls
glutethimide (Doriden):	gorilla pills, GB's, Cibas, D
chloral hydrate (Noctec):	Peter, Mickey
triazolam (Halcion):	sleepers
flurazepam (Dalmane):	sleepers
temazepam (Restoril):	sleepers

Antianxiety Agents

diazepam (Valium):	V's (color designates strength)
chlordiazepoxide (Librium):	green & whites, roaches
meprobamate (Equanil; Miltown):	dolls
oxazepam (Serax)	
alprazolam (Xanax)	
lorazepam (Ativan)	

Julien (1981) outlines several principles that apply fairly uniformly to all CNS depressants.

1. *The effects of CNS depressants are additive with one another and with the behavioral state of the user.* For example, when these drugs are used in combination with each other or in combination with alcohol, the depressive effects are compounded. These intense depressive effects are often unpredictable and can even be fatal. Similarly, a person who is mentally depressed or physically fatigued may have an exaggerated response to a dose of the drug that would only slightly affect a person in a normal or excited state.

2. *There is no specific antagonist that will specifically block the action of the CNS depressants.* CNS stimulants may temporarily arouse the individual, but what is needed is a drug that actually displaces the depressant from its receptors in the brain, thus immediately terminating the action of the depressant. This would save thousands of lives each year of people who attempt suicide with CNS depressants.

3. *Low doses of CNS depressants produce initial excitatory response.* CNS depressants relieve inhibitions and induce a feeling of euphoria. This is believed to occur because, at low doses, inhibitory synapses in the brain are depressed slightly earlier than are excitatory synapses. At higher doses, however, excitatory synapses are also depressed, and sleep follows.

4. *CNS depressants are capable of producing physiological dependency.* If large doses of CNS depressants are repeatedly administered over a prolonged duration, a period of hyperexcitability occurs on withdrawal of the drug. The response can be quite severe, even leading to convulsions and death.

5. *CNS depressants are capable of producing psychological dependence.* CNS depressants have the potential to generate within the individual a psychic drive for periodic or continuous administration of the drug to achieve a maximum level of functioning or feeling of well-being.

6. *Cross tolerance and cross dependence may exist between various CNS depressants.* Cross tolerance is exhibited when one drug results in a lessened response to another drug. Cross dependence is a condition in which one drug can prevent withdrawal symptoms associated with physical dependence on a different drug.

HISTORICAL ASPECTS

Anxiety and insomnia, two of the most common human afflictions, were treated during the 19th century with opiates, bromide salts, chloral hydrate, paraldehyde, and alcohol (Blum, 1984). Because the opiates were known to produce physical dependence, the bromides carried the risk of chronic bromide poisoning, and chloral hydrate and paraldehyde had an objectionable taste and smell, alcohol became the prescribed depressant drug of choice. However, some people refused to use alcohol either because they did not like the taste or for moral reasons. (Also some people tended to take more than was prescribed.) So a search for a better sedative drug continued.

Although barbituric acid was first synthesized in

1864, it was not until 1903 that the first barbiturate derivative (barbital) was introduced into medicine as a sedative drug (Julien, 1981). The second barbiturate to be introduced was phenobarbital (Luminol) in 1912. Since that time, more than 2500 barbiturate derivatives have been synthesized, but of these only about 15 remain in medical use (Drug Enforcement Administration [DEA], 1979). Illicit use of the drugs for recreational purposes grew throughout the 1930s and 1940s.

Efforts to create depressant medications that were not barbiturate derivatives accelerated. By the mid-1950s, the market for depressants had been expanded by the appearance of the nonbarbiturates glutethimide, ethchlorvynol, methyprylon, and meprobamate. Introduction of the benzodiazepines occurred around 1960 with the marketing of chlordiazepoxide (Librium), followed shortly by its derivative diazepam (Valium). The use of these drugs, and others within their group, has grown so rapidly that they have become some of the most widely prescribed medications in clinical use today. Their margin of safety is greater than that of other depressants (DEA, 1979). However, prolonged use of excessive doses is likely to result in physical and psychological dependence, with a characteristic syndrome of withdrawal that can be very severe (see Chapter 16 for detailed discussion of the withdrawal syndrome).

PATTERNS OF USE/ABUSE

Estimates place the number of users of prescription CNS depressants at between 20 and 25 million (Blum, 1984). Approximately 300 tons of barbiturates alone are consumed in the United States annually. Among frequent users, several significant variables have been observed in the pattern of CNS depressant usage. They include:

Age. Frequency of sedative-hypnotic use increases with age and occurs most often among persons aged 60 and older. The use of antianxiety agents is greater among those between ages 30 and 60.

Sex. Women are almost twice as likely to use tranquilizers as men. However, men report use of alcohol more often than women.

Marital status. Persons who are separated or divorced report frequent use more often than married or never-married persons.

Race. Whites are more likely to use barbiturates than nonwhites.

Socioeconomic status. Persons from the middle socioeconomic classes are most likely to use barbiturates.

Education. Persons with higher levels of education are more likely to be regular users of barbiturates than those with less education (Chambers et al, 1972).

Physicians, especially general practitioners, remain the major source of CNS depressants for all age groups; however, the numbers of illicit sources continue to grow (Blum, 1984). Approximately 500,000 of the millions of users of CNS depressants can be considered abusers, that is, their use is nonspecific, excessive in amount or duration of time, serves to obscure real causes while treating symptoms, or is not beneficial (Blum, 1984).

The *DSM-III-R* (APA, 1987) reports on two patterns of development of dependence and abuse. The first pattern is one of an individual whose physician originally prescribed the CNS depressant as treatment for anxiety or insomnia. Independently, the individual has increased the dosage or frequency from that which was prescribed. Use of the medication is justified on the basis of treating symptoms, but as tolerance grows, more and more of the medication is required to produce the desired effect. Substance-seeking behavior is evident as the individual seeks prescriptions from several physicians to maintain sufficient supplies.

The second pattern, which the *DSM-III-R* reports is more frequent than the first, involves young people in their teens or early 20s who, in the company of their peers, use substances that were obtained from illegal sources. The initial objective is to achieve a feeling of euphoria. The drug is generally used intermittently during recreational gatherings. This pattern of intermittent use leads to regular use and extreme levels of tolerance. Combining use with other substances is not uncommon. Physical and psychological dependence leads to intense substance-seeking behaviors, most often through illegal channels.

EFFECTS ON THE BODY

The sedative-hypnotic compounds induce a general depressant effect. That is, they depress the activity of the brain, the nerves, the muscles, and the heart tissue. They reduce the rate of metabolism in a variety of tissues throughout the body, and in general, they depress any system that uses energy (Julien, 1981). Large doses are required to produce these effects. In lower doses, these drugs appear to be more selective in their depressant action. Specifically, in lower doses, these drugs appear to exert their action on the centers within the brain that are concerned with arousal, for example, the ascending reticular activating system, in the reticular formation, and the diffuse thalamic projection system.

As stated previously, the sedative-hypnotics are capable of producing all levels of CNS depression from mild sedation to death. The level is determined by dosage and potency of the drug used. In Figure 17.1, a continuum of the CNS depressant effects is presented to demonstrate how increasing doses of sedative-hypnotic drugs affect behavioral depression.

The primary action of sedative-hypnotics is on nervous tissue. However, large doses may have an effect on other organ systems. Following is a discussion of the physiological effects of large doses of barbiturates (Harvey, 1975).

The Effects on Sleep and Dreaming With the barbiturates, the amount of sleep time spent in dreaming is decreased. Some investigators believe that this decrease (or absence) of rapid-eye-movement sleep with loss of dreaming may be harmful and may even be capable of precipitating psychotic episodes in some individuals (Julien, 1981). Ray (1972) has stated, "When an individual who has been using barbiturates regularly as a sleeping pill suddenly stops using them, he (or she) may overdream or even have nightmares."

Respiratory Depression In large doses, barbiturates depress the respiratory centers in the medulla portion of the brainstem. Death can occur from barbiturate-induced respiratory depression.

Cardiovascular Effects Hypotension may be a problem with large doses. Only a slight decrease in blood pressure is noted with normal oral dosage.

Renal Function In doses high enough to produce anesthesia, barbiturates may suppress urine function. At the usual sedative-hypnotic dosage, however, there is no evidence that they have any direct action on the kidneys.

Hepatic Effects The barbiturates may produce jaundice with doses large enough to produce acute intoxication. Preexisting liver disease may predispose an individual to additional liver damage with excessive barbiturate use.

Body Temperature High doses of barbiturates can greatly decrease body temperature. It is not significantly altered with normal dosage levels.

Sexual Functioning Like alcohol, these other CNS depressants have a tendency to produce a biphasic response. There is an initial increase in libido, supposedly from the primary disinhibitory effects of the drug. This initial response is then followed by a decrease in the ability to maintain erection.

CNS Stimulant Abuse and Dependence

A PROFILE OF THE SUBSTANCE

The CNS stimulants are identified by the behavioral stimulation and psychomotor agitation that they induce. They differ widely in their molecular structures and in their mechanisms of action. The degree of CNS stimulation caused by a certain drug depends on both the area in the brain or spinal cord that is affected by the drug and the cellular mechanism fundamental to the increased excitability (Byers, 1991).

Groups within this category are classified according to similarities in mechanism of action. The *psychomotor stimulants* induce stimulation by augmentation or potentiation of the neurotransmitters norepinephrine, epinephrine, or dopamine. The *general cellular stimulants* (caffeine and nicotine) exert their action directly on cellular activity. Caffeine inhibits the enzyme phosphodiesterase, allowing increased levels of cAMP (a chemical substance that promotes increased rates of cellular metabolism). Nicotine stimulates ganglionic synapses. This results in increased acetylcholine, which stimulates nerve impulse transmission to the entire autonomic nervous system.

Following is a selected list of drugs included in these categories. Generic names are followed in parentheses by the trade names. Common street names for each category are also included.

PSYCHOMOTOR STIMULANTS

Amphetamines

amphetamine sulfate
(Benzedrine):   bennies, splash, peaches

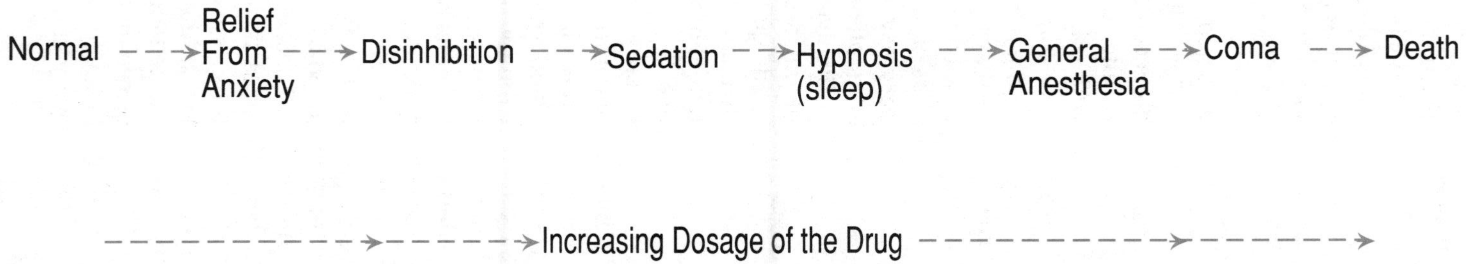

Normal ---→ Relief
From ---→ Disinhibition ---→ Sedation ---→ Hypnosis ---→ General ---→ Coma ---→ Death
Anxiety (sleep) Anesthesia

←--- Increasing Dosage of the Drug ---→

Figure 17.1 Continuum of behavioral depression.

Amphetamines (Continued)

dextroamphetamine
(Dexedrine):   dexies, uppers, diet pills
methamphetamine   meth, speed, water,
(Desoxyn):   crystal
l-amphetamine +
d-amphetamine
(Biphetamine):   black beauties, speed

Nonamphetamine Stimulants

phenmetrazine
(Preludin):   diet pills
methylphenidate
(Ritalin):   speed, uppers
pemoline (Cylert)

Cocaine

cocaine hydrochloride: coke, blow, toot, snow
                              lady, flake

GENERAL CELLULAR STIMULANTS

Caffeine

coffee, tea, colas,
chocolate: java, mud, brew, cocoa

Nicotine

cigarettes, cigars, pipe   weeds, fags, butts, chaw,
tobacco, snuff: cancer sticks

The two most prevalent and widely used stimulants are caffeine and nicotine. Caffeine is readily available in every supermarket and grocery store as a common ingredient in coffee, tea, colas, and chocolate. Nicotine is a primary substance found in tobacco products. When used in moderation, these stimulants tend to relieve fatigue and increase alertness (DEA, 1979). They have become a generally accepted part of our culture.

The more potent stimulants, because of their potential for physiological dependency, are under regulation by the Controlled Substances Act. These controlled stimulants are available for therapeutic purposes by prescription only. They are also clandestinely manufactured in vast quantities for distribution on the illicit market (DEA, 1979).

HISTORICAL ASPECTS

Cocaine is the most potent stimulant derived from natural origin. It is extracted from the leaves of the coca plant, which has been cultivated in the Andean highlands of South America since prehis-

toric times. Natives of the region chew the leaves of the plant for refreshment and relief from fatigue.

The coca leaves must be mixed with lime to release the cocaine alkaloid. The chemical formula for the pure form of the drug was obtained in 1860. Physicians began using the drug as an anesthetic in eye, nose, and throat surgeries. These therapeutic uses are now obsolete. In recent years, however, it has been used in the United States in a morphine-cocaine elixir designed to relieve the suffering associated with terminal illness (DEA, 1979).

Cocaine has achieved a degree of popularity as an acceptable recreational drug. It is illicitly distributed as a white crystalline powder, often mixed with other ingredients to increase its volume and therefore create more profits. The drug is most commonly "snorted," and chronic users may manifest symptoms that resemble the congested nose of a common cold. The intensely pleasurable effects of the drug create the potential for extraordinary psychological dependency.

Amphetamine was first prepared in 1887. Various derivatives of the drug soon followed. Clinical use of the drug began in 1927. Amphetamines were used quite extensively for medical purposes through the 1960s. Recognition of their abuse potential has sharply decreased use in clinical practice. Today, they are only prescribed to treat narcolepsy, a rare disorder resulting in an uncontrollable desire for sleep, hyperactivity disorders in children, and in certain cases of obesity. Clandestine production of amphetamines for distribution on the illicit market has become a thriving business.

The earliest history of caffeine is unknown and shrouded by legend and myth. Caffeine was first discovered in coffee in 1820 and 7 years later in tea. Both beverages have been widely accepted and enjoyed as a "pick-me-up" by many cultures.

Tobacco was used by the aborigines from remote times. Introduced in Europe in the middle 16th century, its use grew rapidly and it soon became prevalent in the Orient. Tobacco came to America with the settlement of the earliest colonies. Today, it is grown in many countries of the world, and tobacco products are used extensively within virtually every culture.

PATTERNS OF USE/ABUSE

Because of their pleasurable effects, CNS stimulants have a high abuse potential. Approximately 30 million Americans admit to having tried some form of cocaine, and about 1 million are so addicted to the drug that they will do *anything* to get it (House, 1990). Many individuals who abuse or are dependent on CNS stimulants began using the substance for the appetite-suppressant effect in an attempt at weight control (APA, 1987). Higher and higher doses are consumed in an effort to maintain the pleasurable effects. With continued use, the pleasurable effects diminish, and there is a corresponding increase in dysphoric effects. There is a persistent craving for the substance, however, even in the face of unpleasant adverse effects from the continued drug taking.

CNS stimulant abuse and dependence are usually characterized by either episodic or chronic daily, or almost daily, use. Individuals who use the substances on an episodic basis often "binge" on the drug with very high dosages followed by a day or two of recuperation. This recuperation period is characterized by extremely intense and unpleasant symptoms (called a "crash").

The daily user may take large or small doses and may use several times a day, or only at a specific time during the day. The amount consumed usually increases over time as tolerance occurs. Chronic users tend to rely on CNS stimulants to feel more powerful, more confident, and more decisive. They often fall into a pattern of taking "uppers" in the morning and "downers," such as alcohol or sleeping pills, at night.

The average American consumes two cups of coffee—or about 200 mg of caffeine—per day. Twenty to thirty percent of the U.S. population ingests 500 to 600 mg of caffeine per day (Pilette, 1983). At this level of daily caffeine consumption, symptoms of anxiety, insomnia, and depression are not uncommon. It is also at this level that caffeine dependence and withdrawal can occur. Caffeine consumption is prevalent among children as well as adults. Table 17.2 lists some common sources of caffeine.

Next to caffeine, nicotine, an active ingredient in tobacco, is the most widely used psychoactive substance in our society (Julien, 1981). About 55 million Americans smoke cigarettes (Kaplan & Sadock, 1985). Since 1964, when the results of the first public health report on smoking were issued, the total percentage of adult smokers has been on the decline. However, the percentage of women and teenage smokers has continued to increase (Kaplan & Sadock, 1985). Approximately 300,000 people die

Table 17.2 COMMON SOURCES OF CAFFEINE	
Source	**Caffeine Content**
Food and Beverages:	
5–6 oz brewed coffee	90–125 mg
5–6 oz instant coffee	60–90 mg
5–6 oz decaffeinated coffee	3 mg
5–6 oz brewed tea	70 mg
5–6 oz instant tea	45 mg
8–12 oz cola drinks	60 mg
5–6 oz cocoa	20 mg
8 oz chocolate milk	2–7 mg
1 oz chocolate bar	22 mg
Prescription medications:	
APC's (aspirin, phenacetin,	
caffeine)	32 mg
Cafergot	100 mg
Darvon compound	32 mg
Fiorinal	40 mg
Migral	50 mg
Over-the-counter analgesics:	
Anacin, Empirin, Midol, Vanquish	32 mg
Excedrin	60 mg
Over-the-counter stimulants:	
No Doz tablets	100 mg
Vivarin	200 mg
Caffedrine	250 mg

Source: Adapted from Kaplan and Sadock (1985), Pilette (1983), Blum (1984), and Bennett and Woolf (1991).

annually because of tobacco use, and an estimated 10 million Americans suffer from smoking-related chronic diseases (Department of Health, Education, and Welfare [DHEW], 1988).

EFFECTS ON THE BODY

The CNS stimulants are a group of pharmacologic agents that are capable of exciting the entire nervous system. This is accomplished by increasing the activity or augmenting the capability of the neurotransmitter agents known to be directly involved in bodily activation and behavioral stimulation. Physiological responses vary markedly according to the potency and dosage of the drug.

Central Nervous System Effects Stimulation of the CNS results in tremor, restlessness, anorexia, insomnia, agitation, and increased motor activity. Amphetamines, nonamphetamine stimulants, and cocaine produce increased alertness, decrease in fatigue, elation and euphoria, and subjective feelings of greater mental agility and muscular power. Chronic use of these drugs may result in compulsive behavior, paranoia, hallucinations, and aggressive behavior (Blum, 1984).

Cardiovascular/Pulmonary Effects   Amphetamines are capable of inducing an increase in both systolic and diastolic blood pressure, increased heart rate, and cardiac arrhymias (Blum, 1984). A relaxation of bronchial smooth muscle is effected.

Cocaine intoxication can result in a rise in myocardial demand for oxygen, an increase in heart rate, and severe vasoconstriction that can result in myocardial infarction, ventricular fibrillation, and sudden death (House, 1990). Inhaled cocaine can cause pulmonary hemorrhage, chronic bronchiolitis, and pneumonia. Nasal rhinitis is a result of chronic cocaine snorting.

Caffeine ingestion can result in increased heart rate, palpitations, extrasystoles, arrhythmias, and in very large doses, cardiac standstill (Pilette, 1983). Caffeine induces dilation of pulmonary and general systemic blood vessels, and constriction of cerebral blood vessels.

Nicotine is capable of increasing heart rate and blood pressure and stimulating the heart muscle. Blood flow to the heart and to skeletal muscle is increased (Julien, 1981).

Gastrointestinal and Renal Effects   Gastrointestinal effects of amphetamines are somewhat unpredictable (Blum, 1984); however, a decrease in gastrointestinal tract motility commonly results in constipation (Bennett & Woolf, 1991). Contraction of the bladder sphincter makes urination difficult. Caffeine exerts a diuretic effect on the kidneys. Nicotine stimulates the hypothalamus to release antidiuretic hormone, reducing the excretion of urine. Because nicotine increases the tone and activity of the bowel, it may occasionally induce diarrhea (Julien, 1981).

Most CNS stimulants induce a small rise in metabolic rate and produce various degrees of anorexic effects. Amphetamines and cocaine can effect a rise in body temperature.

Sexual Functioning   CNS stimulants apparently promote the coital urge in both men and women (Blum, 1984). Women, more than men, report that stimulants make them feel sexier and have more orgasms. In fact, some men may experience sexual dysfunction with stimulants. For the majority of individuals, however, these drugs exert a powerful aphrodisiac effect, and may be one reason for relapse or continued abuse of the substance (Bennett & Woolf, 1991).

Opioid Abuse and Dependence

A PROFILE OF THE SUBSTANCE

The term *opioid* refers to a group of compounds that includes opium, opium derivatives, and synthetic substitutes. Opioids exert both a sedative and an analgesic effect, and their major medical uses are for the relief of pain, the treatment of diarrhea, and the relief of coughing. These drugs have addictive qualities, that is, they are capable of inducing tolerance and physiological and psychological dependence.

Opioids are popular drugs of abuse in that they sensitize an individual to both psychological and physiological pain, and induce a sense of euphoria. Lethargy and indifference to the environment are common manifestations.

Opioid abusers generally spend much of their time nourishing their habit. Individuals who are opioid dependent are seldom able to hold a steady job that will support their need. They must therefore secure funds from friends, relatives, or whomever they have not yet alienated with their dependency-related behavior. Obtaining funds by illegal means is not uncommon. The three most common criminal methods are burglary, prostitution, and the dealing of drugs (Blum, 1984).

Methods of administration of opioid drugs include oral, snorting, smoking, and by subcutaneous, intramuscular, and intravenous injection. Following is a selected list of opioid substances. Generic names are followed in parentheses by the trade names. Common street names for each category are also included.

Opioids of Natural Origin

opium (ingredient in various antidiarrheal agents):	black, poppy, tar, big O
morphine (Astramorph):	M, white stuff, Miss Emma
codeine (an ingredient in various analgesics and cough suppressants):	terp, robo, romo, syrup

Opioid Derivatives

heroin:	H, horse, junk, brown, smack, scag, TNT, Harry
hydromorphone (Dilaudid):	DL's, 4's, lords, little D
oxycodone (in Percodan):	perks, perkies
hydrocodone (Hycodan)	

Synthetic Opiatelike Drugs

meperidine (Demerol)	
methadone (Dolophine):	dollies, done
propoxyphene (Darvon):	pinks and grays
pentazocine (Talwin):	T's

Under close supervision, opioids are indispensable in the practice of medicine. They are the most effective agents known for the relief of intense pain. They also induce a pleasurable effect on the CNS that promotes their abuse. The physiological and psychological dependence that occurs with opioids, as well as the development of profound tolerance, contribute to the addict's ongoing quest for more of the substance, regardless of the means.

HISTORICAL ASPECTS

Opium is the Greek word for "juice." It is produced from the milky exudate of the unripe seed capsules of the poppy plant (Kaplan & Sadock, 1985). References to the use of opiates have been found in the Egyptian, Greek, and Arabian cultures as early as 3000 B.C. (Julien, 1981). The drug became widely used both medicinally and recreationally throughout Europe during the 16th and 17th centuries. Most of the opium supply came from China, where the drug was introduced by Arabic traders in the late 17th century. Morphine, the primary active ingredient of opium, was isolated in 1803 by the European chemist Frederich Serturner. Since that time, morphine, rather than crude opium, has been used throughout the world for the medical treatment of pain and diarrhea (Julien, 1981). This process was facilitated in 1953 by the development of the hypodermic syringe, which made it possible to deliver the undiluted morphine quickly into the body for rapid relief from pain (Blum, 1984).

This development also created a new variety of opiate user in the United States: one who was able to self-administer the drug by injection. During this time, there was also a large influx of Chinese immigrants into the United States, who introduced opium smoking to this country. By the early part of the 20th century, opium addiction was widespread.

In response to the concerns over widespread addiction, the U.S. government passed the Harrison Narcotic Act in 1914. This legislation created strict controls on the accessibility of opiates. Until that time, these substances had been freely available to the public without a prescription. The Harrison Act banned the use of opiates for other than medicinal purposes and drove the use of heroin underground. To this day, the beneficial uses of these substances are widely acclaimed within the medical profession, but the illicit trafficking of the drugs for recreational purposes continues to resist most efforts aimed at control.

PATTERNS OF USE/ABUSE

The *DSM-III-R* (APA, 1987) describes two behavioral patterns by which opioid dependence and abuse develop. The first occurs in the individual who has obtained the drug by prescription from a physician for the relief of a medical problem. Abuse and dependency occur when the individual increases the amount and frequency of use, justifying the behavior as symptom treatment. He or she becomes obsessed with obtaining more and more of the substance, seeking out several physicians to replenish and maintain supplies.

The second pattern of behavior associated with abuse and dependency of opioids occurs among individuals who use the drugs for recreational purposes and obtain them from illegal sources. Opioids may be used alone to induce the euphoric effects or in combination with stimulants or other drugs to enhance the euphoria or to counteract the depressant effects of the opioid. Tolerance develops and dependency occurs, leading the individual to procure the substance by whatever means is required in an effort to support the habit. Blum (1984) states:

> "The classic user (of opioids) was once a young, ghetto male, wearing long sleeves to cover the needle marks. He was unemployed, malnourished, had a short attention span, and of course, noticeable miosis. The major exceptions were members of the medical profession who became dependent on Demerol (or morphine) rather than heroin, and generally attempted to keep working to maintain their proximity to hospital supplies.
>
> Now increasing numbers of young people on all social levels are becoming involved with opioids. Some are students; others work, deal drugs, or steal. However, despite this increase in the number of users, there are still relatively few users of illicit opioids, compared with the tremendous number of people using other drugs."

EFFECTS ON THE BODY

Opiates are sometimes classified as *narcotic analgesics*. They exert their major effects primarily on the CNS, the eye, and the gastrointestinal tract (Julien, 1981). Chronic morphine use or acute morphine toxicity is manifested by a syndrome of sedation, chronic constipation, decreased respiratory rate, and pinpoint pupils. Intensity of symptoms is largely dose dependent. The following physiological effects are common with opioid use.

Central Nervous System All opioids, opioid derivatives, and synthetic opioidlike drugs affect the CNS. Common manifestations include euphoria, mood changes, and mental clouding (Bennett & Woolf, 1991). Other common CNS effects include drowsiness and pain reduction. Pupillary constriction occurs in response to stimulation of the oculomotor nerve. CNS depression of the respiratory centers within the medulla results in respiratory depression. The antitussive response is due to suppression of the cough center within the medulla. The nausea and vomiting commonly associated with opiate ingestion are related to the stimulation of the centers within the medulla that trigger this response.

Gastrointestinal Effects These drugs exert a profound effect on the gastrointestinal tract. Both stomach and intestinal tone are increased, while peristaltic activity of the intestines is diminished. These effects lead to a marked decrease in the movement of food through the gastrointestinal tract. This is a notable therapeutic effect in the treatment of severe diarrhea. In fact, no drugs have yet been developed that are more effective than the opioids for this purpose. However, constipation, and even fecal impaction, may be a serious problem for the chronic opioid user.

Cardiovascular Effects In therapeutic doses, opioids have minimal effect on the action of the heart. Morphine is used extensively to relieve pulmonary edema and the pain of myocardial infarction in cardiac patients (Blum, 1984; Bennett & Woolf, 1991). At high doses, opioids induce hypotension, which may be caused by direct action on the heart or by opioid-induced histamine release.

Sexual Functioning A number of studies with opioids, particularly heroin and methadone, have indicated that these drugs cause decreased libido (in both men and women), retarded ejaculation, impotence, and orgasm failure (Blum, 1984). Sexual side effects from opioids appear to be largely influenced by dosage.

Hallucinogen Abuse and Dependence

A PROFILE OF THE SUBSTANCE

Hallucinogenic substances are capable of distorting an individual's perception of reality. They have the ability to alter sensory perception, induce hallucinations, and for this reason have been referred to as "mind expanding" (Julien, 1981). Some of the manifestations have been likened to a psychotic break, although the hallucinations experienced by a schizophrenic are most often auditory, while substance-induced hallucinations are usually visual (Holbrook, 1991). Perceptual distortions have been reported by some users as a sense of depersonalization (observing oneself having the experience), as one of being at peace with self and the universe, and as spiritual in nature. Others, who describe their experiences as "bad trips," report feelings of panic and a fear of dying or going insane. These feelings of terror can recur at any time, even without the drug, and the experience can have lasting effects (Blum, 1984). These adverse reactions are referred to as "flashbacks."

Recurrent use can produce tolerance, encouraging users to resort to higher and higher dosages. No evidence of physical dependence is detectable when the drug is withdrawn; however, recurrent use appears to induce a psychological dependence that varies according to the drug, the dose, and the individual user (DEA, 1979). Hallucinogens are highly unpredictable in the effects they may induce each time they are used.

Many of the hallucinogenic substances have structural similarities. Some are produced synthetically, while others are natural products of plants and fungi. Following is a list of hallucinogens within these categories, classified according to their chemical composition. Common street names for each category are also included.

Naturally Occurring Hallucinogens

Mescaline (the primary active ingredient of the peyote cactus)	cactus, mesc, mescal, half moon, big chief, bad seed, peyote
Psilocybin and psilocyn (active ingredients of psilocybe mushrooms)	magic mushroom, God's flesh, rooms

Naturally Occurring Hallucinogens (Continued)

Ololiuqui (morning glory seeds)	heavenly blue, pearly gates, flying saucers

Synthetic Compounds

Lysergic acid diethylamide [LSD]: (synthetically produced from a fungal substance found on rye or a chemical substance found in morning glory seeds)	acid, cube, big D, California sunshine, microdots, blue dots, sugar, orange wedges, peace tablets, purple haze, cupcakes
Dimethyltryptamine [DMT] and diethyltryptamine [DET] (chemical analogues of tryptamine)	businessman's trip (DMT)
2,5-dimethoxy-4-methylamphetamine [STP, DOM]:	STP = "serenity, tranquility, peace"
Phencyclidine [PCP]:	angel dust, hog, peace pill, rocket fuel
Methylene-dioxyamphetamine [MDMA]	XTC, ecstasy, Adam
Methoxy-amphetamine [MDA]	Love drug

HISTORICAL ASPECTS

Hallucinogens have been used as part of religious ceremonies and at social gatherings by Native Americans for more than 2,000 years (Schuckit, 1979). Use of the peyote cactus as part of religious ceremonies in the southwestern part of the United States still occurs today, although this ritual use has greatly diminished.

LSD was first synthesized in 1938 by Dr. Albert Hoffman (Holbrook, 1991). It was used as a clinical research tool to investigate the biochemical etiology of schizophrenia. It soon, however, reached the illicit market, and its abuse began to overshadow the research effort.

The abuse of hallucinogens reached a peak in the late 1960s, waned during the 1970s, and returned to favor in the 1980s with the so-called designer drugs (MDMA, MDA). One of the most commonly abused hallucinogens today is phencyclidine, even though many of its effects are perceived as undesirable. A number of deaths have been directly attributed to the use of phencyclidine, as well as numerous accidental deaths that have occurred due to overdose and to the behavioral changes the drug precipitates (Holbrook, 1991).

Several therapeutic uses of LSD have been proposed, including the treatment of chronic alcoholism and the reduction of intractable pain such as occurs in malignant disease and in phantom limb sensations (McKenry & Salerno, 1989). A great deal more research is required, however, regarding the therapeutic uses of LSD. At this time, there is no real evidence that speaks to the safety and efficacy of the drug in humans.

PATTERNS OF USE/ABUSE

Use of hallucinogens is generally episodic. Because cognitive and perceptual abilities are so markedly affected by these substances, the user must set aside time from normal daily activities for indulging in the consequences. The *DSM-III-R* (APA, 1987) reports that in a study conducted from 1981 to 1983, approximately 0.3 percent of the adult population in the United States had abused hallucinogens at some time in their lives. The use of LSD does not lead to the development of either physical or psychological dependence (Holbrook, 1991). However, tolerance does develop to a high degree and very rapidly. In fact, an individual who uses LSD repeatedly for a period of 3 to 4 days may develop complete tolerance to the drug. Recovery from the tolerance does occur very rapidly (in 2 to 3 days), so that the individual is able to achieve the desired effect from the drug repeatedly and often.

Phencyclidine is usually taken episodically, in binges that can last for several days. However, some chronic users take the substance on a daily basis (APA, 1987). Physical dependence does not occur with phencyclidine; however, psychologic dependence characterized by craving for the drug has been reported in chronic users, as has the slow development of tolerance (Holbrook, 1991). Tolerance apparently only develops with frequent use, such as on a daily basis.

Psilocybin is an ingredient of the psilocybe mushroom indigenous to the United States and Mexico. Ingestion of these mushrooms produces an effect similar to LSD but of a shorter duration. This hallucinogenic chemical can now be produced synthetically.

Mescaline is the only hallucinogenic compound

used legally for religious purposes today by members of the Native American Church of the United States. It is the primary active ingredient of the peyote cactus. Neither physical nor psychological dependence has been reported to occur with the use of mescaline, although tolerance does develop slowly with repeated use (Holbrook, 1991).

Among the very potent hallucinogens of the current drug culture are those which are categorized as derivatives of amphetamines. These include STP, DOM, MDMA, and MDA. At lower doses, these drugs produce the "high" associated with CNS stimulants. At higher doses, hallucinogenic effects occur. These drugs have been in existence for many years, but were only *rediscovered* in the mid-1980s. Due to the rapid increase in recreational use, the Drug Enforcement Agency imposed an emergency classification of MDMA as a Schedule I drug in 1985.

EFFECTS ON THE BODY

The effects produced by the various hallucinogenics are highly unpredictable. The variety of effects may be related to dosage, the mental state of the individual, and the environment in which the substance is used. Some common effects have been reported (Kauffman et al, 1985):

Physiological Effects

- Nausea and vomiting
- Chills
- Pupil dilation
- Increased pulse, blood pressure, and temperature
- Mild dizziness
- Trembling
- Loss of appetite
- Insomnia
- Sweating
- A slowing of respirations
- Elevation in blood sugar

Psychological Effects

- Heightened response to color, texture, and sounds
- Heightened body awareness
- Distortion of vision
- Sense of slowing of time
- All feelings magnified: love, lust, hate, joy, anger, pain, terror, despair, and so forth

- Fear of losing control
- Paranoia, panic
- Euphoria, bliss
- Projection of self into dreamlike images
- Serenity, joy, and peace
- Depersonalization
- Derealization
- Increased libido

The effects of hallucinogens are not always pleasurable for the user. Two types of toxic reactions are known to occur. The first is the *panic reaction*, or "bad trip." Symptoms include an intense level of anxiety, fear, and stimulation. The individual is hallucinating and is fearful of going insane. Paranoia and acute psychosis may be evident.

The second type of toxic reaction to hallucinogens is the *flashback*. This phenomenon refers to the transient, spontaneous repetition of a previous LSD-induced experience that occurs in the absence of the substance. The incidence of these reactions is not known, but they have been estimated to occur in as high as 5 percent of users (Schuckit, 1979).

Cannabis Abuse and Dependence

A PROFILE OF THE SUBSTANCE

Cannabis is second only to alcohol as the most widely abused drug in the United States. The major psychoactive ingredient of this class of substances is delta-9-tetrahydrocannabinol (THC). It is naturally occurring in the plant *Cannabis sativa*, which grows readily in warm climates. Marijuana, the most prevalent type of cannabis preparation, is composed of the dried leaves, stems, and flowers of the plant. Hashish is a more potent concentrate of the resin derived from the flowering tops of the plant. Hash oil is a very concentrated form of THC made by boiling hashish in a solvent and filtering out the solid matter (Holbrook, 1991). Cannabis products are usually smoked in the form of loosely rolled cigarettes. They may also be administered orally but are reported to be about three times more potent when smoked (DEA, 1979).

All the cannabis drugs act as CNS depressants (McKenry & Salerno, 1989). By depressing higher brain centers, they release lower centers from inhibitory influences. There has been some controversy in the past over the classification of these substances. They are not narcotics, although they are legally classified as controlled substances. They are not hallucinogens, although in very high dosages they can induce these symptoms. They are not sedative-hypnotics, although they most closely resemble these substances. Like sedative-hypnotics, their action occurs in the ascending reticular activating system. With increasing dosage, they can produce increasing levels of sedation, hypnosis, and anesthesia.

Both tolerance and physical dependence have been reported to develop with the chronic use of marijuana (Holbrook, 1991). Tolerance tends to be lost rapidly, so it may never be evident in the casual or infrequent user. The capacity to lead to psychological dependence is not nearly as strong as that of either tobacco or alcohol (Kaplan & Sadock, 1985).

Following are common categories of cannabinols. Street names for each category are also included.

Marijuana: joint, weed, pot, grass, Mary Jane, Texas tea, locoweed, MJ, hay, stick
Hashish: hash, bhang, ganja, charas

HISTORICAL ASPECTS

Products of the plant *Cannabis sativa* have been used therapeutically for nearly 5,000 years (Blum, 1985). Cannabis was first employed in China and India as an antiseptic and an analgesic. Its use later spread to the Middle East, Africa, and Eastern Europe.

In the United States, medical interest arose in the use of cannabis during the early part of the 19th century. Many articles were published espousing its use for many and varied reasons. The drug was almost as commonly used for medicinal purposes as aspirin is today and could be purchased without a prescription in any drug store. It was purported to have antibacterial and anticonvulsant capabilities, to decrease intraocular pressure, decrease pain, help in the treatment of asthma, increase appetite, and generally raise one's morale (Schuckit, 1979).

The drug grew out of favor primarily because of the huge variation in potency within batches of medication due to the variations in the THC content of different plants. Other medications were favored for their greater degree of solubility and faster onset of action than cannabis products. In the late 1920s, an association between marijuana and crimi-

nal activity was reported (Holbrook, 1991). A federal law put an end to its legal use in 1937. In the 1960s, marijuana became the symbol of the "antiestablishment" generation, at which time it reached its peak as a drug of abuse. It still enjoys that prominence today.

Research continues in regard to the possible therapeutic uses of cannabis. It has been shown to be an effective agent for relieving intraocular pressure in patients with glaucoma. However, the long-term safety and efficacy of these drugs has not been established, nor is there sufficient evidence to indicate that they contribute to preservation of visual function in these patients (Blum, 1985).

The use for which cannabis products appear to have the most promising future is in the treatment of nausea and vomiting that accompanies cancer chemotherapy. It has been shown in a number of studies to be effective for this purpose when other antinausea medications fail.

There are advocates within the United States today who praise the therapeutic usefulness and support the legalization of the cannabinoids. Blum (1985) predicts that if marijuana were legalized, more than 1 million Americans would probably be smoking pot daily by 2001, including more children, at earlier ages. He also suggests that the potency of the cannabis used would increase.

A great deal more research is required to determine the long-term effects of the drug. Until results indicate otherwise, it is safe to assume that the harmful effects of the drug largely outweigh the benefits.

PATTERNS OF USE/ABUSE

The *DSM-III-R* (APA, 1987) reports that in a study conducted from 1981 to 1983, approximately 4 percent of the adult population in the United States had used cannabis at some time in their lives. Approximately 18 million Americans use it on a regular basis, such as several times a week to several times a month (Morganthau, 1988). Cannabis is commonly used in combination with other substances, particularly alcohol and cocaine (APA, 1987). The overall use of marijuana continues to grow yearly, with the 12- to 25-year-old age group showing the highest prevalence (Blum, 1985).

Many people incorrectly regard cannabis as a substance of low abuse potential. This lack of knowledge has promoted use of the substance by some individuals who believe it is harmless. Tolerance, although it tends to decline rapidly, does occur with chronic use. As tolerance develops, physical dependence also occurs, resulting in a mild withdrawal syndrome on cessation of drug use. The syndrome is characterized by irritability, restlessness, anorexia, insomnia, sweating, nausea, vomiting, and diarrhea (Spence, 1987b).

One controversy that exists regarding marijuana is whether or not its use leads to the use of other illicit drugs. Although there is no conclusive evidence that shows there is a definite connection, the issue cannot simply be dismissed. It is logical to consider that the same factors that influenced use of the marijuana might also predispose the individual to try other illicit drugs.

EFFECTS ON THE BODY

Following is a summary of some of the effects that have been attributed to marijuana in recent years. Undoubtedly, as research continues, evidence of additional physiological and psychological effects will be made available.

Cardiovascular Effects Cannabis ingestion induces tachycardia and orthostatic hypotension (Holbrook, 1991). With the decrease in blood pressure, myocardial oxygen supply is decreased. Tachycardia in turn increases oxygen demand.

Respiratory Effects Marijuana produces a greater amount of "tar" than its equivalent weight in tobacco. Because of the method by which marijuana is smoked—that is, the smoke is held in the lungs for as long as possible to achieve the desired effect—larger amounts of tar are deposited in the lungs, promoting deleterious effects to the lungs.

Although the initial reaction to the marijuana is bronchodilatation, thereby facilitating respiratory function, chronic use results in obstructive airway disorders (Holbrook, 1991). Frequent marijuana users often have laryngitis, bronchitis, cough, and hoarseness. Although thus far there is no direct evidence to link marijuana smoking with lung cancer, analysis of marijuana smoke has shown that it contains greater amounts of carcinogens than are present in tobacco smoke (Blum, 1985).

Reproductive Effects Some studies have shown a decrease in levels of serum testosterone and abnormalities in sperm count, motility, and structure correlated with heavy marijuana use (Blum, 1985).

In women, heavy marijuana use has been correlated with failure to ovulate, difficulty with lactation, and an increased risk of reproductive loss.

Central Nervous System Effects Acute CNS effects of marijuana are dose related. Many people report a feeling of being "high"—or the alcohol equivalent of being "drunk." Symptoms include feelings of euphoria, relaxed inhibitions, disorientation, depersonalization, and relaxation. At higher doses, sensory alterations may occur, including impairment in judgment of time and distance, recent memory, and learning ability. Physiologic symptoms may include tremors, muscle rigidity, and conjunctival redness. Toxic effects are generally characterized by panic reactions. Very heavy usage has been shown to precipitate an acute psychosis that is self-limited and short-lived once the drug is removed from the body (Blum, 1984).

Heavy, long-term cannabis use is also associated with a syndrome called *amotivational syndrome.* When this syndrome occurs, the individual is totally preoccupied with using the substance. Symptoms include lethargy, apathy, social and personal deterioration, and lack of motivation. This syndrome appears to be more common in countries in which the most potent preparations are used, and where the substance is more freely available than it is in the United States.

Sexual Functioning Marijuana is reported to enhance the sexual experience in both men and women. The intensified sensory awareness and the subjective slowness of time perception are believed to increase sexual satisfaction. Marijuana also enhances the sexual functioning by releasing inhibitions for certain activities that would normally be restrained.

Table 17.3 includes a summary of the drugs of abuse, their symptoms of use and overdose, possible therapeutic uses, and trade and common names by which they may be referred. The dynamics of substance use disorders using the Transactional Model of Stress/Adaptation is presented in Figure 17.2.

APPLICATION OF THE NURSING PROCESS

Assessment

In the preintroductory phase of relationship development, the nurse must examine his or her feelings about working with a patient who abuses sub-

Table 17.3 DRUGS OF ABUSE

Class of Drugs	Symptoms of Use	Therapeutic Uses	Symptoms of Overdose	Trade Names	Common Names
CNS DEPRESSANTS Alcohol	Relaxation, loss of inhibitions, lack of concentration, drowsiness, slurred speech, sleep	Antidote for methanol consumption; ingredient in many pharmacologic concentrates	Nausea, vomiting; shallow respirations; cold, clammy skin; weak, rapid pulse; coma; possible death	Ethyl alcohol, beer, gin, rum, vodka, bourbon, whiskey, liqueurs, wine, brandy, sherry, champagne	Booze, alcohol, liquor, drinks, cocktails, highballs, nightcaps, moonshine, white lightening, firewater
Other (barbiturates and non-barbiturates)	Same as alcohol	Relief from anxiety and insomnia; as anticonvulsants and anesthetics	Anxiety, fever, agitation, hallucinations, disorientation, tremors, delirium, convulsions, possible death	Seconal, Nembutal, Amytal,	Red birds, yellow birds, blue birds.
				Valium, Librium	Blues/yellows; green & whites
				Noctec	Mickies
				Equanil, Miltown	Downers
CNS STIMULANTS Amphetamines and related drugs	Hyperactivity, agitation, euphoria, insomnia, loss of appetite	Management of narcolepsy, hyperkinesia, and weight control	Cardiac arrhythmias, headache, convulsions, hypertension, rapid heart rate, coma, possible death	Dexedrine, Didrex, Tenuate, Preludin, Ritalin, Plegine, Cylert, Ionamin, Sanorex	Uppers, pep pills, wakeups, bennies, eye-openers, speed, black beauties, sweet A's
Cocaine	Euphoria, hyperactivity, restlessness, talkativeness, increased pulse, dilated pupils	Topical anesthetic	Hallucinations, convulsions, pulmonary edema, respiratory failure, coma, cardiac arrest, possible death	Cocaine hydrochloride	Coke, flake, snow, dust, happy dust, gold dust, girl, cecil, C, toot, blow, crack
OPIOIDS	Euphoria, lethargy, drowsiness, lack of motivation	As analgesics; methadone in substitution therapy; heroin has no therapeutic use	Shallow breathing, slowed pulse, clammy skin, pulmonary edema, respiratory arrest, convulsions, coma, possible death	Heroin	Snow, stuff, H, harry, horse
				Morphine	M, morph, Miss Emma
				Codeine	Schoolboy
				Dilaudid	Lords
				Demerol	Doctors
				Dolophine	Dollies
				Percodan	Perkies
				Talwin	T's
				Opium	Big O, black stuff
HALLUCINOGENS	Visual hallucinations, disorientation, confusion, paranoid delusions, euphoria, anxiety, panic, increased pulse	LSD has been proposed in the treatment of chronic alcoholism, and in the reduction of intractable pain	Agitation, extreme hyperactivity, violence, hallucinations, psychosis, convulsions, possible death	LSD	Acid, cube, big D
				PCP	Angel dust, Hog crystal
				Mescaline	Mesc
				DMT	Businessman's trip
				STP	Serenity and peace

(*continued*)

Table 17.3 CONTINUED

Class of Drugs	Symptoms of Use	Therapeutic Uses	Symptoms of Overdose	Trade Names	Common Names
CANNABINOLS	Relaxation, talkativeness, lowered inhibitions, euphoria, mood swings	Marijuana has been used for relief of nausea and vomiting associated with antineoplastic chemotherapy and to reduce eye pressure in glaucoma patients	Fatigue, paranoia, delusions, hallucinations, possible psychosis	Cannabis Hashish	Marijuana, pot, grass, joint, Mary Jane, MJ Hash, rope, Sweet Lucy

stances. If these behaviors are viewed as morally wrong and the nurse has internalized these attitudes from very early in life, it may be difficult to suppress judgmental feelings. The role that alcohol or other substances has played (or plays) in the life of the nurse will most certainly affect the way in which he or she approaches interaction with the substance-abusing patient.

How are attitudes examined? Some individuals may have sufficient ability for introspection to be able to recognize on their own whether they have unresolved issues related to substance abuse. For others, it may be more helpful to discuss these issues in a group situation, where insight may be gained from feedback regarding the perceptions of others.

Whether alone or in a group, the nurse may gain a greater understanding about attitudes and feelings related to substance abuse by responding to the following types of questions. The questions are specific to alcohol but could be adapted for any substance.

What are my drinking patterns?
If I drink, why do I drink? When, where, and how much?
If I don't drink, why is it that I abstain?
Am I comfortable with my drinking patterns?
If I decided not to drink anymore, would that be a problem for me?
What did I learn from my parents about drinking?
Have my attitudes changed as an adult?
What are my feelings about people who become intoxicated?

Does it seem more acceptable for some individuals than for others?
Do I ever use terms like "sot," "drunk," or "boozer" to describe some individuals who overindulge yet overlook it in others?
Do I ever overindulge myself?
Has the use of alcohol (by myself or others) affected my life in any way?
Do I see alcohol/drug abuse as a sign of weakness? A moral problem? An illness?

Unless nurses fully understand and accept their own attitudes and feelings, they cannot be empathetic toward patients' problems. Patients in recovery need to know they are accepted for themselves, regardless of past behaviors. Nurses must be able to separate the patient from the behavior and to accept that individual with unconditional positive regard.

ASSESSMENT TOOLS

Nurses are often the individuals who perform the admission interview. A variety of assessment tools are appropriate for use on chemical dependency units. A nursing history and assessment tool was presented in Chapter 6 of this text. With some adaptation, it is an appropriate instrument for creating a data base on patients who abuse substances. Table 17.4 presents a drug history and assessment that could be used in conjunction with the general biopsychosocial assessment.

Other screening tools exist for determining whether an individual has a problem with sub-

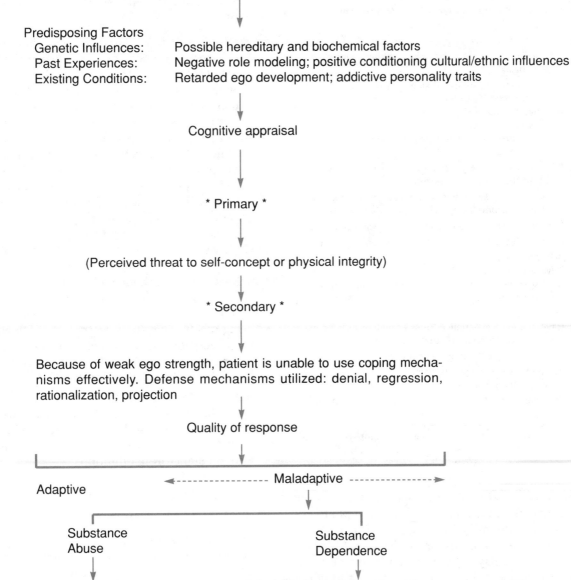

Precipitating Event
(Any event sufficiently stressful to threaten an already weak ego;
the precipitating event for the dependent person may be the onset of withdrawal symptoms)

Predisposing Factors
  Genetic Influences: Possible hereditary and biochemical factors
  Past Experiences: Negative role modeling; positive conditioning cultural/ethnic influences
  Existing Conditions: Retarded ego development; addictive personality traits

Cognitive appraisal

* Primary *

(Perceived threat to self-concept or physical integrity)

* Secondary *

Because of weak ego strength, patient is unable to use coping mechanisms effectively. Defense mechanisms utilized: denial, regression, rationalization, projection

Quality of response

Adaptive   ◄------------- Maladaptive -------------►

Substance   Substance
Abuse   Dependence

1. Uses substances knowing   1. Inability to control or stop use.
   use causes problems in one   2. Uses greater amounts to
   or more aspects of life.   achieve effects.
2. Uses substances in physically   3. Uses substances knowing use
   hazardous situations.   causes problems in one or more
                                       aspects of life.
                                    4. Develops withdrawal symptoms
                                       if ceases or cuts down on use.
                                    5. Takes substance to relieve or
                                       avoid withdrawal symptoms.

Figure 17.2 The dynamics of substance use disorders using the Transactional Model of Stress/Adaptation.

Table 17.4   DRUG HISTORY AND ASSESSMENT*

1. When you were growing up, did anyone in your family drink alcohol or take other kinds of drugs?
2. If so, how did the substance use affect the family situation?
3. When did you have your first drink/drugs?
4. How long have you been drinking/taking drugs on a regular basis?
5. What is your pattern of substance use?
   a. When do you use substances?
   b. What do you use?
   c. How much do you use?
   d. Where are you and with whom when you use substances?
6. When did you have your last drink/drug? What was it and how much did you consume?
7. Does using the substance(s) cause problems for you? Describe. Include family, friends, job, school, other.
8. Have you ever experienced injury due to substance use?
9. Have you ever been arrested or incarcerated for drinking/drugs?
10. Have you ever tried to stop drinking/drugs? If so, what was the result? Did you experience any physical symptoms, such as tremors, headache, insomnia, sweating, seizures?
11. Have you ever experienced loss of memory for times when you have been drinking/taking drugs?
12. Describe a typical day in your life for me.
13. Are there any changes you would like to make in your life? If so, what?
14. What plans or ideas do you have for seeing that these changes occur?

*To be used in conjunction with general biopsychosocial nursing history and assessment tool (see Chapter 6).

stances. Two such tools developed by the APA for the diagnosis of alcoholism include the Michigan Alcoholism Screening Test and the CAGE Questionnaire. These tools are presented in Tables 17.5 and 17.6. Some psychiatric units administer these surveys to all patients who are admitted, in an effort to determine if there is a secondary alcoholism problem in addition to the psychiatric problem for which the patient is being admitted (sometimes called dual diagnosis). It would be possible to adapt these tools to use in diagnosing problems with other drugs as well.

Nursing Diagnoses

The next step in the nursing process is to identify appropriate nursing diagnoses by analyzing the data collected during the assessment phase. The individual who abuses or is dependent on substances will undoubtedly have many unmet physical and emotional needs. Possible nursing diagnoses for patients with substance use disorders include:

Ineffective denial related to weak, underdeveloped ego evidenced by "I don't have a problem with (substance). I can quit any time I want to."
Ineffective individual coping related to inadequate coping skills and weak ego evidenced by use of substances as coping mechanism
Altered nutrition: Less than body requirements/ Fluid volume deficit related to drinks or takes drugs instead of eating evidenced by loss of weight, pale conjunctiva and mucous membranes, poor skin turgor, electrolyte imbalance, anemias (and other signs and symptoms of malnutrition/dehydration)
High risk for infection related to malnutrition and altered immune condition
Self-esteem disturbance related to weak ego, lack of positive feedback evidenced by criticism of self and others, and use of substances as coping mechanism (self-destructive behavior)
Knowledge deficit (effects of substance abuse on the body) related to denial of problems with substances evidenced by abuse of substances

NOTE: Problems related to the acute phases of substance abuse and dependence (intoxication and withdrawal) were addressed in Chapter 16. These problems relate more specifically to substance rehabilitation.

Planning/Implementation

Table 17.7 provides a plan of care for the patient with substance use disorder. Selected nursing diagnoses are presented, along with goals of care and appropriate nursing interventions for each. Rationale is provided in italics.

Implementation with patients who abuse substances is a long-term process, often beginning with detoxification and progressing to total abstinence. Smith et al (1984) identified the following common major treatment objectives for hospitalized patients with substance use disorders.

Short-Term Objectives
1. Support withdrawal from substances and prevent physical complications.
2. Monitor toxic state, provide physical nursing

Table 17.5 MICHIGAN ALCOHOLISM SCREENING TEST

Answer the following questions by placing an X under *yes* or *no.**	Yes	No
1. Do you enjoy a drink now and then?	0	0
2. Do you feel you are a normal drinker? (By normal we mean you drink less than or as much as most people.)		2
3. Have you ever awakened the morning after some drinking the night before and found that you could not remember a part of the evening?	2	
4. Does your wife, husband, parent, or other near relative ever worry or complain about your drinking?	1	
5. Can you stop drinking without a struggle after one or two drinks?		2
6. Do you ever feel guilty about your drinking?	1	
7. Do friends or relatives think you are a normal drinker?		2
8. Are you able to stop drinking when you want to?		2
9. Have you ever attended a meeting of Alcoholics Anonymous (AA)?	5	
10. Have you gotten into physical fights when drinking?	1	
11. Has your drinking ever created problems between you and your wife, husband, a parent, or other relative?	2	
12. Has your wife, husband, or another family member ever gone to anyone for help about your drinking?	2	
13. Have you ever lost friends because of your drinking?	2	
14. Have you ever gotten into trouble at work or school because of drinking?	2	
15. Have you ever lost a job because of drinking?	2	
16. Have you ever neglected your obligations, your family, or your work for 2 or more days in a row because you were drinking?	2	
17. Do you drink before noon fairly often?	1	
18. Have you ever been told you have liver trouble? Cirrhosis?	2	
19. After heavy drinking have you ever had delirium tremens (DT's) or severe shaking or heard voices or seen things that really weren't there?	(5 DT's)	
20. Have you ever gone to anyone for help about your drinking?	5	
21. Have you ever been in a hospital because of drinking?	5	
22. Have you ever been a patient in a psychiatric hospital or on a psychiatric ward of a general hospital where drinking was part of the problem that resulted in hospitalization?	2	
23. Have you ever been seen at a psychiatric or mental health clinic or gone to any doctor, social worker, or clergyman for help with any emotional problem, where drinking was part of the problem?	2	
24. Have you ever been arrested for drunk driving, driving while intoxicated, or driving under the influence of alcoholic beverages? (If yes, how many times?_____)	2 ea	
25. Have you ever been arrested, or taken into custody, even for a few hours, because of other drunk behavior? (If yes, how many times?_____)	2 ea	

*Items are scored under the response that would indicate a problem with alcohol.

Method of scoring: 0–3 points = no problem with alcohol
                                        4 points = possible problem with alcohol
                                        5 or more = indicates problem with alcohol

Source: From Selzer, M. L. (1971), with permission.

care, and administer substitution medication as ordered.

3. Provide psychological support and promote a restful environment.

Intermediate Objectives

1. Interpret symptoms, course of treatment, and expected outcomes for patient and family.

2. Promote understanding of substance abuse and dependency and participation in treatment program.

Long-Term Objectives

1. Encourage participation in the treatment program and promote understanding of underlying problems associated with substance use.

Table 17.6 THE CAGE QUESTIONNAIRE
1. Have you ever felt you should *C*ut down on your drinking?
2. Have people *A*nnoyed you by criticizing your drinking?
3. Have you ever felt bad or *G*uilty about your drinking?
4. Have you ever had a drink first thing in the morning to steady your nerves or get rid of a hangover (*E*ye-opener)?

Scoring: 2 or 3 "yes" answers strongly suggests a problem with alcohol
Source: From Mayfield, D. et al (1974), with permission.

2. Monitor for signs of acute stress or possible resumption of substance use.
3. Assist patient to explore alternative coping strategies to achieve satisfaction (see Table 17.8).
4. Assist with plans for follow-up therapy.

Evaluation

The final step of the nursing process involves reassessment to determine if the nursing interven-

Table 17.7 CARE PLAN FOR PATIENT WITH SUBSTANCE USE DISORDER		
Nursing Diagnoses	**Objectives**	**Nursing Interventions**
Ineffective denial related to weak, underdeveloped ego evidenced by statements indicating no problem with substance use.	Patient will verbalize acceptance of responsibility for own behavior and acknowledge association between substance use and personal problems.	Develop trust. Convey an attitude of acceptance. Ensure that patient understands it is not the *person* but the *behavior* that is unacceptable. *Unconditional acceptance promotes dignity and self-worth, qualities that this individual has been trying to achieve with substances.* Correct any misconceptions, such as, "I don't have a drinking problem. I can quit any time I want to." Do this in a matter-of-fact, nonjudgmental manner. *These interventions help the patient see the condition as an illness that requires help.* Identify recent maladaptive behaviors or situations that have occurred in the patient's life, and discuss how use of substances may be a contributing factor. Say, "The lab report shows your blood alcohol level was 250 when you were involved in that automobile accident." *The first step in decreasing use of denial is for patient to see the relationship between substance use and personal problems. To confront issues with a caring attitude preserves self-esteem.* Do not allow patient to rationalize or blame others for behaviors associated with substance use. *This only serves to prolong the denial.*
Ineffective individual coping related to inadequate coping skills and weak ego evidenced by use of substances as coping mechanism	Patient will be able to verbalize adaptive coping mechanisms to use, instead of substance abuse, in response to stress.	Set limits on manipulative behavior. Administer consequences when limits are violated. Obtain routine urine samples for laboratory analysis of substances. *Because of weak ego and delayed development, patient is unable to establish own limits or delay gratification. Patient may obtain substances from various sources while in the hospital.* Explore options available to assist with stress rather than resorting to substance use (see Table 17.8). Practice these techniques. *Because gratification has been closely tied to oral needs, it is unlikely that patient is aware of more adaptive coping strategies.* Give positive reinforcement for ability to delay gratification and respond to stress with adaptive coping strategies. *Because of weak ego, patient needs lots of positive feedback to enhance self-esteem and enhance ego development.*

(continued)

Table 17.7 CONTINUED

Nursing Diagnoses	Objectives	Nursing Interventions
Altered nutrition: Less than body requirements/Fluid volume deficit related to use of substances instead of eating evidenced by loss of weight, pale conjunctiva and mucous membranes, poor skin turgor, electrolyte imbalance, anemias (and/or other signs and symptoms of malnutrition/dehydration)	Patient will be free of signs/ symptoms of malnutrition/dehydration.	Parenteral support may be required initially *to correct fluid and electrolyte imbalance, hypoglycemia, and some vitamin deficiencies.* Encourage cessation of smoking *in an effort to repair gastrointestinal damage.* Consult dietition. Determine the number of calories required based on body size and level of activity. Document intake and output and calorie count and weigh patient daily *to maintain ongoing nutritional assessment.* Ensure that amount of protein in diet is correct for individual patient condition. Protein intake should be adequate to maintain nitrogen equilibrium but should be drastically decreased or eliminated if there is potential for hepatic coma. *Diseased liver may be incapable of properly metabolizing proteins, resulting in an accumulation of ammonia in the blood that circulates to the brain and can result in altered consciousness.* Sodium may need to be restricted *if fluid retention (e.g., ascites and edema) is a problem.* Provide foods that are nonirritating to patients with esophageal varices, *to avoid irritation and bleeding of these swollen blood vessels.* Provide small frequent feeding of patient's favorite foods. Supplement nutritious meals with multiple vitamin and mineral tablet.

tions have been effective in achieving the intended goals of care. Evaluation of the patient with substance use disorder may be accomplished by using information gathered from the following reassessment questions.

Has detoxification occurred without complications? Is patient still in denial? Does he or she accept responsibility for own behavior? Has patient acknowledged a personal problem with substances? Has a correlation been made between personal problems and the use of substances? Does patient still make excuses or blame others for use of substances? Has patient remained substance-free during hospitalization? Does patient cooperate with treatment? Does patient refrain from manipulative behavior and violation of limits? Is patient able to verbalize alternative adaptive coping strategies to substitute for substance use? Has the use of these strategies been demonstrated? Does positive reinforcement encourage repetition of these adaptive behaviors? Has nutritional status been restored? Does patient consume diet adequate for size and level of activity? Is patient able to discuss importance of adequate nutrition? Has patient remained free of infection during hospitalization? Is patient able to verbalize the effects of substance abuse on the body? Does patient verbalize that he or she *wants* to recover and lead a life free of substances?

THE IMPAIRED NURSE

Substance abuse/dependency is a problem that has the potential for impairment in an individual's social, occupational, psychologic, or physical functioning. This becomes an especially serious problem when the impaired person is responsible for the lives of others on a daily basis. Approximately 40,000 alcoholic nurses work in the United States, and narcotic addiction among nurses is 30 to 100 times greater than it is in the general population (Jefferson & Ensor, 1982). A survey of 44 state boards of nursing revealed that 67 percent of cases handled by the boards were related to substance abuse (Sullivan, Bissell, & Williams, 1988).

Table 17.8 MOTIVES FOR, AND ALTERNATIVES TO, THE USE OF DRUGS

Level of Experience	Examples of Motives for Taking Drugs	Examples of Possible Alternatives to Taking Drugs
Physical	Desire for physical satisfaction; physical relaxation; relief from sickness; desire for more energy; maintenance of physical dependency	Athletics; dance; exercise; hiking; diet; health training; carpentry or outdoor work.
Sensory	Desire to stimulate sight, sound, touch, taste; need for sensual-sexual stimulation; desire to magnify sensorium	Sensory awareness training; sky diving; experiencing sensory beauty of nature; lovemaking; swimming; running; mountaineering
Emotional	Relief from psychological pain; attempt to solve personal perplexities; relief from bad mood; escape from anxiety; desire for emotional insight; liberation of feeling; emotional relaxation	Individual counseling; group therapy; instruction in psychology of personal development; sensitivity training
Interpersonal	To gain peer acceptance; to break through interpersonal barriers; to "communicate," especially nonverbally; defiance of authority figures; cement two-person relationships; relaxation of interpersonal inhibition; solve interpersonal hangups	Sensitivity and encounter groups; group therapy; instruction in social customs; confidence training; social-interpersonal counseling; emphasis on assisting others in distress via education
Social/Cultural/ Environmental	To promote social change; find identifiable subculture; tune out intolerable environmental conditions (e.g., poverty); change awareness of the masses	Social service; community action in positive social change; helping the poor, aged, infirm, young; tutoring handicapped; ecology action
Political	To promote political change; identify with antiestablishment subgroup; to change drug legislation; out of desperation with the social-political order; to gain wealth, affluence, or power	Political service; political action; nonpartisan projects such as ecological lobbying; field work with politicians and public officials
Intellectual	To escape mental boredom; out of intellectual curiosity; to solve cognitive problems; to gain new understanding in the world of ideas; to study better; to research one's own awareness; for science	Intellectual excitement through reading; or through discussion; creative games and puzzles; self-hypnosis; training in concentration; synectics—training in intellectual breakthroughs; memory training
Creative/Aesthetic	To improve creativity in the arts; to enhance enjoyment of art already produced (e.g., music); to enjoy imaginative mental productions	Nongraded instruction in producing and/or appreciating art, music, drama, crafts, handiwork, cooking, sewing, gardening, writing, singing, and so forth.
Philosophical	To discover meaningful values; to grasp the nature of the universe; to find meaning in life; to help establish personal identity; to organize a belief structure	Discussions, seminars, courses in the meaning of life; study of ethics, morality, the nature of reality; relevant philosophical literature; guided exploration of value systems
Spiritual/Mystical	To transcend orthodox religion; to develop spiritual insights; to reach higher levels of consciousness; to have divine visions; to communicate with God; to augment yogic practices; to get a spiritual shortcut; to attain enlightenment; to attain spiritual powers	Exposure to nonchemical methods of spiritual development; study of world religions; introduction to applied mysticism, meditation; yogic techniques
Miscellaneous	Adventure, risk, drama, "kicks," unexpressed motives; prodrug general attitudes	"Outward Bound" survival training; combinations of alternatives above; pronaturalness attitudes; brainwave training; meaningful employment

Sources: Cohen (1972) and Julien (1981).

For years, the impaired nurse was protected, promoted, transferred, ignored, or fired. These types of responses promoted the growth of the problem. A humane system of intervention and treatment is necessary to redeem the future for the chemically dependent nurse, while significantly reducing cost and risk for health-care employers (Sullivan et al, 1988).

How does one identify the impaired nurse? It is still easiest to overlook what "might" be a problem. Denial, on the part of the impaired nurse as well as nurse colleagues, is still the strongest defense for dealing with substance abuse problems. Some states have mandatory reporting laws that require observers to report substance-abusing nurses to the board of nursing (Sullivan et al, 1988). They are difficult laws to enforce, and hospitals are not always compliant with mandatory reporting. Some hospitals may choose not to report to the state board of nursing if the impaired nurse is actively seeking treatment and if the nurse is not placing patients in danger.

Murphy and Violette (1985) have identified some clues for identifying substance impairment in nurses. They are not easy to detect and will vary according to the substance being used. The impaired nurse may appear happy or sad, may have an increased appetite or no appetite at all. He or she may be verbal and energetic, or slow thinking with impaired concentration. This nurse may volunteer to work additional shifts and have an excellent work attendance record (since work is the source of substance supply). However, the impaired nurse may leave the floor a lot or spend a great deal of time in the restroom. When an impaired nurse is on duty, there may be more accidents, more incidents reported, and more patients who complain of unrelieved pain and insomnia, even though many narcotic analgesics and sedatives have been documented as administered. As the impairment progresses, clues may be reflected by inaccurate drug counts, increased vial breakage and drug wastage, and discrepancies in documentation. Lapses in memory may occur, and personal appearance and job performance will likely be affected.

If suspicious behavior occurs, it is important to keep careful, objective records. Confrontation with the impaired nurse will undoubtedly result in hostility and denial. Confrontation should occur in the presence of a supervisor or other nurse and should include the offer of assistance in seeking treatment. If a report is made to the state board of nursing, it should be a factual documentation of specific events and actions, not a diagnostic statement of impairment.

What will the state board do? Sullivan et al (1988) identify three ways in which a state board may respond to a nurse's impaired practice.

1. They may refuse to restore or grant a license.
2. They may rely on a host of experts to testify about whether the nurse's addiction poses a hazard, thus providing some degree of assurance of patient safety as well as someone with whom to share the responsibility if the nurse fails.
3. They may institute or cooperate with a strict and thorough monitoring system designed to discover relapse. Strict monitoring is expensive and intrusive, but it can reduce the public's risk to an acceptable level.

Several state boards of nursing have passed diversionary laws that allow impaired nurses to avoid disciplinary action by agreeing to seek treatment. Some of these state boards administer the treatment programs themselves, while others refer to community resources or state nurses' association assistance programs.

In 1982, the American Nurses' Association House of Delegates adopted a national resolution to provide assistance to impaired nurses. Since that time, approximately 33 state nurses' associations have developed (or are developing) programs for nurses who are impaired by substances or psychiatric illness (Kirkwood, 1985). The individuals who administer these efforts are nurse members of the state associations, as well as nurses who are in recovery themselves. For this reason, they are called peer assistance programs.

The peer assistance programs strive to intervene early, to reduce hazards to patients, and to increase prospects for the nurse's recovery. Most states either provide a hot-line number that the impaired nurse or intervening colleague may call or phone numbers of peer assistance committee members, which are made available for the same purpose. Typically, a contract is drawn up detailing the method of treatment, which may be obtained from various sources, such as employee assistance programs, Alcoholics Anonymous, Narcotics Anonymous, private counseling, or outpatient clinics. Guidelines for monitoring the course of treatment are established. Peer support is provided through regular contact with the impaired nurse, usually for a period of 2 years. Peer assistance programs serve to assist impaired nurses to recognize their impairment, to obtain necessary treatment, and to regain accountability within their profession.

CO-DEPENDENCY

Co-dependence is a term that has been given much attention in the last 10 years. The concept arose out of a need to define the dysfunctional behaviors that are evident among members of the family of a chemically dependent person. The term has been expanded to include all individuals from families that harbor secrets of physical or emotional abuse, other cruelties or pathological conditions—families that admonish their members, "Don't talk, don't trust, don't feel" (Black, 1982). This inability to relate results in unmet needs for autonomy and self-esteem, and a profound sense of powerlessness. The co-dependent person is able to achieve a sense of control only through fulfilling the needs of others. Cermak (1986) has stated, "Power through sacrifice of self lies at the core of co-dependence."

A number of authors have proposed various definitions for co-dependence. Examples include the following:

"An exaggerated dependent pattern of learned behaviors, beliefs, and feelings that make life painful. It is a dependence on people and things outside the self, along with neglect of the self to the point of having little self-identity." (Smalley, 1984)

"A dysfunctional pattern of living learned from our family of origin as well as our culture, producing arrested identity development and resulting in an overreaction to things outside of us and an underreaction to things inside of us. Left untreated, it can deteriorate into an addiction." (Friel & Friel, 1988)

"A recognizable pattern of personality traits, predictably found within most members of chemically dependent families, which are capable of creating sufficient dysfunction to warrant the diagnosis of Mixed Personality Disorder as outlined in *DSM-III*." (Cermak, 1986)

The traits associated with co-dependent personality are widespread. The *DSM-III-R* (APA, 1987) states that personality traits only become disorders when they are "inflexible and maladaptive and cause either significant impairment in social or occupational functioning or significant subjective distress." To date, no diagnostic criteria exist for the diagnosis of co-dependent personality disorder. Cermak (1986) has proposed the following criteria in the style of *DSM-III*:

A. Continued investment of self-esteem in the ability to control both oneself and others in the face of serious adverse consequences.
B. Assumption of responsibility for meeting others' needs to the exclusion of acknowledging one's own.
C. Anxiety and boundary distortions around intimacy and separation.
D. Enmeshment in relationships with personality disordered, chemically dependent, other co-dependent, or impulse disordered individuals.
E. Three or more of the following:
   1. Excessive reliance on denial
   2. Constriction of emotions (with or without dramatic outbursts)
   3. Depression
   4. Hypervigilance
   5. Compulsions
   6. Anxiety
   7. Substance abuse
   8. Has been (or is) the victim of recurrent physical, [emotional], or sexual abuse
   9. Stress-related medical illnesses
   10. Has remained in a primary relationship with an active substance abuser [or individual with other pathological condition] for at least 2 years without seeking outside help.
   (NOTE: Bracketed items added by author.)

An individual who is co-dependent is confused about his or her own identity. In a relationship, the co-dependent person derives self-worth from that of the partner, whose feelings and behaviors determine how the co-dependent should feel and behave. For the co-dependent to feel good, his or her partner must be happy and behave in appropriate ways. If the partner is not happy, the co-dependent feels responsible for *making* him or her happy (Cermak, 1986). The co-dependent's home life is fraught with stress. Ego boundaries are weak, and behaviors are often enmeshed with those of the pathological partner. Denial that problems exist is common. Feelings are kept in control, and anxiety may be released in the form of stress-related illnesses or compulsive behaviors, such as eating, spending, working, or use of substances.

The Co-Dependent Nurse

Hall and Wray (1989) have identified certain characteristics associated with co-dependency that they apply to nursing. A shortage of nurses combined with the increasing ranks of seriously ill patients may result in nurses providing care and fulfilling everyone's needs but their own. Also, a disproportionate percentage of mental health workers come from chemically dependent homes or backgrounds, which puts them at risk for having any unresolved co-dependent tendencies activated (Cermak, 1986). Hall and Wray identify the following classic characteristics of the co-dependent nurse:

1. *Caretaking.* This occurs when nurses attempt to meet others' needs to the point of neglecting their own. They are attracted to people who need them, yet resent receiving so little in return. Their emotional needs go unmet, yet they continue to deny that these needs exist.
2. *Perfectionism.* Low self-esteem and fear of failure drive co-dependent nurses to strive for an unrealistic level of achievement. They are highly critical of self and others. They reject praise from others and achieve personal satisfaction only out of feeling needed.
3. *Denial.* Co-dependent nurses refuse to acknowledge that any personal problems or painful issues exist. This is often facilitated through use of compulsive behaviors, such as work or spending, or addictions, such as food or substances.
4. *Poor communication.* Co-dependent nurses rarely express their true feelings. Their interactive style often reflects a tendency to say and do what they believe others want, to preserve harmony and maintain control.

Treating Co-Dependence

Cermak (1986) has identified four stages in the recovery process for individuals with co-dependent personality. They include:

Stage I: The survival stage. In this first stage, co-dependent persons must begin to let go of the denial that problems exist or that their personal capabilities are unlimited. This initiation of abstinence from blanket denial may be a very emotional and painful period.

Stage II: The re-identification stage. Re-identification occurs when the individuals are able to glimpse their true selves through a break in the denial system. They accept the label of co-dependent and take responsibility for their own dysfunctional behavior. Co-dependents tend to enter re-identification only after being convinced that it is more painful not to. They accept their limitations and are ready to face the issues of co-dependence.

Stage III: The core issues stage. In this stage, the recovering co-dependent must face the fact that relationships cannot be managed by force of will. Each partner must be independent and autonomous. The goal of this stage is to detach from the struggles of life that exist due to prideful and willful efforts to control those things that are beyond the individual's power to control.

Stage IV: The re-integration stage. This is a stage of self-acceptance and willingness to change. They relinquish the power *over others* that was not rightfully theirs, but they reclaim the *personal* power that they do possess. Integrity is achieved out of awareness, honesty, and being in touch with one's spiritual consciousness. Control is achieved through self-discipline and self-confidence.

TREATMENT MODALITIES FOR SUBSTANCE USE DISORDERS

Alcoholics Anonymous

Alcoholics Anonymous (AA) is a major self-help organization for the treatment of alcoholism. It was founded in 1935 by a stockbroker named Bill Wilson and a physician, Dr. Bob Smith, both alcoholics, who discovered that they could remain sober through mutual support. This they accomplished not as professionals, but as peers who were able to share their common experiences. Soon they were working with other alcoholics, who in turn worked with others. The movement grew, and remarkably, individuals who had been treated unsuccessfully by professionals were able to maintain sobriety through helping one another (Curlee-Salisbury, 1986).

Today there are AA chapters in virtually every community in the United States. The self-help groups are based on the concept of peer support — acceptance and understanding from others who have experienced the same problems in their lives. The only requirement for membership is a desire on the part of the alcoholic person to stop drinking (Estes et al, 1980). Each new member is assigned a support person from whom he or she may seek assistance when the temptation to drink occurs.

According to the most recent survey by the General Service Office of Alcoholics Anonymous in 1989 (AA, 1990), changing trends in the membership are becoming apparent. The numbers of female and younger (30 and below) members are increasing, as are the numbers of members addicted to more than one substance. Female membership has grown from 22 percent in 1968 to 35 percent in 1989. Members 30 years old and younger, who comprised 7 percent of the membership in 1968, now make up 22 percent. The 1989 survey reported that 46 percent of the membership now claim addiction to at least one other drug besides alcohol.

The sole purpose of AA is to help members stay sober. When sobriety has been achieved, they in turn are expected to help other alcoholic persons. The "Twelve Steps" that embody the philosophy of AA provide specific guidelines on how to attain and maintain sobriety. These "Twelve Steps" are presented in Table 17.9.

Alcoholics Anonymous accepts alcoholism as an illness and promotes total abstinence as the only cure, emphasizing that the alcoholic person can never safely return to social drinking. They encourage the members to seek sobriety, taking one day at a time. The "Twelve Traditions," which are statements of principles that govern the organization, are presented in Table 17.10.

Alcoholics Anonymous has been the model for various other self-help groups associated with abuse/dependency problems. Some of these groups and the memberships for which they are organized are listed in Table 17.11. Nurses need to be fully and accurately informed about available self-help groups as an important and necessary treatment resource on the health-care continuum so that they can use them as a referral source for pa-

Table 17.9 THE TWELVE STEPS OF ALCOHOLICS ANONYMOUS

1. We admitted we were powerless over alcohol—that our lives have become unmanageable.
2. Came to believe that a Power greater than ourselves could restore us to sanity.
3. Made a decision to turn our will and our lives over to the care of God as we understood Him.
4. Made a searching and fearless moral inventory of ourselves.
5. Admitted to God, to ourselves, and to another human being the exact nature of our wrongs.
6. Were entirely ready to have God remove all these defects of character.
7. Humbly asked Him to remove our shortcomings.
8. Made a list of all persons we had harmed and became willing to make amends to them all.
9. Made direct amends to such people whenever possible except when to do so would injure them or others.
10. Continued to take personal inventory and when we were wrong promptly admitted it.
11. Sought through prayer and meditation to improve our conscious contact with God as we understood Him, praying only for knowledge of His will for us and the power to carry that out.
12. Having a spiritual awakening as the result of these steps, we tried to carry this message to alcoholics and to practice these principles in all our affairs.

Source: From Alcoholics Anonymous (1953).

tients with substance use disorders (Estes et al., 1980).

Alcohol Deterrent Therapy

Disulfiram (Antabuse) is a drug that can be administered to individuals who abuse alcohol as a deterrent to drinking. Ingestion of alcohol while disulfiram is in the body results in a syndrome of symptoms that can produce a good deal of discomfort for the individual. It can even result in death if the blood alcohol level is high. The reaction varies according to the sensitivity of the individual and how much alcohol was ingested.

Antabuse works by inhibiting the enzyme aldehyde dehydrogenase, thereby blocking the oxidation of alcohol at the stage that acetaldehyde is converted to acetate. This results in an accumulation of acetaldehyde in the blood, which is thought

Table 17.10 THE TWELVE TRADITIONS OF ALCOHOLICS ANONYMOUS

1. Our common welfare should come first; personal recovery depends upon AA unity.

2. For our group purpose there is but one ultimate authority—a loving God as He may express Himself in our group conscience. Our leaders are but trusted servants; they do not govern.

3. The one requirement for AA membership is a desire to stop drinking.

4. Each group should be autonomous except in matters affecting other groups or AA as a whole.

5. Each group has but one primary purpose—to carry its message to the alcoholic who still suffers.

6. An AA group ought never endorse, finance, or lend the AA name to any related facility or outside enterprise, lest problems of money, property, and prestige divert us from our primary purpose.

7. Every AA group ought to be fully self-supporting, declining outside contributions.

8. Alcoholics Anonymous should remain forever nonprofessional, but our service centers may employ special workers.

9. Alcoholics Anonymous, as such, ought never be organized; but we may create service boards of committees directly responsible to those they serve.

10. Alcoholics Anonymous has no opinion on outside issues; hence, the Alcoholics Anonymous name ought never be drawn into public controversy.

11. Our public relations policy is based on attraction rather than promotion; we need always maintain personal anonymity at the level of press, radio, and films.

12. Anonymity is the spiritual foundation of all our traditions, ever reminding us to place principles before personalities.

Source: From Alcoholics Anonymous (1953).

Table 17.11 ADDICTION SELF-HELP GROUPS

Group	Membership
Adult Children of Alcoholics	Adults who grew up with an alcoholic in the home
Al-Anon	Families of alcoholics
Alateen	Adolescent children of alcoholics
Children Are People	School-age children with an alcoholic family member
Cocaine Anonymous	Cocaine addicts
Families Anonymous	Parents of children who abuse substances
Fresh Start	Nicotine addicts
Narcotics Anonymous	Narcotics addicts
Nar-Anon	Families of narcotics addicts
Overeaters Anonymous	Food addicts
Pills Anonymous	Polysubstance addicts
Potsmokers Anonymous	Marijuana smokers
Smokers Anonymous	Nicotine addicts
Women for Sobriety	Female alcoholics

to produce the symptoms associated with the disulfiram-alcohol reaction. These symptoms persist as long as alcohol is being metabolized. The rate of alcohol elimination does not appear to be affected (Townsend, 1990).

Symptoms of disulfiram-alcohol reaction can occur within 5 to 10 minutes of ingestion of alcohol. Mild reactions can occur at blood alcohol levels as low as 5 to 10 mg/dl. Symptoms are fully developed at approximately 50 mg/dl, and may include flushed skin, throbbing in the head and neck, respiratory difficulty, dizziness, nausea and vomiting, sweating, hyperventilation, tachycardia, hypoten-

sion, weakness, blurred vision, and confusion. With a blood alcohol level of approximately 125 to 150 mg/dl, severe reactions can occur, including respiratory depression, cardiovascular collapse, arrhythmias, myocardial infarction, acute congestive heart failure, unconsciousness, convulsions, and death.

Disulfiram should not be administered until it has been ascertained that the patient has abstained from alcohol for at least 12 hours. If disulfiram is discontinued, it is important for the patient to understand that the sensitivity to alcohol may last for as long as 2 weeks. Consuming alcohol or alcohol-containing substances during this 2-week period could result in the disulfiram-alcohol syndrome of symptoms.

The patient on disulfiram therapy should be aware of the great number of alcohol-containing substances. These products, such as liquid cough and cold preparations, vanilla extract, aftershave lotions, colognes, mouthwash, nail polish removers, and isopropyl alcohol, if ingested or even rubbed on the skin, are capable of producing the syndrome of symptoms described. The individual must read labels carefully, and must inform any doctor, dentist, or other health-care professional from whom assistance is sought that he or she is taking disulfiram. In addition, it is important that the patient carry a card explaining participation in disulfiram therapy, possible consequences of the therapy, and symptoms that may indicate an emergency situation.

Obviously, the patient must be assessed carefully before beginning disulfiram therapy. A thorough medical screening is performed prior to initiation of therapy. Written informed consent is generally required. The drug is contraindicated for patients who are at high risk for alcohol ingestion. It is also contraindicated for psychotic patients and patients with severe cardiac, renal, or hepatic disease.

Disulfiram therapy is not a cure for alcoholism. It provides a measure of control for the individual who desires to avoid impulse drinking. Patients on disulfiram therapy are encouraged to seek other assistance with their problem, such as AA or other support group, to aid in the recovery process.

Other Treatment Modalities

COUNSELING

Counseling on a one-to-one basis is often used to help the substance-abusing patient. The relationship is goal-directed, and the length of the counseling may vary from weeks to years. The focus is on current reality, active development of a working treatment relationship, environmental manipulation, and strengthening ego assets (Estes et al, 1980). The counselor must be warm, kind, and nonjudgmental, yet able to set limits firmly.

Weinberg (1986) identifies the following stages in the counseling relationship:

Stage I: Assessment. In this stage, factual data are collected to determine that the patient does indeed have a problem with substances; that is, substances are regularly impairing effective functioning in a significant life area.

Stage II: Problem recognition and acceptance. In this stage, the person accepts that the use of substances causes problems in significant life areas and that he or she is not able to prevent it from occurring. The patient states a desire to make changes. During this stage, the denial

defense must be eliminated. The strength of the denial system is determined by the duration and extent of substance-related adverse effects in the person's life. Thus, those individuals with rather minor substance-related problems of recent origin have less difficulty with this stage than those with long-term extensive impairment. Also in Stage II, the individual works to gain self-control and abstain from substances.

Stage III: Sobriety and beyond. The question that is discussed in this stage of counseling is: During the times that you usually used substances, what will you do now instead? The patient must have a concrete and workable plan for getting through the early weeks of abstinence. Anticipatory guidance through role play helps the individual practice how he or she will respond when substances are readily obtainable and the impulse to partake is strong.

Counseling will often include the family or specific family members. In family counseling, the therapist tries to help each member see how he or she has affected, and been affected by, the substance abuse behavior. Family strengths are mobilized, and they are encouraged to move in a positive direction. Referrals are often made to self-help groups, such as Al-Anon, Nar-Anon, Alateen, Families Anonymous, and Adult Children of Alcoholics.

GROUP THERAPY

Group therapy with substance abusers has long been regarded as a powerful agent of change. Vannicelli (1986) identifies three unique opportunities that group work can provide for substance abusers:

1. To share and to identify with others who are going through similar problems
2. To understand their own attitudes about substance use and their defenses about giving up the substance by confronting similar attitudes and defenses in others
3. To learn to communicate needs and feelings more directly.

Some groups may be task-oriented education groups in which the leader is charged with presenting material associated with substance abuse and its various effects on the person's life. Other educational groups that may be helpful with individuals who abuse substances include assertiveness techniques and relaxation training. Teaching groups differ from psychotherapy groups, whose focus is more on helping individuals understand and manage difficult feelings and situations and gain understanding about where they fit in with the difficulties they experience (Vannicelli, 1986).

Therapy groups and self-help groups such as AA are complementary to each other. While the self-help group focus is on achieving and maintaining sobriety, in the therapy group the individual may learn more adaptive ways of coping, how to deal with problems that may have arisen or were exacerbated by the former substance use, and ways to improve quality of life and to function more effectively without substances.

SUMMARY

An individual is considered to be dependent on a substance when he or she is unable to control its use, even knowing that it interferes with normal functioning; when more and more of the substance is required to produce the desired effects; and when characteristic withdrawal symptoms develop upon cessation or drastic decrease in use of the substance. Abuse is considered when there is continued use of the substance despite having a persistent or recurrent problem that is caused or exacerbated by use of the substance, or when the substance is used in physically hazardous situations.

The etiology of substance use disorders is unknown. Various contributing factors have been implicated, such as genetics, biochemical changes, developmental influences, personality factors, social learning, conditioning, and cultural and ethnic influences.

Six classes of substances are presented in terms of a profile of the substance, historical aspects, patterns of use and abuse, and effects on the body. These six classes include alcohol, other CNS depressants, CNS stimulants, opioids, hallucinogens, and cannabinols.

The nursing process is presented as the vehicle for delivery of care of the patient with substance use disorder. The nurse must first examine his or her own feelings regarding substance use, both personally and by others. Only the nurse who can be accepting and nonjudgmental of substance abuse behaviors will be effective in working with these patients.

Substance abuse by members of the nursing profession is discussed. Many state boards of nursing and state nurses' associations have established avenues for peer assistance to provide help to impaired members of the profession.

Individuals who are reared in families with chemically dependent persons learn patterns of dysfunctional behavior that carry over into adult life. These dysfunctional behavior patterns have been termed *co-dependency*. Co-dependent persons sacrifice their own needs for the fulfillment of others' to achieve a sense of control. Many nurses also have co-dependent traits.

Treatment modalities for substance use disorders include self-help groups, deterrent therapy, individual counseling, and group therapy. Treatment modalities are implemented on an inpatient basis or in outpatient settings, depending on the severity of the impairment.

REVIEW QUESTIONS
Self-Examination/Learning Exercise

*Select the answer that is **most** appropriate for each of the following questions.*

Dan, age 32, has been admitted for inpatient treatment of his alcoholism. He began drinking when he was 15 years old. Through the years, the amount of alcohol he consumes has increased. He and his wife report that for the last 5 years he has consumed at least a pint of bourbon a day. He also drinks beer and wine. He has been sneaking drinks at work, and his effectiveness has started to decline. His boss has told him he must seek treatment or be fired. This is his second week in treatment. The first week he experienced an uncomplicated detoxification.

1. Dan states, "I don't have a problem with alcohol. I can handle my booze better than anyone I know. My boss is a jerk! I haven't missed any more days than my co-workers." The nurse's best response is:
   a. "Maybe your boss is mistaken, Dan."
   b. "You are here because your drinking was interfering with your work, Dan."
   c. "Get real, Dan! You're a boozer and you know it!"
   d. "Why do you think your boss sent you here, Dan?"

2. The defense mechanism that Dan is using is:
   a. Denial
   b. Projection
   c. Displacement
   d. Rationalization

3. Dan's drinking buddies come for a visit, and when they leave, the nurse smells alcohol on Dan's breath. Which of the following would be the best intervention with Dan at this time?
   a. Search his room for evidence.
   b. Ask, "Have you been drinking alcohol, Dan?"
   c. Send a urine specimen from Dan to the laboratory for drug screening.
   d. Tell Dan, "These guys cannot come to the unit to visit you again."

4. Dan's wife is afraid that he will lose his job. She says, "It's all my fault. If I were a better wife, he wouldn't drink so much. If I had just kept him home from work that day and called in sick for him, maybe this wouldn't have happened." The nurses *best* response is:
   a. "Why didn't you call for him?"
   b. "You've done too much already, Mrs. Smith."
   c. "Dan has to suffer the consequences of his own behavior, Mrs. Smith."
   d. "Why do you say it's all your fault?"

5. Dan begins attendance at AA meetings. Which of the statements by Dan reflects the purpose of this organization?
   a. "They claim they will help me stay sober."
   b. "I'll dry out in AA, then I can have a social drink now and then."
   c. "AA is only for people who have reached the bottom."
   d. "If I lose my job, AA will help me find another."

6. To become a member of AA, Dan must *first*
   a. Resolve to abstain from alcohol and help others do so.
   b. Admit he is powerless over alcohol and that he needs help.
   c. Make amends to the people he has harmed while under the influence of alcohol.
   d. Ask God to help him overcome his shortcomings.

The following general questions relate to substance abuse.

7. From which of the following symptoms might the nurse identify a chronic cocaine user?
   a. Clear, constricted pupils
   b. Red, irritated nostrils
   c. Muscle aches
   d. Conjunctival redness

8. A patient who is addicted to heroin is likely to experience which of the following symptoms of withdrawal?
   a. Increased heart rate and blood pressure
   b. Tremors, insomnia, and seizures
   c. Incoordination and unsteady gait
   d. Nausea/vomiting, diarrhea, and diaphoresis

9. A polysubstance abuser makes the statement, "The green and whites do me good after speed." How might the nurse interpret the statement?
   a. The patient abuses amphetamines and sedative/hypnotics.
   b. The patient abuses alcohol and cocaine.
   c. The patient is psychotic.
   d. The patient abuses narcotics and marijuana.

10. With an overdose of barbiturates, death would *most likely* occur from:
   a. Kidney failure
   b. Cardiac arrest
   c. Respiratory depression
   d. Cerebral hemorrhage

REFERENCES

Ahlstrom-Laakso, S. (1976). European drinking habits. In Everett et al. (Eds.), *Cross-cultural approaches to the study of alcohol.* The Hague: Mouton.

Alcoholics Anonymous. (1953). *Twelve steps and twelve traditions.* New York: Alcoholics Anonymous World Services, Inc.

Alcoholics Anonymous. (1990). *Analysis of the 1989 survey of the membership of AA.* New York: Alcoholics Anonymous World Services, Inc.

American Psychiatric Association. (1987). Diagnostic and statistical manual of mental disorders, (3rd ed., rev.) Washington, DC: American Psychiatric Association.

Baker, J. M. (1982). Alcoholism and the American Indian. In N. J. Estes and M. E. Heineman (Eds), *Alcoholism: development, consequences, and interventions* (ed. 2). St. Louis: CV Mosby.

Barnes, G. E. (1980). Characteristics of the clinical alcoholic personality. *Journal of Studies on Alcohol, 41,* pp. 894–910.

Bennett, E. G. & Woolf, D. (1991). *Substance abuse: Pharmacologic, developmental, and clinical perspectives* (ed 2.). Albany, NY: Delmar Publishers, Inc.

Black, C. (1982). *It will never happen to me.* Denver: M.A.C., Printing and Publications Division.

Blum, K. (1984). *Handbook of abusable drugs.* New York: Gardner Press, Inc.

Bratter, T. E. & Forrest G. G. (1985). *Alcoholism and substance abuse.* New York: The Free Press.

Byers, V. L. (1991). Central nervous system stimulants. In M. M. Kuhn (Ed.), *Pharmacotherapeutics: A nursing process approach* (ed 2.). Philadelphia: FA Davis Company.

Cermak, T. L. (1986). *Diagnosing and treating co-dependence.* Minneapolis: Johnson Institute Books.

Chambers, C. D. et al. (1972). Barbiturate use, misuse and abuse. *J Drug Issues, 2,* p. 15.

Cohen, A. Y. (1972). The journey beyond trips: Alternative to drugs. In Smith, D. E. & G. R. Gay (Eds.), *It's so good, don't even try it once: Heroin in perspective.* Englewood Cliffs, NJ: Prentice-Hall.

Cosper, R. (1979). Drinking as conformity; A critique of the sociological literature on occupational differences in drinking. *Journal of Studies on Alcohol, 40,* pp. 868–891.

Curlee-Salisbury, J. (1986). Perspectives on Alcoholics Anonymous. In N. J. Estes & M. E. Heinemann, (Eds.), *Alcoholism: Development, consequences, and interventions* (ed 3.). St. Louis: CV Mosby.

Department of Health, Education, and Welfare. (1988). *Nicotine addiction.* Washington, DC: US Government Printing Office.

Drug Enforcement Administration. (1979). *Drugs of abuse.* Washington, DC: US Department of Justice.

Estes, N. J. & Heinemann, M. E. (1986). *Alcoholism: Development, consequences, and interventions* (ed 3.). St. Louis: CV Mosby.

Estes, N. J., Smith-DiJulio, K., & Heinemann, M. E. (1980). *Nursing diagnosis of the alcoholic person.* St. Louis: CV Mosby.

Freud, S. (1959). *Collected papers of Sigmund Freud.* J. Ernest (Ed.), New York: Basic Books.

Friel, J. & Friel, L. (1988). *Adult children: Secrets of dysfunctional families.* Deerfield Beach, FL: Health Communications, Inc.

Goodwin, D. W., Schulinger, F., Hermansen, L., Guze, S. B. and Winoker, G. (1973). Alcohol problems in adoptees raised apart from alcoholic biological parents. *Arch Gen Psychiatry, 28,* pp. 238–243.

Hall, S. F. & Wray, L. M. (1989, November). Codependency: Nurses who give too much. *AJN, 89*(11), pp. 1456–1460.

Harvey, S. C. (1975). Hypnotics and sedatives: The barbiturates. In L. S. Goodman and A. G. Gilman (Eds.), *The pharmacological basis of therapeutics.* New York: Macmillan.

Holbrook, J. M. (1991). Hallucinogens. In E. G. Bennett & D. Woolf (Eds.), *Substance abuse* (ed. 2). Albany, NY: Delmar Publishers Inc.

House, M. A. (1990, April). Cocaine. *AJN, 90*(4), pp. 41–45.

Jefferson, L. V. & Ensor, B. E. (1982, April). Help for the helper: Confronting a chemically-impaired colleague. *AJN,* pp. 574–577.

Jellinek, E. M. (1952). Phases of alcohol addiction. *QJ Stud Alcohol, 13,* pp. 673–584.

Julien, R. M. (1981). *A primer of drug action* (ed 3.). San Francisco: WH Freeman and Company.

Kaij, L. (1960). *Alcoholism in twins.* Stockholm: Almqvist and Wiksell.

Kaplan, H. I. & Sadock, B. J. (1985). *Modern synopsis of comprehensive textbook of psychiatry* (ed 4.). Baltimore: Williams & Wilkins.

Kauffman, J. E. et al. (1985). The biological basics: Drugs and their effects. In Bratter & Forrest (Eds.), *Alcoholism and substance abuse.* New York: The Free Press.

Keller, M. (1979). A historical overview of alcohol and alcoholism. *Cancer Res, 39,* pp. 2822–2829.

Kirkwood, K. R. (1985, August). Addicted nurses: Clues to the hidden problem. *RN, 48*(8), pp. 16–19.

Leigh, G. (1985). Psychosocial factors in the etiology of substance abuse. In T. E. Bratter & G. G. Forrest (Eds.), *Alcoholism and substance abuse: Strategies for clinical intervention.* New York: The Free Press.

Madden, J. S. (1984). *A guide to alcohol and drug dependence* (ed 2.). Bristol, England: John Wright & Sons Ltd.

Mayfield, D., McLeod, G., and Hall, P. (1974). The CAGE questionnaire: Validation of a new alcoholism screening instrument. *American Journal of Psychiatry, 131:*1121–1123.

McKenry, L. M. & Salerno, E. (1989). *Pharmacology in nursing.* St. Louis: CV Mosby.

Milkman, H. & Frosch, W. (1980). Theory of drug use. In Lettieri et al. (Eds.), *Theories on drug abuse: Selected contemporary perspectives.* Rockville, MD: National Institute on Alcohol Abuse and Alcoholism.

Morganthau, T. (1988, March 28). The drug gang. *Newsweek,* pp. 20–25, 27.

Murphy, S. S. & Violette, R. W. (1985, August). More clues to drug abuse. *RN, 48*(8), pp. 19–21.

National Institute on Alcohol Abuse and Alcoholism (1971). *Alcohol: Some questions and answers.* Washington, DC: US Department of Health, Education, and Welfare.

Pilette, W. L. (1983, August). Caffeine: Psychiatric grounds for concern. *J Psychosoc Nurs, 21*(8), pp. 19–24.

Ray, O. S. (1972). *Drugs, society and human behavior.* St. Louis: CV Mosby.

Schuckit, M. A. (1979). *Drug and alcohol abuse: A clinical guide to diagnosis and treatment.* New York: Plenum Medical Book Company.

Seltzer, M. L. (1971). The Michigan Alcoholism Screening Test: The quest for a new diagnostic instrument. *American Journal of Psychiatry, 127:*1653–1658.

Smalley, S. (1984). Paper presented at the Conference of International Doctors in AA. Minneapolis, MN.

Smith, S. F. Karasik, D. A. and Meyer, B. J. (1984). *Psychiatric and psychosocial nursing.* Los Altos, CA: National Nursing Review, Inc.

Spence, W. R. (1987a). *The medical consequences of alcoholism.* Waco, TX: Health Edco, Inc.

Spence, W. R. (1987b). *Substance abuse identification guide.* Waco, TX: Health Edco, Inc.

Sullivan, E., Bissell, L., & Williams, E. (1988). *Chemical dependency in nursing: The deadly diversion.* Menlo Park, CA: Addison-Wesley.

Townsend, M. C. (1990). *Drug guide for psychiatric nursing.* Philadelphia: FA Davis.

Vannicelli, M. (1986). Group psychotherapy with alcoholics: Special techniques. In N. J. Estes & M. E. Hinemann (Eds.), *Alcoholism: Development, consequences, and interventions* (ed 3.). St. Louis: CV Mosby.

Weinberg, J. R. (1986). Counseling the person with alcohol problems. In N. J. Estes & M. E. Heinemann (Eds.), *Alcoholism: Development, consequences, and interventions* (ed 3.). St. Louis: CV Mosby.

Westermeyer, J. & Baker, J. M. (1986). Alcoholism and the American Indian. In N. J. Estes & M. E.

Heinemann (Eds.), *Alcoholism: Development, consequences, and interventions* (ed. 3.). St. Louis: CV Mosby.

BIBLIOGRAPHY

Brodsley, L. (1982, December). Avoiding a crisis: The assessment, *AJN*, pp. 1865–1871.

Cohn, L. (1982, December). The hidden diagnosis. *AJN*, pp. 1863–1864.

Department of Health, Education, and Welfare. (1979). *Smoking and health.* Washington, DC: US Government Printing Office.

Goodwin, D. W. (1988). *Is alcoholism hereditary?* New York: Ballantine Books.

Heinemann, M. E. & Estes, N. J. (1976, May). Assessing alcoholic patients. *AJN*, *76*(5), pp. 785–789.

Jaffe, S. (1982, April). Help for the helper: First-hand views of recovery. *AJN*, pp. 578–579.

Lehmann, W. X. (1979, December). Marijuana alert: Enemy of youth. *Reader's Digest*, *115*(692), pp. 144–146.

Mann, P. (1979, December). Marijuana alert: Brain and sex damage. *Reader's Digest*, *115*(692), pp. 139–144.

Miller, H. (1990, May). Addiction in a coworker: Getting past the denial. *AJN*, *90*(5), pp. 72–75.

Naegle, M. A. (1983, June). The nurse and the alcoholic: Redefining an historically ambivalent relationship. *J Psychosoc Nurs*, *21*(6), pp. 17–24.

National Council on Alcoholism. (1972, August). Criteria for the diagnosis of alcoholism. *Am J Psychiatry*, *129*(2), pp. 127–185.

Steele, O. M. (1986, January). What happens when you drink too much? *Psychology Today*, *20*(1), pp. 48–52.

Townsend, M. C. (1991). *Nursing diagnoses in psychiatric nursing: A pocket guide for care plan construction* (ed 2.). Philadelphia: FA Davis.

18

SCHIZOPHRENIC, DELUSIONAL, AND RELATED PSYCHOTIC DISORDERS

KEY TERMS

delusions
hallucinations
double-bind communication
catatonia
paranoia
religiosity
magical thinking
associative looseness
neologism
clang association
word salad
circumstantiality
tangentiality
perseveration
illusion
echolalia
echopraxia
autism
waxy flexibility
anhedonia
social skills training
neuroleptic

OBJECTIVES

After reading this chapter, the student will be able to:

1. Discuss the concepts of schizophrenic, delusional, and related psychotic disorders.
2. Identify predisposing factors in the development of these disorders.
3. Describe various types of schizophrenic, delusional, and related psychotic disorders.
4. Identify symptomatology associated with these disorders and use this information in patient assessment.
5. Formulate nursing diagnoses and goals of care for patients with schizophrenic, delusional, and related psychotic disorders.
6. Describe appropriate nursing interventions for behaviors associated with these disorders.
7. Describe relevant criteria for evaluating nursing care of patients with schizophrenic, delusional, and related psychotic disorders.
8. Discuss various modalities relevant to treatment of schizophrenic, delusional, and related psychotic disorders.

INTRODUCTION

The term *schizophrenia* was coined in 1908 by the Swiss psychiatrist Eugen Bleuler. The word was derived from the Greek "skhizo" (split) and "phren" (mind) (Birchwood et al, 1989).

Over the years, much debate has surrounded the concept of schizophrenia. Various definitions of the disorder have evolved, and numerous treatment strategies have been proposed, but none have proven to be uniformly effective or sufficient.

Although the controversy lingers, two general factors appear to be gaining acceptance among clinicians. The first is that schizophrenia is probably not a homogeneous disease entity with a single cause but results from a variable combination of genetic predisposition, biochemical dysfunction, physiologic factors, and psychosocial stress. The second factor is that there is not now and probably never will be a single treatment that cures the disorder. Instead, effective treatment requires a comprehensive, multidisciplinary effort, including pharmacotherapy, living skills and social skills training, rehabilitation, family therapy, and extensive social support (Bellack, 1984).

Of all the mental illnesses responsible for suffering in society, schizophrenia probably causes more lengthy hospitalizations, more chaos in family life, more exorbitant costs to individuals and governments, and more fears than any other. Because it is such an enormous threat to life and happiness and because its causes are an unsolved puzzle, it has been studied more than any other mental disorder (Tsuang, 1982).

This chapter explores various theories of predisposing factors that have been implicated in the development of schizophrenia. Symptomatology associated with different diagnostic categories of the disorder is discussed. Nursing care is presented in the context of the five steps of the nursing process. Various dimensions of medical treatment are explored.

NATURE OF THE DISORDER

Perhaps no psychological disorder is more crippling than schizophrenia. Characteristically, disturbances in thought processes, perception, and affect invariably result in a severe deterioration of social and occupational functioning (Hollandsworth, 1990).

Approximately 1 percent of the population will develop schizophrenia during the course of a lifetime (Birchwood et al, 1989). Societal economic costs are estimated in billions of dollars per year. Symptoms generally appear in late adolescence or early adulthood, although they may occur in middle or late adult life (American Psychiatric Association [APA], 1987). Some studies have indicated that symptoms occur earlier in men than in women. The premorbid personality usually indicates social and sexual maladjustment or schizoid, paranoid, or borderline personality characteristics (Cutting, 1985; APA, 1987).

This premorbid behavior is often a predictor in the pattern of development of schizophrenia, which can be viewed in four phases:

Phase I — The schizoid personality. The *Diagnostic and Statistical Manual of Mental Disorders*, ed. 3. revised (*DSM-III-R*) (APA, 1987) describes these individuals as indifferent to social relationships and having a very limited range of emotional experience and expression. They do not enjoy close relationships and prefer to be "loners." They appear cold and aloof. Not all individuals who demonstrate the characteristics of schizoid personality will progress to schizophrenia. However, most individuals with schizophrenia show evidence of having had these characteristics in the premorbid condition.

Phase II — The prodromal phase. Characteristics of this phase include social withdrawal; impairment in role functioning; behavior that is peculiar or eccentric; neglect of personal hygiene and grooming; blunted or inappropriate affect; disturbances in communication; bizarre ideas; unusual perceptual experiences; and lack of initiative, interests, or energy. The length of this phase is highly variable and may last for many years before deteriorating to the schizophrenic state (APA, 1987).

Phase III — Schizophrenia. In the active phase of the disorder, psychotic symptoms are prominent. Following are the *DSM-III-R* (APA, 1987) diagnostic criteria for schizophrenia:

A. Presence of characteristic psychotic symptoms in the active phase: either (1), (2), or (3) for at least 1 week (unless the symptoms are successfully treated):
   (1) Two of the following:
       (a) Delusions
       (b) Prominent hallucinations (throughout the day for several days or several times a week for several weeks, each hallucinatory experience not being limited to a few brief moments)
       (c) Incoherence or marked loosening of associations
       (d) Catatonic behavior
       (e) Flat or grossly inappropriate affect
   (2) Bizarre delusions (i.e., involving a phenomenon that the person's culture would regard as totally implausible, e.g., thought broadcasting, being controlled by a dead person)
   (3) Prominent hallucinations of a voice with content having no apparent relation to depression or elation, or a voice keeping up a running commentary on the person's behavior or thoughts, or two or more voices conversing with each other.
B. During the course of the disturbance, functioning in such areas as work, social relations, and self-care is markedly below the highest level achieved before onset of the disturbance (or, when the onset is in childhood or adolescence, failure to achieve expected level of social development)
C. Schizoaffective disorder and mood disorder with psychotic features have been ruled out
D. Continuous signs of the disturbance for at least 6 months. The 6-month period must include an active phase (of at least 1 week) during which there were psychotic symptoms. For example, 6

months of prodromal symptoms with 1 week of active psychotic symptoms.

Phase IV—Residual phase. Schizophrenia is characterized by periods of remission and exacerbation. A residual phase usually follows an active phase of the illness. Symptoms during the residual phase are similar to those of the prodromal phase, with flat affect and impairment in role functioning being prominent. Residual impairment often increases between episodes of active psychosis.

A return to full premorbid functioning is not common (APA, 1987). However, several factors have been associated with a positive prognosis. They include absence of premorbid personality disturbance or impairment in social functioning, abrupt onset of symptoms precipitated by a stressful event (as opposed to gradual insidious onset of symptoms), and onset in midlife.

PREDISPOSING FACTORS

The cause of schizophrenia is still uncertain. Most likely no single factor can be implicated in the etiology, rather the disease results from a combination of influences including genetics, biochemical dysfunction, physiological, psychological, and environmental factors.

Genetic Influences

The body of evidence for genetic vulnerability to schizophrenia is growing. Studies show that relatives of schizophrenics have a much higher probability of developing the disease than the general population. Whereas the lifetime risk for developing schizophrenia is about 1 percent in most population studies, the sibling or offspring of an identified patient has about 10 percent risk of developing schizophrenia (Gottesman, 1978).

How schizophrenia is inherited is uncertain. No reliable biological marker has as yet been found (Cutting, 1985). It is unknown which genes are important in the vulnerability to schizophrenia, or whether one or many genes are implicated. Some individuals may have a strong genetic link to the illness, while in others there may be only a weak ge-

netic basis. This theory gives further credence to the notion of multiple causation.

TWIN STUDIES

The rate of schizophrenia among monozygotic (identical) twins is three times that of dizygotic (fraternal) twins, and lies between 35 and 60 times that of the general population (Gottesman & Shields, 1982). Identical twins reared apart have the same rate of development of the illness as those reared together. Because in about half of the cases only one of a pair of monozygotic twins develops schizophrenia, some investigators believe environmental factors interact with the genetic ones.

ADOPTION STUDIES

In studies conducted by both American and Danish investigators, children born in schizophrenic families, but adopted and reared by nonschizophrenic families, were more likely to develop the illness than the comparison control groups (Tsuang, 1982). From the same studies, children born of nonschizophrenic parents, but reared by schizophrenic parents, did not suffer more often from schizophrenia than those of the control group. These findings provide additional evidence for the genetic basis of schizophrenia.

Biochemical Influences

The oldest and most thoroughly explored theoretical approach to the explanation of schizophrenia is that which attributes a pathogenic role to abnormal brain biochemistry (Birchwood et al, 1989). Notions of a "chemical disturbance" in the explanation for insanity were suggested by some theorists as early as the midnineteenth century.

THE DOPAMINE HYPOTHESIS

This theory suggests that schizophrenia (or schizophreniclike symptoms) may be caused by an excess of dopamine-dependent neuronal activity in the brain (Hollandsworth, 1990). This excess activity may be related to increased production or release of the substance at nerve terminals, increased receptor sensitivity, or reduced activity of dopamine antagonists (Birchwood et al, 1989).

Pharmacological support for this hypothesis exists. Amphetamines have been found to increase levels of dopamine, manifesting schizophrenialike symptoms in healthy volunteers (Tsuang, 1982). The neuroleptics (e.g., chlorpromazine or haloperidol) lower brain levels of dopamine by blocking dopamine receptors, thus reducing the schizophrenic symptoms induced by amphetamines.

Postmortem studies of schizophrenic brains have reported a significant increase in the average number of dopamine receptors in approximately two-thirds of the brains studied. This suggests that an increased dopamine response may not be important in *all* schizophrenic patients. Patients with acute manifestations (e.g., delusions and hallucinations) respond with greater efficacy to neuroleptic drugs than do patients with chronic manifestations (e.g., apathy, poverty of ideas, and loss of drive). The current position, in terms of the dopamine hypothesis, is that manifestations of acute schizophrenia may be related to increased numbers of dopamine receptors in the brain and respond to neuroleptic drugs that block these receptors. Manifestations of chronic schizophrenia are probably unrelated to numbers of dopamine receptors, and neuroleptic drugs are unlikely to be effective in treating these chronic symptoms.

OTHER BIOCHEMICAL HYPOTHESES

Various other biochemicals have been implicated in the predisposition to schizophrenia. Abnormalities in the neurotransmitters norepinephrine, serotonin, acetylcholine, and gamma-aminobutyric acid, and the neuroregulators, such as prostaglandins and endorphins, have been suggested. The body may manufacture a hallucinogen or psychotomimetic that usurps the usual neurotransmitter or neuroregulator pathways in the brains of schizophrenics (Cutting, 1985).

Physiological Influences

A number of physical factors of possible etiological significance have been identified in the medical literature, although their specific mechanisms in the implication of schizophrenia are unclear.

VIRAL INFECTION

In postmortem studies, Stevens (1982) reported observations of degenerative changes within the neurons and an increase in the supporting glial cells of schizophrenic brains. These structural changes are similar to those characteristically reported in infectious inflammatory diseases, such as viral encephalitis. Stevens considered these changes in the schizophrenic brains to be consistent with a "healed inflammatory" process.

ANATOMICAL ABNORMALITIES

Some studies have shown a significant enlargement in cerebral ventricular size in the brains of schizophrenics. In one study, Weinberger et al (1979) reported 53 percent of those with chronic schizophrenia having ventricular sizes more than two standard deviations larger than the mean of the controls. Dilation of cortical sulci and fissures were also observed. Together, these abnormalities may represent brain atrophy.

Functional cerebral asymmetries of the brain occur normally as they relate to language comprehension and speech production. Computerized studies with schizophrenic populations have suggested that some individuals with the disorder exhibit a reversal of the normal anatomical asymmetry (Birchwood et al, 1989). The significance of these results in the etiology of schizophrenia is unclear, however, because of the relatively few studies that have addressed this issue to date.

HISTOLOGICAL CHANGES

Scheibel (1991) and his associates at UCLA have studied cerebral changes at the microscopic level. In studying brains of schizophrenic patients, they found a "disordering" or disarray of the pyramidal cells in the area of the hippocampus. This they compared to the normal alignment of the cells in the brains of nonschizophrenic patients. They have hypothesized that this alteration in hippocampal cells occurs during the second trimester of pregnancy and may be related to an influenza virus encountered by the mother during this period. Further research is required to determine the possible link between this birth defect and the development of schizophrenia.

PHYSICAL CONDITIONS

Cutting (1985) cites various studies that report a well-established, positive link between schizophrenia and the following conditions: epilepsy (particularly temporal lobe), Huntington's chorea, birth trauma, head injury in adulthood, alcohol abuse, cerebral tumor (particularly in the limbic system), cerebrovascular accidents, systemic lupus erythematosus, myxedema, parkinsonism, and Wilson's disease.

Psychological Influences

Early conceptualizations of schizophrenia focused on family relationship factors as major influences in the development of the illness. In the past decade, researchers have cast doubt on these theories and are focusing their studies more in terms of schizophrenia as a brain disorder. Can family interaction patterns cause schizophrenia? Cutting (1985) states: "These purely psychological causes are *theoretically* possible, even if difficult to prove in practice."

MOTHER-CHILD RELATIONSHIP

Early theorists characterized the mothers of schizophrenics as cold, overprotective, and domineering (Birchwood et al, 1989). They were thought to have arrested the ego development of the child, who upon encountering the real world in adolescence or early adulthood was unable to deal with the demands and forced to retreat into a form of thinking characteristic of early childhood. Freud (1961) coined the term *primary process thinking* to describe the narcissism and fantasy associated with schizophrenic thought processes.

Sullivan (1953), who did much of his work with schizophrenic patients, believed that the illness stemmed from a parent-child relationship fraught with intense anxiety. He described three components of the self-system (the good me, the bad me, and the not me) which are determined by one's early interpersonal experiences. (see Chapter 3, for a discussion of Sullivan's theory.) The intense anxiety produces feelings of horror, awe, dread, and loathing, leading the child to deny these feelings in an effort to relieve anxiety. These feelings, having then been denied, become "not me," but someone else. This withdrawal from emotions, or the "not me" portion of the self-system, is the basis for the later development of schizophrenia.

Mahler et al (1975) describe the important phases in the separation-individuation process of the infant from the maternal figure. In phase 2 (age 1 to 5 months), which is called the symbiotic phase, there is a type of "psychic fusion" of mother and child. The child does not view the self as separate but as an extension of the mother, who serves to fulfill every need. Fixation in this stage of development has been implicated in the predisposition to adult schizophrenia.

Erikson (1963) described eight stages of human development during which individuals struggle with various crises, the resolution of which contribute to emotional growth. In the first stage, which Erikson called "trust vs. mistrust," the task is to develop trust in the mothering figure that is then generalized to other interpersonal relationships. Nonachievement and fixation at this level result in suspiciousness of others, dissatisfaction with the self, isolation, and difficulty with interpersonal relationships. This occurs when the child is rejected and deprived of nurturing and love from the primary caregiver — experiences that have been associated with vulnerability to serious mental disturbances in later life.

DYSFUNCTIONAL FAMILY SYSTEM

Bowen (1978) describes the development of schizophrenia as it evolves out of a dysfunctional family system. When a conflictual marital relationship exists, a great deal of anxiety may be experienced within the family. Out of a need to reduce the anxiety, one parent (usually the mother) may become emotionally overinvested in the child. Her anxiety decreases out of her attachment to the child, and the problems within the marriage relationship, although unresolved, become stabilized. A symbiotic relationship may develop between mother and child (the psychic fusion, as described by Mahler) — a relationship so intense that they may report thinking the same thoughts or expressing the same emotions. The child remains totally dependent on the parent into adulthood and is unable to respond to the demands of adult functioning.

DOUBLE-BIND COMMUNICATION

Bateson et al (1956) identified a pattern of communication that has been implicated in the development of schizophrenia. Communication between parents and offspring was described as frequently contradictory and placed the child in a "double-bind." Double-bind communication may occur when a statement is made and succeeded by a contradictory statement. It also occurs when a statement is made accompanied by nonverbal expression that is inconsistent with the verbal communication. These incompatible communications may interfere with ego development, thereby causing the individual to generate false ideas and exhibit extreme mistrust of all communications (Birchwood et al, 1989).

Double-bind communications give mixed messages and create confusion in the receiver.

Examples
1. Mother says, "I'm really happy you are going to the school dance tonight, Sally. I'll just stay here at home all alone."
2. Johnny falls and hurts his hand. Mother says, "Come and let Mommy kiss it for you." When Johnny goes to his Mother she says, "Don't be a baby! Big boys don't cry! Shut up. You're not hurt!"
3. Jack, who is 27 years old, has never lived away from home. His parents have told him he should get his own apartment. When his parents go on a trip, his Mother leaves prepared food for each day they will be gone and ensures that Jack's clothes have been washed and ironed before they leave.

Environmental Influences

SOCIOCULTURAL FACTORS

Many studies have been conducted that have attempted to link schizophrenia to social class. Indeed epidemiological statistics have shown that greater numbers of individuals from the lower socioeconomic classes experience symptoms associated with schizophrenia than those from the higher socioeconomic groups (Wiersma et al, 1983). Explanations for this occurrence refer to the conditions associated with living in poverty, such as congested housing accommodations, inade-

quate nutrition, absence of prenatal care, few resources for dealing with stressful situations, and feelings of hopelessness for changing their lifestyle of poverty.

Some studies have attempted to refute this hypothesis and view the link between low socioeconomic status and schizophrenia as merely a shift downward due to the patient's difficulty maintaining stable employment and relationships (Birchwood et al, 1989). These statistics may relate to the schizophrenic's tendency for social isolation, and the segregation of self from others in areas accessible to one who has experienced a passive downward shift in social status due to characteristics of the disease process itself. Proponents of this notion view poor social conditions as a consequence rather than a cause of schizophrenia.

STRESSFUL LIFE EVENTS

Studies have been conducted in an effort to determine whether psychotic episodes may be precipitated by stressful life events. The strongest evidence for the role of stressful life events in schizophrenia comes from the research of Brown and Birley (1968). In the individuals they studied, it was found that stressful events were most likely to have occurred in the 3-week period just prior to the onset of symptoms. Other investigators have supported the hypothesis that stressful life events can precipitate schizophrenic symptoms in a genetically predisposed individual (Goldstein, 1987; Liberman et al, 1984).

Birchwood et al (1989) suggest that an individual's response to stressful life events may vary as a function of (1) the number or severity of life events and (2) the degree of vulnerability to the impact of life stress. They suggest that one's degree of vulnerability may be increased by a high level of autonomic arousal, an impoverished capacity to cope with stressful experiences, or a lack of support and ties with other people, including family.

THE TRANSACTIONAL MODEL

The etiology of schizophrenia remains unclear. No single theory or hypothesis has been postulated that substantiates a clear-cut explanation for the disease. Indeed, it seems the more research that is conducted, the more evidence is compiled to support the concept of multiple causation. The transactional model recognizes the combined effects of biological, psychological, and environmental influences on an individual's susceptibility to psychotic illness. Liberman et al (1984) support the concept of multiple causation. They state:

"Schizophrenic symptoms and impaired functioning occur when noxious social events combine with preexisting vulnerability to produce states of sensory overload, hyperarousal, and impaired processing of social stimuli. The appearance or increase in characteristic schizophrenic symptoms may occur in a susceptible individual when:

1. The underlying biological vulnerability increases.
2. Stressful life events intervene that overwhelm the individual's coping in social and instrumental roles.
3. The individual's social support network weakens or diminishes.
4. Previously acquired social problem-solving skills diminish due to disuse, reinforcement of the sick role, loss of motivation, or social isolation."

The dynamics of schizophrenia using the Transactional Model of Stress/Adaptation are presented in Figure 18.1.

TYPES OF SCHIZOPHRENIC AND OTHER PSYCHOTIC DISORDERS

The *DSM-III-R* (APA, 1987) identifies various types of schizophrenic and other psychotic disorders. Differential diagnosis is made according to the total symptomatic clinical picture presented.

Disorganized Schizophrenia

This type of schizophrenia was previously called *hebephrenic schizophrenia*. Onset of symptoms is usually before age 25, and the course is commonly chronic. Behavior is markedly regressive and primitive. Contact with reality is extremely poor. Affect is flat or grossly inappropriate, often with periods of silliness and incongruous giggling. Facial grimaces and bizarre mannerisms are common, and communication is consistently incoherent. Personal appearance is generally neglected, and social impairment is extreme.

Catatonic Schizophrenia

This type of schizophrenia is characterized by marked abnormalities in motor behavior and may be manifested in the form of stupor or excitement (Kaplan & Sadock, 1985).

Catatonic stupor is characterized by extreme psychomotor retardation. The individual exhibits a pronounced decrease in spontaneous movements and activity. Mutism (i.e., absence of speech) is common, and negativism (i.e., an apparently motiveless resistance to all instructions or attempts to be moved) may be evident. Waxy flexibility may be exhibited. This term describes a type of "posturing," or voluntary assumption of bizarre positions, in which the individual may remain for long periods. Efforts to move the individual may be met with rigid bodily resistance.

Catatonic excitement is manifested by a state of extreme psychomotor agitation. The movements are frenzied and purposeless, and are usually accompanied by continuous incoherent verbalizations and shouting. Patients in catatonic excitement urgently require physical and medical control, since they are often destructive and violent to others, and their dangerous excitement can cause them to injure themselves or to collapse from complete exhaustion (Kaplan & Sadock, 1985).

Catatonic schizophrenia was very common only a few decades ago. However, since the advent of antipsychotic medications for use in psychiatry, the illness is now rare in Europe and North America (APA, 1987).

Paranoid Schizophrenia

This disorder is characterized mainly by the presence of delusions of persecution or grandeur and auditory hallucinations related to a single theme. The individual is often tense, suspicious, and guarded, and may be argumentative, hostile, and aggressive. Onset of symptoms is usually later (perhaps in the late 20s or 30s), and less regression of mental faculties, emotional response, and behavior is seen than in the other subtypes of schizophrenia (Kaplan & Sadock, 1985). Social impairment may be minimal, and some evidence suggests that prognosis, particularly with regard to occupational functioning and capacity for independent living, is promising (APA, 1987).

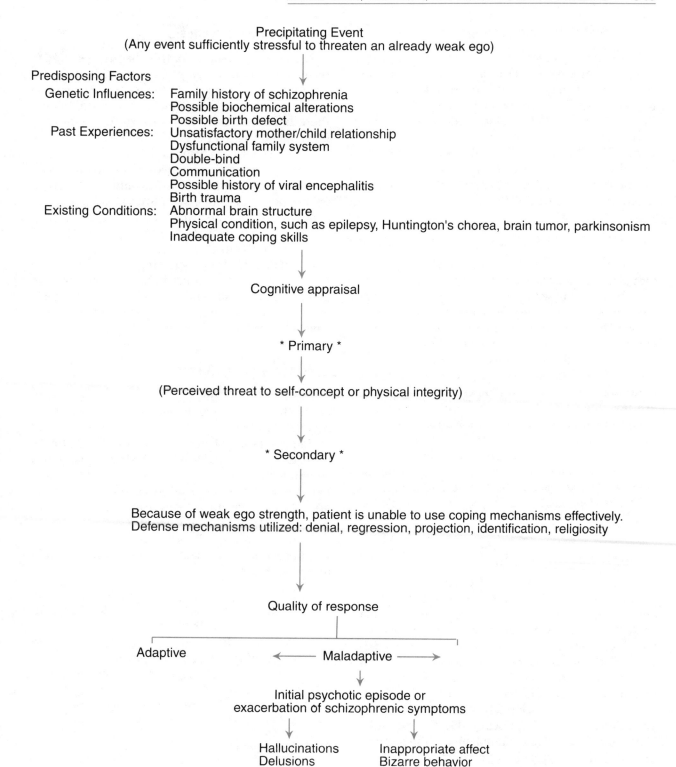

Figure 18.1   The dynamics of schizophrenia using the transactional model of stress/adaptation.

Undifferentiated Schizophrenia

Sometimes, patients with schizophrenic symptoms do not meet the criteria for any of the subtypes, or they may meet the criteria for more than one subtype. These individuals may be given the diagnosis of undifferentiated schizophrenia. The behavior is clearly psychotic, that is, there is evidence of delusions, hallucinations, incoherence, and bizarre behavior. However, the symptoms cannot be easily classified into any of the previously listed diagnostic categories.

Residual Schizophrenia

This diagnostic category is used when the individual has a history of at least one previous episode of schizophrenia with prominent psychotic symptoms. Residual schizophrenia occurs in an individual who has a chronic form of the disease and is the stage that follows an acute episode (prominent delusions, hallucinations, incoherence, bizarre behavior, violence). In the residual stage, there is continuing evidence of the illness, although there are no prominent psychotic symptoms. Residual symptoms may include social isolation, eccentric behavior, impairment in personal hygiene and grooming, blunted or inappropriate affect, poverty of or overelaborate speech, illogical thinking, or apathy. Residual schizophrenia is sometimes referred to as *ambulatory schizophrenia* (Kaplan & Sadock, 1985).

Schizoaffective Disorder

This disorder is manifested by schizophrenic behaviors, with a strong element of symptomatology associated with the mood disorders, either mania or depression. The patient may appear depressed, with psychomotor retardation and suicidal ideation; or, symptoms may include euphoria, grandiosity, and hyperactivity. The decisive factor in the diagnosis of schizoaffective disorder, however, is the presence of characteristic schizophrenic symptoms (Kaplan & Sadock, 1985). For example, in addition to the dysfunctional mood, the individual exhibits bizarre delusions, prominent hallucinations, incoherent speech, catatonic behavior, or blunted or inappropriate affect. The prognosis for schizoaffective disorder is generally better than that for other schizophrenic disorders, but worse than that for mood disorders alone (APA, 1987).

Brief Reactive Psychosis

The essential feature of this disorder is sudden onset of psychotic symptoms following a severe psychosocial stressor. These symptoms last at least a few hours, but no more than 1 month, and there is an eventual full return to the premorbid level of functioning (APA, 1987). The stressor is of sufficient severity to bring about emotional turmoil or overwhelming perplexity or confusion in the individual. This diagnosis applies only if the individual has never exhibited symptoms characteristic of a schizophrenic disorder (including prodromal symptoms or schizoid/schizotypal personality disorder) prior to onset of the current symptoms. Evidence of impaired reality testing may include incoherent speech, delusions, hallucinations, bizarre behavior, and disorientation. When the diagnosis must be made without waiting for the expected recovery, it is qualified as "provisional."

Schizophreniform Disorder

The essential features of this disorder are identical to those of schizophrenia, with the exception that the duration, including prodromal, active, and residual phases, is less than 6 months (APA, 1987). If the diagnosis is made while the individual is still symptomatic, but has been so for less than 6 months, it is qualified as "provisional." The diagnosis is changed to schizophrenia if the clinical picture persists beyond 6 months.

Schizophreniform disorder is thought to have a good prognosis if at least two of the following features are present:

1. Onset of prominent psychotic symptoms within 4 weeks of first noticeable change in usual behavior or functioning
2. Confusion, disorientation, or perplexity at the height of the psychotic episode
3. Good premorbid social and occupational functioning
4. Absence of blunted or flat affect

Delusional Disorder

This disorder was previously called *paranoid disorder*. The name was changed to delusional disorder, which more closely describes the essential feature of persistent, nonbizarre delusions. Hallucinations, if present at all, are not prominent, and behavior, apart from the delusions, is not bizarre. The type of delusional disorder is based on the predominant delusional theme, although it is not uncommon for an individual with the disorder to present with more than one delusional theme (APA, 1987).

EROTOMANIC TYPE

With this type of delusion, the individual believes that someone, usually of a higher status, is in love with him or her. Famous persons are often the subjects of erotomanic delusions. Sometimes the delusion is kept secret, but some individuals may follow, contact, or otherwise try to pursue the object of their delusion.

GRANDIOSE TYPE

Individuals with grandiose delusions have irrational ideas regarding their own worth, talent, knowledge, or power. They may believe that they have a special relationship with a famous person, or even assume the identity of a famous person (believing that the actual person is an imposter). Grandiose delusions of a religious nature may lead to assumption of the identity of a great diety or religious leader.

JEALOUS TYPE

The content of jealous delusions centers around the theme that the person's sexual partner is unfaithful. The idea is irrational and without cause, but the deluded individual searches for evidence to justify the belief. The sexual partner is confronted (and sometimes physically attacked) regarding the imagined infidelity. The imagined "lover" of the sexual partner may also be the object of the attack. Attempts to restrict the autonomy of the sexual partner in an effort to stop the imagined infidelity are common.

PERSECUTORY TYPE

In persecutory delusions, which are the most common type, individuals believe they are being malevolently treated in some way. Frequent themes include being conspired against, cheated, spied upon, followed, poisoned or drugged, maliciously maligned, harassed, or obstructed in the pursuit of long-term goals (APA, 1987). The individual may obsess about and exaggerate a slight rebuff (either real or imagined) until it becomes the focus of a delusional system. Repeated complaints may be directed to legal authorities, lack of satisfaction from which may result in violence toward the object of the delusion.

SOMATIC TYPE

Individuals with somatic delusions believe they have some physical defect, disorder, or disease. The *DSM-III-R* (APA, 1987) identifies the most common types of somatic delusions as those in which the individual believes that he or she:

1. Emits a foul odor from the skin, mouth, rectum, or vagina
2. Has an infestation of insects in or on the skin
3. Has an internal parasite
4. Has misshapen and ugly body parts
5. Has dysfunctional body parts

Induced Psychotic Disorder

The characteristic feature of this disorder is "a delusional system that develops in a second person as a result of a close relationship with another person who already has a psychotic disorder with prominent delusions" (APA, 1987). The person with the primary delusional disorder is usually the dominant person in the relationship, and the delusional thinking is gradually imposed upon the more passive partner. This occurs within the context of a long-term, close relationship, and when the couple has been socially isolated from other people. The course is usually chronic, and is more common in women than in men.

APPLICATION OF THE NURSING PROCESS

Background Assessment Data

In the first step of the nursing process, the nurse gathers a data base from which nursing diagnoses are derived and a plan of care is formulated. This first step of the nursing process is extremely important, for without an accurate assessment, problem identification, objectives of care, and outcome criteria cannot be accurately determined.

Assessment of the schizophrenic patient may be a complex process, based on information gathered from a number of sources. Schizophrenic patients in an acute episode of their illness are seldom able to make a significant contribution to their history. Data may be obtained from family members, if possible; old records, if available; or from other individuals who have been in a position to report on the progression of the patient's behavior.

The *DSM-III-R* (APA, 1987) identifies disturbances in eight areas of functioning: content of thought, form of thought, perception, affect, sense of self, volition, impaired interpersonal functioning and relationship to the external world, and psychomotor behavior. Within these areas of functioning, the initial assessment of the schizophrenic patient is made. Additional impairments may occur outside the limits of these eight areas. Following are some important behaviors associated with these areas of functioning with which the nurse must be familiar to obtain an adequate assessment of the schizophrenic patient. Additional features are also included.

CONTENT OF THOUGHT

Delusions   Delusions are false personal beliefs that are inconsistent with the person's intelligence or cultural background. The individual continues to have the belief in spite of obvious proof that it is false or irrational. Delusions are subdivided according to their content. Some of the more common ones include:

Delusion of persecution. The individual feels threatened and believes that others intend harm or persecution toward him or her in some way. (e.g., "The FBI has 'bugged' my room and intend to kill me." "I can't take a shower in this bathroom. The nurses have put a camera in there so that they can watch everything I do.")

Delusion of grandeur. The individual has an exaggerated feeling of importance, power, knowledge, or identity. (e.g., "I am Jesus Christ.")

Delusion of reference. All events within the environment are referred by the psychotic person to himself or herself. (e.g., "Someone is trying to get a message to me through the articles in this magazine [or newspaper; or TV program]. I must break the code so that I can receive the message.") Ideas of reference are less rigid

than delusions of reference. An example of an idea of reference would be irrational thinking that one is being talked about or laughed at by other people.

Delusion or control or influence. The individual believes certain objects or persons have control over his or her behavior. (e.g., "The dentist put a filling in my tooth. I now receive transmissions through the filling that control what I think and do.")

Somatic delusion. The individual has a false idea about the functioning of his or her body. (e.g., "I'm 70 years old and I will be the oldest person ever to give birth. The doctor says I'm not pregnant, but I know I am.")

Nihilistic delusion. The individual has a false idea that the self, a part of the self, others, or the world is nonexistent. (e.g., "The world no longer exists." "I have no heart.")

Religiosity   This is an excessive demonstration of or obsession with religious ideas and behavior. Because individuals vary greatly in their religious beliefs and level of spiritual commitment, this symptom is often difficult to assess. The schizophrenic patient may use religious ideas in an attempt to provide rational meaning and structure to his or her behavior. Religious preoccupation in this vein may therefore be considered a manifestation of the illness. However, patients who derive comfort from their religious beliefs should not be discouraged from employing this means of support (e.g., the individual who believes the voice he hears is God, and incessantly searches the Bible for interpretation).

Paranoia   This condition is characterized by extreme suspiciousness of others and of their actions or perceived intentions. (e.g., "I won't eat this food. I know it has been poisoned.")

Magical Thinking   The person believes that his or her thoughts or behaviors have control over specific situations or people. (e.g., The mother who believed if she scolded her son in any way he would be taken away from her.) Magical thinking is common in children. (e.g., "Step on a crack and you break your mother's back." "An apple a day keeps the doctor away.")

FORM OF THOUGHT

Associative Looseness   Thinking is characterized by speech in which ideas shift from one unrelated subject to another. The individual is unaware that the topics are unconnected. When associative looseness is severe, speech may be incoherent (APA, 1987). (e.g., "We wanted to take the bus, but the airport took all the traffic. Driving is the ticket when you want to get somewhere. No one needs a ticket to heaven. We have it all in our pockets.")

Neologisms   The psychotic person invents new words that are meaningless to others but have symbolic meaning to himself or herself. (e.g., "She wanted to give me a ride in her new uniphorum.")

Concrete Thinking   Concreteness, or literal interpretations of the environment, represents a regression to an earlier level of cognitive development. Abstract thinking is very difficult. (e.g., The schizophrenic patient would have great difficulty describing the abstract meaning of sayings such as "I'm climbing the walls," or "It's raining cats and dogs.")

Clang Associations   Choice of words is governed by sounds. Clang associations often take the form of rhyming. (e.g., "It is very cold. I am cold and bold. The gold has been sold.")

Word Salad   A word salad is a group of words that are put together in a random fashion, without any logical connection. (e.g., "Most forward action grows life double plays circle uniform.")

Circumstantiality   The individual is delayed in reaching the point of a communication due to unnecessary and tedious details. The point or goal is usually met but only with numerous interruptions by the interviewer to keep the person on track of the topic being discussed.

Tangentiality   Tangentiality differs from circumstantiality in that the person never really gets to the point of the communication. Unrelated topics are introduced, and the original discussion is lost.

Mutism   This is an individual's inability or refusal to speak.

Perseveration   The individual persistently repeats the same word or idea in response to different questions.

PERCEPTION

Hallucinations   Hallucinations, or false sensory perceptions not associated with real external stimuli (Kaplan & Sadock, 1985), may involve any of the five senses. The *DSM-III-R* (APA, 1987) describes the following examples:

Auditory. A false perception of sound. Most commonly they are of voices, but the individual may report clicks, rushing noises, music, and so forth. Command hallucinations may place the individual or others in a potentially dangerous situation. "Voices" that issue commands for violence to self or others may or may not be heeded by the psychotic person.

Visual. A false visual perception. They may consist of formed images, such as people, or of unformed images, such as flashes of light.

Tactile. A false perception of the sense of touch, often of something on or under the skin. One specific tactile hallucination is *formication*, the sensation that something is crawling on or under the skin.

Gustatory. A false perception of taste. Most commonly, gustatory hallucinations are described as unpleasant tastes.

Olfactory. A false perception of the sense of smell.

Illusions   Misperceptions of real external stimuli (APA, 1987).

AFFECT

Affect describes the behavior associated with an individual's feeling state or emotional tone.

Inappropriate Affect   Affect is inappropriate when the individual's emotional tone is incongruent with the circumstances. (e.g., A young woman laughs when told of the death of her mother.)

Bland or Flat Affect   Affect is described as bland when the emotional tone is very weak. The individual with flat affect appears to be void of emotional tone (or feeling response).

Apathy   The schizophrenic patient often demonstrates an indifference to or disinterest in the environment. The bland or flat affect is a manifestation of the emotional apathy.

SENSE OF SELF

Sense of self describes the uniqueness and individuality a person feels. Because of extremely weak ego boundaries, the schizophrenic lacks this feeling of uniqueness and experiences a great deal of confusion regarding his or her identity.

Echolalia   The patient with schizophrenia may

repeat words that he or she hears. This is an attempt to identify with the person speaking. (e.g., Nurse: "John, it's time for lunch." Patient may respond: "It's time for lunch. It's time for lunch." or sometimes, "Lunch, lunch, lunch, lunch.")

Echopraxia The patient may purposelessly imitate movements made by others.

Identification (on an Unconscious Level) and Imitation (on a Conscious Level) These ego defense mechanisms are used by schizophrenics in their confusion regarding their self-identity. Because they have difficulty knowing where their ego boundaries end and another person's begin, their behavior often takes on the form of that which they see in the other person.

Depersonalization The schizophrenic's unstable self-identity may lead to feelings of unreality. (e.g., Feeling that one's extremities have changed in size; or a sense of seeming to perceive oneself from a distance [APA, 1987].)

VOLITION

Volition has to do with impairment in the schizophrenic's ability to initiate goal-directed activity. This may take the form of inadequate interest, drive, or ability to follow a course of action to its logical conclusion (APA, 1987).

Emotional Ambivalence Ambivalence in the schizophrenic refers to the coexistence of opposite emotions toward the same object, person, or situation. These opposing emotions may interfere with the person's ability to make even a very simple decision (e.g., whether to have coffee or tea with lunch). Underlying the ambivalence in the schizophrenic patient is the difficulty he or she has in fulfilling a satisfying human relationship. This difficulty is based on the *need-fear dilemma*—the simultaneous need for and fear of intimacy.

IMPAIRED INTERPERSONAL FUNCTIONING AND RELATIONSHIP TO THE EXTERNAL WORLD

Some patients with acute schizophrenia cling to others, intrude upon strangers, and fail to recognize that excessive closeness makes other people uncomfortable and likely to pull away (APA, 1987). Impairment in social functioning may also be reflected in social isolation, emotional detachment, and lack of regard for social convention.

Autism Autism describes the condition created by the person with schizophrenia who focuses inward on a fantasy world, while distorting or excluding the external environment.

Deteriorated Appearance Personal grooming and self-care activities may become minimal. The schizophrenic patient may appear disheveled and untidy, and may need to be reminded of the need for personal hygiene.

PSYCHOMOTOR BEHAVIOR

Anergia A deficiency of energy. The individual with schizophrenia may lack sufficient energy to carry out activities of daily living or to interact with others.

Waxy Flexibility Waxy flexibility describes a condition by which the schizophrenic patient passively yields all moveable parts of the body to any efforts made at placing them in certain positions (Kaplan & Sadock, 1985). For example, once placed in position, the arm, leg, or head remains in that position for long periods, regardless of how uncomfortable it is for the patient.

Posturing This symptom is manifested by the voluntary assumption of inappropriate or bizarre postures.

Pacing and Rocking Pacing back and forth and body rocking (a slow, rhythmic, backward-and-forward swaying of the trunk from the hips, usually while in a sitting position) are common psychomotor behaviors of the schizophrenic patient (Kaplan & Sadock, 1985).

ASSOCIATED FEATURES

Anhedonia The inability to experience or even imagine any pleasant emotion (Kaplan & Sadock, 1985). This is a particularly distressing symptom that compels some patients to attempt suicide.

Regression The retreat to an earlier level of development. Regression, a primary defense mechanism of schizophrenia, is a dysfunctional attempt to reduce anxiety. It provides the basis for changes in cognition, perception, affect, relationships, and behavior seen in the schizophrenic (Haber et al, 1987).

Nursing Diagnoses

From analysis of the assessment data, appropriate nursing diagnoses are formulated for the psychotic patient and his or her family. From these identified problems, accurate planning of nursing care is executed. Possible nursing diagnoses for patients with psychotic disorders include:

Alteration in thought processes related to inability to trust, panic anxiety, possible hereditary or biochemical factors, evidenced by delusional thinking; inability to concentrate; impaired volition; inability to problem solve, abstract, or conceptualize; extreme suspiciousness of others.

Sensory-perceptual alteration: Auditory/visual related to panic anxiety, extreme loneliness and withdrawal into the self, evidenced by inappropriate responses, disordered thought sequencing, rapid mood swings, poor concentration, disorientation.

Social isolation related to inability to trust, panic anxiety, weak ego development, delusional thinking, regression, evidenced by withdrawal, sad, dull affect, need-fear dilemma, preoccupation with own thoughts, expression of feelings of rejection or of aloneness imposed by others.

High risk for violence: Self-directed or directed at others related to extreme suspiciousness, panic anxiety, catatonic excitement, rage reactions, command hallucinations evidenced by overt and aggressive acts, goal-directed destruction of objects in the environment, self-destructive behavior or active aggressive suicidal acts.

Impaired verbal communication related to panic anxiety, regression, withdrawal, disordered, unrealistic thinking evidenced by loose association of ideas, neologisms, word salad, clang association, echolalia, verbalizations that reflect concrete thinking, poor eye contact.

Self-care deficit related to withdrawal, regression, panic anxiety, perceptual or cognitive impairment, inability to trust, evidenced by difficulty carrying out tasks associated with hygiene, dressing, grooming, eating, toileting.

Ineffective family coping: Disabling related to highly ambivalent family relationships, impaired family communication, evidenced by neglectful care of the patient in regard to basic human needs or illness treatment, extreme denial or prolonged overconcern regarding patient's illness.

Altered health maintenance related to disordered thinking, delusions, evidenced by reported or observed inability to take responsibility for meeting basic health practices in any or all functional pattern areas.

Impaired home maintenance management related to regression, withdrawal, lack of knowledge/resources, impaired physical or cognitive functioning, evidenced by unsafe, unclean, disorderly home environment.

Planning/Implementation

Table 18.1 provides a plan of care for the patient with schizophrenic disorder. Selected nursing diagnoses are presented, along with goals of care and appropriate nursing interventions for each. Rationale is provided in italics.

Some institutions are using a case management model to coordinate care (see Chapter 6). In case management models, the plan of care may take the form of a critical pathway. Table 18.2 depicts an example of a critical pathway of care for a patient experiencing an exacerbation of schizophrenic psychosis.

OUTCOME CRITERIA

The following criteria may be used for measurement of outcomes in the care of the schizophrenic patient.

The patient:

1. demonstrates ability to relate satisfactorily with others.
2. recognizes distortions of reality.
3. perceives self realistically.
4. demonstrates the ability to perceive the environment correctly.
5. maintains anxiety at a manageable level.
6. relinquishes need for delusions and hallucinations.
7. demonstrates ability to trust others.
8. uses appropriate verbal communication in interactions with others.
9. performs self-care activities independently.

Evaluation

In the final step of the nursing process, a reassessment is conducted to determine if the nursing actions have been successful in achieving the objectives of care. Evaluation of the nursing actions for the patient with schizophrenic psychosis may be facilitated by gathering information using the following types of questions.

Table 18.1	CARE PLAN FOR THE PATIENT WITH SCHIZOPHRENIC PSYCHOSIS	
Nursing Diagnoses	**Objectives**	**Nursing Interventions**
Alteration in thought processes related to inability to trust, panic anxiety, possible hereditary or biochemical factors, evidenced by delusional thinking; inability to concentrate; impaired volition; inability to problem solve, abstract, or conceptualize; extreme suspiciousness of others.	Patient will eliminate pattern of delusional thinking. Patient will demonstrate trust in others.	Convey acceptance of patient's need for the false belief, but that you do not share the belief. *Patient must understand that you do not view the idea as real.* Do not argue or deny the belief. Use *reasonable doubt* as a therapeutic technique: "I find that hard to believe." *Arguing or denying the belief serves no useful purpose, as delusional ideas are not eliminated by this approach, and the development of a trusting relationship may be impeded.* Reinforce and focus on reality. Discourage long ruminations about the irrational thinking. Talk about real events and real people. *Discussions that focus on the false ideas are purposeless and useless, and may even aggravate the psychosis.* If patient is highly suspicious, the following interventions may help: a. *To promote trust:* use same staff as much as possible; be honest and keep all promises. b. *To prevent the patient from feeling threatened:* avoid physical contact; avoid laughing, whispering, or talking quietly where patient can see but cannot hear what is being said; provide canned food with can opener or serve food family style; avoid competitive activities; use assertive, matter-of-fact, yet friendly approach.
Sensory-perceptual alteration: Auditory/Visual related to panic anxiety, extreme loneliness and withdrawal into the self, evidenced by inappropriate responses, disordered thought sequencing, rapid mood swings, poor concentration, disorientation.	Patient will be able to define and test reality, eliminating the occurrence of hallucinations.	Observe patient for signs of hallucinations (listening pose, laughing or talking to self, stopping in midsentence). *Early intervention may prevent aggressive response to command hallucinations.* Avoid touching the patient without warning. *Patient may perceive touch as threatening and may respond in an aggressive manner.* An attitude of acceptance will encourage the patient to share the content of the hallucination with you. *This is important to prevent possible injury to the patient or others from command hallucinations.* Do not reinforce the hallucination. Use "the voices" instead of words like "they" that imply validation. Let patient know that you do not share the perception. Say, "Even though I realize the voices are real to you, I do not hear any voices speaking." *Patient must accept the perception as unreal before hallucinations can be eliminated.* Help the patient understand the connection between anxiety and hallucinations. *If patient can learn to interrupt escalating anxiety, hallucinations may be prevented.* Try to

(*continued*)

Table 18.1 CONTINUED		
Nursing Diagnoses	**Objectives**	**Nursing Interventions**
		distract the patient away from the hallucination. *Involvement in interpersonal activities and explanation of the actual situation will help bring the patient back to reality.*
Social isolation related to inability to trust, panic anxiety, weak ego development, delusional thinking, regression, evidenced by withdrawal, sad, dull affect, need-fear dilemma, preoccupation with own thoughts, expression of feelings of rejection or of aloneness imposed by others.	Patient will voluntarily spend time with other patients and staff members in group activities on the unit.	Convey an accepting attitude by making brief, frequent contacts. Show unconditional positive regard. *This increases feelings of self-worth and facilitates trust.* Offer to be with patient during group activities that he or she finds frightening or difficult. *The presence of a trusted individual provides emotional security for the patient.* Give recognition and positive reinforcement for patient's voluntary interactions with others. *Positive reinforcement enhances self-esteem and encourages repetition of acceptable behaviors.*
Potential for violence: Self-directed or directed at others related to extreme suspiciousness, panic anxiety, catatonic excitement, rage reactions, command hallucinations, evidenced by overt and aggressive acts, goal-directed destruction of objects in the environment, self-destructive behavior or active aggressive suicidal acts.	Patient will not harm self or others.	Maintain low level of stimuli in patient's environment (low lighting, few people, simple decor, low noise level). *Anxiety level rises in stimulating environment. Individuals may be perceived as threatening by a suspicious, agitated patient.* Observe patient's behavior frequently. Do this while carrying out routine activities, *to avoid creating suspiciousness in the individual. Close observation is necessary so that intervention can occur if required to ensure patient's (and others') safety.* Remove all dangerous objects from patient's environment, *so that in an agitated, confused state, he or she may not use them to harm self or others.* Redirect violent behavior with physical outlets for the anxiety. *Physical exercise is a safe and effective way of relieving pent-up tension.* Staff should maintain a calm attitude toward patient. *Anxiety is contagious and can be transmitted from staff to patient.* Have sufficient staff available to indicate a show of strength to patient if it becomes necessary. *This shows the patient evidence of control over the situation and provides some physical security for staff.* Administer tranquilizing medications as ordered by physician. If patient is not calmed by "talking down" or by medication, use of mechanical restraints may be necessary. *The avenue of the "least restrictive alternative" must be selected when planning interventions for a violent patient.*

(*continued*)

Table 18.1 CONTINUED

Nursing Diagnoses	Objectives	Nursing Interventions
Impaired verbal communication related to panic anxiety, regression, withdrawal, disordered, unrealistic thinking, evidenced by loose association of ideas, neologisms, word salad, clang association, echolalia, verbalizations that reflect concrete thinking, poor eye contact.	Patient will be able to communicate appropriately and comprehensibly by discharge.	Attempt to decode incomprehensible communication patterns. Seek validation and clarification by stating, "Is it that you mean . . .?" or "I don't understand what you mean by that. Would you please clarify it for me?" *These techniques reveal how the patient is being perceived by others, while the responsibility for not understanding is accepted by the nurse. Facilitate trust and understanding* by maintaining staff assignments as consistently as possible. The technique of VERBALIZING THE IMPLIED is used with the patient who is mute (unable or unwilling to speak). Example: "That must have been a very difficult time for you when your mother left. You must have felt very alone." *This approach conveys empathy and may encourage the patient to disclose painful issues.* Anticipate and fulfill patient's needs until functional communication pattern returns. Orient patient to reality as required. Call the patient by name. Validate those aspects of communication that help differentiate between what is real and unreal.
Self-care deficit related to withdrawal, regression, panic anxiety, perceptual or cognitive impairment, inability to trust, evidenced by difficulty carrying out tasks associated with hygiene, dressing, grooming, eating, toileting	Patient will demonstrate ability to meet self-care needs independently.	Provide assistance with self-care needs as required. Some patients who are severely withdrawn may require total care. *Patient safety and comfort are nursing priorities.* Encourage patient to perform independently as many activities as possible. Provide positive reinforcement for independent accomplishments. *Independent accomplishment and positive reinforcement enhance self-esteem and promote repetition of desirable behaviors.* Use concrete communication to show patient what is expected. Example: "Pick up the spoon, scoop some mashed potatoes into it, and put it in your mouth." *Because concrete thinking prevails, explanations must be provided at the patient's concrete level of comprehension.* Creative approaches may need to be taken with the patient who is not eating because he or she has suspicions of being poisoned (e.g., allow patient to open own canned or packaged foods; family-style serving may also be an option). If toileting needs are not being met, establish structured schedule to help patient fulfill these needs until he or she is able to do so independently.

(continued)

Table 18.1 CONTINUED

Nursing Diagnoses	Objectives	Nursing Interventions
Ineffective family coping: Disabling related to highly ambivalent family relationships, impaired family communication, evidenced by neglectful care of the patient in regard to basic human needs or illness treatment, extreme denial or prolonged overconcern regarding patient's illness.	Family will identify more adaptive coping strategies for dealing with patient's illness and treatment regimen.	Identify level of family functioning. Assess communication patterns, interpersonal relationships between members, role expectations, problem-solving skills, and availability of outside support systems. *These factors will help to identify how successful the family is in dealing with stressful situations, and areas where assistance is required.* Provide information for the family about the patient's illness, what will be required in the treatment regimen, and long-term prognosis. *Knowledge and understanding about what to expect may facilitate the family's ability to successfully integrate the schizophrenic patient into the system.* With family members, practice how to respond to bizarre behavior and communication patterns, and in the event that the patient becomes violent. *A plan of action will assist the family to respond adaptively in the face of what they may consider to be a crisis situation.*

Table 18.2 CRITICAL PATHWAY OF CARE FOR PATIENT WITH SCHIZOPHRENIC PSYCHOSIS

Estimated Length of Stay: 14 days — Variations from designated pathway should be documented in progress notes

Nursing Diagnoses and Categories of Care	Time Dimension	Goals and/or Actions	Time Dimension	Goals and/or Actions	Time Dimension	Discharge Outcome
Alteration in thought processes/ sensory-perceptual alteration			Day 7	Patient is able to differentiate between what is real and what is not real.	Day 14	Patient experiences no delusional thinking or hallucinations
Referrals	Day 1	Psychiatrist Psychologist Social worker Clinical nurse specialist Music therapist Occupational therapist Recreational therapist			Day 14	Discharge with follow-up appointments as required.

(*continued*)

Table 18.2 CONTINUED

Estimated Length of Stay: 14 days—Variations from designated pathway should be documented in progress notes

Nursing Diagnoses and Categories of Care	Time Dimension	Goals and/or Actions	Time Dimension	Goals and/or Actions	Time Dimension	Discharge Outcome
Diagnostic studies	Day 1 Day 3–5	Drug screen CT scan, MRI, PET, EEG (These may be ordered to examine structure and function of the brain.)				
Additional assessments	Day 1 Day 1	VS every shift Assess for: delusions, hallucinations, loose associations, inappropriate affect, excitement/ stupor, panic anxiety, suspiciousness	Day 2–14 Day 2–5	Ongoing assessments Establish trust with at least one person.	Day 2–14 Day 14	VS daily if stable No evidence of delusions, hallucinations, loose associations, inappropriate affect, excitement/ stupor, panic anxiety, suspiciousness.
Medications	Day 1	Antipsychotic medication (scheduled and prn). May need order for concentrate and injectable form. Antiparkinsonian medication (prn)	Day 1–14	Assess for effectiveness and side effects of medications.	Day 14	Patient is discharged with medications.
Patient education			Day 7 Day 10	Discuss correlation between increased anxiety and psychotic symptoms. Discuss ways to de-escalate anxiety. Discuss importance of taking medications regularly, even when feeling well. Discuss possible side effects of medications and when to see the doctor.	Day 12–13 Day 14	Reinforce teaching. Patient verbalizes understanding of information presented prior discharge.

(continued)

Table 18.2 CONTINUED

Estimated Length of Stay: 14 days — Variations from designated pathway should be documented in progress notes

Nursing Diagnoses and Categories of Care	Time Dimension	Goals and/or Actions	Time Dimension	Goals and/or Actions	Time Dimension	Discharge Outcome
Potential for violence: Self-directed or directed at others	Day 1	Environment is made safe for patient and others.	Ongoing	Patient does not harm self or others.	Day 14	Patient is discharged without harm to self or others.
Referrals	Day 1	Alert hostility management team of the admission of a potentially violent patient. For relaxation therapy: Music therapist Clinical nurse specialist Stress management specialist Psychiatrist: May give order for mechanical restraints to be used if needed.			Day 14	Discharge with follow-up appointments as required.
Additional assessments	Day 1	Assess for signs of impending violent behavior: increase in psychomotor activity; angry affect; verbalized persecutory delusions or frightening hallucinations.	Day 2–14	Ongoing assessments		
Medications	Day 1	Prn antipsychotic medications when signs of agitation begin.	Day 1–14	Use of medications, isolation/seclusion, or mechanical restraints. If patient refuses medications, administer following application of restraints.	Day 14	Patient is discharged with medications.

(continued)

Table 18.2 CONTINUED

Estimated Length of Stay: 14 days — Variations from designated pathway should be documented in progress notes

Nursing Diagnoses and Categories of Care	Time Dimension	Goals and/or Actions	Time Dimension	Goals and/or Actions	Time Dimension	Discharge Outcome
Patient education			Day 3–12	Teach relaxation techniques; discuss activities in which patient could participate to relieve pent-up tension; discuss signs and symptoms of escalating anxiety.	Day 12–13 Day 14	Reinforce teaching. Patient verbalizes understanding of information presented prior to discharge.

Has the patient established trust with at least one staff member? Is the anxiety level maintained at a manageable level? Is delusional thinking still prevalent? Is hallucinogenic activity evident? Does patient share content of hallucination, particularly if commands are heard? Is the patient able to interrupt escalating anxiety with adaptive coping mechanisms? Is the patient easily agitated? Is the patient able to interact with others appropriately? Does the patient voluntarily attend therapy activities? Is verbal communication comprehensible? Is patient compliant with medication? Does patient verbalize importance of taking medication regularly and on a long-term basis? Does patient verbalize understanding of possible side effects and when to seek assistance from the physician? Does patient spend time with others rather than isolating self? Is patient able to carry out all activities of daily living independently? Is patient able to verbalize resources from whom he or she may seek assistance outside the hospital? Does the family have information regarding support groups in which they may participate and from which they may seek assistance in dealing with their ill member? If patient lives alone, does he or she have a source for assistance with home maintenance and health management?

TREATMENT MODALITIES FOR SCHIZOPHRENIC AND OTHER PSYCHOTIC DISORDERS

Psychological Treatments

INDIVIDUAL PSYCHOTHERAPY

Arieti (1976) describes the approach to individual psychotherapy for schizophrenia as:

> "Psychotherapy aims at re-establishing the bond of human relatedness with the patient, attacking psychotic symptoms, understanding the psychodynamic history, and helping the patient unfold towards new nonpsychotic patterns of living."

Strauss (1983) suggests that "reality-oriented individual therapy" is the most suitable approach to individual psychotherapy with schizophrenics. The primary focus in all cases must reflect efforts to decrease anxiety and increase trust.

Establishing a relationship is often particularly difficult, for the schizophrenic is desperately lonely yet defends against closeness and trust, and is likely to become suspicious, anxious, hostile, or regressed when someone attempts to draw close (Kaplan & Sadock, 1985). Successful intervention may be achieved with honesty, simple directness, and a manner that respects the patient's privacy and human dignity. Exaggerated warmth and professions of friendship are likely to be met with confusion and suspiciousness.

Once a therapeutic interpersonal relationship has been established, reality orientation is maintained through exploration of the patient's behavior within relationships. Education is provided to help the patient identify sources of real or perceived danger and ways of reacting appropriately. Methods for improving interpersonal communication, emotional expression, and frustration tolerance are attempted.

Individual psychotherapy with schizophrenic patients is seen as a long-term endeavor that requires from a therapist exquisite patience and freedom from the need to prove oneself by effecting change (Gomes-Schwartz, 1984). Some cases report treatment durations of many years before patients regain some degree of independent functioning.

GROUP THERAPY

A number of studies on the efficacy of group therapy in the treatment of schizophrenia have reported meager but positive results, particularly with outpatients, and when combined with drug treatment (Cutting, 1985; Kaplan & Sadock, 1985). Kaplan and Sadock (1985) state,

> "Results are more likely to be positive when treatment focuses on real-life plans, problems, and relationships; on social and work roles and interaction; on cooperation with drug therapy and discussion of the side effects; or on some practical recreational or work activity."

Group therapy in inpatient settings is less productive. Inpatient treatment usually occurs when symptomatology and social disorganization are at their most intense. At this time, the least amount of stimuli possible is most beneficial for the patient. Because group therapy is, in fact, a multistimuli situation frequently high in intensity, it may be counterproductive early in treatment (Keith & Matthews, 1984).

Group therapy with schizophrenics has been most useful over the long-term course of the illness. The social interaction, sense of cohesiveness, identification, and reality testing achieved within the group setting have proven to be highly therapeutic processes for these individuals (Kaplan & Sadock, 1985).

BEHAVIOR THERAPY

Behavior modification cannot cure schizophrenia in the sense of reversing the assumed biological or psychological defect (Kaplan & Sadock, 1985). It has, however, had a history of qualified success in reducing the frequency of bizarre, disturbing, and deviant behaviors and increasing appropriate behaviors.

Liberman (1970) has summarized the behavior modification features that have led to the most positive results as follows:

1. Clear definition and measurement of goals
2. Attachment of clear positive and negative consequences to adaptive and maladaptive behavior
3. Reinforcement for making small steps
4. Use of instructions and prompts to elicit the desired behavior

Token economies (see Chapter 15) are used as the rewards, which can then be exchanged for previously agreed upon privileges. Some skepticism exists regarding the effectiveness of token economies. The chief drawback has been the inability to generalize to the community setting once the patient has been discharged (Cutting, 1985). Because of this, some behavioralists have turned their attention instead to social skills training.

SOCIAL SKILLS TRAINING

Social skills training has become one of the most widely used psychosocial interventions in the treatment of schizophrenia. Bellack (1984) defines a social skill as the use of

> ". . . eye contact, interpersonal distance, voice intonation, posture, etc., with appropriate variation as to sex, age, status, degree of familiarity, and the cultural background of the interpersonal partner, as well as with the context of the interaction."

Social dysfunction is a hallmark of schizophrenia. Indeed, impairment in social functioning is included as one of the defining diagnostic criteria for schizophrenia in the *DSM-III-R* (APA, 1987). Considerable attention is now being given to enhancement of social skills in these patients.

Focus of the educational procedure in social skills training is on role play. A series of brief scenarios are selected. These should be typical of situations patients experience in their daily lives and be graduated in terms of level of difficulty (Bellack, 1984). The therapist may serve as a role model for some behaviors. For example, "See how I sort of nod my head up and down and look at your face while you talk." The therapist's demonstration is followed by the patient's role playing. Immediate feedback is provided regarding the patient's presentation. Only by countless repetitions does the response gradually become smooth and effortless.

Progress is geared toward the patient's needs and limitations. The focus is on small units of behavior, and the training proceeds in a very gradual manner. Highly threatening issues are avoided, and emphasis is placed on functional skills that are relevant to daily living and are likely to secure positive reinforcement for the patient (Bellack, 1984).

Social Treatment

MILIEU THERAPY

Some clinicians believe that milieu therapy can be an appropriate treatment for the schizophrenic. In general, research supports the greater efficacy of psychotropic medication at all levels of care, and indications are that milieu therapy is more successful if used in conjunction with drug therapy.

Kaplan and Sadock (1985) state:

"Milieu therapy is enhanced by group meetings of patients and staff, separately and together, that focus on social functioning, rather than on psychopathology. In general, a therapeutic community encourages self-reliance and rewards the patient progressively for efforts toward social readaptation. The patient is expected to participate in planning his or her own treatment program and in helping other patients, and to assume responsibility in unit affairs and the outside world."

Research studies have indicated that schizophrenics treated with milieu therapy alone require longer hospital stays than those treated with drugs and behavior therapy. Other economic considerations, such as the need for a high staff-to-patient ratio, in addition to the longer admission, will likely limit the use of milieu therapy in the treatment of schizophrenia.

FAMILY THERAPY

Some therapists treat schizophrenia as an illness not of the patient alone, but of the entire family. Even when families appear to cope well, there is a notable impact on the mental health status of relatives. In one study by Hawks (1975), 50 percent of relatives stated that their own mental health had been adversely affected in the process of coping with the patient's mental disorder.

As health-care workers have become increasingly aware of the expanded role of family in the aftercare of schizophrenic relatives, interest has been renewed in family intervention programs designed to support the family system, prevent relapse, and foster the social recovery of the patient (Goldstein, 1984). These psychoeducational programs treat the family as a resource rather than a stress, with the focus on concrete problem solving and specific helping behaviors for coping with stress. Many of these programs recognize a biological basis for the illness and the impact that stress has on the patient's ability to function. By providing the family with information about the illness and suggestions for effective coping, psychoeducational programs serve to reduce the likelihood of the patient's relapse and the possible emergence of mental illness in previously nonaffected relatives.

Anderson et al (1980) outlined several goals and strategies in family therapy for schizophrenic patients. The goals include:

1. To increase family members' understanding of the illness
2. To reduce family stress
3. To enhance social networks for family interaction
4. To diminish long-term issues contributing to family stress

Strategies for intervention with families include:

1. Connection with, and introduction to, the family
2. Teaching survival skills for living with a schizophrenic
3. Monitoring the application of these skills
4. Continued treatment or disengagement

Family therapy typically consists of a brief program of family education about schizophrenia and a more extended program of family contact designed to reduce overt manifestations of conflict and to alter patterns of family communication and problem solving. The response to this type of therapy has been very dramatic. Goldstein (1984) reports on various research studies that indicate that some form of extended family intervention, together with a program of regular pharmacotherapy, can make a substantial contribution to the reduction of relapse in recently discharged schizophrenic patients, even with those who have been chronically ill for a number of years.

Organic Treatment

PSYCHOPHARMACOLOGY

Chlorpromazine (Thorazine) was first introduced in the United States in 1952. At that time, it was used in conjunction with barbiturates in surgical anesthesia. With increased use, the drug's psychic properties were recognized, and by 1954, it was marketed as an antipsychotic medication in the United States. The manufacture and sale of other antipsychotic drugs followed in rapid succession (see Chapter 12 for a detailed discussion of antipsychotic medications).

Antipsychotic medications are very effective in treating the symptoms of schizophrenia. Unfortunately, substantiated evidence of long-term recovery with antipsychotic medications is notably lacking. The most optimistic estimates suggest that approximately 10 percent of the patients fail to respond to drugs and remain chronically ill inside psychiatric hospitals for much of their lives. About 30 percent experience partial recovery; these people remain outside the hospital and are employed much of the time, but they still need some help in caring for themselves. Approximately 30 percent do not recover completely, but they are not obviously ill. Their occupational level may have decreased because of their illness, or they may be social isolates. The remaining 30 percent appear to recover completely. These people are almost continuously employed and stay out of institutions. Some are married. It is not obvious that they had previously suffered from schizophrenia (Lickey & Gordon, 1983).

Schatzberg & Cole (1986) state:

". . . although psychotropic drugs exert profound and beneficial effects on cognition, mood, and behavior, they often do not change the underlying disease process, which is frequently highly sensitive to intrapsychic, intrapersonal, and psychosocial stressors."

The efficacy of antipsychotic medications is enhanced by adjunct psychosocial therapy. Because the psychotic manifestations of the illness subside with use of the drugs, patients are generally more cooperative with the psychosocial therapies.

Antipsychotic drugs, also called neuroleptics or major tranquilizers, are effective in the treatment of acute and chronic manifestations of schizophrenia, as well as in maintenance therapy to prevent exacerbation of schizophrenic symptoms. However, because of a number of unpleasant and even dangerous side effects, the advisability of long-term use may be questionable. Common side effects include anticholinergic manifestations (dry mouth, blurred vision, constipation, urinary retention), nausea, gastrointestinal upset, skin rash, sedation, orthostatic hypotension, photosensitivity, decreased libido, retrograde ejaculation, gynecomastia, amenorrhea, weight gain, reduction in seizure threshold, agranulocytosis, extrapyramidal symptoms (pseudoparkinsonism, akinesia, akathisia, dystonia, oculogyric crisis), tardive dyskinesia, and neuroleptic malignant syndrome.

Antiparkinsonian agents may be prescribed to counteract the extrapyramidal symptoms associated with antipsychotic medications. These drugs are cholinergic blockers, producing the same anticholinergic side effects as the antipsychotic medications. Some physicians routinely prescribe the antiparkinsonian drug to be given on a scheduled basis with the antipsychotic medication. Some prefer to order the drug on a prn basis to be administered only if the neurological symptoms appear, thus reducing the compounded anticholinergic effects of the two drugs together. When the drug is given prn, it is extremely important for the nurse to be able to recognize the symptoms associated with extrapyramidal side effects so that he or she can administer the antiparkinsonian drug without delay (see Chapter 12 for a detailed discussion of antiparkinsonian drugs).

For those patients with schizophrenia who do not respond to antipsychotic medications, various other pharmacological options have been tried, albeit with little benefit to the patient. Schatzberg and Cole (1986) discuss trials with the following medication alternatives:

1. Reserpine: most often used as an antihypertensive; very slow onset of action; has produced tardive dyskinesia early in therapy in some individuals.
2. Lithium carbonate: can ameliorate schizophrenic symptoms or suppress episodic violence in schizophrenic patients but is seldom an adequate drug therapy alone.
3. Carbamazepine: ameliorates symptoms in some treatment-resistant psychotic patients but alone is not an adequate therapy for schizophrenia.
4. Valium: in high dosages, was shown to control psychotic symptoms in paranoid schizophrenics for up to 4 weeks. Follow-up data are not available.
5. Propranolol: may be useful in controlling temper outbursts in aggressive or violent psychotic patients.

The advent of antipsychotic medications in the 1950s was hailed as a medical breakthrough for psychiatry. At last the physician could do something substantive for the schizophrenic patient. No one knows exactly how the antipsychotic effect is achieved, or why it takes several weeks for these effects to be observed. Scientists cannot yet explain why patients do not become tolerant to antipsychotics, or why discontinuing the drug does not make the disease worse than it was before treatment (Lickey & Gordon, 1983). But by studying the action of antipsychotic drugs, progress has been made toward understanding what is wrong with the schizophrenic brain. Continual refinement of the research methods and investigation of other transmitter systems may reveal more precisely how the schizophrenic brain differs from the healthy one.

SUMMARY

Of all mental illness, schizophrenia undoubtedly results in the greatest amount of personal, emotional, and social costs. It presents an enormous threat to life and happiness, yet it remains a puzzle to the medical community. In fact, for many years there was little agreement regarding a definition of the concept of schizophrenia. The *DSM-III-R* (APA, 1987) identifies specific criteria for the diagnosis of the disorder. These criteria were presented in this chapter.

The initial symptoms of schizophrenia most often occur in early adulthood, and development of the disorder can be viewed in four phases: the schizoid personality, the prodromal phase, the active phase of schizophrenia, and the residual phase.

The cause of schizophrenia remains unclear. Research continues, and many contemporary psychiatrists are giving more credence to the biological theories and are placing less emphasis on psychosocial influences. The transactional view, however, supports the idea that no single factor can be implicated in the etiology, but that the disease most likely results from a combination of influences including genetics, biochemical dysfunction, and physiological, psychological, or environmental factors.

Various types of schizophrenic and related psychotic disorders have been identified. They are differentiated by their total picture of clinical symptomatology. They include disorganized schizophrenia, catatonic schizophrenia, paranoid schizophrenia, undifferentiated schizophrenia, residual schizophrenia, schizoaffective disorder, brief reactive psychosis, schizophreniform disorder, delusional disorder, and induced psychotic disorder.

Care of the patient with schizophrenic psychosis was presented in the context of the five steps of the nursing process. Nursing assessment is based on knowledge of symptomatology related to thought content and form, perception, affect, sense of self, volition, impaired interpersonal functioning and relationship to the external world, and psychomotor behavior. Nursing diagnoses were formulated from the assessment data, and a plan of care was developed. A critical pathway of care for the schizophrenic patient was included as a guideline for nurses who follow a program of case management. Guidelines for evaluation of patient outcomes were presented.

Various treatment modalities for the schizophrenic patient were discussed. They include individual psychotherapy, group therapy, behavior therapy, social skills training, milieu therapy, family therapy, and psychopharmacology. For the majority of patients, the most effective treatment appears to be a combination of psychotropic medication and psychosocial therapy.

REVIEW QUESTIONS
Self-Examination/Learning Exercise

*Select the answer that is **most** appropriate for each of the following questions.*

Tony, a 20-year-old college dropout who had become increasingly withdrawn, suspicious, and isolated during the past 2 months since his return from an out-of-state college, is brought to the emergency room. His family reports that he has been looking at them strangely as if he didn't know them, refusing to talk to anyone, spending a lot of time in his room alone, refusing all help. The father brought the patient to the hospital against his will following a verbal argument in the course of which the patient had attempted to stab the father with a kitchen knife. The father had successfully subdued him and had removed the weapon. On arrival at the emergency room, the patient was agitated and exhibiting acutely psychotic symptoms. He reports that "they" told him to kill his father before his father kills him. Verbalizations are often incoherent. Affect is flat, and he continuously scans the environment. He is admitted to the psychiatric unit with a diagnosis of schizophreniform disorder, provisional.

1. The *initial* nursing intervention for Tony is to:
   a. give him an injection of chlorpromazine (Thorazine).
   b. ensure a safe environment for him and others.
   c. place him in restraints.
   d. order him a nutritious diet.

2. The primary goal in working with Tony would be to:
   a. promote interaction with others.
   b. decrease his anxiety and increase trust.
   c. improve his relationship with his parents.
   d. encourage participation in therapy activities.

3. Orders from the physician include 100 mg chlorpromazine (Thorazine) STAT and then 50 mg bid; 2 mg benztropine (Cogentin) bid prn. For what reason is the order for chlorpromazine given?
   a. To reduce extrapyramidal symptoms
   b. To prevent neuroleptic malignant syndrome
   c. To decrease psychotic symptoms
   d. To induce sleep

4. Benzotropine was ordered on a prn basis. Which of the following assessments by the nurse would convey a need for this medication?
   a. The patient's level of agitation increases.
   b. The patient complains of a sore throat.
   c. The patient's skin has a yellowish cast.
   d. The patient develops tremors and a shuffling gait.

5. Tony begins to tell the nurse about how the CIA is looking for him and will kill him if they find him. The most appropriate response by the nurse is:
   a. "That's ridiculous, Tony. No one is going to hurt you."
   b. "The CIA isn't interested in people like you, Tony."
   c. "Why do you think the CIA wants to kill you?"
   d. "I find that very hard to believe, Tony."

6. Tony's belief about the CIA is an example of a:
   a. Delusion of persecution
   b. Delusion of reference
   c. Delusion of control or influence
   d. Delusion of grandeur

7. Tony tilts his head to the side, stops talking in midsentence, and listens intently. The nurse recognizes with these signs that Tony is likely experiencing:
   a. Somatic delusions
   b. Catatonic stupor
   c. Auditory hallucinations
   d. Pseudoparkinsonism

8. The most appropriate nursing intervention for the symptom described above is:
   a. Ask the patient to describe his physical symptoms.
   b. Ask the patient to describe what he is hearing.
   c. Administer a dose of benztropine.
   d. Call the physician for additional orders.

9. Should Tony suddenly become aggressive and violent on the unit, which of the following approaches would be *best* for the nurse to use *first?*
   a. Provide large motor activities to relieve Tony's pent-up tension.
   b. Administer a large dose of sedative to keep Tony calm.
   c. Call for sufficient help to control the situation in a safe manner.
   d. Convey to Tony that his behavior is unacceptable and will not be permitted.

10. Tony and his parents attend a weekly family therapy group. The primary focus of this type of group is:
    a. to discuss concrete problem solving and adaptive behaviors for coping with stress.
    b. to introduce the family to others with the same problem.
    c. to keep the patient and family in touch with the health-care system.
    d. to promote family interaction with the identified patient.

REFERENCES

American Psychiatric Association. (1987). *Diagnostic and statistical manual of mental disorders* (3rd ed., rev.). Washington, DC: American Psychiatric Association.

Anderson, C. M. et al. (1980). Family treatment of adult schizophrenic patients: A psychoeducational approach. *Schizophrenia Bulletin, 6,* 490–505.

Arieti, S. (1976). The psychotherapeutic approach to schizophrenia. In Kemali et al. (Eds.), *Schizophrenia today.* Oxford: Pergamon Press.

Bateson, G. et al (1956). Towards a theory of schizophrenia. *Behavioral Science, 1,* 251–264.

Bellack, A. S. (1984). *Schizophrenia: Treatment, management, and rehabilitation.* Orlando, FL: Grune & Stratton.

Birchwood, M. J. et al. (1989). *Schizophrenia: An integrated approach to research and treatment.* New York: New York University Press.

Bowen, M. (1978). A family concept of schizophrenia. In M. Bowen (Ed.), *Family therapy in clinical practice.* New York: Aronson.

Brown G. W. & Birley, J. (1968). Crises and life changes and the onset of schizophrenia. *Journal of Health and Social Behavior. 9,* 203–214.

Cutting, J. (1985). *The psychology of schizophrenia.* New York: Churchill Livingstone.

Erikson, E. (1963). *Childhood and society* (2nd ed.). New York: WW Norton & Co.

Freud, S. (1961). The ego and the id. In *Standard edition of the complete psychological works of Freud, vol XIX*. London: The Hogarth Press.

Goldstein, M. J. (1987). Psychosocial issues. *Schizophrenia Bulletin, 13*(1)157–172.

Goldstein, M. J. (1984). Family intervention programs. In A. S. Bellack (Ed.), *Schizophrenia: Treatment, management, and rehabilitation*. Orlando, FL: Grune & Stratton.

Gomes-Schwartz, B. (1984). Individual psychotherapy of schizophrenia. In A. S. Bellack (Ed.), *Schizophrenia: Treatment, management, and rehabilitation*. Orlando, FL: Grune & Stratton.

Gottesman, I. I. (1978). Schizophrenia and genetics: Where are we? Are you sure? In L. C. Wynne et al. (Eds.), *The nature of schizophrenia: New approaches to research and treatment*. New York: John Wiley & Sons.

Gottesman, I. I. & Shields, J. (1982). *Schizophrenia: The epigenetic puzzle*. Cambridge, England: Cambridge University Press.

Haber, J., Hoskins, P.P., Leach, A. M., and Sideleau, B. F. (1987). *Comprehensive psychiatric nursing* (3rd ed.). New York: McGraw-Hill.

Hawks, D. (1975). Community care: An analysis of assumptions. *Br J Psychiatry, 127,* 276–283.

Hollandsworth, J. G. (1990). *The physiology of psychological disorders*. New York: Plenum Press.

Kaplan, H. I. & Sadock, B. J. (1985). *Modern synopsis of comprehensive textbook of psychiatry* (4th ed.). Baltimore: Williams & Wilkins.

Keith, S. J. & Matthews, S. (1984). Group psychotherapy. In A. S. Bellack (Ed.), *Schizophrenia: Treatment, management, and rehabilitation*. Orlando, FL: Grune & Stratton.

Liberman, R. P. (1970). Behavior modification with chronic mental patients. *J Chron Dis, 23,* 803–812.

Liberman, R. P. et al. (1984). The nature and problem of schizophrenia. In A. S. Bellack (Ed.), *Schizophrenia: Treatment, management, and rehabilitation*. Orlando, FL: Grune & Stratton.

Lickey, M. E. & Gordon, B. (1983). *Drugs for mental illness: A revolution in psychiatry*. New York: WH Freeman and Company.

Mahler, M, Pine, F. and Bergman, A. (1975). *The psychological birth of the human infant*. New York: Basic Books.

Schatzberg, A. F. & Cole, J. O. (1986). *Manual of clinical psychopharmacology*. Washington, DC: American Psychiatric Press.

Scheibel, A. B. (1991, Summer). Schizophrenia: Cells in disarray. *Journal of the California Alliance for the Mentally Ill, 2*(4), 9–10.

Stevens, J. R. (1982). Neuropathology of schizophrenia. *Arch Gen Psychiatry, 39,* 1131–1139.

Strauss, J. S. (1983). The evolution of psychotherapeutic approaches for affective and schizophrenic disorders. In M. R. Zales (Ed.), *Affective and schizophrenic disorders*. New York: Brunner/Mazel.

Sullivan, H. S. (1953). *The interpersonal theory of psychiatry*. New York: WW Norton & Co.

Tsuang, M. T. (1982). *Schizophrenia: The facts*. New York: Oxford University Press.

Weinberger, D. R. et al. (1979). Lateral cerebral ventricular enlargement in chronic schizophrenia. *Arch Gen Psychiatry, 36,* 735–739.

Wiersma, D. et al. (1983). Social class and schizophrenia. *Psychol Med (13):* 141–150.

BIBLIOGRAPHY

Altshuler, L. (1991, Summer). Neuroanatomy in schizophrenia and affective disorder. *Journal of the California Alliance for the Mentally Ill, 2*(4), 27–30.

Bleuler, E. (1966). *Dementia praecox or the group of schizophrenias (1908)*. J. Zinkin (Trans.) New York: International University Press.

Chapman, T. (1991, June). The nurse's role in neuroleptic medications. *J Psychosoc Nurs, 29*(6), 6–8.

Dzurec, L. C. (1990, August). How do they see themselves? Self-perception and functioning for people with chronic schizophrenia. *J Psychosoc Nurs, 28*(8), 10–14.

Feinberg, I. (1991, Summer). Synaptic pruning and the adolescent brain. *Journal of the California Alliance for the Mentally Ill, 2*(4), 22–24.

Field, W. E. (1985, January). Hearing voices. *J Psychosoc Nurs, 23*(1), 8–14.

Jernigan, T. L. (1991, Summer). When and why does schizophrenia develop? *Journal of the California Alliance for the Mentally Ill, 2*(4), 25–26.

Kahn, E. M. (1984, July). Psychotherapy with chronic schizophrenics. *J Psychosoc Nurs, 22*(7), 20–25.

Malone, J. A. (1990, August). Schizophrenia research update: Implications for nursing. *J Psychosoc Nurs, 28*(8), 4–9.

Mednick, S. A. (1991, Summer). Fetal neural development and adult schizophrenia. *Journal of the California Alliance for the Mentally Ill, 2,* 6–8.

Peschel, E. & Peschel, R. (1991, Summer). Neurobiological disorders. *Journal of the California Alliance for the Mentally Ill, 2*(4), 4.

Smith, S. F., Karasik, D. A. and Meyer, B. J. (1984). *Psychiatric and psychosocial nursing.* Los Altos, CA: National Nursing Review.

Stevenson, S. (1991, September). Heading off violence with verbal de-escalation. *J Psychosoc Nurs 29*(9), 6–10.

Townsend, M. C. (1991). *Nursing diagnoses in psychiatric nursing: A pocket guide for care plan construction* (2nd ed.). Philadelphia: FA Davis.

Wirshing, W. C. (1991, Summer). Searching the brain: Trying to see neurobiological disorders. *Journal of the California Alliance for the Mentally Ill, 2*(4), 2–3.

Wirshing, W. C. (1991, Summer). Schizophrenia, neuroleptics, and brain rust: Speculations from the research fringe. *Journal of the California Alliance for the Mentally Ill, 2*(4), 31–34.

MOOD DISORDERS

KEY TERMS
anticipatory grieving
altruistic suicide
anomic suicide
bereavement overload
bipolar disorder
cognitive therapy
cyclothymia
delayed grief
delirious mania
dysthymia
egoistic suicide
tyramine
exaggerated grief
grief
hypomania
mania
melancholia
mood
mourning
postpartum depression
prolonged grief
psychomotor retardation

OBJECTIVES

After reading this chapter, the student will be able to:

1. Recount historical perspectives of mood disorders.
2. Discuss epidemiological statistics related to mood disorders.
3. Differentiate between normal and maladaptive responses to loss.
4. Describe various types of mood disorders.
5. Identify predisposing factors in the development of mood disorders.
6. Discuss implications of depression related to developmental stage.
7. Identify symptomatology associated with mood disorders and use this information in patient assessment.
8. Formulate nursing diagnoses and goals of care for patients with mood disorders.
9. Describe appropriate nursing interventions for behaviors associated with mood disorders.
10. Describe relevant criteria for evaluating nursing care of patients with mood disorders.
11. Discuss various modalities relevant to treatment of mood disorders.
12. Discuss epidemiological statistics and risk factors related to suicide.
13. Describe predisposing factors implicated in the etiology of suicide.
14. Differentiate between facts and fables regarding suicide.
15. Apply the nursing process to individuals exhibiting suicidal behavior.

INTRODUCTION

Depression is likely the oldest and still one of the most frequently described psychiatric illnesses. Symptoms of depression have been described almost as far back as there is evidence of written documentation.

An occasional bout with the "blues," a feeling of sadness or downheartedness, is common among healthy people and considered to be a normal, healthy response to everyday disappointments in life. These episodes are short-lived as the individual adapts to the loss, change, or failure (real or perceived) that has been experienced. Pathological depression occurs when adaptation is ineffective.

This chapter focuses on the consequences of dysfunctional grieving, as it is manifested by mood disorders. Mood describes an individual's sustained emotional tone, which significantly influences behavior, personality, and perception. Mood disorders are classified as depressive or bipolar.

A historical perspective and epidemiological statistics related to mood disorders are presented. Predisposing factors that have been implicated in the etiology of mood disorders provide a framework for studying the dynamics of depression and bipolar disorder. A discussion of the normal grief process precedes an explanation of the maladaptive response.

The implications of depression relevant to individuals of various developmental stages is discussed. An explanation of the symptomatology is presented as background knowledge for assessing the patient with mood disorder. Nursing care is described in the context of the nursing process, and critical pathways of care are included as guidelines for use in a case management approach. Suicide as a coping strategy closely associated with mood disorders is discussed. Various medical treatment modalities are explored.

HISTORICAL PERSPECTIVE

Many ancient cultures (e.g., Babylonian, Egyptian, Hebrew) have believed in the supernatural or divine origin of depression and mania (Georgotas & Cancro, 1988). The Old Testament states in the Book of Samuel that King Saul's depression was inflicted by an "evil spirit" sent from God to "torment" him.

A clearly nondivine point of view regarding depressive and manic states was held by the Greek medical community from the 5th century B.C. through the 3rd century A.D. This represented the thinking of Hippocrates, Celsus, and Galen, among others. They strongly rejected the idea of divine origin, and considered the brain as the seat of all emotional states (Georgotas & Cancro, 1988). Hippocrates believed that melancholia was caused by an excess of black bile, a heavily toxic substance produced in the spleen or intestine, which affected the brain.

During the Renaissance period, several new theories evolved. Depression was viewed by some as being the result of obstruction of vital air circulation, excessive brooding, or helpless situations beyond the patient's control. These strong emotions of depression and mania were reflected in major literary works of the time, including Shakespeare's *King Lear*, *Macbeth*, and *Hamlet*.

In the 19th century, the definition of mania was narrowed down from the concept of total madness to that of a disorder of affect and action (Berrios, 1988). The old notion of melancholia was refurnished with meaning, and emphasis was placed on the primary affective nature of the disorder. Finally, an introduction was made to the possibility of an alternating pattern of affective symptomatology associated with the disorders.

Contemporary thinking has been shaped to a great deal by the works of Sigmund Freud, Emil Kraepelin, and Adolf Meyer. Evolving from these early 20th century models, current ideas about mood disorders are generally placed within frames of reference that represent the intrapsychic, behavioral, and biological perspectives (Whybrow, Akiskal, & McKinney, 1984). These various perspectives lend support to the notion of multiple causation in the development of mood disorders.

EPIDEMIOLOGY

Current estimates suggest that 10 to 14 million Americans are afflicted with some form of major affective disorder. Recent studies indicate that as many as 1 in 10 Americans may experience, at some point in their lives, the severity of mood disturbance associated with an affective disorder (Charney & Weissman, 1988). Additional statistics include those by the World Health Organization (WHO), which has established the worldwide annual prevalence rate for depression at 3 percent to 5 percent—approximately 100 million people (WHO, 1977). This preponderance has led to the perception of depression by some researchers as "the common cold of psychiatric disorders," and this generation as an "age of melancholia."

Gender

Studies indicate that the incidence of depressive disorder is higher in women than it is in men by about 2 to 1. The incidence of bipolar disorder is roughly equal, with a ratio of women to men of 1.2 to 1.

Age

Several studies have shown that the incidence of depression is higher in young women and has a tendency to decrease with age. The opposite has been found in men, with the prevalence of depressive symptoms being lower in younger men and increasing with age (Boyd & Weissman, 1982). Studies regarding the incidence of bipolar disorder are inconsistent. Some studies indicate that the incidence rises until the age of 35, then gradually declines (Myers et al, 1984; Weissman et al, 1988). Others suggest that the incidence of mania consistently increases with age and that half of the new cases occur in those older than age 50 (Spicer et al, 1973).

Social Class

Studies relating mood disorders to social class were reported by Charney and Weissman (1988). Results have indicated an inverse relationship between social class and report of depressive symptoms. Bipolar disorder appears to occur more frequently among the higher social classes, especially professionals and the highly educated.

Race

Studies have shown no consistent relationship between race and affective disorder. One problem encountered in reviewing racial comparisons has

to do with the socioeconomic class of the race being investigated. Sample populations of nonwhite patients are many times predominantly lower class and are often compared to white populations from middle and upper social classes. Other studies suggest a second problematic factor in the study of racial comparisons. Nonwhite patients (particularly African-Americans and Hispanics) may be more likely to be misdiagnosed as schizophrenic, instead of bipolar manic, than whites. Bell and Mehta (1980) suggested that this misdiagnosis may result from language barriers between patients and physicians who are unfamiliar with cultural aspects of nonwhite patients' language and behavior.

Marital Status

The highest incidence of depressive symptoms has been indicated in single and divorced persons (Charney & Weissman, 1988). Gender differences reveal lowest rates of depressive symptoms among married men, with the highest rates being reported by married women and single men. No consistent relationship has been revealed between marital status and bipolar disorder.

Seasonality

A number of studies have examined seasonal patterns associated with mood disorders. These studies have revealed two prevalent periods of seasonal involvement: one in the spring (March, April, and May) and one in the fall (September, October, and November). This pattern tends to parallel the seasonal pattern for suicide, which shows a large peak in the spring and a smaller one in October (Goodwin & Jamison, 1990).

THE GRIEF RESPONSE

Loss can be defined as "an experience in which an individual relinquishes a connection to a valued object." The *object* may be animate or inanimate, a relationship or situation, or even a change or a failure (real or perceived). Following are examples of some notable forms of loss.

1. A significant other, through death, divorce, or separation for any reason.

2. Illness or hospitalization can represent a loss for an individual due to the many changes that may be incurred, as well as the possible fears associated with threat to physiological integrity.

3. A decrease in self-esteem can be experienced as a loss in the event that one is unable to meet self-expectations or the expectations of others (or even if these expectations are only *perceived* by the individual as unfulfilled).

4. Personal possessions symbolize familiarity and security in a person's life. Separation from these familiar and personally valued external objects represents a loss of material extensions of the self.

Some texts differentiate the terms *mourning* and *grief* by describing mourning as the "psychological process (or stages) through which the individual passes on the way to successful adaptation to the loss of a valued object." *Grief* is defined as the "subjective states that accompany mourning, or the emotional work involved in the mourning process." For purposes of this text, grief work and the process of mourning will be collectively referred to as the *grief response*.

Stages of Grief

Behavior patterns associated with the grief response include many individual variations. However, sufficient similarities have been observed to warrant characterization of grief as a syndrome that has a predictable course with an expected resolution (Kaplan & Sadock, 1985). A number of theorists, including Kübler-Ross (1969), Bowlby (1961), and Engel (1964), have described behavioral stages through which individuals advance in their progression toward resolution. A number of variables influence one's progression through the grief process. Some individuals may reach acceptance, only to revert to an earlier stage; some may never complete the sequence; and indeed, some may never progress beyond the initial stage. A comparison of the similarities among these three models is presented in Table 19.1.

ELISABETH KÜBLER-ROSS

These well-known stages of the grief process were identified by Kübler-Ross in her extensive work with dying patients. Behaviors associated with each of these stages can be observed in individuals experiencing the loss of any object of personal value.

Stage I. Denial In this stage the individual does not acknowledge that the loss has occurred. Verbal expression may reflect ideas of, "No, it can't be true!" or "It's just not possible." This stage may offer the individual some protection against the psychological pain of reality.

Stage II. Anger This is the stage during which reality sets in. Feelings associated with this stage include sadness, guilt, shame, helplessness, and hopelessness. Self-blame or blaming of others may lead to feelings of anger toward self and others. The anxiety level may be elevated, and the individual may experience confusion and a decreased ability to function independently. He or she may be preoccupied with an idealized image of the lost object. Numerous somatic complaints are common.

Stage III. Bargaining At this stage in the dying process, the individual attempts to strike a bargain with God for a second chance, or for more time. The person acknowledges the loss, or impending loss, but holds out hope for additional alternatives, as evidenced by statements such as, "If only I could . . ." or "If only I had . . ."

Stage IV. Depression In this stage, the individual mourns for that which has been or will be lost. This is a very painful stage during which the individual must confront feelings associated with having lost an object of value (called *reactive* depression). An example might be the individual who is mourning a change in body image. Feelings associated with an impending loss (called *preparatory* depression) are also confronted. Examples include permanent life-style changes related to the altered body image or even an impending loss of life itself. Regression, withdrawal, and social isolation may be observed behaviors associated with this stage. Therapeutic intervention should be available, but not imposed, and with guidelines for implementation based on patient readiness.

Stage V. Acceptance At this time, the individual has worked through the behaviors associated with the other stages, and accepts or is resigned to the loss. Anxiety decreases and methods for coping without the lost object have been established. There is less preoccupation with what has been lost and increasing interest in other aspects of the environment. If this is an impending death of self, the

Table 19.1 STAGES OF THE NORMAL GRIEF RESPONSE:

A Comparison of Models by Elisabeth Kübler-Ross, John Bowlby, and George Engel

STAGES				
Kübler-Ross	Bowlby	Engel	Possible Time Dimension	Behaviors
I. Denial	I. Numbness/Protest	I. Shock/Disbelief	Occurs immediately upon experiencing the loss. Usually lasts no more than 2 weeks.	Individual refuses to acknowledge that the loss has occurred.
II. Anger	II. Disequilibrium	II. Developing awareness	In most cases, begins within hours of the loss. Peaks within 2 to 4 weeks.	Anger is directed toward self or others. Ambivalence and guilt may be felt toward the lost object.
III. Bargaining				The individual fervently seeks alternatives to improve current situation.
		III. Restitution		Attends to various rituals associated with the culture in which the loss has occurred.
IV. Depression	III. Disorganization and despair	IV. Resolution of the loss	A year or more	The actual work of grieving. Preoccupation with the lost object. Feelings of helplessness and loneliness occur in response to realization of the loss. Feelings associated with the loss are confronted.
V. Acceptance	IV. Reorganization	V. Recovery		Resolution is complete. The bereaved person experiences a reinvestment in new relationships and new goals. In the case of the terminally ill person, he or she expresses a readiness to die.

individual is ready to die. The person may become very quiet and withdrawn, seemingly void of feelings. These behaviors represent an attempt to facilitate the passage by slowly disengaging from the environment.

JOHN BOWLBY

John Bowlby hypothesized four stages in the grief process. He implies that these behaviors can be observed in all individuals who have experienced the loss of a valued object, even in babies as young as 6 months of age (Bowlby, 1973).

Stage I. Numbness or Protest This stage is characterized by a feeling of shock and disbelief that the loss has occurred. Reality of the loss is not acknowledged.

Stage II. Disequilibrium During this stage, the individual has a profound urge to recover the lost object. Behaviors associated with this stage include a preoccupation with the lost object, intense weeping and expressions of anger toward self and others, and feelings of ambivalence and guilt toward the lost object.

Stage III. Disorganization and Despair Feelings of despair occur in response to the realization that the loss has occurred. Activities of daily living become increasingly disorganized, and behavior is characterized by restlessness and aimlessness. Efforts to regain productive patterns of behavior are ineffective and the individual experiences fear, helplessness, and hopelessness. Somatic complaints are common. Perceptions of visualizing or being in the presence of the lost object may occur. Social isolation is common and the individual may feel a great deal of loneliness.

Stage IV. Reorganization The individual accepts or becomes resigned to the loss. New goals and patterns of organization are established. The individual begins a reinvestment in new relationships and indicates a readiness to move forward within the environment. Grief subsides and recedes into valued remembrances.

GEORGE ENGEL

Stage I. Shock and Disbelief The initial reaction to a loss is a stunned, numb feeling and refusal by the individual to acknowledge the reality of the loss. Engel (1964) states that this stage is an attempt on the part of the individual to protect the self "against the effects of the overwhelming stress by raising the threshold against its recognition or against the painful feelings evoked thereby."

Stage II. Developing Awareness This stage begins within minutes to hours of the loss. Behaviors associated with this stage include excessive crying and regression to a state of helplessness and childlike manner. Awareness of the loss creates feelings of emptiness, frustration, anguish, and de-

spair. Anger may be directed toward the self or to others in the environment who are held accountable for the loss.

Stage III. Restitution In this stage, the various rituals associated with loss within a culture are performed. Examples include funerals, wakes, special attire, a gathering of friends and family, and religious practices customary to the spiritual beliefs of the bereaved. Participation in these rituals is believed to assist the individual to accept the reality of the loss and facilitates the recovery process.

Stage IV. Resolution of the Loss This stage is characterized by a preoccupation with the lost object. The concept of the lost object is idealized, and the individual may even imitate admired qualities of that which has been lost. Preoccupation with the lost object gradually decreases during a period of a year or more, and the individual eventually begins to make a reinvestment of feelings in others within the environment.

Stage V. Recovery Obsession with the lost object has ended and the individual is able to go on with his or her life.

Length of the Grief Process

Stages of grief allow bereaved persons an orderly approach to the resolution of mourning. Each stage presents tasks that must be overcome through a painful experiential process. Engel (1964) has stated that successful resolution of the grief response is thought to have occurred when a bereaved individual is able "to remember comfortably and realistically both the pleasures and disappointments of the lost [object]." Length of the grief process is exceedingly individual and can last for a number of years without being maladaptive. The acute phase of normal grieving usually lasts 6 to 8 weeks — longer in older adults — but complete resolution of the grief response may take up to 3 years (Thompson et al, 1986).

Smith et al (1984) have identified the following factors that influence the eventual outcome of the grief response:

1. The importance of the lost object as a source of support.
2. The degree of dependency on the relationship with the lost object. The greater the degree of

dependency, the more difficult is the task of resolution.

3. The degree of ambivalence felt toward the lost object. A love-hate relationship may instill feelings of guilt that can interfere with the work of mourning.

4. The number and nature of other meaningful relationships the mourner has. Letting go of the attachment to the lost object is facilitated by support from significant others.

5. The number and nature of previous grief experiences. Grief is cumulative, and if previous losses have not been resolved, each succeeding grief response becomes more difficult.

6. The age of a lost person is influential. The loss of a child usually has a more profound effect on the survivor than that of an elderly parent.

7. Health of the mourner at the time of the loss. The state of one's physical and psychological condition influences the capacity to cope with the stress of the loss.

8. The degree of preparation for the loss. The experience of *anticipatory grieving* is thought to facilitate the grief response that occurs at the time of the actual loss.

Anticipatory Grief

Anticipatory grieving is the initiation and actual process of grieving that takes place when anticipating a significant loss, before the significant loss actually takes place (Thompson et al, 1986). In anticipatory grieving, the stages of grief and the feelings and behaviors associated with them are very similar to those experienced in normal grieving. One dissimilar aspect relates to the fact that conventional grief tends to diminish in intensity with the passage of time. Conversely, anticipatory grief may increase in intensity as the expected loss becomes more imminent.

Although anticipatory grief is thought to facilitate the actual mourning process following the loss, there may be some problems. In the case of a dying person, difficulties can arise when the family members complete the process of anticipatory grief and detachment from the dying person occurs prematurely. Feelings of loneliness and isolation are experienced by the dying person as the psychological pain of imminent death is faced without family support. Another example of difficulties associated

with premature completion of the grief response is described by Kaplan and Sadock (1985):

> "Once anticipatory grief has been expended, it may be difficult to reestablish the prior relationship, as has been demonstrated with the return from combat or concentration camps of persons previously thought to be dead."

Anticipatory grieving may serve as a defense for some individuals to ease the burden of loss when it actually occurs. It may prove to be less functional for others who, because of interpersonal, psychological, or sociocultural variables, are unable in advance of the actual loss to express the intense feelings that accompany the grief response.

MALADAPTIVE RESPONSES TO LOSS

When, then, is the grieving response considered to be maladaptive? Lindemann (1944) described two types of pathological grief reactions: the delayed reaction and the distorted reaction. Most theorists agree that resolution has failed to occur when the grief process has been delayed, inhibited, prolonged, or exaggerated.

Delayed or Inhibited Grief

Delayed or inhibited grief refers to the absence of evidence of grief when it ordinarily would be expected (Kaplan & Sadock, 1985). Many times, cultural influences effect the delayed response, such as the expectation to keep a "stiff upper lip."

Delayed or inhibited grief is potentially pathological because the person is simply not dealing with the reality of the loss. He or she remains fixed in the denial stage of the grief process, sometimes for many years. When this occurs, the grief response may be triggered, sometimes many years later, when the individual experiences a subsequent loss. Sometimes the grief process is triggered spontaneously or in response to a seemingly insignificant event. Overreaction to another person's loss may be one manifestation of delayed grief.

The recognition of delayed grief is critical because, depending on the profoundness of the loss, the failure of the mourning process may prevent assimilation of the loss and thereby delay a return to satisfying living (Ruark & Gonda, 1988). Delayed grieving most commonly occurs due to ambivalent feelings toward the lost object, outside pressure to resume normal function, or to perceived lack of internal and external resources to cope with a profound loss.

Prolonged Grief

The grief response is considered to be pathologically prolonged if there has been no resumption of normal activities of daily living within 4 to 8 weeks of a loss (Ruark & Gonda, 1988). The prolonged grief pattern has been associated with self-blame on the part of the bereaved, difficulty accepting the loss, sudden and untimely loss, and a history of a passive clinging type of relationship with the one who has died (Parkes, 1975).

Stories abound in the literature of bereaved individuals who establish shrines to their dead and conduct rituals that perpetuate the grieving process. Other evidences of prolonged grief may include an intensification, rather than diminishment, of the behaviors associated with normal grieving; development of physical symptoms similar to those experienced by the deceased person before death; progressive social isolation and interrupted interpersonal relationships with friends and relatives; and participation in activities that are detrimental to one's social or economic existence (Shives, 1990).

Exaggerated Grief Response

Lindemann (1944) described a distorted grief reaction in which all of the symptoms associated with normal grieving are exaggerated out of proportion. Feelings of sadness, helplessness, hopelessness, powerlessness, anger, and guilt as well as numerous somatic complaints render the individual dysfunctional in terms of management of daily living. Horowitz and associates (1980) describe this pathological grief reaction as:

". . . the intensification of grief to the level where the person is overwhelmed, resorts to maladaptive behavior, or remains interminably in the state of grief without progression of the mourning process toward completion."

When the distorted grief reaction occurs, the individual remains fixed in the anger stage of the grief response. This anger may be directed toward others in the environment to whom the individual may be attributing the loss. However, many times the anger is turned inward on the self. When this occurs, depression is the result. Depressive mood disorder is a type of distorted grief reaction.

Normal versus Maladaptive Grieving

Several authors have identified one crucial difference between normal and maladaptive grieving: the loss of self-esteem. Henderson and Nite (1978) state, "The loss of self-esteem that almost invariably occurs in depression is not present with normal grief." Regarding depression, Brown, Harris, and Copeland (1977) have stated:

"We believe that what is crucial in determining whether the specific feelings of hopelessness develop into the three feelings that the world is meaningless, the self is worthless, and the future hopeless is a person's ongoing self-esteem."

Becker (1964) also expounds upon this major difference between normal grieving and a maladaptive response (depression). He states, "It is the threat to self-esteem, or the threat of reduction in self-esteem, which ultimately precipitates the depression."

TYPES OF MOOD DISORDERS

The *Diagnostic and Statistical Manual of Mental Disorders*, ed 3., revised (*DSM-III-R*) (American Psychiatric Association [APA], 1987) describes the essential feature of these disorders as a disturbance of mood, accompanied by a full or partial manic or depressive syndrome, that is not due to any other physical or mental disorder. Mood disorders are classified under two major categories: depressive disorders and bipolar disorders.

Depressive Disorders

MAJOR DEPRESSION, SINGLE EPISODE OR RECURRENT

This disorder is characterized by depressed mood or loss of interest or pleasure in usual activities and pastimes (APA, 1987). Evidence of impaired social and occupational functioning has existed for at least 2 weeks. There is no history of manic behavior. Major depression is described as recurrent when two or more episodes of depressed mood have occurred, each separated by at least 2 months of return to more or less usual functioning.

Major depression may be further classified as follows:

1. *With psychotic features.* The impairment of reality testing is evident. The individual experiences delusions or hallucinations.
2. *Melancholic type.* A typically severe form of major depressive episode. Symptoms are exaggerated. There is a loss of interest or pleasure in all activities. The individual has experienced previous major depressive episodes followed by complete recovery. History reveals a good response to antidepressant or other somatic therapy.
3. *Chronic.* This classification applies when the current episode has lasted 2 consecutive years without a period of 2 months or longer in which there have been no depressive symptoms.
4. *Seasonal pattern.* This diagnosis indicates that there has been at least a 3-year pattern of onset of depressive disorder beginning between the early part of October and the end of November and ending between mid-February and mid-April. Full remissions occur in between these periods.

The *DSM-III-R* diagnostic criteria for major depression are presented in Table 19.2.

DYSTHYMIA

This disorder is also identified by the *DSM-III-R* as depressive neurosis. Characteristics of this mood disturbance are similar to, if somewhat milder than, those ascribed to major depression. There is no evidence of psychotic symptoms. The essential feature is a chronic depressed mood (or possibly an irritable mood in children or adolescents), for most of the day more days than not, for at least 2 years (1 year for children and adolescents).

Table 19.2 DIAGNOSTIC CRITERIA FOR MAJOR DEPRESSION

A. At least five of the following symptoms have been present during the same 2-week period and represent a change from previous functioning; at least one of the symptoms is either (1) depressed mood or (2) loss of interest or pleasure.
1. Depressed mood (or can be irritable mood in children and adolescents) most of the day, nearly every day, as indicated either by subjective account or observation by others
2. Markedly diminished interest or pleasure in all, or almost all, activities most of the day, nearly every day (as indicated either by subjective account or observation by others of apathy most of the time)
3. Significant weight loss or weight gain when not dieting (e.g., more than 5 percent of body weight in a month), or decrease or increase in appetite nearly every day (in children, consider failure to make expected weight gains)
4. Insomnia or hypersomnia nearly every day
5. Psychomotor agitation or retardation nearly every day (observable by others, not merely subjective feelings of restlessness or being slowed down)
6. Fatigue or loss of energy nearly every day
7. Feelings of worthlessness or excessive or inappropriate guilt (which may be delusional) nearly every day (not merely self-reproach or guilt about being sick)
8. Diminished ability to think or concentrate, or indecisiveness, nearly every day (either by subjective account or as observed by others)
9. Recurrent thoughts of death (not just fear of dying), recurrent suicidal ideation without a specific plan, or a suicide attempt or a specific plan for committing suicide

B. 1. It cannot be established that an organic factor initiated and maintained the disturbance.
2. The disturbance is not a normal reaction to the death of a loved one (uncomplicated bereavement).

C. Has never had a manic episode or an unequivocal hypomanic episode.

D. Specify if single or recurrent episode.

E. Specify if:
1. with psychotic features
2. Melancholic type
3. Chronic
4. Seasonal pattern

Source: American Psychiatric Association (1987) with permission.

Dysthymia may be further classified as:

1. *Secondary type.* This classification indicates that the dysthymia is a consequence of a preexisting, chronic, nonmood disorder, such

Table 19.3 DIAGNOSTIC CRITERIA FOR DYSTHYMIA

A. Depressed mood (or can be irritable mood in children and adolescents) for most of the day, more days than not, as indicated either by subjective account or observation by others, for at least 2 years (1 year for children and adolescents).

B. Presence, while depressed, of at least two of the following:
   1. Poor appetite or overeating
   2. Insomnia or hypersomnia
   3. Low energy or fatigue
   4. Low self-esteem
   5. Poor concentration or difficulty making decisions
   6. Feelings of hopelessness

C. During a 2-year period (1-year for children and adolescents) of the disturbance, never without the symptoms in A for more than 2 months at a time.

D. No evidence of an unequivocal major depressive episode during the first 2 years (1 year for children and adolescents) of the disturbance.

E. Has never had a manic or hypomanic episode.

F. No evidence of psychotic symptoms or organic etiology, such as side effect of various medications.

G. Specify if:
   1. Primary or secondary type
   2. Early or late onset

Source: American Psychiatric Association (1987) with permission.

as anorexia nervosa, somatization disorder, psychoactive substance dependence, anxiety disorder, or rheumatoid arthritis.

2. *Primary type.* This diagnosis applies to cases of dysthymia that are apparently not related to a preexisting chronic disorder.

3. *Early onset.* Identifies cases of dysthymia that develop before the age of 21.

4. *Late onset.* Identifies cases of dysthymia that develop at or after age 21.

The *DSM-III-R* diagnostic criteria for dysthymia are presented in Table 19.3.

Bipolar Disorders

Bipolar disorders are characterized by mood swings from profound depression to extreme euphoria (mania), with intervening periods of normalcy. Delusions or hallucinations may or may not be a part of the clinical picture, and onset of symptoms may reflect a seasonal pattern.

BIPOLAR DISORDER, MIXED

This diagnosis applies to a full symptomatic picture of both manic and major depressive episodes intermixed or rapidly alternating every few days. Psychotic features may or may not be present.

BIPOLAR DISORDER, DEPRESSED

Diagnostic criteria for bipolar disorder, depressed are identical to those described for major depression, with one addition. The patient must have a history of one or more manic episodes.

BIPOLAR DISORDER, MANIC

This diagnosis applies when the predominant mood is elevated, expansive, or irritable. The disturbance is sufficiently severe to cause marked impairment in occupational functioning or in usual social activities or relationships with others, or to require hospitalization to prevent harm to self or others. Motor activity is excessive and frenzied. Psychotic features may or may not be present. A milder degree of symptomatology is often called *hypomania*. Hypomania is not severe enough to cause marked impairment in social or occupational functioning or to require hospitalization.

The *DSM-III-R* criteria for bipolar disorder, manic are presented in Table 19.4.

CYCLOTHYMIA

The essential feature of this disorder is a chronic mood disturbance of at least 2 years' duration, involving numerous episodes of hypomania and depressed mood of insufficient severity or duration to meet the criteria for bipolar disorder. The individual is never without hypomanic or depressive symptoms for more than 2 months. The *DSM-III-R* criteria for cyclothymia are presented in Table 19.5.

DEPRESSIVE DISORDERS

Predisposing Factors

BIOLOGICAL THEORIES

Genetics Affective illness has been the subject of considerable research on the relevance of hered-

Table 19.4 DIAGNOSTIC CRITERIA FOR BIPOLAR DISORDER, MANIC

A. A distinct period of abnormally and persistently elevated, expansive, or irritable mood.

B. During the period of mood disturbance, at least three of the following symptoms have persisted (four if the mood is only irritable) and have been present to a significant degree:
   1. Inflated self-esteem or grandiosity
   2. Decreased need for sleep (e.g., feels rested after only 3 hours of sleep)
   3. More talkative than usual or pressure to keep talking
   4. Flight of ideas or subjective experience that thoughts are racing
   5. Distractibility (i.e., attention too easily drawn to unimportant or irrelevant external stimuli)
   6. Increase in goal-directed activity (either socially, at work or school, or sexually) or psychomotor agitation
   7. Excessive involvement in pleasurable activities that have a high potential for painful consequences (e.g., the person engages in unrestrained buying sprees, sexual indiscretions, or foolish business investments)

C. Mood disturbance sufficiently severe to cause marked impairment in occupational functioning or in usual social activities or relationships with others, or to necessitate hospitalization to prevent harm to self or others.

D. No evidence of organic etiology.

E. Specify with or without psychotic features.

F. Specify, if seasonal pattern.

Source: American Psychiatric Association (1987) with permission.

Table 19.5 DIAGNOSTIC CRITERIA FOR CYCLOTHYMIA

A. For at least 2 years (1 year for children and adolescents), presence of numerous hypomanic and depressive episodes that did not meet the criteria for bipolar disorder, manic, or major depressive disorder.

B. During a 2-year period (1 year in children and adolescents) of the disturbance, never without hypomanic or depressive symptoms for more than 2 months at a time.

C. No clear evidence of a major depressive or manic episode during the first 2 years of the disturbance (or 1 year in children or adolescents).

D. No evidence of psychotic symptoms or organic etiology.

Source: American Psychiatric Association (1987) with permission.

itary factors. A genetic link has been suggested in numerous studies; however, no definitive mode of genetic transmission has yet to be demonstrated.

Twin Studies Twin studies suggest a genetic factor in the illness, since about 65 percent of monozygotic twins are concordant for the illness. (NOTE: Concordance refers to twins who are both affected with the illness.) Only about 14 percent of dizygotic twins are concordant (Nurnberger & Gershon, 1982). Similar results (67 percent concordance) were revealed in studies of monozygotic twins raised apart.

Family Studies Most family studies have shown that major depression is 1.5 to 3 times more common among first-degree biological relatives of people with the disorder than among the general population (APA, 1987). Indeed, the evidence to support an increased risk of depressive disorder in individuals with positive family history is quite compelling. Random environmental factors could not cause the concentration of illness that is seen within families (Nurnberger & Gershon, 1982).

Adoption Studies Further support for heritability as an etiological influence in depression are studies of the adopted offspring of affectively ill biological parents. Cadoret (1978) showed that these adopted offspring presented with significantly more depressive disorders in adulthood than adoptees whose biological parents were well or had other psychiatric conditions.

Biochemical Influences

Biogenic Amines It has been hypothesized that depressive illness may be related to a deficiency of the neurotransmitters norepinephrine, serotonin, and dopamine, at functionally important receptor sites in the brain (Janowsky et al, 1988). Historically, the biogenic amine hypothesis of mood disorders grew out of associations between serendipitous observations of the clinical effects of certain drugs and the neurochemical effects of these drugs in animal brains (Zis & Goodwin, 1982). The catecholamine norepinephrine has been identified as a key component in the mobilization of the body to deal with stressful situations. Neurons that contain serotonin are critically involved in the regulation of such diverse functions as sleep, temperature, pain sensitivity, appetite, locomotor activity, neuroendocrine secretions, and mood (Janowsky et al,

1988). Tryptophan, the amino acid precursor of serotonin, has been shown to enhance the efficacy of antidepressant medications and, on occasion, to be effective as an antidepressant itself. The level of dopamine in the mesolimbic system of the brain is thought to exert a strong influence over human mood and behavior. A diminished supply of these biogenic amines inhibits the transmission of impulses from one neuronal fiber to another, causing a failure of the cells to fire or become charged.

More recently, the biogenic amine hypothesis has been expanded to include another neurotransmitter, acetylcholine. Since it is known that cholinergic agents do have profound effects on mood, electroencephalogram, sleep, and neuroendocrine function, it has been suggested that the problem in depression and mania is an imbalance between the biogenic amines and acetylcholine (Hollandsworth, 1990).

The precise role that any of the neurotransmitters plays in the etiology of depression is unknown. As the body of research grows, there is no doubt that increased knowledge regarding the biogenic amines will contribute to a greater capacity for understanding and treating affective illness.

Neuroendocrine Disturbances

Neuroendocrine disturbances may play a role in the pathogenesis or persistence of depressive illness. This notion has arisen in view of the marked disturbances in mood observed with the administration of certain hormones or in the presence of spontaneously occurring endocrine disease (Stokes, 1988).

Hypothalamic-Pituitary-Adrenocortical Axis In patients who are depressed, the normal system of hormonal inhibition fails, resulting in a hypersecretion of cortisol. This elevated serum cortisol is the basis for the dexamethasone suppression test that is sometimes used to determine if an individual has somatically treatable depression.

Hypothalamic-Pituitary-Thyroid Axis Thyrotropin-releasing factor (TRF) from the hypothalamus stimulates the release of thyroid-stimulating hormone (TSH) from the anterior pituitary gland. In turn, TSH stimulates the thyroid gland. Diminished TSH response to administered TRF is observed in approximately 25 percent of depressed persons. This laboratory test has future potential for identifying patients at high risk for affective illness.

Physiological Influences

Depressive symptoms that occur as a consequence of a nonmood disorder or as an adverse effect of certain medications is called a *secondary* depression. Secondary depression may be related to medication side effects, neurological disorders, electrolyte disturbances, hormonal disorders, nutritional deficiencies, and other physiological conditions (Field, 1985).

Medication Side Effects A number of drugs, either alone or in combination with other medications, can produce a depressive syndrome. Most common among these drugs are those that have a direct effect on the central nervous system. Examples of these include the anxiolytics, antipsychotics, and sedative-hypnotics. Certain antihypertensive medications, such as propranolol and reserpine, have been known to produce depressive symptoms. Depressed mood may also occur with any of the following medications (Hollandsworth, 1990):

Antiparkinsonians:	levodopa; amantadine
Hormones:	estrogen, progesterone
Corticosteroids:	cortisone
Antituberculars:	cycloserine
Antineoplastics:	vincristine; vinblastine
Antiulcers:	cimetidine

Neurological Disorders An individual who has suffered a cardiovascular accident (CVA) may experience a despondency unrelated to the severity of the CVA. These are true mood disorders, and antidepressant drug therapy may be indicated. Brain tumors, particularly in the area of the temporal lobe, often present with the symptoms of depression. Agitated depression may be part of the clinical picture associated with Alzheimer's disease. Agitation and restlessness may also represent an underlying depression in the individual with multiple sclerosis.

Electrolyte Disturbances Excessive levels of sodium bicarbonate or calcium can produce symptoms of depression, as can deficits in magnesium and sodium. Potassium is also implicated in the syndrome of depression. Symptoms have been observed with excesses of potassium in the body, as well as in instances of potassium depletion.

Hormonal Disorders Depression is associated with dysfunction of the adrenal cortex and is commonly observed in both Addison's disease and

Cushing's syndrome. Other endocrine conditions that may result in symptoms of depression include hypoparathyroidism and hyperparathyroidism and hypothyroidism and hyperthyroidism.

Nutritional Deficiencies   Various dietary deficiencies that may produce symptoms of depression include deficiencies of vitamin B_1 (thiamine), vitamin B_6 (pyridoxine), vitamin B_{12}, niacin, vitamin C, iron, folic acid, zinc, and protein (Field, 1985; Hollandsworth, 1990).

Other Physiological Conditions   Other conditions that have been associated with secondary depression include collagen disorders, such as systemic lupus erythematosus and polyarteritis nodosa; cardiovascular disease, such as cardiomyopathy, congestive heart failure, and myocardial infarction; infections, such as encephalitis, hepatitis, mononucleosis, pneumonia, and syphilis; and metabolic disorders, such as diabetes mellitus and porphyria.

PSYCHOSOCIAL THEORIES

Psychoanalytic Theories   Freud presented his classic paper "Mourning and Melancholia" in 1917. He defined the distinguishing features of melancholia as:

> ". . . a profoundly painful dejection, cessation of interest in the outside world, loss of the capacity to love, inhibition of all activity, and a lowering of the self-regarding feelings to a degree that finds utterances in self-reproaches and self-revilings, and culminates in a delusional expectation of punishment."

He observed that melancholia occurs after the loss of a loved object, either actually by death or emotionally by rejection, or the loss of some other abstraction of value to the individual. Freud indicated that in melancholic patients, the lost object becomes identified with the ego by a process of incorporation or introjection and that the hostility that was felt for the rejecting or disappointing object becomes experienced as directed against the ego, with which the object is now identified (Mendelson, 1982).

Freud believed that the potential melancholic experienced ambivalence in love relationships. He postulated, therefore, that once the loss had been incorporated into the self (ego), the hostile part of the ambivalence that had been felt for the lost object is then turned inward against the ego.

Klein (1940) viewed the predisposition to depression as stemming from the quality of the mother-infant relationship. She postulated that the 'depressive position' occurred as a normal stage in development when the child began to realize that whole love objects were comprised of both 'good' and 'bad' parts. At this point, the child is aware of his or her own ambivalence in relationships with others. However, until the child is able to integrate these feelings and become confident of the mother's love, each disappointment, each frustration, each separation is interpreted as the loss of a good object. These losses are related to the child's own destructive fantasies, and are accompanied by feelings of sadness, guilt, and regret. Klein believed that those children who never received sufficient love to achieve a sense of security from the mothering figure were always predisposed to return to the depressive position: to feelings of loss, sadness, guilt, and low self-esteem. In other words, they became particularly susceptible to depressive episodes throughout their life.

Learning Theory   The model of "learned helplessness" arises out of Seligman's (1973) experiments with dogs. The animals were exposed to electrical stimulation from which they could not escape. Later, when they were given the opportunity to avoid the traumatic experience, they reacted with helplessness and made no attempt to escape. A similar state of helplessness exists in humans who have experienced numerous failures (either real or perceived). The individual abandons any further attempt to succeed. Seligman theorized that learned helplessness predisposes individuals to depression by imposing a feeling of lack of control over their life situation. McKinney and Moran (1982) state:

> "Negative expectations about the effectiveness of one's own efforts in bringing about the control of one's own environment leads to passivity and diminished initiation of responses."

Object Loss Theory   The theory of object loss (Bowlby, 1973) suggests that depressive illness occurs if the person is abandoned by, or otherwise separated from, a significant other during the first 6 months of life. Since during this period the mother represents the child's main source of security, she is therefore the 'object.' The response occurs not only with a physical loss. The effect is the same if the mother is emotionally absent, failing to provide a secure base for the child (Freden, 1982). This absence of attachment leads to feelings of helplessness and despair that contribute to lifelong patterns of depression in response to loss.

Spitz (1946) described behaviors that he observed in infants who were responding to maternal deprivation during the first year of life. He identified the reaction as 'anaclitic depression,'' which included behaviors such as excessive crying, anorexia, withdrawal, psychomotor retardation, stupor, and a generalized impairment in the normal process of growth and development. According to White (1977), many researchers confirm that loss in adult life afflicts people much more severely in the form of depression if the subjects have suffered early childhood loss.

Cognitive Theory Beck et al (1979) have proposed a theory suggesting that the primary disturbance in depression is cognitive rather than affective. The underlying cause of the depressive affect is seen as cognitive distortions that result in negative, defeated attitudes. Beck identifies three cognitive distortions that he believes serve as the basis for depression:

1. Negative expectations of the environment
2. Negative expectations of the self
3. Negative expectations of the future

These cognitive distortions arise out of a defect in cognitive development, and the individual feels inadequate, worthless, and rejected by others. Outlook for the future is one of pessimism and hopelessness.

Cognitive theorists believe that depression is the product of negative thinking. This is in contrast to the other theorists, who suggest that negative thinking occurs when an individual is depressed. Cognitive therapy focuses on helping the individual to alter mood by changing the way he or she thinks. The individual is taught to control negative thought distortions that lead to pessimism, lethargy, procrastination, and low self-esteem.

THE TRANSACTIONAL MODEL

The etiology of depression remains unclear. No single theory or hypothesis has been postulated that substantiates a clear-cut explanation for the disease. Evidence continues to mount in support of multiple causation. The transactional model recognizes the combined effects of genetic, biochemical, and psychosocial influences on an individual's susceptibility to depression. The dynamics of depression using the Transactional Model of Stress/Adaptation are presented in Figure 19.1.

Developmental Implications

CHILDHOOD

It has only been within the past 15 years that there has been a consensus among investigators in the field that major depressive disorder is an entity in children and adolescents that can be identified using criteria similar to those used for adults and that can be assessed using similar instruments (Geller & Carr, 1988). Depression manifests itself differently in childhood than in adulthood, which has led to considerable confusion in defining the concept of childhood depressive disorders. Herskowitz (1988) states:

"A child doesn't have to be sad to be depressed. You have to look and see what is the child's prevailing mood. It could be anger or irritability. There don't have to be tears."

Herskowitz described the following symptoms specific to preschoolers:

1. Appearing bored, angry, or sad
2. Crying for no apparent reason
3. Needing to rest, or seeming tired or listless
4. Being rejected by or rejecting others
5. Seeming cranky or irritable
6. Being moody; changeable
7. Restless; fidgety; constantly on the move
8. Fighting with others
9. Excessive talking

Other symptoms of childhood depression may include hyperactivity, delinquency, school problems, psychosomatic complaints, sleeping and eating disturbances, social isolation, and suicidal thoughts or actions.

Children may become depressed for various reasons. In many depressed children, there is a genetic predisposition toward the condition, which is then precipitated by a stressful situation. Common precipitating factors include physical or emotional detachment by the primary caregiver, parental separation or divorce, death of a loved one (person or

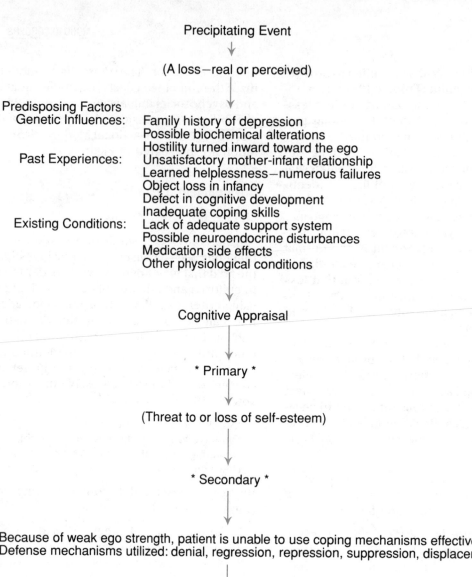

Precipitating Event
↓
(A loss—real or perceived)
↓

Predisposing Factors
Genetic Influences: Family history of depression
                        Possible biochemical alterations
                        Hostility turned inward toward the ego
Past Experiences: Unsatisfactory mother-infant relationship
                        Learned helplessness—numerous failures
                        Object loss in infancy
                        Defect in cognitive development
                        Inadequate coping skills
Existing Conditions: Lack of adequate support system
                        Possible neuroendocrine disturbances
                        Medication side effects
                        Other physiological conditions
↓

Cognitive Appraisal
↓

* Primary *
↓

(Threat to or loss of self-esteem)
↓

* Secondary *
↓

Because of weak ego strength, patient is unable to use coping mechanisms effectively.
Defense mechanisms utilized: denial, regression, repression, suppression, displacement, isolation
↓

Quality of response

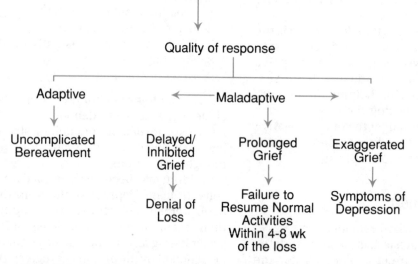

Adaptive   Maladaptive

Uncomplicated   Delayed/   Prolonged   Exaggerated
Bereavement   Inhibited   Grief   Grief
                   Grief
                     ↓   ↓   ↓
                   Denial of   Failure to   Symptoms of
                   Loss   Resume Normal   Depression
                                   Activities
                                   Within 4-8 wk
                                   of the loss

Figure 19.1 The dynamics of depression using the transactional model of stress/adaptation.

pet), a move, academic failure, or physical illness. In any event, the common denominator is loss.

The focus of therapy with depressed children is to alleviate the child's symptoms and strengthen the child's coping and adaptive skills, with the hope of possibly preventing future psychological problems. Some studies have shown that untreated childhood depression may lead to subsequent problems in adolescence and adult life (Sargent, 1989). Most children are treated on an outpatient basis. Hospitalization of the depressed child usually occurs only if he or she is actively suicidal, when the home environment precludes adherence to a treatment regimen, or if the child needs to be separated from the home for psychosocial deprivation.

Parental and family therapy are commonly used to help the younger depressed child. Recovery is facilitated by emotional support and guidance to family members. Children older than age 8 usually participate in family therapy. In some situations, individual treatment may be appropriate for older children. Medications, such as antidepressants or lithium, can be important in the treatment of children, especially for the more serious and recurrent forms of depression.

Adolescence

Depression may be even harder to recognize in an adolescent than in a younger child. Feelings of sadness, loneliness, anxiety, and hopelessness associated with depression may be perceived as the normal emotional stresses of growing up. Therefore, many young people whose symptoms are attributed to the "normal adjustments" of adolescence do not get the help they need. Depression is a major cause of suicide among teens. During the past three decades, suicide among adolescents has increased 300 percent (Sargent, 1989), and it is second only to automobile and other accidents as the leading cause of death among youths aged 15 to 24 (Department of Health and Human Services, 1983).

Common symptoms of depression in the adolescent are inappropriately expressed anger, aggressiveness, running away, delinquency, social withdrawal, sexual acting out, substance abuse, restlessness, and apathy. Loss of self-esteem, sleeping and eating disturbances, and psychosomatic complaints are also common.

Bipolar disorder, which often emerges during adolescence, is manifested by episodes of impulsivity, irritability, and loss of control, sometimes alternating with periods of withdrawal. These behaviors are often confused with the emotional cycles of adolescence, delaying necessary treatment.

What, then, is the indicator that differentiates affective disorder from the typical stormy behavior of adolescence? The clue is revealed by a visible manifestation of *behavioral change that lasts for several weeks*. For example: the normally outgoing and extroverted adolescent who has become withdrawn and antisocial; the good student who previously received consistently high marks but is now failing and skipping classes; the usually self-confident teenager who is now inappropriately irritable and defensive with others.

Adolescents become depressed for all the same reasons that were discussed in childhood depression. Rosenn (1982) states:

> "It has been suggested that repeated childhood losses cause disturbances in early ego development. The biologic and psychosocial drive towards autonomy during adolescence overly taxes the teenager's defenses. When actual separation from the real or surrogate parents (e.g., girlfriend or boyfriend) is threatened, the usual defensive network may break down."

This threat of imminent abandonment by parents or closest peer relationship is thought to be the most frequent immediate precipitant to adolescent suicide.

Treatment of the depressed adolescent is often conducted on an outpatient basis. Geller and Carr (1988) suggest the following guidelines for hospitalization of depressed adolescents:

1. When the adolescent is suicidal and the family cannot set up the appropriate precautions at home.
2. When the psychosocial situation precludes adherence to a treatment regimen (i.e., The family is unable to keep therapy appointments or administer medications as required at home).
3. When the adolescent, because of depressive stupor or marked anorexia, is unable to sustain his or her own biological needs.
4. When the adolescent's anger is excessive and

imposes a risk of harm to younger siblings in the home.

Antidepressant or lithium therapy, in addition to supportive psychosocial intervention, is the common modality for treatment of adolescent mood disorders. Various treatments may have to be attempted to determine the one that is most effective.

Senescence

Depression is the most common psychiatric disorder of the elderly, who make up approximately 12 percent of the general population of the United States (Georgotas & McCue, 1988). This is not surprising considering the disproportionate value our society places on youth, vigor, and uninterrupted productivity. These societal attitudes continually nurture the feelings of low self-esteem, helplessness, and hopelessness that become more pervasive and intensive with advanced age. Further, the aging individual's adaptive coping strategies may be seriously challenged by major stressors, such as financial problems, physical illness, changes in bodily functioning, and an increasing awareness of approaching death. The problem is often intensified by the numerous losses individuals experience during this period in life, such as spouse, friends, children, home, and independence. A phenomenon called *bereavement overload* occurs when individuals experience so many losses in their lives that they are not able to resolve one grief response before another one begins. Bereavement overload predisposes elderly individuals to depressive illness.

About 25 percent of the successful suicides in the United States are by elderly individuals (Georgotas & McCue, 1988). The risk of suicide increases with advanced age to approximately four times that of the general population at the seventh decade of life.

Symptoms of depression in the elderly are not very different from those in younger adults. However, depressive syndromes are often confused by other illnesses associated with the aging process. Symptoms of depression are often misdiagnosed as senile dementia, when in fact the memory loss, confused thinking, or apathy symptomatic of senility actually may be due to depression. The early awakening and reduced appetite typical of depression are common among many older persons who are not depressed. Compounding this situation is the fact that many medical conditions, such as endocrinological, neurological, nutritional, and metabolic disorders, often present with classic symptoms of depression. Many medications commonly used by the elderly, such as antihypertensives, corticosteroids, and analgesics, can also produce a depressant effect.

On the other hand, depression does accompany many of the illnesses that afflict older persons, such as Parkinson's disease, cancer, arthritis, and the early stages of Alzheimer's disease. Treating depression in these situations can reduce unnecessary suffering and help afflicted individuals cope with their medical problems (Sargent, 1989).

The most effective treatment of depression in the elderly individual is thought to be a combination of psychosocial and biologic approaches (Georgotas & McCue, 1988). Antidepressant medications are administered with age-related physiologic changes in absorption, distribution, elimination, and brain receptor sensitivity in mind. Due to these changes, plasma concentrations of these drugs can reach very high levels despite moderate oral doses.

Electroconvulsive therapy (ECT) still remains one of the safest and most effective treatments for major depression in the elderly (Georgotas & McCue, 1988). The response to ECT appears to be slower with advancing age, and the therapeutic effects are of limited duration. However, it may be considered the treatment of choice for the elderly individual who is an acute suicidal risk or who is unable to tolerate antidepressant medications.

Other therapeutic approaches include interpersonal, behavioral, group, and family psychotherapies. Appropriate treatment of the depressed elderly individual can bring relief from suffering, and offer a new lease on life with a feeling of renewed productivity.

Postpartum Depression

The severity of depression in the postpartum period varies from a feeling of the "blues," to moderate depression, to melancholia. Approximately 50 percent of women who give birth experience the "blues" following delivery. The incidence of moderate (neurotic) depression is about 10 percent and that of severe or psychotic depression (melancholia) is 0.5 percent (Pitt, 1982).

Symptoms of the "maternity blues" include tearfulness, despondency, anxiety, and subjectively impaired concentration appearing in the early puerperium. Typically, the condition appears on the third or fourth day postpartum and lasts for only a day or two.

Symptoms of moderate postpartum depression have been described as depressed mood varying from day to day, with more bad days than good, tending to be worse toward evening and associated with fatigue, irritability (especially toward the spouse and any other children), disturbance of appetite (usually anorexia), early insomnia, and loss of libido (Pitt, 1982). In addition, there is excessive worry about the condition and comfort of the baby. These symptoms begin somewhat later than those described in the "maternity blues," and take from a few weeks to several months to abate.

Postpartum melancholia, or depressive psychosis, is characterized by depressed mood, agitation, indecision, lack of concentration, guilt, and an abnormal attitude toward bodily functions. There may be lack of interest in, or rejection of, the baby, or a morbid fear that it may be harmed. Risks of suicide and infanticide should not be overlooked. These symptoms generally develop within 2 weeks following delivery. Response to treatment is slow, with a tendency for relapse.

The etiology of postpartum depression remains unclear. "Maternity blues" may be associated with hormonal changes, tryptophan metabolism, or alterations in membrane transport during the early postpartum period. Besides being exposed to these same somatic changes, the woman who experiences moderate-to-severe symptoms probably possesses a vulnerability to depression related to heredity, upbringing, early life experiences, personality, or social circumstances. Pitt (1982) reported on the results of two studies, one of which found a close association between postpartum depression and loss of a parent before age 11. The second reported a relationship between postpartum depression and women who had had insufficient contact with their mothers during childhood.

Treatment of postpartum depression varies with the severity of the illness. Psychotic depression may be treated with tricyclic antidepressants, along with supporting psychotherapy, group therapy, and possibly family therapy. Moderate depression may be relieved with supportive psychotherapy and continuing assistance with home management until the symptoms subside. "Maternity blues" usually need no treatment beyond a word of comfort and reassurance from the physician that these feelings are common and will soon pass.

APPLICATION OF THE NURSING PROCESS TO DEPRESSIVE DISORDERS

Background Assessment Data

Symptomatology of depression can be viewed on a continuum according to severity of the illness. All individuals become depressed from time to time. These are the transient symptoms that accompany the everyday disappointments of life. Examples include failing an exam, or breaking up with one's boyfriend or girlfriend. Transient symptoms of depression subside relatively quickly, as the individual advances toward other goals and achievements.

Mild depressive episodes occur when the grief process is triggered in response to the loss of a valued object. This can occur with the loss of a loved one, pet, friend, home, or significant other. As one is able to work through the stages of grief, the loss is accepted, symptoms subside, and activities of daily living are resumed within a few weeks time. If this does not occur, grief is prolonged or exaggerated, and symptoms intensify.

Moderate depression occurs when grief is prolonged or exaggerated. The individual becomes fixed in the anger stage of the grief response, and the anger is turned inward on the self. All of the feelings associated with normal grieving are exaggerated out of proportion, and the individual is unable to function without assistance. Dysthymia is an example of moderate depression.

Severe depression is an intensification of the symptoms associated with the moderate level. The individual who is severely depressed may also demonstrate a loss of contact with reality. This level is associated with a complete lack of pleasure in all activities, and ruminations about suicide are common. Major depression is an example of severe depression.

A continuum of depression is presented in Figure 19.2.

Symptoms of depression can be described as alterations in four spheres of human functioning: affective, behavioral, cognitive, and physiologic. Alterations within these spheres differ according to the degree of severity of symptomatology.

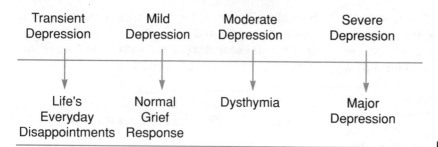

Figure 19.2 A continuum of depression.

TRANSIENT DEPRESSION

Symptoms at this level of the continuum are not necessarily dysfunctional. Alterations include:

1. *Affective:* sadness, dejection, downhearted, a case of the "blues"
2. *Behavioral:* some crying may occur
3. *Cognitive:* some difficulty getting mind off of one's disappointment
4. *Physiological:* may feel tired and listless

MILD DEPRESSION

Symptoms at the mild level of depression are identified by those associated with normal grieving. Alterations include:

1. *Affective:* denial of feelings, anger, anxiety, guilt, helplessness, hopelessness, sadness, despondency
2. *Behavioral:* tearfulness, regression, restlessness, agitation, withdrawal
3. *Cognitive:* preoccupation with the loss, self-blame, ambivalence, blaming others
4. *Physiological:* anorexia or overeating, insomnia or hypersomnia, headache, backache, chest pain, or other symptoms associated with the loss of significant other

MODERATE DEPRESSION

This level of depression represents a more problematic disturbance. Symptoms associated with dysthymia include:

1. *Affective:* feelings of sadness, dejection, helplessness, powerlessness, hopelessness; outlook is gloomy and pessimistic; low self-esteem; difficulty experiencing pleasure in activities.
2. *Behavioral:* physical movements are slowed (i.e., psychomotor retardation); posture may be slumped; speech is slowed; verbalizations are limited, and may consist of ruminations about life's failures or regrets; social isolation with a focus on the self is common; use of substances may increase; self-destructive behavior may be evident; decreased interest in personal hygiene and grooming is common.
3. *Cognitive:* thinking processes are retarded; the person has difficulty concentrating and directing attention; thoughts may be obsessive and repetitive, and generally portray pessimism and negativism; verbalizations and behavior may reflect suicidal ideation
4. *Physiological:* anorexia or overeating; insomnia or hypersomnia; sleep disturbances; amenorrhea; decreased libido; headaches; backaches; chest pain; abdominal pain; level of energy is low; feels tired and listless; generally feel their best early in the morning and continually feel worse as the day progresses (Note: This may have to do with the diurnal variation in the level of neurotransmitters that affect mood and level of activity.)

SEVERE DEPRESSION

Severe depression is characterized by an intensification of the symptoms described for moderate depression. Examples of severe depression include major depression and bipolar disorder, depressed. Symptoms include:

1. *Affective:* feelings are of total despair, hopelessness, and worthlessness; affect is flat (unchanging); in fact, they may appear to be void

of emotional tone; feelings of nothingness and emptiness prevail; apathy; loneliness; sadness; inability to feel pleasure

2. *Behavioral:* psychomotor retardation is so severe that physical movement may literally come to a standstill; or psychomotor behavior may be manifested by rapid, agitated, purposeless movements; posture is slumped; sitting usually takes the form of a curled-up position; walking is slow and rigid; communication is virtually nonexistent; when verbalizations do occur, they may reflect delusional thinking; personal hygiene and grooming go unattended; social isolation is common, with virtually no inclination toward interaction with others.

3. *Cognitive:* delusional thinking prevails; delusions of persecution and somatic delusions are common; the individual is confused, indecisive, and unable to concentrate; hallucinations can reflect misinterpretations of the environment; excessive self-deprecation, self-blame, and thoughts of suicide (Note: Because of the low energy level and retarded thought processes, the individual is unable to follow through on suicidal ideas. However, the desire is strong at this level.)

4. *Physiological:* a general slowdown of the entire body is reflected in sluggish digestion, constipation, and urinary retention; amenorrhea; impotence; diminished libido; anorexia; weight loss; may have difficulty falling asleep and when they do, may wake very early in the morning; feels worse early in the morning and somewhat better as the day progresses (Note: As with moderate depression, this may reflect the diurnal variation in the level of neurotransmitters that affect mood and activity.)

Nursing Diagnoses

From the assessment data, the nurse then formulates the appropriate nursing diagnoses for the depressed patient. From these identified problems, care planning is executed, nursing actions are implemented, and relevant criteria for evaluation are established. Possible nursing diagnoses for depressed patients include:

High risk for self-directed violence related to depressed mood, feelings of worthlessness, anger turned inward on the self, misinterpretations of reality.

Dysfunctional grieving related to real or perceived loss, bereavement overload, evidenced by denial of loss, inappropriate expression of anger, idealization of or obsession with the lost object, inability to carry out activities of daily living.

Self-esteem disturbance related to learned helplessness, feelings of abandonment by significant other, impaired cognition fostering negative view of self, evidenced by expressions of worthlessness, hypersensitivity to slight or criticism, negative, pessimistic outlook.

Powerlessness related to dysfunctional grieving process, life-style of helplessness, evidenced by feelings of lack of control over life situation, overdependence on others to fulfill needs.

Spiritual distress related to dysfunctional grieving over loss of valued object evidenced by anger toward God, questions meaning of own existence, unable to participate in usual religious practices

Social isolation/impaired social interaction related to developmental regression, egocentric behaviors, fear of rejection or failure of the interaction, evidenced by being uncommunicative, withdrawn, seeking to be alone, dysfunctional interaction with peers, family, or others.

Altered thought processes related to withdrawal into the self, underdeveloped ego, punitive superego, impaired cognition fostering negative perception of self or environment, evidenced by delusional thinking, confusion, difficulty concentrating, impaired problem-solving ability.

Altered nutrition, less than body requirements related to depressed mood, loss of appetite, or lack of interest in food, evidenced by weight loss, poor muscle tone, pale conjunctiva and mucous membranes, poor skin turgor, weakness.

Sleep pattern disturbance related to depressed mood, anxiety, fears, evidenced by difficulty falling asleep, awakening earlier or later than desired, verbal complaints of not feeling well rested.

Self-care deficit (hygiene, grooming) related to depressed mood, feelings of worthlessness, evidenced by uncombed hair, disheveled clothing, offensive body odor.

Planning/Implementation

Table 19.6 provides a plan of care for the depressed patient. Selected nursing diagnoses are presented, along with goals or care and appropriate nursing interventions for each. Rationale is provided in italics.

Some institutions are using a case management model to coordinate care (see Chapter 6, for more detailed explanation). In case management models, the plan of care may take the form of a critical pathway. Table 19.7 depicts an example of a critical pathway of care for a depressed patient.

Table 19.6 CARE PLAN FOR THE DEPRESSED PATIENT

Nursing Diagnoses	Objectives	Nursing Interventions
High risk for self-directed violence related to depressed mood, feelings of worthlessness, anger turned inward on the self, misinterpretations of reality.	Patient will not harm self.	Ask patient directly: "Have you thought about harming yourself in any way? If so, what do you plan to do? Do you have the means to carry out this plan?" *The risk of suicide is greatly increased if the patient has developed a plan and particularly if means exist for the patient to execute the plan.* Create a safe environment for the patient. Remove all potentially harmful objects from patient's access (sharp objects, straps, belts, ties, glass items, alcohol). Supervise closely during meals and medication administration. Perform room searches as deemed necessary. *Patient safety is a nursing priority.* Formulate a short-term verbal or written contract that the patient will not harm self. When time is up, make another, and so forth. Secure promise that patient will seek out staff when feeling suicidal. *A degree of the responsibility for his or her safety is given to the patient. Increased feelings of self-worth may be experienced when patient feels accepted unconditionally regardless of thoughts or behavior.* Encourage patient to express honest feelings, including anger. Provide hostility release if needed. *Depression and suicidal behaviors may be viewed as anger turned inward on the self. If this anger can be verbalized in a nonthreatening environment, the patient may be able to eventually resolve these feelings.*
Dysfunctional grieving related to real or perceived loss, bereavement overload, evidenced by denial of loss, inappropriate expression of anger, idealization of or obsession with lost object, inability to carry out activities of daily living.	Patient will be able to verbalize normal behaviors associated with grieving and begin progression toward resolution by discharge.	Assess stage of fixation in grief process. *Accurate baseline data is required to plan accurate care.* Develop trust. Show empathy, caring, and unconditional positive regard. *These interventions provide the basis for a therapeutic relationship.* Explore feelings of anger and help patient direct them toward the intended object or person. Promote the use of large motor activities for relieving pent-up tension. *Until patient can recognize and accept personal feelings regarding the loss, grief work cannot progress. Physical exercise is a safe and effective way of relieving internalized anger.* Teach normal behaviors associated with grieving *to prevent feelings of guilt generated by these responses.* Help patient with honest review of relationship with lost object. *Only when patient is able to see both positive and negative aspects related to the lost object will the grieving process be complete.*

(continued)

Table 19.6 CONTINUED

Nursing Diagnoses	Objectives	Nursing Interventions
Self-esteem disturbance related to learned helplessness, feelings of abandonment by significant other, impaired cognition fostering negative view of self, evidenced by expressions of worthlessness, hypersensitivity to slights or criticism, negative and pessimistic outlook.	Patient will be able to attempt new activities without fear of failure. Patient will be able to verbalize positive aspects about self.	Be accepting of patient and spend time with him or her even though pessimism and negativism may seem objectionable. Focus on strengths and accomplishments and minimize failures. *These interventions contribute toward feelings of self-worth.* Promote attendance in therapy groups that offer patient simple methods of accomplishment. Encourage patient to be as independent as possible. *Success and independence promote feelings of self-worth.* Encourage patient to recognize areas of change and provide assistance toward this effort. *Patient will need assistance with problem-solving.* Teach assertiveness and communication techniques, *the use of which can serve to enhance self-esteem.*
Powerlessness related to dysfunctional grieving process, life-style of helplessness, evidenced by feelings of lack of control over life situation, overdependence on others to fulfill needs.	Patient will be able to problem solve ways to take control of life situation.	Allow patient to participate in goal setting and decision making regarding own care. *Providing patient with choices will increase his or her feelings of control.* Ensure that goals are realistic and that patient is able to identify areas of life situation that are realistically under his or her control, *to avoid setting patient up for further failures.* Encourage patient to verbalize feelings about areas that are not within his or her ability to control. *Verbalization of unresolved issues may help patient accept what cannot be changed.*
Spiritual distress related to dysfunctional grieving over loss of valued object, evidenced by anger toward God, questioning of meaning of own existence, inability to participate in usual religious practices.	Patient will express achievement of support and personal satisfaction from spiritual practices.	Be accepting and nonjudgmental when patient expresses anger and bitterness toward God. Stay with patient. *The nurse's presence and nonjudgmental attitude increase the patient's feelings of self-worth and promote trust in the relationship.* Encourage patient to ventilate feelings related to meaning of own existence in the face of current loss. *Patient may believe he or she cannot go on living without lost object. Catharsis can provide relief and put life back into realistic perspective.* Encourage patient as part of grief work to reach out to previously used religious practices for support. Encourage patient to discuss these practices and how they provided support in the past. *Patient may find comfort in religious rituals with which he or she is familiar.* Ensure patient that he or she is not alone when feeling inadequate in the search for life's answers. *Validation of patient's feelings and assurance that they are shared by others offers reassurance and an affirmation of acceptability.* Contact spiritual leader of patient's choice, if he or she requests.

Table 19.7 CRITICAL PATHWAY OF CARE FOR THE DEPRESSED PATIENT

Estimated Length of Stay: 14 days—Variations from designated pathway should be documented in progress notes

Nursing Diagnoses and Categories of Care	Time Dimension	Goals and/or Actions	Time Dimension	Goals and/or Actions	Time Dimension	Discharge Outcome
High risk for self-directed violence	Day 1	Environment is made safe for patient.	Ongoing	Patient does not harm self.	Day 14	Patient is discharged without harm to self.
Referrals	Day 1	Psychiatrist: May give order to isolate if risk is great or may do ECT. For relaxation therapy: Music therapist Clinical nurse specialist Stress management specialist			Day 14	Discharge with follow-up appointments as required.
Additional assessments	Day 1	Suicidal assessment: • ideation • gestures • threats • plan • means • anxiety level • thought disorder	Day 2–14	Ongoing assessments	Day 14	Patient discharged. Denies suicidal ideations.
	Day 1	Secure no-suicide contract				
Medications	Day 1	Antidepressant medication, as ordered. Prn antianxiety agents	Day 1–14	Assess for effectiveness and side effects of medications. Be alert for sudden lifts in mood.	Day 14	Discharged with antidepressant medications.
Patient education	Day 3–12	Teach relaxation techniques. Discuss resources outside the hospital from whom patient may seek assistance when feeling suicidal.	Day 12–13	Reinforce teaching	Day 14	Discharge with verbalized understanding of instruction given.

(*continued*)

Table 19.7   CONTINUED

Estimated Length of Stay: 14 days—Variations from designated pathway should be documented in progress notes

Nursing Diagnoses and Categories of Care	Time Dimension	Goals and/or Actions	Time Dimension	Goals and/or Actions	Time Dimension	Discharge Outcome
Dysfunction grieving	Day 1	Assess stage of fixation in grief process.			Day 14	Discharge with evidence of progression toward resolution of grief.
Referrals	Day 1	Psychiatrist Psychologist Social worker Clinical nurse specialist Music therapist Occupational therapist Recreational therapist Chaplain			Day 14	Discharge with follow-up appointments as required.
Diagnostic studies		Any of the following tests *may* be ordered:				
	Day 1	Drug screen				
	Day 2–3	Urine test for norepinephrine and serotonin Dexamethasone-suppression test A measure of TSH response to administered thyrotropin-releasing hormone Serum and urine studies for nutritional deficiencies.				
Medications	Day 1	Antidepressant medication, as ordered. Prn antianxiety agent.	Day 1–14	Assess for effectiveness and side effects of medications.	Day 14	Patient is discharged with medications.

(continued)

Table 19.7 CONTINUED

Estimated Length of Stay: 14 days—Variations from designated pathway should be documented in progress notes

Nursing Diagnoses and Categories of Care	Time Dimension	Goals and/or Actions	Time Dimension	Goals and/or Actions	Time Dimension	Discharge Outcome
Diet	Day 1	If antidepressant medication is MAO inhibitor: Low tyramine			Day 14	Patient has experienced no symptoms of hypertensive crisis.
Additional assessments	Day 1 Day 1	VS every shift Assess: ● mental status ● mood, affect ● thought disorder ● communication patterns ● level of interest in environment ● participation in activities ● weight	Day 2–14 Day 2–14	VS daily if stable Ongoing assessment	Day 14	Mood and affect appropriate. No evidence of thought disorders. Participates willingly and appropriately in activities.
Patient education	Day 1	Orient to unit	Day 8 Day 12–13	Discuss importance of taking medications regularly, even when feeling well or if feeling medication is not helping. Discuss possible side effects of medication and when to see the doctor. Teach which foods to eliminate from diet if on MAO inhibitor. Reinforce teaching.	Day 14	Patient is discharged. Verbalizes understanding of information presented prior to discharge.

OUTCOME CRITERIA

The following criteria may be used for measurement of outcomes in the care of the depressed patient.

The patient:
1. has experienced no physical harm to self.
2. discusses the loss with staff and family members.
3. no longer idealizes or obsesses about the lost object.
4. sets realistic goals for self.
5. is no longer afraid to attempt new activities.
6. is able to identify aspects of self-control over life situation.
7. expresses personal satisfaction and support from spiritual practices.
8. interacts willingly and appropriately with others.
9. is able to maintain reality orientation.
10. is able to concentrate, reason, and solve problems.
11. eats a well-balanced diet with snacks to prevent weight loss and maintain nutritional status
12. sleeps 6 to 8 hours per night and verbalizes feeling well rested.
13. bathes, washes and combs hair, and dresses in clean clothing without assistance.

Evaluation of Care for the Depressed Patient

In the final step of the nursing process, a reassessment is conducted to determine if the nursing actions have been successful in achieving the objectives of care. Evaluation of the nursing actions for the depressed patient may be facilitated by gathering information using the following types of questions.

Has self-harm to the individual been avoided? Have suicidal ideations subsided? Does the individual know where to seek assistance outside the hospital when suicidal thoughts occur? Has the patient discussed the recent loss with staff and family members? Is he or she able to verbalize feelings and behaviors associated with each stage of the grieving process and recognize own position in the process? Has obsession with and idealization of the lost object subsided? Is anger toward the lost object expressed appropriately? Does patient set realistic goals for self? Is he or she able to verbalize positive aspects about self, past accomplishments, and future prospects? Can the patient identify areas of life situation over which he or she has control? Is patient able to participate in usual religious practices and feel satisfaction and support from them? Is patient seeking out interaction with others in an appropriate manner? Does patient maintain reality orientation with no evidence of delusional thinking? Is he or she able to concentrate and make decisions concerning own self-care? Is patient selecting and consuming foods sufficiently high in nutrients and calories to maintain weight and nutritional status? Does patient sleep without difficulty and wake feeling rested? Does patient show pride in appearance by attending to personal hygiene and grooming? Have somatic complaints subsided?

BIPOLAR DISORDER, MANIC

Predisposing Factors

BIOLOGICAL THEORIES

Genetics

Twin Studies Twin studies have indicated that if one twin has bipolar disorder, the other twin is four to five times more likely to also have the disorder if the twins are identical than if they are fraternal (Kelsoe, 1991). Since identical twins have identical genes and fraternal twins share only approximately half their genes, this is strong evidence that genes play a major role in the etiology.

Family Studies Family studies have shown that if one member of a family has bipolar disorder, then the other members are 7 to 10 times more likely to also have bipolar disorder than in the general population (Kelsoe, 1991). This has also been shown to be the case in studies of children born to parents with bipolar disorder who were adopted at birth and reared by adoptive parents without evidence of the disorder. These results strongly indicate that genes play a role separate from that of the environment. Kelsoe adds:

> "It is important to understand that if an individual inherits a gene for bipolar disorder, they have only about a 50% to 80% chance of ever having a mood disorder. Hence, it is a predisposition or susceptibility that is inherited."

Biochemical Influences

Biogenic Amines Early studies have associated symptoms of depression with a functional deficiency of norepinephrine and dopamine, and mania with a functional excess of these amines. The neurotransmitter serotonin appears to remain low in both states (Goodwin & Jamison, 1990). These conclusions have been substantiated by the effects of neuroleptic drugs that influence the levels of these biogenic amines to produce the desired effect.

Electrolytes Some studies have indicated that bipolar illness is accompanied by increased intracellular sodium and calcium. These electrolyte imbalances may be related to abnormalities in cellular membrane function in bipolar disorder. A possible deficiency in the membrane-bound sodium pump has been suggested as an explanation for the increased intracellular sodium. The link between increased intracellular calcium and symptoms of bipolar disorder may be indicated by the drugs known as calcium channel blockers. These medications inhibit the influx of calcium into the cell and have been shown to have antimanic, and possibly antidepressant and anticycling, properties (Goodwin & Jamison, 1990).

Physiologic Influences

Brain Lesions Studies have shown that depressions tend to be associated with lesions in the left frontotemporal or right parieto-occipital quadrants (Goodwin & Jamison, 1990). The most common affective sequelae of brain lesions involve poststroke depressions, the severity of which increases the closer the damage is to the left frontal pole. Secondary maniclike symptoms appear to be associated with right frontotemporal or left parieto-occipital lesions.

Medication Side Effects Certain medications used to treat somatic illnesses have been known to trigger a manic response. The most common of these are the steroids, frequently used to treat chronic illness, such as multiple sclerosis and lupus. Some cases whose first episode of mania was encountered during steroid therapy have reported spontaneous recurrence of manic symptoms years later (Kaplan & Sadock, 1985). Amphetamines and tricyclic antidepressants also have the potential for initiating a manic episode.

PSYCHOSOCIAL THEORIES

Psychoanalytic Theories Freud (1957) believed that depression and mania were maladaptive responses to loss. He suggested that the lost object became merged with the ego, and the rage felt for having been rejected or abandoned was then directed inward against the self. In this way, the individual is able to remain unaware of the unacceptable anger against the love object. Freud assumed that in mania the lost object is rapidly relinquished (though he could not explain why), and a vast amount of psychic energy becomes free to be invested upon the self and the surrounding world (Aleksandrowicz, 1980). In this model, mania is viewed as a denial of depression.

Klein (1940) viewed depression as a developmental phase, occurring toward the end of the first year of life caused by weaning and gradual weakening of the deep bond between the infant and the mothering figure. Mania is viewed as a denial of, or defense against, the depression, and represents a reactivation of the corresponding infantile state.

Theory of Family Dynamics A study by Cohen et al (1954) found that the individual with bipolar disorder most likely began life in a loving, nurturing environment. All physical and emotional needs were fulfilled by the primary caregiver, who assumed the image of "goodness" in the mind of the infant. As the child developed and became increasingly independent, some of the nurturing was withdrawn. The child, who has not yet achieved object constancy by this time, is unable to incorporate the concepts of both "good" and "bad" in the primary caregiver. A feeling of ambivalence develops toward the primary caregiver as the child learns the necessity of fulfilling expectations to gain affection, even at the expense of negating his or her own needs and desires.

As the child matures, he or she has a tendency to be particularly sensitive, and to crave approval, support, and affection from others. Gibson et al (1959) found that the childhood family of the manic-depressive had been characterized by a striving for social prestige, and that as a child the patient had borne the brunt of this, with heavy pressure on him or her from one or both of the parents to succeed in social life. The family showed little interest in the child in his or her own right, but only in the role as carrier of prestige. Parental approval depended not on "who you are" but on "what you do" (Freden, 1982). Expectations were often unrealistic, and the child's social and psychological life became greatly restricted, resulting in the development of rigid behavior patterns. A love-hate relationship is established as resentment toward the parents continues to grow, even though there is a strong desire and continued effort on the part of the child to please them.

The child's ego development is disrupted in this dysfunctional family system, and the adult bipolar patient's gratification and security are strongly tied to unfulfilled needs for approval. The depressive and manic episodes are precipitated by a loss in which the patient feels rejected, rebuked, or not appreciated (Aleksandrowicz, 1980). The loss need not be a conspicuous and obviously stressful life event. Cohen et al (1954) pointed out that even a change in the patient's appraisal of existing relationships may be subjectively experienced as loss of love.

Because there is weak ego development, the response to loss is directed by influences from the id or the superego components of the personality. If the superego becomes punitive, the individual turns anger inward on the self, and experiences depression. When the depression subsides, the ego may still be too weak to control the impulsive, excessive behavior dominated by the id, and the symptoms of mania are manifested (Aleksandrowicz, 1980).

THE TRANSACTIONAL MODEL

The etiology of bipolar disorder remains uncertain. Most likely it results from an interaction between genetic and environmental determinants. Aleksandrowicz (1980) states:

> "At our present state of knowledge, it is pure speculation to consider the failure of mood regulation to be primarily a psychological or biological defect, to be genetically determined or related to early environment. We begin to realize now that it is not an either-or issue. Environmental influences can have lasting biological effects, and innate qualities affect the environment in which one is developing."

The transactional model takes these various etiological influences, as well as those associated with past experiences, existing conditions, and the individual's perception of the event, into consideration. Figure 19.3 depicts the dynamics of bipolar disorder, manic using the Transactional Model of Stress/Adaptation.

APPLICATION OF THE NURSING PROCESS TO BIPOLAR DISORDER, MANIC

Background Assessment Data

Goodwin and Jamison (1990) described symptoms of manic states according to three stages: hypomania, acute mania, and delirious mania. Symptoms of mood, cognition and perception, and activity and behavior are presented for each stage.

STAGE I. HYPOMANIA

At this stage, the disturbance is not sufficiently severe to cause marked impairment in social or occupational functioning or to require hospitalization (APA, 1987).

Mood The mood of a hypomanic person is cheerful and expansive. However, there is an underlying irritability that surfaces rapidly when the person's wishes and desires go unfulfilled. The nature of the hypomanic person is very volatile and fluctuating.

Cognition and Perception Perceptions of the self are exalted—ideas of great worth and ability. Thinking is flighty, with a rapid flow of ideas. Perception of the environment is heightened, but the individual is so easily distracted by irrelevant stimuli, that goal-directed activities are difficult.

Activity and Behavior The hypomanic individual exhibits increased motor activity. They are perceived as being very extroverted and sociable, and because of this they attract numerous acquaintances. However, they lack the depth of personality and warmth to formulate close friendships. They do a great deal of talking and laughing, usually very loudly, and often inappropriately. Increased libido is common. Some individuals experience anorexia and weight loss. The exalted self-perception leads some hypomanics to engage in inappropriate behaviors, such as calling the President, or charging huge amounts of purchases without the resources to pay.

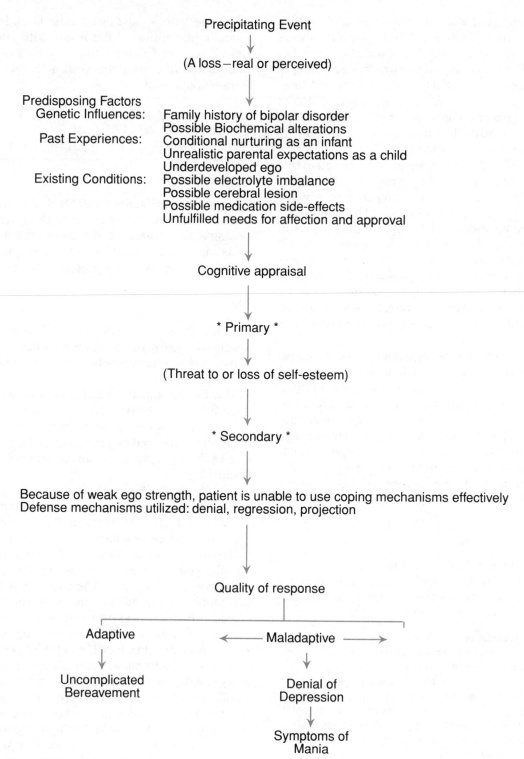

Figure 19.3 The dynamics of bipolar disorder, manic using the transactional model of stress/adaptation.

STAGE II. ACUTE MANIA

Symptoms of acute mania may be viewed as a progression in intensification of those experienced in hypomania, or they may be manifested directly. Most individuals experience marked impairment in functioning and require hospitalization.

Mood Acute mania is characterized by euphoria and elation. The person appears to be on a continuous "high." However, the mood is always subject to frequent variation, easily changing to irritability and anger or even to sadness and crying.

Cognition and Perception Cognition and perception become fragmented and often psychotic in acute mania. Rapid thinking proceeds to racing and disjointed thinking (flight of ideas) and may be manifested by a continuous flow of accelerated, pressured speech (loquaciousness), with abrupt changes from topic to topic. When flight of ideas is severe, speech may be disorganized and incoherent. Distractibility becomes all-pervasive. Attention can be diverted by even the smallest of stimuli. Paranoid and grandiose delusions are common, as are illusions and hallucinations (Goodwin & Jamison, 1990).

Activity and Behavior Psychomotor activity is excessive. Sexual interest in increased. There is poor impulse control, and the individual who is normally discreet may become socially and sexually uninhibited. Excessive spending is common. They have the ability to manipulate others to carry out their wishes and if things go wrong they can skillfully project responsibility for the failure onto others (Janowsky et al, 1974). Energy seems inexhaustible, and the need for sleep is diminished. They may go for many days without sleep and still not feel tired. Hygiene and grooming may be neglected. Dress may be disorganized, flamboyant, or bizarre, with excessive make-up or jewelry.

STAGE III. DELIRIOUS MANIA

Delirious mania is a grave form of the disorder characterized by severe clouding of consciousness and representing an intensification of the symptoms associated with acute mania (Goodwin & Jamison, 1990). The symptoms of delirious mania have become relatively rare since the availability of antipsychotic medication.

Mood The mood of the delirious person is very labile. Commonly the individual changes from ti-midity and feelings of despair to unrestrained merriment and ecstasy to irritability and indifference (Kraepelin, 1921). Panic anxiety may be evident.

Cognition and Perception Cognition and perception are characterized by a clouding of consciousness, with accompanying confusion, disorientation, and sometimes stupor. Other common manifestations include religiosity, delusions of grandeur or persecution, and auditory or visual hallucinations. The individual is extremely distractible and incoherent.

Activity and Behavior Psychomotor activity is frenzied and characterized by agitated, purposeless movements. The safety of these individuals is at stake unless this activity is curtailed. Exhaustion, injury to self or others, and eventually death could occur without intervention.

Nursing Diagnoses

From the assessment data, nursing diagnoses are formulated from which the plan of care is derived. Possible nursing diagnoses for the patient with bipolar disorder, manic include:

High risk for injury related to extreme hyperactivity evidenced by increased agitation and lack of control over purposeless and potentially injurious movements

High risk for violence: Self-directed or directed at others related to manic excitement, delusional thinking, hallucinations

Altered nutrition: Less than body requirements related to refusal or inability to sit still long enough to eat evidenced by loss of weight, amenorrhea

Altered thought processes related to unresolved grief—denial of depression, evidenced by delusions of grandeur and persecution

Sensory-perceptual alteration related to unresolved grief—denial of depression, possible sleep deprivation, evidenced by auditory and visual hallucinations

Impaired social interaction related to egocentric and narcissistic behavior evidenced by inability to develop satisfying relationships and manipulation of others for own desires

Sleep pattern disturbance related to excessive hyperactivity and agitation, evidenced by difficulty falling asleep and sleeping only short periods

Planning/Implementation

Table 19.8 provides a plan of care for the manic patient. Selected nursing diagnoses are presented, along with goals of care and appropriate nursing interventions for each. Rationale is provided in italics.

Some institutions are using a case management model to coordinate care (see Chapter 6 for more detailed explanation). In case management models, the plan of care may take the form of a critical pathway. Table 19.9 depicts an example of a critical pathway of care for a manic patient.

OUTCOME CRITERIA

The following criteria may be used for measurement of outcomes in the care of the manic patient.

Table 19.8 CARE PLAN FOR THE MANIC PATIENT

Nursing Diagnoses	Objectives	Nursing Interventions
High risk for injury related to extreme hyperactivity evidenced by increased agitation and lack of control over purposeless and potentially injurious movements.	Patient will not experience injury.	Reduce environmental stimuli. Assign private room with simple decor, on quiet unit if possible. Keep lighting and noise level low. *Patient is extremely distractible and responses to even the slightest stimuli are exaggerated. A milieu unit may be too stimulating.* Remove hazardous objects and substances (including smoking materials). *Rationality is impaired, and patient may harm self inadvertently.* Stay with patient *to offer support and provide feeling of security* as agitation grows and hyperactivity increases. Provide physical activities *to help relieve pent-up tension.* Administer tranquilizing medication as ordered by physician. *Antipsychotics are common and are very effective for providing rapid relief from symptoms of hyperactivity.*
High risk for violence: Self-directed or directed at others related to manic excitement, delusional thinking, hallucinations.	Patient will not harm self or others.	Maintain low level of stimuli in patient's environment *to minimize anxiety, agitation, and suspiciousness.* Observe patient's behavior at least every 15 minutes *so that intervention can occur if required to ensure patient's (and others') safety.* Ensure that all sharp objects, glass or mirrored items, belts, ties, smoking materials have been removed from patient's environment *so that they may not be used to harm self or others.* Redirect violent behavior with physical outlets *for relieving pent-up tension and hostility.* Maintain and convey a calm attitude to patient. Respond matter-of-factly to verbal hostility. *Anxiety is contagious and can be transmitted from staff to patient.* Have sufficient staff to indicate a show of strength to patient if necessary. *This conveys evidence of control over the situation and provides some physical security for staff.* Offer tranquilizing medication. If patient refuses, use of mechanical restraints may be necessary. *Patient should be offered an avenue of the "least restrictive alternative."* Medication may then be administered following application of mechanical restraints. Observe patient every 15 minutes *to ensure that needs for circulation, nutrition, hydration, and elimination are met.* Remove restraints gradually, one at a time, *to minimize potential for injury to patient and staff*

(continued)

Table 19.8 CONTINUED

Nursing Diagnoses	Objectives	Nursing Interventions
Altered nutrition: Less than body requirements related to refusal or inability to sit still long enough to eat, evidenced by weight loss, amenorrhea.	Patient will exhibit no signs or symptoms of malnutrition.	Provide high-protein, high-calorie, nutritious finger foods and drinks that can be consumed "on the run" *because patient has difficulty sitting still long enough to eat a meal.* Have juice and snacks on unit at all times. *Nutritious intake is required on a regular basis to compensate for increased caloric requirements due to hyperactivity.* Maintain accurate record of intake, output, calorie count, and weight. Monitor daily laboratory values. *These are important nutritional assessment data.* Provide favorite foods *to encourage eating.* Supplement diet with vitamins and minerals *to improve nutritional status.* Walk or sit with patient while he or she eats *to offer support and to encourage patient to eat food that will maintain physical wellness.*
Impaired social interaction related to egocentric and narcissistic behavior, evidenced by inability to develop satisfying relationships and manipulation of others for own desires.	Patient will interact with others on the unit in an appropriate manner by discharge.	Recognize that manipulative behaviors help to reduce feelings of insecurity by increasing feelings of power and control. *Understanding the motivation behind the behavior may facilitate greater acceptance of the individual.* Set limits on manipulative behaviors. Explain what is expected and the consequences if limits are violated. Terms of the limitations must be agreed upon by all staff who will be working with the patient. *Consequences for violation of limits must be consistently administered, or behavior will not be eliminated.* Ignore attempts by patient to argue, bargain, or charm his or her way out of the limit setting. *Lack of feedback may decrease these behaviors.* Give positive reinforcement for nonmanipulative behaviors *to enhance self-esteem and promote repetition.* Discuss consequences of patient's behavior and how attempts are made to attribute them to others. *Patient must accept responsibility for own behavior before adaptive change can occur.* Help patient identify positive aspects about self, recognize accomplishments, and feel good about them. *As self-esteem is increased, patient will feel less need to manipulate others for own gratification.*

The patient:
1. exhibits no evidence of physical injury.
2. has not harmed self or others.
3. is no longer exhibiting signs of physical agitation.
4. eats a well-balanced diet with snacks to prevent weight loss and maintain nutritional status.
5. verbalizes an accurate interpretation of the environment.
6. verbalizes that hallucinatory activity has ceased.
7. accepts responsibility for own behaviors.
8. does not manipulate others for gratification of own needs.
9. interacts appropriately with others.
10. is able to fall asleep within 30 minutes of retiring.
11. is able to sleep 6 to 8 hours per night without medication.

Table 19.9 CRITICAL PATHWAY OF CARE FOR THE MANIC PATIENT

Estimated Length of Stay: 14 days—Variations from designated pathway should be documented in progress notes

Nursing Diagnoses and Categories of Care	Time Dimension	Goals and/or Actions	Time Dimension	Goals and/or Actions	Time Dimension	Discharge Outcome
High risk for injury/violence	Day 1	Environment is made safe for patient and others.	Ongoing	Patient does not harm self or others.	Day 14	Patient has not harmed self or others.
Referrals	Day 1	Psychiatrist Clinical nurse specialist Internist (may need to determine if symptoms are caused by other illness or medication side effects) Neurologist (may want to check for brain lesion) Alert hostility management team			Day 14	Discharge with follow-up appointments as required.
Diagnostic studies	Day 1	Drug screen Electrolytes Lithium level	Day 5 Day 10	Lithium level Lithium level	Day 14	Lithium level and discharge with instructions to return monthly to have level drawn.
Additional assessments	Day 1 Ongoing Ongoing	VS q4h Restraints prn Assess for signs of impending violent behavior: Increase in psychomotor activity, angry affect, verbalized persecutory delusions, or frightening hallucinations.	Day 2–14	Ongoing assessments		

(continued)

Table 19.9 CONTINUED

Estimated Length of Stay: 14 days—Variations from designated pathway should be documented in progress notes

Nursing Diagnoses and Categories of Care	Time Dimension	Goals and/or Actions	Time Dimension	Goals and/or Actions	Time Dimension	Discharge Outcome
Medications	Day 1	Antipsychotic medications, scheduled and prn. Lithium carbonate 600 mg tid or qid	Day 2–14	Administer medications as ordered and observe for effectiveness and side effects.	Day 14	Patient is discharged on maintenance dose lithium carbonate.
Patient education			Day 9	Teach about lithium: Continue to take medication even when feeling okay. Teach signs and symptoms of toxicity. Emphasize importance of monthly blood levels.	Day 14	Patient is discharged with written instructions and verbalizes understanding of material presented.
			Day 12	Reinforce teaching.		
Altered nutrition: Less than body requirements					Day 14	Nutritional condition and weight have stabilized.
Referrals	Day 1	Consult dietitian	Day 1–14	Fulfill nutritional needs		
Diet	Day 1	High-protein, high-calorie, nutritious finger foods. Juice and snacks as tolerated.	As mania subsides	Regular diet with foods of patient's choice.		
Diagnostic studies	Day 1	Chemistry profile Urinalysis	Day 2–13	Repeat of selected diagnostic studies as required.		

(*continued*)

Table 19.9 CONTINUED

Estimated Length of Stay: 14 days—Variations from designated pathway should be documented in progress notes

Nursing Diagnoses and Categories of Care	Time Dimension	Goals and/or Actions	Time Dimension	Goals and/or Actions	Time Dimension	Discharge Outcome
Additional assessments	Day 1–14	Weight I&O Skin turgor Color of mucous membranes				
Medications	Day 1–14	Multiple vitamin/mineral tab				
Patient education			Day 9	Principles of nutrition; foods for maintenance of wellness; adequate sodium; 6–8 glasses of water/day. Contact dietitian if weight gain becomes a problem.	Day 12–14	Patient demonstrates ability to select appropriate foods for healthy diet and verbalizes understanding of material presented.
			Day 12	Reinforce teaching.		

Evaluation of Care for the Manic Patient

In the final step of the nursing process, a reassessment is conducted to determine if the nursing actions have been successful in achieving the objectives of care. Evaluation of the nursing actions for the manic patient may be facilitated by gathering information using the following types of questions.

Has the individual avoided personal injury? Has violence to patient or others been prevented? Has agitation subsided? Have nutritional status and weight been stabilized? Is patient able to select foods to maintain adequate nutrition? Have delusions and hallucinations ceased? Is patient able to interpret the environment correctly? Is patient able to make decisions about own self-care? Have hygiene and grooming improved? Is behavior socially acceptable? Is patient able to interact with others in a satisfactory manner? Has patient stopped manipulating others to fulfill own desires? Is patient able to sleep 6 to 8 hours per night and awaken feeling rested? Does patient understand importance of maintenance lithium therapy? Does patient understand that symptoms may return if lithium is stopped? Can patient verbalize early signs of lithium toxicity? Does he or she understand the necessity for monthly blood level checks?

TREATMENT MODALITIES FOR MOOD DISORDERS

Psychological Treatments

INDIVIDUAL PSYCHOTHERAPY

For Depression Research has documented both the importance of close and satisfactory attachments in the prevention of depression and the role of disrupted attachments in the development of depression (Klerman, 1988). With this concept in mind, interpersonal psychotherapy (IPT) focuses on the patient's current interpersonal relations. Interpersonal psychotherapy with the depressed person proceeds through the following phases and interventions (Klerman, 1988):

Phase I. During the first phase, the patient is assessed to determine the extent of the illness. Complete information is then given to the individual regarding the nature of depression, symptom pattern, frequency, clinical course, and alternative treatments. If the level of depression is severe, IPT has been shown to be more effective if conducted in combination with antidepressant medication. The patient is encouraged to continue working and participation in regular activities during therapy. A mutually agreeable therapeutic contract is negotiated.

Phase II. Treatment at this phase focuses on helping the patient resolve dysfunctional grief reactions. This may include resolving the ambivalence with the lost relationship, serving as a temporary substitute for the lost relationship, and assistance with establishing new relationships. Other areas of treatment focus may include interpersonal disputes between the patient and a significant other, difficult role transitions at various developmental life cycles, and correction of interpersonal deficits that may interfere with the patient's ability to initiate or sustain interpersonal relationships.

Phase III. During the final phase of IPT the therapeutic alliance is terminated. With emphasis on reassurance, clarification of emotional states, improvement of interpersonal communication, testing of perceptions, and performance in interpersonal settings, IPT has been successful in helping depressed persons recover enhanced social functioning.

For Mania Manic patients traditionally have been difficult candidates for psychotherapy. They form a therapeutic relationship easily because they are eager to please and grateful for the therapist's interest. However, the relationship tends to remain shallow and rigid (Aleksandrowicz, 1980). However, recent reports indicate that psychotherapy

(in conjunction with lithium maintenance treatment) and counseling may indeed be useful with these individuals (Klerman, 1982).

Aleksandrowicz (1980) states:

". . . the manic patient should receive adequate biological treatment. Once the mood is stabilized the patient and therapist should decide whether psychological exploration is needed. Attempts to control severe mood swings by psychological means alone are of questionable value, and may even be risky. On the other hand, there is clinical evidence that in some patients skillfully conducted psychotherapy helps to avert the recurrence or reduce the severity of manic attacks."

GROUP THERAPY

For Depression and Mania Group therapy forms an important dimension of multimodal treatment of the manic or depressed patient (Spitz, 1988). Once an acute phase of the illness is passed, groups can provide an atmosphere in which individuals may discuss issues in their lives that cause, maintain, or arise out of having a serious affective disorder. The element of peer support provides a feeling of security as troublesome or embarrassing issues are discussed and resolved. Some groups have other specific purposes, such as helping to monitor medication-related issues or as an avenue for promoting education related to affective disorder and its treatment.

Support groups help members gain a sense of perspective on their condition and tangibly encourage them to link up with others who have common problems. A sense of hope is conveyed when the individual is able to see that he or she is not alone or unique in experiencing affective illness.

Self-help groups offer another avenue of support for the depressed or manic patient. These groups are usually peer-led, and are not meant to substitute for, or compete with, professional therapy. They offer supplementary support that frequently enhances compliance with the medical regimen. Some examples of self-help groups include the National Depressive and Manic-Depressive Association (NDMDA), Depressives Anonymous, Families of Depressives, Manic and Depressive Support Group, Recovery Inc., and New Images for Widows. Though self-help groups are not psychotherapy groups, they do provide important adjunctive support experiences which often have "therapeutic" benefit for participants (Spitz, 1988).

FAMILY THERAPY

For Depression and Mania   The ultimate objective in working with families of patients with mood disorders is to synthesize the available data to formulate a therapeutic plan with two key goals: resolution of the symptoms and restoration or creation of adaptive family function (Spitz, 1988). As with group therapy, the most effective approach appears to be with a combination of psychotherapeutic and psychopharmacologic treatments.

The management of mood disorders within the family context differs very little from approaches used to manage other types of family problems. Paolino and McCrady (1978) have identified the following tasks of family therapy that can be applied with families who have members with mood disorders:

1. specifying problems
2. clarifying each individual's needs and desires
3. redefining the nature of the family's difficulties
4. encouraging recognition of each member's contribution to the discord
5. recognizing and modifying communication patterns, rules, and interactional patterns
6. increasing reciprocity
7. decreasing the use of coercion and blaming
8. increasing cooperative problem solving
9. establishing a positive working relationship between family and therapist
10. increasing each member's ability to express feelings clearly and directly, and to "hear" others accurately

COGNITIVE THERAPY

For Depression and Mania   In cognitive therapy, the individual is taught to control thought distortions that are considered to be a factor in the development and maintenance of mood disorders. In the cognitive model, depression is characterized by a triad of negative distortions related to expectations of the environment, self, and future. The environment and activities within it are viewed as unsatisfying, the self is unrealistically devalued, and the

future is perceived as hopeless. In the same model mania is characterized by a positive cognitive triad —the self is seen as highly valued and powerful, experiences within the environment are viewed as overly positive, and the future is seen as one of unlimited opportunity (Leahy & Beck, 1988).

The general goals in cognitive therapy are to obtain symptom relief as quickly as possible, to assist the patient in identifying dysfunctional patterns of thinking and behaving, and to guide the patient to evidence and logic that effectively tests the validity of the dysfunctional thinking. Therapy focuses on changing "automatic thoughts" that occur spontaneously and contribute to the distorted affect. Examples of "automatic thoughts" in depression include:

1. personalizing: "I'm the only one who failed."
2. all or nothing: "I'm a complete failure."
3. mind reading: "He thinks I'm foolish."
4. discounting positives: "The other questions were so easy. Any dummy could have gotten them right."

Examples of "automatic thoughts" in mania include:

1. personalizing: "She's this happy only when she's with me."
2. all or nothing: "Everything I do is great."
3. mind reading: "She thinks I'm wonderful."
4. discounting negatives: "None of those mistakes are really important."

The patient is asked to describe evidence that both supports and disputes the automatic thought. The logic underlying the inferences is then reviewed with the patient. Another technique involves evaluating what would most likely happen if the patient's automatic thoughts were true. Implications of the consequences are then discussed.

Patients should not become discouraged if one technique seems not to be working. There is no single technique that works with all patients. He or she should be reassured that there are a number of techniques that may be used, and both therapist and patient may explore these possibilities.

Finally, the use of cognitive therapy does not preclude the value of administering medication (Leahy & Beck, 1988). Particularly in the treatment of mania, cognitive therapy should be considered a secondary treatment to pharmacological treatment. Cognitive therapy alone has offered encouraging results in the treatment of depression. In fact, the results of several studies with depressed patients provide evidence that cognitive therapy may be more effective than antidepressant medication in some cases (Lewinsohn & Hoberman, 1982; Wolpert, 1988).

Organic Treatments

PSYCHOPHARMACOLOGY

For Depression The tricyclic antidepressants (TCAs), along with related and newer heterocyclic compounds, such as fluoxetine and bupropion, are the most widely prescribed drugs used to treat depression (Goodwin & Jamison, 1990). Since the initial discovery of their antidepressant properties, the tricyclic drugs have been subjected to hundreds of controlled trials, and their efficacy in treating depressive illness is now firmly established (see Chapter 12 for a detailed discussion of antidepressant medications).

A subsiding of symptoms may not occur for up to four weeks after beginning therapy with TCAs. It is important, therefore, for patients to understand that even though it may seem the medication is now producing the desired effects, he or she must continue taking it for at least a month to determine efficacy. The greater effectiveness of one TCA over another with any given patient is not yet fully understood. Choice of drug may be based on symptoms. For example, anxious patients may be started on TCAs with high sedative properties and patients with psychomotor retardation on those with the least sedative properties. When possible, selection of the appropriate drug is based on a history of previous responses to antidepressant therapy.

Common side effects of the TCAs and related drugs include sedation, tachycardia, dry mouth, constipation, urinary retention, blurred vision, orthostatic hypotension, lowering of the seizure threshold, weight gain, and changes in sexual functioning. Elderly individuals may be particularly sensitive to these medications, and adjustments in dosage must be considered. TCAs are absolutely contraindicated in cases of severe heart disease and untreated narrow-angle glaucoma (Kragh-Sorensen, 1988).

Monoamine oxidase (MAO) inhibitors have a unique place in the history of antidepressant medications. They were originally used in the treatment of tuberculosis. Evidence that individuals who were treated with the medication experienced a sense of well-being, without bacteriologic improvement, led to the discovery of their enzyme inhibition properties and the subsequent hypothesis that monoamines have a function in regulating mood (Schildkraut, 1965).

Following the initial enthusiasm about MAO inhibitors, they fell into relative disuse for nearly two decades because of a perceived poor risk-to-benefit ratio (Kurtz & Robinson, 1988). They have now regained widespread acceptance as a viable alternative to TCAs, as it has been shown that some individuals respond more beneficially to MAOIs than to any other antidepressant medication.

The greatest concern with using MAO inhibitors is the potential for hypertensive crisis, which is considered a medical emergency. Hypertensive crisis occurs in patients on MAO inhibitor therapy who consume foods and/or drugs high in tyramine content (Table 19.10). Typically, symptoms develop within two hours after ingestion of a food or drug high in tyramine, and include severe occipital and/or temporal pounding headaches with occasional photophobia. Sensations of choking, palpitations, and a feeling of "dread" are common. Marked systolic and diastolic hypertension occurs, sometimes with neck stiffness (Kurtz & Robinson, 1988). In addition to hypertensive crisis, side effects are similar to those associated with the TCAs.

A "second generation" of antidepressants have been marketed since the early 1970s. These include maprotiline (Ludiomil), amoxapine (Asendin), trazodone (Desyrel), bupropion (Wellbutrin), fluoxetine (Prozac), and sertraline (Zoloft). While most of these new antidepressants were initially touted as being better than drugs used in the past, accumulated evidence and experience have usually dampened this initial enthusiasm (McCue & Georgotas, 1988).

Maprotiline, although found to be as effective as the older antidepressants in treating depressive symptoms, carries an increased risk of seizures and greater toxicity in overdose.

Amoxapine, a derivative of the antipsychotic loxapine, has been shown to be effective for psychotic depression, but has a potential for causing neuroleptic malignant syndrome and tardive dyskinesia.

Trazodone is equally as effective as the older an-

Table 19.10 TYRAMINE-CONTAINING FOODS AND DRUGS: IMPLICATIONS FOR MAOI THERAPY

Foods High in Tyramine Content Must be Avoided	Foods Moderate in Tyramine Content Limited Amounts Allowed	Foods Low in Tyramine Content Permissible
Aged cheeses (cheddar, Camembert, blue cheese)	Avocados	Pasteurized cheeses (cream cheese, cottage cheese, ricotta)
Yeast extract (found in some packaged soups)	Bananas	Distilled spirits (in moderation)
Smoked herring	Ales and beers	
Smoked and processed meats (salami, pepperoni, summer sausage)	Most white wines and champagnes	
Fava beans	Caffeinated coffee	
Red Wines (chianti, burgundy, cabernet sauvignon)	Chocolate	
	Colas	

Drugs Absolutely Contraindicated	Drugs Markedly Potentiated by Tyramine	Drugs Potentiated by Tyramine
Stimulants (amphetamines, cocaine, diet drugs)	Narcotics (meperidine)	Narcotics (morphine, codeine)
Decongestants (sinus, hay fever, and cold tablets)	Sympathomimetics (epinephrine, norepinephrine, dopamine)	Sedatives (barbiturates, alcohol)
Antihypertensives (methyldopa, guanethidine, reserpine)	General anesthetics	Local anesthetics with vasoconstrictors
Antiparkinsonian (L-dopa)		

Source: Kurtz and Robinson (1988).

tidepressants, and with fewer side effects (the most common being sedation). A relatively rare adverse effect that has been observed with trazodone is priapism (prolonged, painful erection). This is a very problematic condition requiring surgical intervention in some patients.

Bupropion has been found to be as effective as the older antidepressants, and has notably fewer anticholinergic and cardiovascular side effects. There have been some difficulties in the past, however, with increased risk of seizures, especially in emaciated patients.

Fluoxetine, one of the newest of the second generation antidepressants, has yet to undergo extensive studies. Initial data indicate that it has fewer anticholinergic and cardiovascular side effects, and is equally as effective in alleviating symptoms of depression as the older antidepressants. Its most common side effects are nervousness, nausea and weight loss. Some recent reports suggest that fluoxetine may be implicated in several cases of suicide, but empirical supportive evidence is lacking.

Sertraline, the latest antidepressant to be mar-keted in the United States, is comparable in its action to fluoxetine. Both of these drugs block the reuptake of serotonin. Sertraline has undergone limited clinical trials which indicated the most common side effects to be GI upset, headache, and insomnia. A significant number of male subjects experienced primary ejaculatory delay. Cardiovascular side effects were minimal.

For Mania Lithium carbonate is the drug of choice for acute manic episodes, as well as for maintenance therapy to prevent or diminish the intensity of subsequent manic episodes. Its mode of action in the control of manic symptoms is unclear. It has also been indicated for treatment of bipolar depression (see Chapter 12 for a detailed discussion of lithium carbonate).

Common side effects of lithium therapy include drowsiness, dizziness, headache, dry mouth, thirst, GI upset, fine hand tremors, pulse irregularities, polyuria, and weight gain. In initiating lithium therapy with an acutely manic individual, physicians commonly order an antipsychotic as well. Because normalization of symptoms with lithium may not be achieved for up to one to three weeks, the antipsychotic medication will serve to calm the excessive hyperactivity of the manic patient until the lithium reaches therapeutic level.

Therapeutic level of lithium carbonate is 1.0 to 1.5 mEq/L for acute mania and 0.6 to 1.2 mEq/L for maintenance therapy. There is a narrow margin between the therapeutic and toxic levels, and lithium levels should be drawn weekly until therapeutic level is reached, then monthly during maintenance therapy (Townsend, 1990). Lithium toxicity is a life-threatening condition and monitoring of lithium levels is critical. The initial signs of lithium toxicity include ataxia, blurred vision, severe diarrhea, persistent nausea and vomiting, and tinnitis. Symptoms intensify as toxicity increases and include excessive output of dilute urine, psychomotor retardation, mental confusion, tremors and muscular irritability, seizures, impaired consciousness, oliguria/anuria, arrhythmias, coma and eventually death.

Pretreatment assessments should include adequacy of renal functioning, as 95 percent of ingested lithium is eliminated via the kidneys (Johnson, 1988). Use of lithium during pregnancy is not recommended due to results of studies that indicate a greater number of cardiac anomalies in babies born to mothers who consumed lithium, particularly in the first trimester.

A number of other medications have been tried on an investigational basis in the treatment of mania, with varying degrees of success. Examples include anticonvulsants (carbamazapine, clonazepam, valproic acid) and calcium channel blockers (verapamil). These drugs have been used as alternate or adjunctive approaches to management of patients with bipolar illness refractory to lithium.

ELECTROCONVULSIVE THERAPY

For Depression and Mania Electroconvulsive therapy (ECT) is the induction of a grand mal (generalized) seizure through the application of electrical current to the brain. The effectiveness of electroconvulsive therapy has been demonstrated with patients who are acutely suicidal. It has also been very effective in the treatment of severe depression, particularly in those patients who are also experiencing psychotic symptoms and those with psychomotor retardation and neurovegetative changes, such as disturbances in sleep, appetite, and energy. It is often considered for treatment only after a trial of therapy with antidepressant medication has proved ineffective.

Episodes of acute mania are occasionally treated with ECT, particularly in instances when the patient does not tolerate or fails to respond to lithium or other drug treatment, or when life is threatened by dangerous behavior or exhaustion (see Chapter 13 for a detailed discussion of electroconvulsive therapy).

SUICIDE

Epidemiological Factors

Approximately 25,000 persons in the United States end their lives each year by suicide. These statistics have established suicide as the fifth leading cause of death among adults and the second leading cause of death among adolescents (Slaby et al, 1986). Many more people attempt suicide than succeed, and countless others seriously contemplate the act without carrying it out. Suicide has indeed become a major health care problem in the United States today.

Over the years there has been some confusion over the reality of various notions regarding suicide. A variety of facts and fables as they relate to suicide are presented in Table 19.11.

Risk Factors

MARITAL STATUS

The suicide rate for single persons is twice that of married persons. Divorced and widowed individuals have rates four to five times greater than those of the married (Slaby et al, 1986).

GENDER

Women attempt suicide more, but more men succeed. Successful suicides number about 70% for men and 30% for women. This has to do with the lethality of the means. While women tend to overdose, men use more lethal means such as firearms. Interestingly, female medical students have suicide rates three to four times that of their non-medical agemates (Slaby et al, 1986).

Table 19.11 FACTS AND FABLES ABOUT SUICIDE	
Fables	**Facts**
People who talk about suicide don't commit suicide. Suicide happens without warning.	Eight out of ten people who kill themselves have given definite clues and warnings about their suicidal intentions. Very subtle clues may be ignored or disregarded by others.
You can't stop a suicidal person. He/she is fully intent on dying.	Most suicidal people are very ambivalent about their feelings regarding living or dying. Most are "gambling with death," and see it as a cry for someone to save them.
Once a person is suicidal, he or she is suicidal forever.	People who want to kill themselves are only suicidal for a limited time. If they are saved from feelings of self-destruction, they can go on to lead normal lives.
Improvement after severe depression means that the suicidal risk is over.	Most suicides occur within about 3 months after the beginning of "improvement," when the individual has the energy to carry out suicidal intentions.
Suicide is inherited or "runs in families."	Suicide is not inherited. It is an individual matter and can be prevented. However, suicide by a close family member increases an individual's risk factor for suicide.
All suicidal individuals are mentally ill, and suicide is the act of a psychotic person.	Although suicidal persons are extremely unhappy, they are not necessarily psychotic nor otherwise mentally ill. They are merely unable at that point in time to see an alternative solution to what they consider an unbearable problem.
Suicidal threats and gestures should be considered manipulative or attention-seeking behavior, and should not be taken seriously.	All suicidal behavior must be approached with the gravity of the potential act in mind. Attention should be given to the possibility that the individual is issuing a cry for help.

(*continued*)

Table 19.11 CONTINUED	
Fables	**Facts**
People usually commit suicide by taking an overdose of drugs.	Gunshot wounds are the leading cause of death among suicide victims.
If a patient has attempted suicide, he or she will not do it again.	Fifty to 80 percent of all people who ultimately kill themselves have a history of a previous attempt.

Sources: Shneidman and Farberow (1965); Freedman et al. (1976); and Slaby et al (1986).

AGE

Suicide risk and age are positively correlated. After adolescence, there is a decline in rates until age 40, at which time they again begin to rise. Rates continue to rise to a peak of 42 per 100,000 per year at age 75 to 79, the highest in any group (Frederick, 1978).

Suicide has been identified as second only to accidents as the leading cause of death among adolescents. High-risk factors associated with adolescent suicide include religion (less likely if Catholic or Jewish), having parents with psychiatric illness (particularly drug/alcohol abuse), a history of suicide in the family, paternal unemployment, and paternal or maternal absence (Slaby et al, 1986).

RELIGION

Protestants have significantly higher rates of suicide than Catholics and Jews (Hipple & Cimbolic, 1979). A strong feeling of cohesiveness within a religious organization seems to be an important factor.

SOCIOECONOMIC STATUS

Individuals in the very highest and lowest social classes have higher suicide rates than those in the middle classes (Hipple & Cimbolic, 1979). With regard to occupation, suicide rates are higher among physicians, business executives, pharmacists, dentists, lawyers, and engineers. Rates are lowest among farm workers and artisans (Slaby et al, 1986).

RACE

Whites have suicide rates higher than those of Blacks. Suicide is a special problem among Native Americans, who have rates 64% higher than whites (Slaby et al, 1986).

OTHER RISK FACTORS

Patients with depressive and manic-depressive illness are far more likely to commit suicide than individuals in any other psychiatric or medical risk group (Goodwin & Jamison, 1990). Self-inflicted death among the seriously depressed has been estimated to be from 70 to 500 times more frequent than in the general population (Slaby et al, 1986). Suicide risk may increase early during treatment with antidepressants as the return of energy brings about an increased ability to act out self-destructive wishes.

Severe insomnia is associated with increased suicide risk even in the absence of depression. Use of alcohol, and particularly a combination of alcohol and barbiturates, increases risk of suicide. Psychosis, particularly with command hallucinations, poses a higher risk. Individuals with a predominantly homosexual orientation have a higher risk, especially if depressed, aging, or alcoholic (Slaby et al, 1986). Affliction with a chronic painful and/or disabling illness increases the risk of suicide.

Higher risk is also associated with a family history of suicide, especially in a same-sex parent, and with previous attempters. Fifty to eighty percent of those who ultimately commit suicide have a history of a previous attempt (Slaby et al, 1986). Loss of a loved one through death or separation and lack of employment or increased financial burden increase risk.

Predisposing Factors: Theories of Suicide

PSYCHOANALYTIC THEORY

Freud (1957) believed that suicide was a response to the intense self-hatred that an individual possessed. The anger had originated toward a love object, but was ultimately turned inward against the self. Freud believed that suicide occurred as a result of an earlier repressed desire to kill someone else. He interpreted suicide to be an aggressive act toward the self that often was really directed toward others.

SOCIOLOGICAL THEORY

Durkheim (1951) studied the individual's interaction with the society in which he or she lived. He believed that the more cohesive the society, and the more that the individual felt an integrated part of the society, the less likely he or she was to commit suicide. Durkheim described three social categories of suicide:

Egoistic suicide identified the response of the individual who felt separate and apart from the mainstream of society. Integration was lacking.

Altruistic suicide is the opposite of egoistic suicide. The individual who is prone to altruistic suicide is excessively integrated into the group. Allegiance to the group is governed by cultural, religious, or political ties.

Anomic suicide occurs in response to changes that occur in an individual's life (e.g., divorce, loss of job) that disrupt feelings of relatedness to the group. An interruption in the customary norms of behavior instills feelings of "separateness," and fears of being without support from the formerly cohesive group.

APPLICATION OF THE NURSING PROCESS TO THE SUICIDAL PATIENT

Assessment

Bassuk et al (1982) outline the following items that should be considered in a suicidal assessment:

DEMOGRAPHICS

The following demographics are assessed:

Age Suicide is highest in persons over age 50. Adolescents are also at high risk.

Gender Males are at higher risk than females.

Race Native Americans > Whites > Blacks.

Marital Status Single, divorced, and widowed are at higher risk than married.

Occupation Professional health care personnel and business executives are at highest risk.

Method Firearms > > overdose of substances.

Religion Protestants are at greater risk than Catholics or Jewish.

Family History Higher risk if has family history of suicide.

PRESENTING SYMPTOMS/ MEDICAL-PSYCHIATRIC DIAGNOSIS

Assessment data must be gathered regarding any psychiatric or physical condition for which the patient is being treated. Depression is the most common disorder which preceeds suicide. Other chronic and terminal physical illnesses have also precipitated suicidal acts.

SUICIDAL IDEAS OR ACTS

How serious is the intent? Does the person have a plan? If so, does he or she have the means? How lethal is the means? These are all questions that must be answered by the person conducting the suicidal assessment.

Individuals may leave both behavioral and verbal clues as to intent of their act. Examples of behavioral clues include giving away prized possessions, getting financial affairs in order, writing suicide notes, or sudden lifts in mood (may indicate a decision to carry out the intent).

Verbal clues may be both direct and indirect. Examples of direct statements include:

"I want to die."
"I'm going to kill myself."

Examples of indirect statements include:

"This is the last time you'll see me."
"I won't be around much longer for the doctor to have to worry with."
"I don't have anything worth living for anymore."

Other assessments include determining whether the individual has a plan, and if so, whether he or she has the means to carry out that plan. If the person states the suicide will be carried out with a gun, does he or she have access to a gun? Bullets? If pills are planned, what kind of pills? Are they accessible?

INTERPERSONAL SUPPORT SYSTEM

Does the individual have support persons on whom he or she can rely during a crisis situation?

Lack of a meaningful network of satisfactory relationships may implicate an individual at high risk for suicide during an emotional crisis.

ANALYSIS OF THE SUICIDAL CRISIS

The Precipitating Stressor Life stresses accompanied by an increase in emotional disturbance include the loss of a loved person either by death or by divorce, problems in major relationships, changes in roles, or serious physical illness. When compared with the general population, suicide attempters have experienced a greater number of situational crises in the previous 6 months, with the peak in the month prior to the suicidal act (Bassuk et al, 1982).

Relevant History Has the individual experienced numerous failures or rejections which would increase his or her vulnerability for a dysfunctional response to the current situation?

Life-Stage Issues The ability to tolerate losses and disappointments is often compromised if they occur during various stages of life in which individuals are struggling with developmental issues (e.g., adolescence, midlife).

PSYCHIATRIC/MEDICAL/FAMILY HISTORY

The individual should be assessed with regard to previous psychiatric treatment for depression, alcoholism, or for previous suicide attempts. Medical history should be obtained to determine presence of chronic, debilitating, or terminal illness. Is there a history of depressive disorder in the family, and has a close relative committed suicide in the past?

COPING STRATEGIES

How has the individual handled previous crisis situations? How does this situation differ from previous ones?

Planning/Implementation

Colvin (1980) suggests that the most important aspect of care for the suicidal person is the provision of a caring, therapeutic environment. She states that the nurse may provide this type of environment by instituting the following eight-point plan:

1. ***Establish a therapeutic relationship.*** A therapeutic relationship conveys acceptance of the individual aside from the unacceptable act of suicide. If even one person is able to establish rapport with the patient, this may well be the best protection against suicide.
2. ***Communicate the potential for suicide to team members.*** This is an around-the-clock team effort. Any clues of potential suicide, no matter how insignificant they may seem, should be reported to all team members, including the physician. Subtle clues may well reveal intent, and after-the-fact is too late to make the determination that the patient was indeed serious about suicide.
3. ***Stay with the person.*** Provide watchful care and give the person a sense of assurance that control will be provided until he or she can regain self-control. The nurse's presence will convey support for the suicidal person throughout the current crisis.
4. ***Accept the person.*** Show unconditional positive regard. That is, convey to the individual: "I care about you and accept you for no other reason than the fact that you are a fellow human being." Unless the suicide potential is extremely acute, don't completely isolate this person from others and strip him or her of all personal possessions. This only serves to intensify feelings of worthlessness. Do, however, make the environment safe. Remove sharp items, belts, ties, smoking materials, and substances with which the individual could harm himself or herself.
5. ***Listen to the person.*** After the patient comes to realize that the nurse is interested in and accepts him or her, the nurse should encourage the patient to identify, examine and share the source of the current emotional pain. The suicide risk may decrease if the individual feels that someone hears and understands what he or she is feeling. Explore with the patient others who might be available to provide comfort. Perhaps communication patterns with significant others may need improvement.
6. ***Secure a no-suicide contract.*** Have the patient promise (verbally or in writing) that he or she will not attempt suicide for a specified length of time. When that time has elapsed, secure another promise. This gives the nurse and other professionals some time to help the patient. This may also offer the patient a sense of relief for getting the idea of suicide out in the open and discussing it in a nonjudgmental environment with a trusted individual.
7. ***Give the person a message of hope.*** The suicidal person views life as hopeless, without any possibility for improvement. He or she undoubtedly has many ambivalent feelings regarding living or dying, but without hope for betterment, sees life as not worth living. After listening to the patient's expression of emotional pain, encourage him or her to accept a message of optimism that life can be better. Discuss possible alternatives available to solve painful issues, and convey to the patient that although the process may be very difficult, a measure of hope does exist.
8. ***Give the person something to do.*** Meaningful activities that release tension and anger can benefit the individual by allowing a medium for expression of hostility and aggression in a constructive manner. Large motor activities, such as volleyball, pounding clay, or repairing, sanding, and refinishing furniture, are best for this. It is also important that the individual resume independent participation in activities of daily living. Activities such as these that promote achievement and a sense of belonging increase feelings of self-worth, as the individual once again becomes involved in the interactions of living.

Evaluation

Evaluation of the suicidal patient is an ongoing process accomplished through continuous reassessment of the patient, as well as determination of goal achievement. Once the immediate crisis has been resolved, extended psychotherapy may be indicated. The long-term goals of individual or group psychotherapy for the suicidal patient would be for him or her to:

1. develop and maintain a more positive self-concept.
2. learn more effective ways to express feelings to others.

3. achieve successful interpersonal relationships.
4. feel accepted by others and achieve a sense of belonging.

A suicidal person feels worthless and hopeless. These goals serve to instill a sense of self-worth, while offering a measure of hope and a meaning for living.

SUMMARY

Depression is one of the oldest recognized psychiatric illnesses that is still prevalent today. It is so common, in fact, that it has been referred to as the "common cold of psychiatric disorders."

Everyone experiences transient feelings of depression from time to time, most commonly in response to a real or perceived loss. Several theorists have described the grief response as it progresses through stages over a predictable period. Grieving is considered to be maladaptive when the response is delayed, prolonged, or exaggerated. Pathological depression is an exaggerated grief response and occurs when an individual experiences a threat to the self-esteem.

The cause of depressive disorders is not entirely known. A number of factors, including genetics, biochemical influences, and psychosocial experiences enter into the development of the disorder. Secondary depression occurs in response to other physiological disorders. Symptoms occur along a continuum according to the degree of severity from transient to severe. The disorder occurs in all developmental levels, including childhood, adolescence, senescence, and during the puerperium.

Bipolar disorder, mania, is a maladaptive response to loss and has been referred to as the "mirror image of depression." Symptoms occur in response to a real or perceived loss, and are considered a denial of depression. Genetic influences have been strongly implicated in the development of the disorder. Various other physiologic factors, such as biochemical and electrolyte alterations, as well as cerebral structural changes, have been implicated. Side effects of certain medications have also been shown to induce symptoms of mania. No one theory can explain the etiology of bipolar disorder, and it is likely that the illness is caused by a combination of biologic and psychosocial factors. Symptoms of bipolar disorder, manic may be observed on a continuum of three phases, each identified by the degree of severity: phase I, hypomania; phase II, acute mania; phase III, delirious mania.

Treatment of mood disorders include individual, group, family, and cognitive therapies. Somatic therapies include psychopharmacology and ECT. Nursing care follows the five steps of the nursing process.

Suicide is the fifth leading cause of death among adults and the second leading cause of death among adolescents in the United States today. Assessment of the suicidal patient implicates the following factors for determining high-risk status: marital status, age, gender, race, occupation, religion, family history, physical condition, support systems, precipitating stressors, coping strategies, seriousness of intent, and lethality and availability of method.

Nursing care is accomplished using the steps of the nursing process. When the immediate crisis has been resolved, the patient may require long-term psychotherapy.

REVIEW QUESTIONS
Self-Examination/Learning Exercise

*Select the answer that is **most** appropriate for each of the following questions.*

Margaret, age 68, was brought to the emergency department of a large regional medical center by her sister-in-law who stated, "She does nothing but sit and stare into space. I can't get her to eat or anything!" Upon assessment, it was found that 6 months ago Margaret's husband of 45 years had died of a massive myocardial infarction. They had no children, and were inseparable. Since her husband's death, Margaret has visited the cemetery every day, changing the flowers often on his grave. She has not removed any of his clothes from the closet or chest of drawers. His shaving materials still occupy the same space in the bathroom. Over the months, Margaret has become more and more socially isolated. She refuses invitations from friends, preferring instead to make her daily trips to the cemetery. She has lost 15 pounds, and her sister-in-law reports that there is very little food in the house. Today she said to her sister-in-law, "I don't really want to live anymore. My life is nothing without Frank." Her sister-in-law became frightened and, with forceful persuasion, was able to convince Margaret she needed to see a doctor.

1. The priority nursing diagnosis for Margaret would be:
   a. Altered nutrition: less than body requirements
   b. Dysfunctional grieving
   c. High risk for self-directed violence
   d. Social isolation

2. The physician orders amitriptyline (Elavil) 20 mg qid for Margaret. After 3 days of taking the medication, Margaret says to the nurse, "I don't think this medicine is doing any good. I don't feel a bit better." What is the most appropriate response by the nurse?
   a. "Cheer up, Margaret. You have so much to be happy about."
   b. "Sometimes it takes a few weeks for the medicine to bring about an improvement in symptoms."
   c. "I'll report that to the physician, Margaret. Maybe he will order something different."
   d. "Try not to dwell on your symptoms, Margaret. Why don't you join the others down in the dayroom?"

After 3 weeks, Margaret's mood improved and she was released from the hospital with directions to continue taking the amitriptyline as ordered. A week later her sister-in-law found Margaret in bed and was unable to awaken her. An empty prescription bottle was by her side. She was revived in the emergency department and transferred to the psychiatric unit in a state of severe depression. The physician determines that electroconvulsive therapy may help Margaret. Consent is obtained.

3. About 30 minutes prior to the first treatment the nurse administers atropine sulfate 0.4 mg IM. Rationale for this order is:
   a. to decrease secretions and increase heart rate.
   b. to relax muscles.
   c. to produce a calming effect.
   d. to induce anesthesia.

4. When Margaret is in the treatment room, the anesthesiologist administers thiopental sodium (Pentothal) followed by IV succinylcholine (Anectine). The purposes of these medications are to:
   a. decrease secretions and increase heart rate.
   b. prevent nausea and induce a calming effect.
   c. minimize memory loss and stabilize mood.
   d. induce anesthesia and relax muscles.

5. After three ECTs, Margaret's mood begins to lift, and she states to the nurse, "I feel so much better, but I'm having trouble remembering some things that happened this last week." The nurse's best response would be:

    a. "Don't worry about that. Nothing important happened."
    b. "Memory loss is just something you have to put up with in order to feel better."
    c. "Memory loss is a side effect of ECT. But it is only temporary. Your memory should return within a few weeks."
    d. "Forget about last week, Margaret. You need to look forward from here."

A year later, Margaret presents in the emergency department, once again accompanied by her sister-in-law. This time Margaret is agitated, pacing, demanding, and speaking very loudly. "I didn't want to come here! My sister-in-law is just jealous, and she's trying to make it look like I'm insane!" Upon assessment, the sister-in-law reports that Margaret has become engaged to a 25-year-old construction worker to whom she has willed her sizable inheritance and her home. Margaret loudly praises her fiance's physique and sexual abilities. She has been spending large sums of money on herself, and giving her fiance $500 a week. The sister-in-law tells the physician, "I know it is Margaret's business what she does with her life, but I'm really worried about her. She is losing weight again. She eats very little, and almost never sleeps. I'm afraid she's going to just collapse!"

6. The priority nursing diagnosis for Margaret is:
    a. Altered nutrition: less than body requirements related to not eating.
    b. High risk for injury related to hyperactivity.
    c. Sleep pattern disturbance related to agitation.
    d. Ineffective individual coping related to denial of depression.

7. One way to promote adequate nutritional intake for Margaret is to:
    a. sit with her during meals to ensure that she eats everything on her tray.
    b. have her sister-in-law bring all her food from home, since she knows Margaret's likes and dislikes.
    c. provide high-calorie, nutritious finger foods and snacks that Margaret can eat "on the run."
    d. tell Margaret that she will be on room restriction until she starts gaining weight.

8. The physician orders lithium carbonate 600 mg tid, and chlorpromazine (Thorazine) 25 mg qid for Margaret. Since lithium is the treatment of choice for mania, what is the physician's rationale for ordering the chlorpromazine?
    a. Thorazine potentiates the effect of lithium carbonate.
    b. To minimize the GI symptoms associated with lithium therapy.
    c. To counteract extrapyramidal symptoms.
    d. To reduce hyperactivity until lithium takes effect.

9. There is a narrow margin between the therapeutic and toxic levels of lithium. Therapeutic range for acute mania is:
    a. 1.0–1.5 mEq/L.
    b. 10–15 mEq/L.
    c. 0.5–1.0 mEq/L.
    d. 5–10 mEq/L.

10. The initial symptoms of lithium toxicity include:
    a. tremors, shuffling gait, drooling, and rigidity.
    b. stiff neck, occipital headache, and increased blood pressure.
    c. ataxia; blurred vision; severe nausea, vomiting, and diarrhea; and tinnitis.
    d. fever, sore throat, malaise, and cardiac arrhythmias.

REFERENCES

Aleksandrowicz, D. R. (1980). Psychoanalytic studies of mania. In R. H. Belmaker & H. M. vanPraag (Eds.), *Mania: An evolving concept.* Jamaica, NY: Spectrum Publications.

American Psychiatric Association. (1987). *Diagnostic and statistical manual of mental disorders* (ed. 3, rev.). Washington, DC: American Psychiatric Association.

Bassuk, E. L., Schoonover, S. C., & Gill, A. D. (Eds.). (1982). *Lifelines: Clinical perspectives on suicide.* New York: Plenum Press.

Beck, A. T., Rush, A. J., Shaw, B. F., and Emery, G. (1979). *Cognitive theory of depression.* New York: Guilford Press.

Becker, E. (1964). *The revolution in psychiatry: The new understanding of man.* Glencoe, IL: Free Press.

Bell, C. C. & Mehta, H. (1980). The misdiagnosis of black patients with manic depressive illness. *J Natl Med Assoc, 72,* 141–145.

Berrios, G. E. (1988). Depressive and manic states during the nineteenth century. In A. Georgotas & R. Cancro (Eds.), *Depression and mania.* New York: Elsevier Science Publishing.

Bowlby, J. (1961). Processes of mourning. *Int J Psychoanal, 42,* 22.

Bowlby, J. (1973). *Attachment and loss: Separation, anxiety, and anger.* New York: Basic Books.

Boyd, J. H. & Weissman, M. M. (1982). Epidemiology. In E. S. Paykel (Ed.), *Handbook of affective disorders.* New York: Guilford Press.

Brown, G. W., Harris, T., & Copeland J. R. (1977). Depression and loss. *Br J Psychiatry, 130,* 1–18.

Cadoret, R. J. (1978). Evidence for genetic inheritance of primary affective disorder in adoptees. *Am J Psychiatry, 134,* 463–466.

Charney, E. A. & Weissman, M. M. (1988). Epidemiology of depressive and manic syndromes. In A. Georgotas & R. Cancro (Eds.), *Depression and mania.* New York: Elsevier Science Publishing.

Cohen, M. B. et al. (1954). An intensive study of twelve cases of manic-depressive psychosis. *Psychiatry 17,* 103–138.

Colvin, L. Depression and suicidal behavior. (1980). In J. Lancaster (Ed.), *Adult psychiatric nursing.* Garden City, NY: Medical Examination Publishing Co.

Department of Health and Human Services. (1983). *Vital statistics of the U.S.* Washington DC: National Center for Health Statistics.

Durkheim, E. (1951). *Suicide: A study of sociology.* Glencoe, IL: Free Press.

Engel, G. (1964). Grief and grieving. *Am J Nurs, 64,* 93.

Field, W. E. (1985). Physical causes of depression. *J Psychosocial Nurs, 23*(10), 6–11.

Freden, L. (1982). *Psychosocial aspects of depression.* Chichester, England: John Wiley and Sons.

Frederick, C. (1978). Current trends in suicidal behavior in the United States. *Am J Psychother 32:* 172–201.

Freedman, A. M. et al. (1976). *Modern synopsis of psychiatry II.* Baltimore: Williams & Wilkins.

Freud, S. (1957). *Mourning and melancholia,* vol. 14 (standard ed.) London: Hogarth Press. (Original work published 1917).

Geller, B. & Carr, L. G. (1988). Similarities and differences between adult and pediatric major depressive disorders. In A. Georgotas & R. Cancro (Eds.), *Depression and mania.* New York: Elsevier Science Publishing.

Georgotas, A. & Cancro, R. (Eds.). (1988). *Depression and mania.* New York: Elsevier Science Publishing.

Georgotas, A. & McCue, R. E. (1988). Depressive and manic states of late life. In A. Georgotas & R. Cancro (Eds.), *Depression and mania.* New York: Elsevier Science Publishing.

Gibson, R. W. et al. (1959). On the dynamics of the manic-depressive personality. *Am J Psychiatry 115,* 1101–1107.

Goodwin, F. K. & Jamison, K. R. (1990). *Manic-depressive illness.* New York: Oxford University Press.

Henderson, V. & Nite, G. (1978). *Principles and practice of nursing* (6th ed.). New York: Macmillan Publishing.

Herskowitz, J. (1988). *Is your child depressed?* New York: Pharos Books.

Hipple, J. & Cimbolic, P. (1979). *The counselor and suicidal crisis.* Springfield, IL: Charles C. Thomas.

Hollandsworth, J. G. (1990). *The physiology of psychological disorders.* New York: Plenum Press.

Horowitz, M. J. et al. (1980). Pathological grief and the activation of latent self-images. *Am J Psychiatry 137*(10), 1157–1162.

Janowsky, D. S. et al. (1974). Interpersonal maneuvers of manic patients. *Am J Psychiatry, 131,* 250–255.

Janowsky, D. S. et al. (1988). Neurochemistry of depression and mania. In A. Georgotas & R. Cancro (Eds.), *Depression and mania.* New York: Elsevier Science Publishing.

Johnson, G. F. S. (1988). Highlights on the main pharmacological treatments for mania. In A. Georgotas & R. Cancro (Eds.), *Depression and mania*. New York: Elsevier Science Publishing.

Kaplan, H. I. & Sadock, B. J. (1985). *Modern synopsis of comprehensive textbook of psychiatry* (4th ed.). Baltimore: Williams & Wilkins.

Kelsoe, J. R. (1991, Summer). Molecular genetics of mood disorders. *Journal of California Alliance for the Mentally Ill, 2*(4), 20–22.

Klein, M. (1948). Mourning and its relation to manic-depressive states. In M. Klein (Ed.), *Contributions to psychoanalysis, 1921–1945*. London: Hogarth Press.

Klerman, G. L. (1982). Practical issues in the treatment of depression and mania. In E. S. Paykel (Ed.), *Handbook of affective disorders*. New York: Guilford Press.

Klerman, G. L. (1988). Principles of interpersonal psychotherapy for depression. In Georgotas & Cancro (Eds.), *Depression and mania*. New York: Elsevier Science Publishing.

Kraepelin, E. (1921). *Manic-depressive insanity and paranoia*. Edinburgh: Churchill-Livingstone.

Kragh-Sorensen, P. (1988). Tricyclic antidepressants. In A. Georgotas & R. Cancro (Eds.), *Depression and mania*. New York: Elsevier Science Publishing.

Kübler-Ross, E. (1969). *On death and dying*. New York: Macmillan.

Kurtz, N. M. & Robinson, D. S. (1988). Monoamine oxidase inhibitors. In A. Georgotas & R. Cancro (Eds.), *Depression and mania*. New York: Elsevier Science Publishing.

Leahy, R. L. & Beck, A. T. (1988). Cognitive therapy of depression and mania. In A. Georgotas & R. Cancro (Eds.), *Depression and mania*. New York: Elsevier Science Publishing.

Lewinsohn, P. M. & Hoberman, H. M. (1982). Behavioral and cognitive approaches. In E. S. Paykel (Ed.), *Handbook of affective disorders*. New York: Guilford Press.

Lindemann (1944). Symptomatology and management of acute grief. *Am J Psychiatry*, 101:141.

McCue, R. E. & Georgotas, A. (1988). Newer generation antidepressants and lithium. In A. Georgotas & R. Cancro (Eds.), *Depression and mania*. New York: Elsevier Science Publishing.

McKinney, W. T. & Moran, E. C. (1982). Animal models. In E. S. Paykel (Ed.), *Handbook of affective disorders*. New York: Guilford Press.

Mendelson, M. (1982). Psychodynamics of depression. In E. S. Paykel (Ed.), *Handbook of affective disorders*. New York: Guilford Press.

Myers, J. K. et al. (1984). Six-month prevalence of psychiatric disorders in three communities: 1980–1982. *Arch Gen Psychiatry, 41*, 959–967.

Nurnberger, J. I. & Gershon, E. S. (1982). Genetics. In E. S. Paykel (Ed.), *Handbook of affective disorders*. New York: Guilford Press.

Paolino, T. J. & McCrady, E. S. (1978). *Marriage and marital therapy: Psychoanalytic, behavioral and systems theory perspectives*. New York: Brunner/Mazel.

Parkes, C. M. (1975). Determinants of outcome following bereavement. *Omega, 6*(4), 303–323.

Pitt, B. (1982). Depression and childbirth. In E. S. Paykel (Ed.), *Handbook of affective disorders*. New York: Guilford Press.

Rosenn, D. W. (1982). Suicidal behavior in children and adolescents. In Bassuk et al. (Eds.), *Lifelines: Clinical perspectives on suicide*. New York: Plenum Press.

Ruark, J. E. & Gonda, T. A. (1988). Grief and mourning. In A. Georgotas & R. Cancro (Eds.), *Depression and mania*. New York: Elsevier Science Publishing.

Sargent, M. (1989). *Depressive illnesses: Treatments bring new hope*. Rockville, MD: National Institute of Mental Health.

Schildkraut, J. J. (1965). The catecholamine hypothesis of affective disorder: A review of supportive evidence. *Am J Psychiatry 122*, 505–518.

Shneidman, E. S. & Farberow, N. L. (1965). *Some facts about suicide*. Washington, DC: Superintendent of Documents.

Seligman, M. E. P. (1973). Fall into helplessness. *Psychology Today, 7*, 43–48.

Shives, L. R. (1990). *Basic concepts of psychiatric-mental health nursing* (2nd ed.). Philadelphia: JB Lippincott.

Slaby, A. E., Lieb, J, & Tancredi, L. (1986). *The handbook of psychiatric emergencies* (3rd ed.). New York: Medical Examination Publishing.

Smith, S. F., Karasik, D. A., & Meyer, B. J. (1984). *Psychiatric and psychosocial nursing*. Los Altos, CA: National Nursing Review.

Spicer, C. C. et al. (1973). Neurotic and psychotic forms of depressive illness: Evidence from age-incidence in a national sample. *Br J Psychiatry, 123*, 535–541.

Spitz, R. A. (1946). Anaclitic depression: An inquiry into the genesis of psychiatric conditions in early childhood, II. *Psychoanal Study Child, 2*, 313–347.

Spitz, H. I. (1988). Principles of group and family therapy for depression and mania. In A. Georgotas & R. Cancro (Eds.), *Depression and mania*. New York: Elsevier Science Publishing.

Stokes, P. E. (1988). Psychoendocrinology of depression and mania. In Georgotas & Cancro (Eds.), *Depression and mania.* New York: Elsevier Science Publishing.

Thompson, J. M., McFarland, G. K., Hirsch, J. E., Tucker, S. M., & Bowers, A. C. (1986). *Clinical nursing.* St. Louis: CV Mosby.

Townsend, M. C. (1990). *Drug guide for psychiatric nursing.* Philadelphia: FA Davis.

Townsend, M. C. (1991). *Nursing diagnosis in psychiatric nursing: A pocket guide for care plan construction* (2nd ed.). Philadelphia: FA Davis.

Weissman, M. M. et al. (1988). Affective disorders in five United States communities. *Psychol Med 18,* 141–153.

White, R. (1977). Current psychoanalytic concepts of depression. In W. Flann (Ed.), *Phenomenology and treatment of depression.* New York: Spectrum.

Whybrow, P. C., Akiskal, H. S., & McKinney, W. T. (1984). *Mood disorders: Toward a new psychobiology.* New York: Plenum Press.

Wolpert, E. A. (1988). Combined therapies for depression and mania. In A. Georgotas & R. Cancro (Eds.), *Depression and mania.* New York: Elsevier Science Publishing.

World Health Organization. (1977). *Manual of the international statistical classification of diseases, injuries, and causes of death* (9th rev.). Geneva: World Health Organization.

Zis, A. P. & Goodwin, F. K. (1982). The amine hypothesis. In E. S. Paykel (Ed.), *Handbook of affective disorders.* New York: Guilford Press.

BIBLIOGRAPHY

Anderson, D. B. (1991). Never too late: Resolving the grief of suicide. *J Psychosoc Nurs, 29*(3), 29–31.

Bailey, D. S., Cooper, S. O., & Bailey, D. R. (1984). *Therapeutic approaches to the care of the mentally ill* (2nd ed.). Philadelphia: FA Davis.

Belmaker, R. H. & vanPraag, H. M. (Eds.). (1980). *Mania: An evolving concept.* Jamaica, NY: Spectrum Publications.

Busteed, E. L. & Johnstone, C. (1983). The development of suicide precautions for an inpatient psychiatric unit. *J Psychosoc Nurs, 21*(5), 15–19.

Capodanno, A. E. & Targum, S. D. (1983, May). Assessment of suicide risk: Some limitations in the prediction of infrequents events. *J Psychosoc Nurs, 21*(5), 11–14.

Chaisson, M., Beutler, L., Yost, E., & Allender, J. (1984). Treating the depressed elderly. *J Psychosoc Nurs, 22*(5) 25–30.

Doenges, M. E., Townsend, M. C., & Moorhouse, M. F. (1989). *Psychiatric care plans: Guidelines for client care.* Philadelphia: FA Davis.

Fitzpatrick, J. J. (1983). Suicidology and suicide prevention: Historical perspectives from the nursing literature. *J Psychosoc Nurs, 21*(5), 20–28.

Gordon, V. C. & Ledray, L. E. (1985). Depression in women: The challenge of treatment and prevention. *J Psychosoc Nurs, 23*(1), 26–34.

Harris, E. (1982, May). The dexamethasone suppression test. *Am J Nurs, 82*(5), 784–785.

Hauser, M. J. (1983). Bereavement outcome for widows. *J Psychosoc Nurs, 21*(9), 22–31.

Hellenbrand, M. (1985). The therapeutic community and the depressed patient: Guidelines for nursing management. *Psychiatric Nursing Forum, 2*(1), 4–12.

Neville, D. & Barnes, S. (1985). The suicidal phone call. *J Psychosoc Nurs, 23*(8), 14–18.

Paykel, E. S. (1982). *Handbook of affective disorders.* New York: Guilford Press.

Rodgers, B. M. (1986). Nursing management of a depressed child with a chronic physical illness. *Psychiatric Nursing Forum, 3*(1), 4–12.

Tuskan, J. J. & Thase, M. E. (1983). Suicides in jails and prisons. *J Psychosoc Nurs, 21*(5), 29–33.

Zerhusen, J. D., Boyle, K., & Wilson, W. (1991). Out of the darkness: Group cognitive therapy for depressed elderly. *J Psychosoc Nurs, 29*(9), 16–21

Anxiety Disorders

OBJECTIVES

After reading this chapter, the student will be able to:

1. Differentiate between the terms *stress, anxiety,* and *fear.*
2. Discuss historical aspects and epidemiological statistics related to anxiety disorders.

3. Differentiate between "normal" anxiety and "psychoneurotic" anxiety.
4. Describe various types of anxiety disorders and identify symptomatology associated with each. Use this information in patient assessment.
5. Identify predisposing factors in the development of anxiety disorders.
6. Formulate nursing diagnoses and goals of care for patients with anxiety disorders.
7. Describe appropriate nursing interventions for behaviors associated with anxiety disorders.
8. Evaluate nursing care of patients with anxiety disorders.
9. Discuss various modalities relevant to treatment of anxiety disorders.

INTRODUCTION

The following is an account by a college professor reflecting upon his irrational fear of public speaking (Beck & Emery, 1985):

"As I stand talking to the audience, I hope that my mind and voice will function properly, that I won't lose my balance, and everything else will function. But, then my heart starts to pound, I feel pressure build up in my chest as though I'm ready to explode, my tongue feels thick and heavy, my mind feels foggy and then goes blank. I can't remember what I have just said or what I am supposed to say. Then I start to choke. I can barely push the words out. My body is swaying; my hands tremble. I start to sweat and I am ready to topple off the platform. I feel terrified and I think that I will probably disgrace myself."

Individuals face anxiety on a daily basis. Anxiety, which provides the motivation for achievement, is a necessary force for survival. The term *anxiety* is often used interchangeably with the word *stress.* They are not the same. Stress, or more properly, a stressor, is an external pressure that is brought to bear upon the individual. Anxiety is the subjective emotional response to that stressor (see Chapter 2, for an overview of anxiety as a psychological response to stress.)

Anxiety may be distinguished from fear in that the former is an emotional process while fear is a cognitive one. Fear involves the intellectual appraisal of a threatening stimulus; anxiety involves the emotional response to that appraisal (Beck & Emery, 1985).

This chapter focuses on disorders that are characterized by exaggerated and often disabling anxiety reactions. Historical aspects and epimediological statistics are presented. Predisposing factors that have been implicated in the etiology of anxiety disorders provide a framework for studying the dynamics of phobias, obsessive-compulsive disorder, generalized anxiety disorder, panic disorder, and post-traumatic stress disorder.

An explanation of the symptomatology is presented as background knowledge for assessing the patient with an anxiety disorder. Nursing care is described in the context of the nursing process, and a critical pathway of care is included as a guideline for use in a case management approach. Various medical treatment modalities are explored.

HISTORICAL ASPECTS

Man has experienced anxiety throughout the ages. Yet anxiety, like fear, was not clearly defined or isolated as a separate entity by psychiatrists or psychologists until the 19th and 20th centuries (Gray, 1978). In fact, what we now know as anxiety was once solely identified by its physiological symptoms, focusing largely on the cardiovascular system. A myriad of diagnostic terms attempted to identify these symptoms. For example, cardiac neurosis, DaCosta's syndrome, irritable heart, nervous tachycardia, neurocirculatory asthenia, soldier's heart, vasomotor neurosis, and vasoregulatory asthenia are just a few of the names under which anxiety has been described through the years (Kaplan & Sadock, 1989).

The term *anxiety neurosis* was first introduced by Freud in 1895. Freud wrote, "I call this syndrome 'anxiety neurosis' because all its components can be grouped round the chief symptom of anxiety" (Freud, 1959). This notion attempted to negate the previous concept of the problem as strictly physical, although it was some time before physicians of internal medicine were ready to accept the psychological implications for the symptoms. In fact, it was not until the years during World War II that the psychological dimensions of these various functional heart conditions were recognized.

For many years, anxiety disorders were viewed as purely psychological or purely biological in nature. During the past 10 years, a number of researchers have begun to focus on the interrelatedness of mind and body. Beck and Emery (1985) state,

"The 'cause' of these psychological disorders may be found to reside in no specific factor but is best viewed as a composite of many interacting factors: genetic, developmental, environmental, and psychological."

EPIDEMIOLOGICAL STATISTICS

Although no empirical evidence exists to indicate that anxiety is on the increase, primary anxiety disorders represent one of the most prevalent mental health problems in the United States today (Uhde & Nemiah, 1989). Statistics vary widely, but most agree that anxiety disorders are more common in women than in men by at least 2 to 1. Prevalence rates have been given at 0.6 to 1.0 per 100 for panic disorder; 1.3 to 2.0 per 100 for obsessive-compulsive disorder; and 2.7 to 5.8 per 100 for agoraphobia (Weissman, 1985). A review of the literature revealed a wide range of reports regarding the prevalence of anxiety disorders in children (2 percent to 43 percent). Some of the studies suggested that the symptoms were more prevalent among girls than boys, among black than white children, and in lower than higher socioeconomic children (Weissman, 1985). Studies of familial patterns suggest that a familial predisposition to anxiety disorders probably exists.

HOW MUCH IS TOO MUCH?

Anxiety is generally considered a normal reaction to a realistic danger or threat to biologic integrity or self-concept. Normal anxiety dissipates when the danger or threat is no longer present.

It is very difficult to draw a precise line between normal and abnormal anxiety. "Normality" is determined by societal standards. What is normal in Chicago, Illinois may not be considered so in Cairo, Egypt. There may even be regional differences within a country, or cultural differences within a region. So what criteria can be used to determine if an individual's anxious response is "normal?"

Beck and Emery (1985) offer the following guidelines. Anxiety is considered abnormal or pathological if:

1. The response is greatly disproportionate to the risk and severity of the danger or threat.
2. The response continues beyond the existence of a potential danger or threat.
3. Intellectual, social, or occupational functioning is impaired.
4. The individual suffers from a psychosomatic effect (e.g., colitis or dermatitis).

APPLICATION OF THE NURSING PROCESS

Classifications of Anxiety Disorders: Background Assessment Data

PANIC DISORDER

This disorder is characterized by recurrent panic attacks, the onset of which are unpredictable, and manifested by intense apprehension, fear, or terror, often associated with feelings of impending doom and accompanied by intense physical discomfort. The symptoms come on unexpectedly, that is, they do not occur immediately before or on exposure to a situation that almost always causes anxiety (as in simple phobia). They are not triggered by situations in which the person is the focus of others' attention (as in social phobia). Organic factors in the role of etiology have been ruled out.

At least four of the following symptoms must be present to identify the presence of a panic attack. When fewer than four symptoms are present, the individual is diagnosed as having a limited symptom attack.

1. Shortness of breath (dyspnea) or smothering sensations
2. Dizziness, unsteady feelings, or faintness
3. Palpitations or accelerated heart rate (tachycardia)

4. Trembling or shaking
5. Sweating
6. Choking
7. Nausea or abdominal distress
8. Depersonalization or derealization
9. Numbness or tingling sensations (paresthesias)
10. Flushes (hot flashes) or chills
11. Chest pain or discomfort
12. Fear of dying
13. Fear of going crazy or of doing something uncontrolled

The attacks usually last minutes, or more rarely, hours. The individual often experiences varying degrees of nervousness and apprehension between attacks. Symptoms of depression are common. The average age of onset is in the late 20s.

Attacks may occur several times a week or even daily (American Psychiatric Association [APA], 1987). The disorder may last for a few weeks or months, or for a number of years. Sometimes the individual experiences periods of remission and exacerbation. In times of remission, the person may have recurrent limited symptom attacks. Panic disorder may or may not be accompanied by agoraphobia.

With Agoraphobia Panic disorder with agoraphobia is characterized by the symptoms described for panic disorder. In addition, the individual experiences a fear of being in places or situations from which escape might be difficult (or embarrassing) or in which help might not be available in the event of a panic attack. This fear severely restricts travel, and the individual may become nearly or completely housebound or unable to leave the house unaccompanied (APA, 1987). Common agoraphobic situations include being outside the home alone, being in a crowd or standing in a line, being on a bridge, and traveling in a bus, train, or car. The condition may be described as mild, moderate, or severe.

GENERALIZED ANXIETY DISORDER

This disorder is characterized by chronic, unrealistic, and excessive anxiety and worry. The symptoms have existed for 6 months or longer and cannot be attributed to specific organic factors, such as caffeine intoxication or hyperthyroidism. The *Diagnostic and Statistical Manual of Mental*

Disorders, ed. 3, revised (DSM-III-R) identifies the following symptoms associated with generalized anxiety disorder.

1. *Motor tension*
   a. Trembling, twitching, or feeling shaky
   b. Muscle tension, aches, or soreness
   c. Restlessness
   d. Easy fatigability
2. *Autonomic hyperactivity*
   a. Shortness of breath or smothering sensations
   b. Palpitations or accelerated heart rate (tachycardia)
   c. Sweating, or cold clammy hands
   d. Dry mouth
   e. Dizziness or lightheadedness
   f. Nausea, diarrhea, or other abdominal distress
   g. Flushes (hot flashes) or chills
   h. Frequent urination
   i. Trouble swallowing or "lump in throat"
3. *Vigilance and scanning*
   a. Feeling keyed up or on edge
   b. Exaggerated startle response
   c. Difficulty concentrating or "mind going blank"
   d. Trouble falling or staying asleep
   e. Irritability

Age at onset is usually in the 20s and 30s. Mild depressive symptoms are common, and the symptoms of generalized anxiety disorder often follow an episode of major depression (APA, 1987). Numerous somatic complaints may be a part of the clinical picture, and patients may have a fear of underlying, life-threatening illness (Uhde & Nemiah, 1989). Generalized anxiety disorder tends to be chronic, with frequent stress-related exacerbations and fluctuations in the course of the illness.

Predisposing Factors to Panic and Generalized Anxiety Disorders

Psychodynamic Theory The psychodynamic view focuses on the inability of the ego to intervene when conflict occurs between the id and the superego, producing anxiety. For various reasons (unsatisfactory parent/child relationship; conditional love or provisional gratification), ego development is delayed. When developmental defects in ego functions compromise the capacity to modulate anxiety, the individual resorts to unconscious mechanisms to resolve the conflict. Overuse or ineffective use of ego defense mechanisms results in maladaptive responses to anxiety (Nemiah, 1971).

Cognitive Theory The main thesis of the cognitive view is that a central process in adaptation is cognition, or information processing (Beck & Emery, 1985). When there is a disturbance in this central mechanism of cognition, there is a consequent disturbance in feeling and behavior. Because of distorted thinking, anxiety is maintained by mistaken or dysfunctional appraisal of a situation. There is a loss of ability to reason regarding the problem, whether it is physical or interpersonal. The individual feels vulnerable in a given situation, and the distorted thinking results in an irrational appraisal, fostering a negative outcome.

Biological Aspects Research investigations into the psychobiological correlation of panic and generalized anxiety disorders are in their infancy. Ongoing investigations require further empirical confirmation. Biological aspects include:

- ***Neuroanatomical.*** Modern theory on the physiology of emotional states places the key in the lower brain centers, including the limbic system, the diencephalon (thalamus and hypothalamus), and the reticular formation. This lower part of the brain, or subcortex, is believed to be responsible for initiating and controlling states of physiological arousal and for the involuntary homeostatic functions (Keable, 1989).
- ***Biochemical.*** Abnormal elevations of blood lactate have been noted in patients with panic disorder. Likewise, infusion of sodium lactate into patient's with anxiety neuroses produced symptoms of panic disorder. Although several laboratories have replicated these findings of increased lactate sensitivity in panic-prone individuals, no conclusive evidence exists relating these findings to direct cause of the disorder (Uhde & Nemiah, 1989).
- ***Medical conditions.*** The following medical conditions have been associated to a greater degree with individuals who suffer panic and generalized anxiety disorders than in the general population.

1. Abnormalities in the hypothalamic-pituitary-adrenal and hypothalamic-pituitary-thyroid axes.

2. Acute myocardial infarction
3. Pheochromocytomas
4. Substance intoxication and withdrawal (cocaine, alcohol, marijuana, opioids)
5. Hypoglycemia
6. Caffeine intoxication
7. Mitral valve prolapse
8. Complex partial seizures

Transactional Model of Stress/Adaptation The etiology of panic and generalized anxiety disorders is most likely influenced by multiple factors. In Figure 20.1, a graphic depiction of this theory of multiple causation is presented in the Transactional Model of Stress/Adaptation.

Nursing Diagnosis, Planning/Implementation Nursing diagnoses are formulated from the data gathered during the assessment phase and with background knowledge regarding predisposing factors to the disorder. Some common nursing diagnoses for patients with panic disorder and generalized anxiety disorder include:

Panic anxiety related to real or perceived threat to biological integrity or self-concept evidenced by any or all of the physical symptoms identified by the *DSM-III-R* as being descriptive of panic or generalized anxiety disorder.

Powerlessness related to impaired cognition evidenced by verbal expressions of no control over life situation and nonparticipation in decision making related to own care or life situation.

In Table 20.1, these nursing diagnoses are presented in a plan of care for the patient with panic disorder or generalized anxiety disorder. Goals of care and appropriate nursing interventions are included for each. Rationales are provided in italics.

Outcome Criteria The following criteria may be used for measurement of outcomes in the care of the patient with panic disorder or generalized anxiety disorder.

The patient:
1. Is able to recognize signs of escalating anxiety.
2. Is able to intervene so that anxiety does not reach the panic level.
3. Is able to discuss long-term plan to prevent panic anxiety when stressful situation occurs.

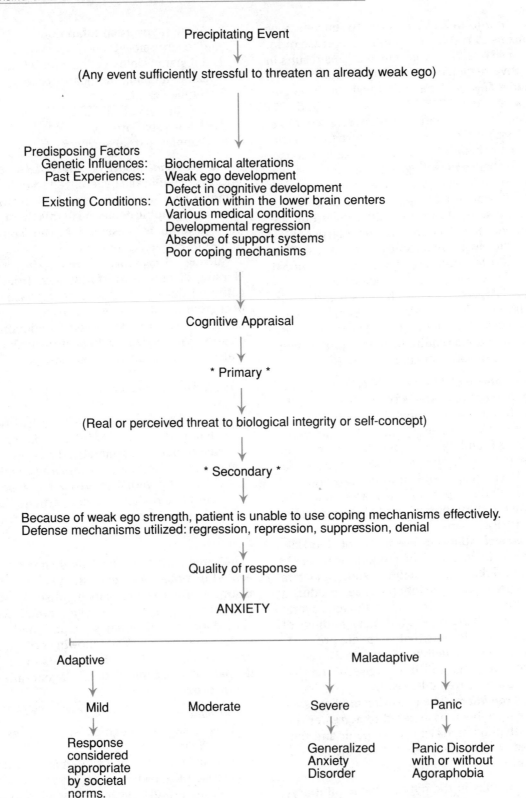

Figure 20.1   The dynamics of panic and generalized anxiety disorders using the transactional model of stress/adaptation.

Table 20.1 CARE PLAN FOR THE PATIENT WITH PANIC DISORDER OR GENERALIZED ANXIETY DISORDER

Nursing Diagnoses	Objectives	Nursing Interventions
Panic anxiety related to real or perceived threat to biological integrity or self-concept evidenced by any or all of the physical symptoms identified by the *DSM-III-R*.	Patient will be able to recognize symptoms of onset of anxiety and intervene before reaching panic level.	**Stay with the patient and offer reassurance of safety and security.** *Patient may fear for life. Presence of trusted individual provides feeling of security and assurance of personal safety.* **Maintain a calm, nonthreatening, matter-of-fact approach.** *Anxiety is contagious and may be transferred from staff to patient or vice versa. Patient develops feeling of security in presence of calm staff person.* **Use simple words and brief messages, spoken calmly and clearly, to explain hospital experiences.** *In an intensely anxious situation, patient is unable to comprehend anything but the most elemental communication.* **Keep immediate surroundings low in stimuli (dim lighting, few people, simple decor).** *A stimulating environment may increase level of anxiety.* **Administer tranquilizing medication, as ordered by physician. Assess for effectiveness and for side effects.** *Antianxiety medication provides relief from the immobilizing effects of anxiety.* **When level of anxiety has been reduced, explore possible reasons for occurrence.** *Recognition of precipitating factor(s) is the first step in teaching patient to interrupt escalation of anxiety.* **Teach signs and symptoms of escalating anxiety, and ways to interrupt its progression (relaxation techniques, deep-breathing exercises, and meditation, or physical exercise, brisk walks, and jogging).** *The first three of these activities result in a physiologic response opposite of the anxiety response. The latter three activities discharge excess energy in a healthful manner.*
Powerlessness related to impaired cognition evidenced by verbal expressions of no control over life situation and nonparticipation in decision making related to own care or life situation.	Patient will be able to effectively problem solve ways to take control of life situation, thereby decreasing feelings of powerlessness and anxiety.	**Allow patient to take as much responsibility as possible for self-care practices.** *Providing choices will increase patient's feeling of control.* Examples include: a. **Allow patient to establish own schedule for self-care activities.** b. **Include patient in setting goals of care.** c. **Provide patient with privacy as need is determined.** d. **Provide positive feedback for decisions made. Respect patient's right to make those decisions independently, and refrain from attempting to influence him or her toward those that may seem more logical.** **Assist patient to set realistic goals.** *Unrealistic goals set the patient up for failure and reinforce feelings of powerlessness.* **Help identify areas of life situation that patient can control.** *Patient's emotional condition interferers with the ability to solve problems. Assistance is required to perceive the benefits and consequences of available alternatives accurately.* **Help patient identify areas of life situation that are not within his or her ability to control. Encourage verbalization of feelings related to this inability** *in an effort to deal with unresolved issues and accept what cannot be changed.*

4. Practices techniques of relaxation daily.
5. Engages in physical exercise three times a week.
6. Performs activities of daily living independently.
7. Expresses satisfaction for independent functioning.
8. Is able to maintain anxiety at manageable level without use of medication.
9. Is able to participate in decision making, thereby maintaining control over life situation.
10. Verbalizes acceptance of life situations over which he or she has no control.

Evaluation Reassessment is conducted to determine if the nursing actions have been successful in achieving the objectives of care. Evaluation of the nursing actions for the patient with panic disorder or generalized anxiety disorder may be facilitated by gathering information using the following types of questions.

Can the patient recognize signs and symptoms of escalating anxiety? Is the patient able to use skills learned to interrupt the escalating anxiety before it reaches the panic level? Can the patient demonstrate the activities most appropriate for him or her that can be used to maintain anxiety at a manageable level (e.g., relaxation techniques, physical exercise)? Is the patient able to maintain anxiety at a manageable level without medication? Can the patient verbalize a long-term plan for preventing panic anxiety in the face of a stressful situation? Does the patient perform activities of daily living independently? Does the patient exercise control over life situation by participating in decision-making process? Is the patient able to name resources outside the hospital from whom he or she can seek assistance during times of extreme stress?

PHOBIAS

Agoraphobia Without History of Panic Disorder Agoraphobia without accompanying panic disorder is less common than the type that precipitates panic attacks. In this disorder, there is a fear of being in places or situations from which escape might be difficult or in which help might not be available in the event of suddenly developing a limited symptom attack (APA, 1987); that is, the individual may experience only a single symptom, but

---

Table 20.2 DIAGNOSTIC CRITERIA FOR AGORAPHOBIA WITHOUT HISTORY OF PANIC DISORDER

A. Agoraphobia: Fear of being in places or situations from which escape might be difficult (or embarrassing) or in which help might not be available in the event of suddenly developing a symptom(s) that could be incapacitating or extremely embarrassing. Examples include dizziness or falling, depersonalization or derealization, loss of bladder or bowel control, vomiting, or cardiac distress. As a result of this fear, the person either restricts travel or needs a companion when away from home, or else endures agoraphobic situations despite intense anxiety. Common agoraphobic situations include being outside the home alone, being in a crowd or standing in a line, being on a bridge, and traveling in a bus, train, or car.

B. Has never met the criteria for panic disorder.

Source: From American Psychiatric Association (1987) with permission.

---

at least fewer than four symptoms, commonly associated with panic attacks. The individual may have experienced the symptom(s) in the past and is preoccupied with fears of their recurrence. The *DSM-III-R* diagnostic criteria for agoraphobia without history of panic disorder are presented in Table 20.2.

Onset of symptoms most commonly occurs in the 20s and 30s and persists for many years. It is diagnosed more commonly in women than in men. Impairment can be very severe. In extreme cases, the individual is unable to leave his or her home without being accompanied by a friend or relative. If this is not possible, the person may become totally confined to his or her home (Kaplan & Sadock, 1989).

Social Phobia Social phobia is characterized by a persistent fear of appearing shameful, stupid, or inept in the presence of others (Kaplan & Sadock, 1989). The individual has extreme concerns about being exposed to possible scrutiny by others and fears that he or she may do something or act in a way that will be humiliating or embarrassing (APA, 1987). In some instances, the fear may be very defined, such as the fear of speaking or eating in a public place, fear of using a public restroom, or fear of writing in the presence of others. In other cases, the social phobia may involve general social situations, such as saying things or answering questions in a manner that would provoke laughter on the part of others (APA, 1987). Exposure to the phobic situation usually results in feelings of panic anxiety, with sweating, tachycardia, and dyspnea.

Onset of symptoms of this disorder usually begins in late childhood or early adolescence, and runs a chronic course. It appears to be more common among men than women (APA, 1987). Impairment will usually interfere with social or occupational functioning, depending on the specific fear. The *DSM-III-R* diagnostic criteria for social phobia are presented in Table 20.3.

Simple Phobia Simple phobias are sometimes referred to as "specific" phobias. The essential feature of this disorder is a persistent fear of a *specific* object or situation, other than the fear of being unable to escape from a situation (agoraphobia) or the fear of being humiliated in social situations (social phobia).

Simple phobia is not usually associated with other psychiatric symptoms or other psychiatric disorders (Goodwin, 1983). The phobic person is no more (or less) anxious than anyone else until exposed to the phobic object or situation. Exposure to the phobic stimulus produces overwhelming symptoms of panic, including palpitations, sweating, dizziness, and difficulty breathing. In fact, these symptoms may occur in response to the individual's merely *thinking* about the phobic stimulus. Invariably, the person recognizes that his or her

fear is excessive or unreasonable, but is powerless to change, even though occasionally the individual must endure the phobic stimulus, while experiencing intense anxiety (APA, 1987).

Phobias may begin at almost any age. Those that begin in childhood often disappear without treatment, but those that begin in or persist into adulthood almost always require assistance with therapy. The disorder is diagnosed more often in women than men.

Even though the disorder is common among the general population, people seldom seek treatment unless the phobia interferes with ability to function. Obviously, the individual who has a fear of snakes, but who lives on the 23rd floor of an urban, high-rise apartment building, is not likely to be bothered by the phobia unless he or she decides to move to an area where snakes are prevalent. On the other hand, a fear of elevators may very well interfere with this individual's daily functioning.

Phobias have been classified according to the phobic stimulus. A list of some of the more common ones appears in Table 20.4. This list is by no means all inclusive. People can become phobic about almost any object or situation, and anyone with a little knowledge of Greek or Latin can produce a phobia classification, thereby making possibilities for the list almost infinite. The *DSM-III-R* diagnostic criteria for simple phobia are presented in Table 20.5.

Table 20.3 DIAGNOSTIC CRITERIA FOR SOCIAL PHOBIA

A. A persistent fear of one or more situations (the social phobic situations) in which the person is exposed to possible scrutiny by others and fears that he or she may do something or act in a way that will be humiliating or embarrassing. Examples include being unable to continue talking while speaking in public, choking on food when eating in front of others, being unable to urinate in a public lavatory, hand trembling when writing in the presence of others, and saying foolish things or not being able to answer questions in social situations.

B. If another disorder is present, the fear in A is unrelated to it, for example, the fear is not of having a panic attack (panic disorder), stuttering (stuttering), trembling (Parkinson's disease), or exhibiting abnormal eating behavior (anorexia nervosa or bulimia nervosa).

C. During some phase of the disturbance, exposure to the specific phobic stimulus (or stimuli) almost invariably provokes an immediate anxiety response.

D. The phobic situation(s) is avoided, or is endured with intense anxiety.

E. The avoidant behavior interferes with occupational functioning or with usual social activities or relationships with others, or there is marked distress about having the fear.

F. The person recognizes that his or her fear is excessive or unreasonable.

G. If the person is younger than age 18, the disturbance does not meet the criteria for avoidant disorder of childhood or adolescence.

Source: From American Psychiatric Association (1987) with permission.

Table 20.4 CLASSIFICATIONS OF SIMPLE PHOBIAS

Classification	Fear
acrophobia	height
ailurophobia	cats
algophobia	pain
anthophobia	flowers
anthropophobia	people
aquaphobia	water
arachnophobia	spiders
astraphobia	lightning
belonophobia	needles
brontophobia	thunder
claustrophobia	closed spaces
cynophobia	dogs
dementophobia	insanity
equinophobia	horses
herpetophobia	lizards, reptiles
mikrophobia	germs
murophobia	mice
mysophobia	dirt, germs, contamination
numerophobia	numbers
nyctophobia	darkness
ophidiophobia	snakes
pyrophobia	fire
siderodromophobia	railways
taphaphobia	being buried alive
thanatophobia	death
trichophobia	hair
triskaidekaphobia	13 persons at a table
xenophobia	strangers
zoophobia	animals

Source: Goodwin (1983).

Table 20.5 DIAGNOSTIC CRITERIA FOR SIMPLE PHOBIA

A. A persistent fear of a circumscribed stimulus (object or situation) other than fear of having a panic attack (as in panic disorder) or of humiliation or embarrassment in certain social situations (as in social phobia).

B. During some phase of the disturbance, exposure to the specific phobic stimulus (or stimuli) almost invariably provokes an immediate anxiety response.

C. The object or situation is avoided or is endured with intense anxiety.

D. The fear or the avoidant behavior significantly interferes with the person's normal routine or with usual social activities or relationships with others, or there is marked distress about having the fear.

E. The person recognizes that his or her fear is excessive or unreasonable.

F. The phobic stimulus is unrelated to the content of the obsessions of obsessive-compulsive disorder or the trauma of post-traumatic stress disorder.

Source: From American Psychiatric Association (1987) with permission.

Predisposing Factors to Phobias

The cause of phobias is unknown. There are, however, various theories that may offer insight into the etiology.

Psychoanalytic Theory Freud believed that phobias develop when a child, feeling normal incestual feelings toward the opposite sex parent (Oedipal complex), becomes frightened of the aggression he fears the same sex parent feels for him (castration anxiety). To protect himself, the child *represses* this fear of hostility from the father and *displaces* it on to something safer and more neutral, which becomes the phobic stimulus. The phobic stimulus becomes the symbol for the father, but the child does not realize this.

Modern-day psychoanalyists believe in the same concept of phobic development, but that castration anxiety is not the sole source of phobias. They believe that other unconscious fears may also be expressed in a symbolic manner as phobias. For example, a female child who was sexually abused by an adult male family friend while he was taking her for a ride in his boat grew up with an intense, irrational fear of all water vessels. Psychoanalytic theory postulates that the fear of the man was repressed and displaced onto boats. Boats became an unconscious symbol for the feared person, but one that the young girl viewed as safer since her fear of boats prevented her from having to confront the real fear.

Learning Theory Classical conditioning in the case of phobias may be explained as follows: a stressful stimulus produces an 'unconditioned' response: fear. When the stressful stimulus is repeatedly paired with a harmless object, eventually the harmless object alone produces a 'conditioned' response: fear. If, to avoid fear, the person avoids the harmless object, the fear becomes a phobia (Goodwin, 1983).

Some learning theorists hold that fears are conditioned responses and thus learned by imposing rewards for appropriate behaviors. What then is the reward if a phobia is learned? Goodwin (1983) states:

"The reward is powerful indeed. Every time a person avoids a phobic situation, he escapes fear. Avoidance may be a nuisance, but it is clearly preferable to panic."

Phobias may also be acquired by direct learning or imitation (modeling). For example, a mother who exhibits fear toward an object will provide a model for the child, who may also develop a phobia toward the same object.

Cognitive Theory Cognitive theorists espouse that anxiety is the product of faulty cognitions or anxiety-inducing self-instructions (Emmelkamp, 1982). Two types of faulty thinking have been investigated: negative self-statements and irrational beliefs. Cognitive theorists believe that some individuals engage in negative and irrational thinking that produce anxiety reactions. The individual begins to seek out avoidance behaviors to prevent the anxiety reactions, and phobias result.

Somewhat related to the cognitive theory is the involvement of locus of control. Johnson and Sarason (1978) suggested that individuals with internal locus of control and those with external locus of control might respond differently to life change. These researchers propose that locus of control orientation may be an important variable in the development of phobias. Emmelkamp (1982) states that persons with an external control orientation experiencing anxiety attacks in a stressful period are likely to mislabel the anxiety and attribute it to external sources (e.g., crowded areas) or to a disease (e.g., heart attack). They may perceive the experienced anxiety as being outside of their control. Figure 20.2 depicts a graphic model of the relationship between locus of control and the development of phobias.

Biological Aspects

- *Temperament.* Goodwin (1983) suggests that some fears are innate. He states,

"These fears even follow a kind of biological timetable. At 6 months, the infant is frightened by loud noises and sudden movements. At age 3, he is frightened by strangers; at 5 by animals. Fear of open spaces and social situations occur (if they occur) much later: in adolescence or early adulthood."

'Innate' does not necessarily mean 'genetic.' Innate fears represent a part of the overall characteristics or tendencies with which one is born that influence how he or she responds throughout life to specific situations. Innate fears usually do not reach phobic intensity but may have the capacity for such development if reinforced by events in later life. For example, a 4-year-old-girl is afraid of dogs. But by age 5, she has overcome her fear and plays with her own dog and the neighbors' dogs without fear. Then, when she is 19, she is bitten by a stray dog and develops a dog phobia.

Life Experiences Certain early experiences may set the stage for phobic reactions later in life. Some researchers believe that phobias, particularly simple phobias, are symbolic of original anxiety-producing objects or situations that have been repressed. Examples include:

1. A child who is punished by being locked in a closet develops a phobia for elevators or other closed places.
2. A child who falls down a flight of stairs develops a phobia for high places.
3. A young woman who, as a child, survived a plane crash in which both her parents were killed, has a phobia of airplanes

Transactional Model of Stress/Adaptation The etiology of phobic disorders is most likely influenced by multiple factors. In Figure 20.3, a graphic depiction of this theory of multiple causation is presented in the Transactional Model of Stress/Adaptation.

Nursing Diagnosis, Planning/Implementation Nursing diagnoses are formulated from the data gathered during the assessment phase and with background knowledge regarding predisposing factors to the disorder. Some common nursing diagnoses for patients with phobias include:

Fear related to causing embarrassment to self in front of others; to being in a place from which one is unable to escape; or to a specific stimulus (simple phobia), evidenced by behavior directed toward avoidance of the feared object/situation.

Social isolation related to fears of being in a place

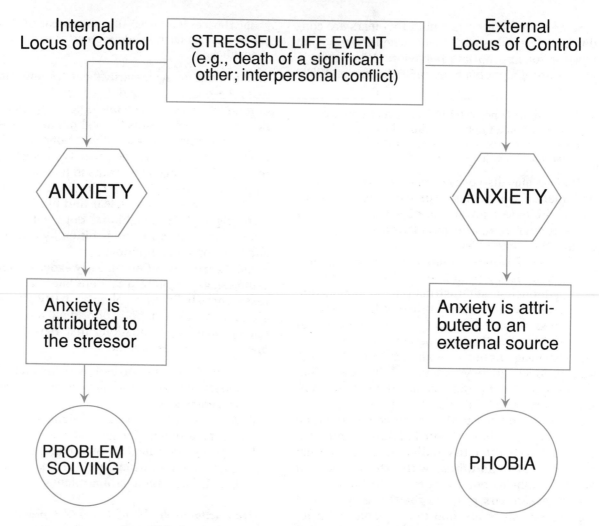

Figure 20.2   Locus of control as a variable in the etiology of phobias.

from which one is unable to escape, evidenced by staying alone; refuses to leave room/home.

In Table 20.6, these nursing diagnoses are presented in a plan of care for the patient with phobic disorder. Goals of care and appropriate nursing interventions are included for each. Rationales are provided in italics.

Outcome Criteria   The following criteria may be used for measurement of outcomes in the care of the patient with phobic disorders.

The patient:
1. Is able to function in the presence of the phobic object/situation without experiencing panic anxiety.
2. Demonstrates techniques that can be used to maintain anxiety at a manageable level.
3. Voluntarily attends group activities and interacts with peers.
4. Discusses feelings that may have contributed to irrational fears.
5. Verbalizes a future plan of action for responding in the presence of the phobic object/situation without resorting to panic anxiety.

Evaluation   Reassessment is conducted to determine if the nursing actions have been successful in achieving the objectives of care. Evaluation of the nursing actions for the patient with a phobic disorder may be facilitated by gathering information using the following types of questions.

Can the patient discuss the phobic object/situation without becoming anxious? Can the patient function in the presence of the phobic object/situa-

Precipitating Event

↓

(Any event sufficienty stressful to threaten an already weak ego)

↓

Predisposing Factors
    Genetic Influences: Locus of control orientation
                            Innate tendencies (temperament)
    Past Experiences: Unresolved fears and/or aggression
                            Conditioned learning
                            Imitative learning
                            Defect in cognitive development
                            Anxiety-producing life experiences
    Existing Conditions: Developmental regression
                            Absence of support systems
                            Poor coping mechanisms

↓

Cognitive Appraisal

↓

* Primary *

↓

(Real or perceived threat to biological integrity or self-concept)

↓

* Secondary *

↓

Because of weak ego strength, patient is unable to use coping mechanisms effectively.
Defense mechanisms utilized: denial, regression, repression, displacement, imitation

↓

Quality of response

↓

ANXIETY

Adaptive		Maladaptive	
↓		↓	↓
Mild	Moderate	Severe	Panic
↓		↓	↓
Response considered appropriate by societal norms.		Agoraphobia Social Phobias Simple Phobias	Symptoms may progress to panic in presence of phobic object/situation

Figure 20.3 The dynamics of phobic disorder using the transactional model of stress/adaptation.

Table 20.6 CARE PLAN FOR PATIENTS WITH PHOBIC DISORDERS

Nursing Diagnoses	Objectives	Interventions
Fear related to causing embarrassment to self in front of others; to being in a place from which one is unable to escape; or to a specific stimulus (simple phobia), evidenced by behavior directed toward avoidance of the feared object or situation.	Patient will be able to function in presence of phobic object or situation without experiencing panic anxiety.	Reassure patient that he or she is safe. *At the panic level of anxiety, patient may fear for own life.* Explore patient's perception of the threat to physical integrity or threat to self-concept. *It is important to understand patient's perception of the phobic object or situation to assist with the desensitization process.* Discuss reality of the situation with patient to recognize aspects that can be changed and those that cannot. *Patient must accept the reality of the situation (aspects that cannot change) before the work of reducing the fear can progress.* Include patient in making decisions related to selection of alternative coping strategies. (Example: Patient may choose either to avoid the phobic stimulus or attempt to eliminate the fear associated with it.) *Allowing the patient choices provides a measure of control and serves to increase feelings of self-worth.* If patient elects to work on elimination of the fear, techniques of desensitization or implosion therapy may be employed. (See explanation of these techniques under "Treatment Modalities" at the end of this chapter.) *Fear is decreased as the physical and psychologic sensations diminish in response to repeated exposure to the phobic stimulus under nonthreatening conditions.* Encourage patient to explore underlying feelings that may be contributing to irrational fears, and explain how *facing these feelings, rather than suppressing them, may result in more adaptive coping abilities.*
Social isolation related to fears of being in a place from which one is unable to escape, evidenced by staying alone; refuses to leave room/home.	Patient will voluntarily participate in group activities with peers.	Convey an accepting attitude and unconditional positive regard. Make brief, frequent contacts. Be honest and keep all promises. *These interventions increase feelings of self-worth and facilitate a trusting relationship.* Attend group activities with patient that may be frightening for him or her. *The presence of a trusted individual provides emotional security.* Be cautious with touch. Allow patient extra space and an avenue for exit if anxiety becomes overwhelming. *A person in panic anxiety may perceive touch as threatening.* Administer tranquilizing medications as ordered by physician. Monitor for effectiveness and adverse side effects. *Antianxiety medications, such as diazepam, chlordiazepoxide, or alprazolam, help to reduce level of anxiety in most individuals, thereby facilitating interactions with others.* Discuss with patient signs and symptoms of increasing anxiety and techniques to interrupt the response (e.g., relaxation exercises, "thought stopping"). *Maladaptive behaviors, such as withdrawal and suspiciousness, are manifested during times of increased anxiety.* Give recognition and positive reinforcement for voluntary interactions with others *to enhance self-esteem and encourage repetition of acceptable behaviors.*

tion without experiencing panic anxiety? Does the patient voluntarily leave room/home to attend group activities? Is the patient able to verbalize the signs and symptoms of escalating anxiety? Is the patient able to demonstrate techniques that he or she may use to prevent the anxiety from escalating to the panic level? Can the patient verbalize the thinking process that promoted the irrational fears? Is the patient capable of creating change in his or her life to confront (or eliminate, or avoid) the phobic situation? Is the patient able to name resources outside the hospital from whom he or she can seek assistance during times of extreme stress?

OBSESSIVE COMPULSIVE DISORDER

The *DSM-III-R* describes this disorder as recurrent obsessions or compulsions sufficiently severe to cause marked distress, be time-consuming, or significantly interfere with the person's normal routine, occupational functioning, or usual social activities or relationships with others (APA, 1987).

Obsessions are defined as unwanted, intrusive, persistent ideas, thoughts, impulses, or images. The most common ones include thoughts of violence, contamination, and doubt.

Compulsions denote unwanted repetitive acts or intentional behavior patterns. They may be performed in response to an obsession or in a stereotyped fashion. The individual recognizes that the behavior is excessive or unreasonable, but because of the feeling of relief from discomfort that it promotes, is compelled to continue the act. The most common compulsions involve hand washing, counting, checking, and touching (APA, 1987).

The *DSM-III-R* diagnostic criteria for obsessive compulsive disorder are presented in Table 20.7.

The disorder is equally common among men and women. It may begin in childhood but more often begins in adolescence or early adulthood. The course is usually chronic and may be complicated by major depression or abuse of substances. Recent studies indicate that the frequency of the disorder is higher in upper-class persons and in those with higher intelligence levels (Kaplan & Sadock, 1989).

Predisposing Factors to Obsessive-Compulsive Disorder

Psychoanalytic Theory Psychoanalytic theorists propose that individuals with obsessive-compul-

---

Table 20.7 DIAGNOSTIC CRITERIA FOR OBSESSIVE COMPULSIVE DISORDER

A. Either obsessions or compulsions:

Obsessions: 1., 2., 3., and 4.:

1. Recurrent and persistent ideas, thoughts, impulses, or images that are experienced, at least initially, as intrusive and senseless (e.g., a parent's having repeated impulses to kill a loved child, a religious person's having recurrent blasphemous thoughts)
2. The person attempts to ignore or suppress such thoughts or impulses or to neutralize them with some other thought or action.
3. The person recognizes that the obsessions are the product of his or her own mind, not imposed from without.
4. If another Axis I disorder is present, the content of the obsession is unrelated to it (e.g., the ideas, thoughts, impulses, or images are not about food in the presence of an eating disorder, about drugs in the presence of a psychoactive substance use disorder, or guilty thoughts in the presence of a major depression).

Compulsions: 1., 2., and 3.:

1. Repetitive, purposeful, and intentional behaviors that are performed in response to an obsession, or according to certain rules or in a stereotyped fashion.
2. The behavior is designed to neutralize or to prevent discomfort or some dreaded event or situation; however, either the activity is not connected in a realistic way with what it is designed to neutralize or prevent, or it is clearly excessive.
3. The person recognizes that his or her behavior is excessive or unreasonable (this may not be true for young children; it may no longer be true for people whose obsessions have evolved into overvalued ideas).

B. The obsessions or compulsions cause marked distress, are time-consuming (take more than an hour a day), or significantly interfere with the person's normal routine, occupational functioning, or usual social activities or relationships with others.

Source: From American Psychiatric Association (1987) with permission.

sive disorder have weak, underdeveloped egos (for any of a variety of reasons: unsatisfactory parent/child relationship, conditional love, or provisional gratification). The psychoanalytic concept views patients with obsessive compulsive disorder as having regressed to developmentally earlier stages of the infantile superego—the harsh, exacting, punitive characteristics which now reappear as part of the psychopathology (Kaplan & Sadock, 1989). Regression to the preoedipal anal-sadistic phase, combined with use of specific ego defense mechanisms (isolation, undoing, displacement, reaction formation), produce the clinical symptoms of obsessions and compulsions. Aggressive impulses (common during the anal-sadistic developmental phase) are channeled into thoughts and behaviors that prevent the feelings of aggression from surfacing and producing intense anxiety fraught with guilt (generated by the punitive superego).

Learning Theory Learning theorists explain obsessive compulsive behavior as a conditioned response to a traumatic event. The traumatic event produces anxiety and discomfort, and the individual learns to prevent the anxiety and discomfort by avoiding the situation with which they are associated. This type of learning is called *passive avoidance* (staying away from the source). When passive avoidance is not possible, the individual learns to engage in behaviors that provide relief from the anxiety and discomfort associated with the traumatic situation. This type of learning is called *active avoidance*, and describes the behavior pattern of the individual with obsessive compulsive disorder (Teasdale, 1974).

According to this classical conditioning interpretation, a traumatic event should mark the beginning of the obsessive compulsive behaviors. However, in a significant number of cases, the onset of the behavior is gradual, and the patients relate the onset of their problems to life stress in general rather than to one or more traumatic events (Emmelkamp, 1982).

Biological Aspects Recent findings suggest that neurobiological disturbances may play a role in the pathogenesis and maintenance of obsessive compulsive disorder (Kaplan & Sadock, 1989). Biological aspects include:

- *Neuroanatomy.* Lesions in various regions of the brain have been implicated in the neurobi-

ology of obsessive compulsive disorder. For example, repetitive stereotyped behavior has been noted in animals with lesions in areas of the hippocampus, orbital gyri, and caudate nuclei. Rachman and Hodgson (1980) view these "organic obsessional compulsive disorders" as psychologically and phenomenologically distinct from obsessive compulsive disorders.

- *Physiology.* Some individuals with obsessive compulsive disorder exhibit nonspecific electroencephalogram changes. Some researchers have hypothesized that obsessive compulsive disorder may represent a nonconvulsive epileptiform disorder (e.g., abnormal discharges in selective brain regions) or an abnormality in left-frontal brain functions (Kaplan & Sadock, 1989).

- *Biochemical.* A number of studies have implicated the neurotransmitter serotonin as influential in the etiology of obsessive compulsive behaviors. Drugs that have been used successfully in alleviating the symptoms of obsessive compulsive disorder are clomipramine and trazodone, both of which are believed to either increase the concentration, or potentiate the effects, of serotonin.

Transactional Model of Stress/Adaptation The etiology of obsessive compulsive disorder is most likely influenced by multiple factors. In Figure 20.4, a graphic depiction of this theory of multiple causation is presented in the Transactional Model of Stress/Adaptation.

Nursing Diagnosis, Planning/Implementation Nursing diagnoses are formulated from the data gathered during the assessment phase and with background knowledge regarding predisposing factors to the disorder. Some common nursing diagnoses for patients with obsessive compulsive disorder include:

Ineffective individual coping related to underdeveloped ego, punitive superego; avoidance learning; possible biochemical changes; evidenced by ritualistic behavior or obsessive thoughts.

Altered role performance related to need to perform rituals, evidenced by inability to fulfill usual patterns of responsibility.

In Table 20.8, these nursing diagnoses are presented in a plan of care for the patient with obses-

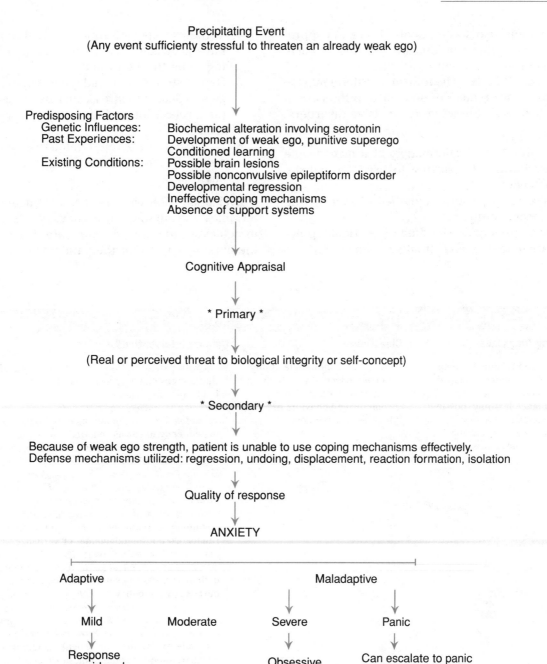

Precipitating Event
(Any event sufficienty stressful to threaten an already weak ego)

Predisposing Factors
  Genetic Influences: Biochemical alteration involving serotonin
  Past Experiences: Development of weak ego, punitive superego
                        Conditioned learning
  Existing Conditions: Possible brain lesions
                        Possible nonconvulsive epileptiform disorder
                        Developmental regression
                        Ineffective coping mechanisms
                        Absence of support systems

Cognitive Appraisal

* Primary *

(Real or perceived threat to biological integrity or self-concept)

* Secondary *

Because of weak ego strength, patient is unable to use coping mechanisms effectively.
Defense mechanisms utilized: regression, undoing, displacement, reaction formation, isolation

Quality of response

ANXIETY

Adaptive   Maladaptive

Mild   Moderate   Severe   Panic

Response   Obsessive   Can escalate to panic
considered   Compulsive   anxiety if unable to
appropriate   Disorder   perform rituals.
by societal
norms.

Figure 20.4 The dynamics of obsessive compulsive disorder using the transactional model of stress/adaptation.

sive compulsive disorder. Goals of care and appropriate nursing interventions are included for each. Rationales are provided in italics.

Outcome Criteria The following criteria may be used for measurement of outcomes in the care of the patient with obsessive compulsive disorder:

The patient:

1. Is able to maintain anxiety at a manageable level without resorting to use of ritualistic behavior.
2. Is able to perform activities of daily living independently.
3. Verbalizes understanding of relationship between anxiety and ritualistic behavior.

4. Verbalizes specific situations that in the past have provoked anxiety and resulted in seeking relief through rituals.
5. Demonstrates more adaptive coping strategies to deal with stress, such as thought stopping, relaxation techniques, and physical exercise.
6. Is able to resume role-related responsibilities due to decreased need for ritualistic behaviors.

Evaluation Reassessment is conducted to determine if the nursing actions have been successful in achieving the objectives of care. Evaluation of the nursing actions for the patient with obsessive

---

Table 20.8 CARE PLAN FOR THE OBSESSIVE COMPULSIVE PATIENT

Nursing Diagnoses	Objectives	Nursing Interventions
Ineffective individual coping related to underdeveloped ego, punitive superego; avoidance learning; possible biochemical changes; evidenced by ritualistic behavior or obsessive thoughts.	Patient will demonstrate ability to cope effectively without resorting to obsessive compulsive behaviors or increased dependency.	Work with patient to determine types of situations that increase anxiety and result in ritualistic behaviors. *Recognition of precipitating factors is the first step in teaching the patient to interrupt the escalating anxiety.* Initially meet the patient's dependency needs as required. Encourage independence and give positive reinforcement for independent behaviors. *Sudden and complete elimination of all avenues for dependency would create intense anxiety on the part of the patient. Positive reinforcement enhances self-esteem and encourages repetition of desired behaviors.* In the beginning of treatment, allow plenty of time for rituals. Do not be judgmental or verbalize disapproval of the behavior. *To deny patient this activity may precipitate panic anxiety.* Support patient's efforts to explore the meaning and purpose of the behavior. *Patient may be unaware of the relationship between emotional problems and compulsive behaviors. Recognition is important before change can occur.* Provide structured schedule of activities for patient, including adequate time for completion of rituals. *Structure provides a feeling of security for the anxious patient.* Gradually begin to limit amount of time allotted for ritualistic behavior as patient becomes more involved in unit activities. *Anxiety is minimized when patient is able to replace ritualistic behaviors with more adaptive ones.* Give positive reinforcement for nonritualistic behaviors. *Positive reinforcement enhances self-esteem and encourages repetition of desired behaviors.* Help patient learn ways of interrupting obsessive thoughts and ritualistic behavior with techniques such as thought stopping, relaxation, and exercise.

(continued)

Table 20.8 CONTINUED

Nursing Diagnoses	Objectives	Nursing Interventions
Altered role performance related to need to perform rituals, evidenced by inability to fulfill usual patterns of responsibility.	Patient will be able to resume role-related responsibilities.	Determine patient's previous role within the family and extent to which this role is altered by the illness. Identify roles of other family members. *This is important assessment data for formulating an appropriate plan of care.* Discuss patient's perception of role expectations. *Determine if patient's perception of his or her role expectations are realistic.* Encourage patient to discuss conflicts evident within the family system. Identify how patient and other family members have responded to this conflict. *Identifying specific stressors, as well as adaptive and maladaptive responses within the system, is necessary before assistance can be provided in an effort to create change.* Explore available options for changes or adjustments in role. Practice through role play. *Planning and rehearsal of potential role transitions can reduce anxiety.* Encourage family participation in the development of plans to effect positive change, and work to resolve the cause of the anxiety from which the patient seeks relief through use of ritualistic behaviors. *Input from the individuals who will be directly involved in the change will increase the likelihood of a positive outcome.* Give patient lots of positive reinforcement for ability to resume role responsibilities by decreasing need for ritualistic behaviors. *Positive reinforcement enhances self-esteem and promotes repetition of desired behaviors.*

compulsive disorder may be facilitated by gathering information using the following types of questions.

Can the patient refrain from performing ritualistic behaviors when anxiety level rises? Is he or she able to demonstrate substitute behaviors to maintain anxiety at a manageable level? Does the patient recognize the relationship between escalating anxiety and the dependence on ritualistic behaviors for relief? Can he or she verbalize situations that occurred in the past during which this strategy was used? Is the patient able to verbalize a plan of action for dealing with these stressful situations in the future? Is the patient able to perform self-care activities independently? Can he or she demonstrate an ability to fulfill role-related responsibilities? Can the patient name resources from whom he or she can seek assistance during times of extreme stress?

POST-TRAUMATIC STRESS DISORDER

Post-traumatic stress disorder (PTSD) is described by the *DSM-III-R* as the development of characteristic symptoms following a psychologically distressing event that is outside the range of usual human experience. These symptoms are not related to common experiences, such as uncomplicated bereavement, marital conflict, or chronic illness. They are associated with events that would be markedly distressing to almost everyone, and are usually experienced with intense fear, terror, and helplessness (APA, 1987). Characteristic symptoms may include a reexperiencing of the traumatic event, a sustained high level of anxiety/arousal, or a general numbing of responsiveness.

The individual may experience the trauma alone or in the presence of others. Examples of some experiences that may produce this type of response include rape, assault, military combat, flood, earthquakes, tornados, car or airplane crashes, fires, bombings, and torture.

Symptoms of depression are common and may be severe enough to warrant a diagnosis of a depressive disorder. In the case of a life-threatening trauma shared with others, survivors often describe painful guilt feelings about surviving when others did not or about the things they had to do to survive (APA, 1987).

The disorder can occur at any age. Symptoms may begin immediately following the trauma, or they may remain latent only to surface months or years later. Substance abuse is common. The *DSM-III-R* diagnostic criteria for PTSD are presented in Table 20.9.

Studies examining the prevalence of PTSD have established a rate of 1 percent among the general U.S. population (Helzer et al, 1987). In a separate study investigating the incidence of combat-related PTSD in veterans of the Vietnam War, the rate was found to be 15 percent (Kulka et al, 1988).

Predisposing Factors to Post-traumatic Stress Disorder

Reports of symptoms and syndromes with PTSD-like features have existed in writing throughout the centuries. In the early part of the 20th century, traumatic neurosis was viewed as the ego's inability to master the degree of trauma that resulted in the disorganization of ego-functioning (Kardiner, 1941). Very little was written about post-traumatic neurosis during the years between 1950 and 1970.

Table 20.9   DIAGNOSTIC CRITERIA FOR POST-TRAUMATIC STRESS DISORDER

A. The person has experienced an event that is outside the range of usual human experience and that would be markedly distressing to almost anyone (e.g., serious threat to one's life or physical integrity; serious threat or harm to one's children, spouse, or other close relatives and friends; sudden destruction of one's home or community; or seeing another person who has recently been, or is being, seriously injured or killed as the result of an accident or physical violence).

B. The traumatic event is persistently reexperienced in at least one of the following ways:
 1. Recurrent and intrusive distressing recollections of the event (in young children, repetitive play in which themes or aspects of the trauma are expressed)
 2. Recurrent distressing dreams of the event
 3. Sudden acting or feeling as if the traumatic event were recurring (includes a sense of reliving the experience, illusions, hallucinations, and dissociative [flashback] episodes, even those that occur upon awakening or when intoxicated)
 4. Intense psychological distress at exposure to events that symbolize or resemble an aspect of the traumatic event, including anniversaries of the trauma

C. Persistent avoidance of stimuli associated with the trauma or numbing of general responsiveness (not present before the trauma), as indicated by at least three of the following:
 1. Efforts to avoid thoughts or feelings associated with the trauma
 2. Efforts to avoid activities or situations that arouse recollections of the trauma
 3. Inability to recall an important aspect of the trauma (psychogenic amnesia)
 4. Markedly diminished interest in significant activities in young children, loss of recently acquired developmental skills, such as toilet training or language skills
 5. Feeling of detachment or estrangement from others
 6. Restricted range of affect (e.g., unable to have loving feelings)
 7. Sense of a foreshortened future (e.g., does not expect to have a career, marriage, or children, or a long life)

D. Persistent symptoms of increased arousal (not present before the trauma) as indicated by at least two of the following:
 1. Difficulty falling or staying asleep
 2. Irritability or outbursts of anger
 3. Difficulty concentrating
 4. Hypervigilance
 5. Exaggerated startle response
 6. Physiological reactivity upon exposure to events that symbolize or resemble an aspect of the traumatic event (e.g., a woman who was raped in an elevator breaks out in a sweat when entering any elevator)

E. Duration of the disturbance of at least 1 month.

F. Specify *delayed onset* if the onset of symptoms was at least 6 months after the trauma.

Source: From American Psychiatric Association (1987) with permission.

This absence was followed in the '70s and '80s with an explosion in the amount of research and writing on the subject. Peterson and colleagues (1991) have stated:

"Clearly, the psychological casualties of the Vietnam War were largely responsible for the renewed interest in post-traumatic neurosis. Most of the early papers on post-traumatic neurosis were about Vietnam veterans."

Indeed, the category of PTSD did not appear until the third edition of the *Diagnostic and Statistical Manual of Mental Disorders* in 1980. The increasingly obvious problems of Vietnam veterans plus clinical work with victims of multiple disasters made clear a need for this post-traumatic stress category in the *DSM-III* (Kaplan & Sadock, 1989).

Psychosocial Theory Green et al (1985) have proposed an etiological model of PTSD that has become widely accepted. This theory seeks to explain why certain persons exposed to massive trauma develop PTSD while others do not. Variables include characteristics that relate to 1) the traumatic experience, 2) the individual, and 3) the recovery environment.

- *The traumatic experience.* Specific characteristics relating to the trauma have been identified as crucial elements in the determination of an individual's long-term response to stress. They include:

1. Severity and duration of the stressor
2. Degree of anticipatory preparation prior to the onset
3. Exposure to death
4. Numbers affected by life threat
5. Degree of control over recurrence
6. Location of where the trauma was experienced (e.g., familiar surroundings, at home, in a foreign country, etc.)

- *Individual characteristics.* Variables that are considered important in determining an individual's response to trauma include:

1. Degree of ego strength
2. Effectiveness of coping resources
3. Presence of preexisting psychopathology
4. Outcomes of previous experiences with stress/trauma
5. Behavioral tendencies (temperament)

6. Current psychosocial developmental stage (Erikson, 1968)
7. Demographic factors (e.g., age, socioeconomic status, education, etc.)

- *The recovery environment.* Green et al (1985) suggest that the quality of the environment in which the individual attempts to work through the traumatic experience is correlated with outcome. Environmental variables include:

1. Availability of social supports
2. The cohesiveness and protectiveness of family and friends
3. The attitudes of society regarding the experience
4. Cultural and subcultural influences

Peterson and associates (1991) suggest that the recovery environment for Vietnam veterans and rape victims has often been less supportive than that for disaster victims or the victims of assault or other crimes.

In research conducted by Wilson and Krauss (1985) using this model with Vietnam combat veterans, the best predictors of PTSD were the severity of the stressor and the degree of psychosocial isolation in the recovery environment.

Learning Theory Learning theorists view negative reinforcement as behavior that leads to a reduction in an aversive experience. This reduction is the reinforcement that enhances the repetition of the behavior. The avoidance behaviors and psychological numbing in response to a trauma are mediated by negative reinforcement (behaviors that decrease the emotional pain of the trauma). Behavioral disturbances, such as anger and aggression, and drug and alcohol abuse, "are conceptualized as behavioral patterns that are functionally reinforced by their capacity to reduce aversive feelings" (Keane et al, 1985).

Cognitive Therapy These models take into consideration the cognitive appraisal of an event and focus on assumptions that an individual makes about the world. Epstein (1990) outlines three fundamental beliefs that most people construct within a personal theory of reality. They include:

1. The world is benevolent and a source of joy.
2. The world is meaningful and controllable.
3. The self is worthy (e.g., lovable, good, and competent).

As life situations occur, some disequilibrium is expected to occur until accommodation for the change has been made and it has become assimilated into one's personal theory of reality. An individual is vulnerable to PTSD when the fundamental beliefs are invalidated by a trauma that cannot be comprehended, and a sense of helplessness and hopelessness prevail. One's appraisal of the environment can be drastically altered.

Biological Aspects Kaplan and Sadock (1989) explain a biological hypothesis for chronic PSTD that suggests reactivation of symptoms stimulated by a situation that resembles the original trauma. This arousal state, which is mediated by the sympathetic nervous system, is central in promoting the return of the traumatic images.

Van der Kolk (1988) has suggested that an endogenous opioid peptide response may assist in the maintenance of chronic PTSD. The hypothesis supports a type of "addiction to the trauma," which is explained in the following manner:

Opioids, including endogenous opioid peptides, have the following psychoactive properties:

1. Tranquilizing action
2. Reduction of rage/aggression
3. Reduction of paranoia
4. Reduction of feelings of inadequacy
5. Antidepressant actions

Van der Kolk suggests that physiological arousal initiated by reexposure to traumalike situations enhances production of endogenous opioid peptides and results in increased feelings of comfort and control. When the stressor terminates, the individual may experience opioid withdrawal, the symptoms of which bear strong resemblance to those of PTSD.

Transactional Model of Stress/Adaptation The etiology of PTSD is most likely influenced by multiple factors. In Figure 20.5, a graphic depiction of this theory of multiple causation is presented in the Transactional Model of Stress/Adaptation.

Nursing Diagnosis, Planning/Implementation Nursing diagnoses are formulated from the data gathered during the assessment phase and with background knowledge regarding predisposing factors to the disorder. Some common nursing diagnoses for patients with PTSD include:

Post-trauma response related to distressing event considered to be outside the range of usual human experience, evidenced by flashbacks, intrusive recollections, nightmares, psychological numbness related to the event, dissociation, or amnesia.

Dysfunctional grieving related to loss of self as perceived prior to the trauma or other actual/perceived losses incurred during/following the event, evidenced by irritability and explosiveness, self-destructiveness, substance abuse, verbalization of survival guilt or guilt about behavior required for survival.

In Table 20.10, these nursing diagnoses are presented in a plan of care for the patient with PTSD. Goals of care and appropriate nursing interventions are included for each. Rationales are provided in italics.

Some institutions are using a case management model to coordinate care (see Chapter 6, for a more detailed explanation). In case management models, the plan of care may take the form of a critical pathway. Table 20.11 depicts an example of a critical pathway of care for a patient with PTSD.

Outcome Criteria The following criteria may be used for measurement of outcomes in the care of the patient with PTSD.

The patient:

1. Is able to acknowledge the traumatic event and the impact it has had on his or her life.
2. Is experiencing fewer flashbacks, intrusive recollections, and nightmares than he or she was on admission (or at the beginning of therapy).
3. Is able to demonstrate adaptive coping strategies (e.g., relaxation techniques, mental imagery, music, art).
4. Is able to concentrate and has made realistic goals for the future.
5. Includes significant others in the recovery process and willingly accepts their support.
6. Verbalizes no ideas or intent for self-harm.
7. Has worked through feelings of survivor's guilt.
8. Gets sufficient sleep so that risk of injury has diminished.
9. Verbalizes community resources from whom he or she may seek assistance in times of stress.
10. Attends support group of individuals who have recovered or are recovering from similar traumatic experiences.

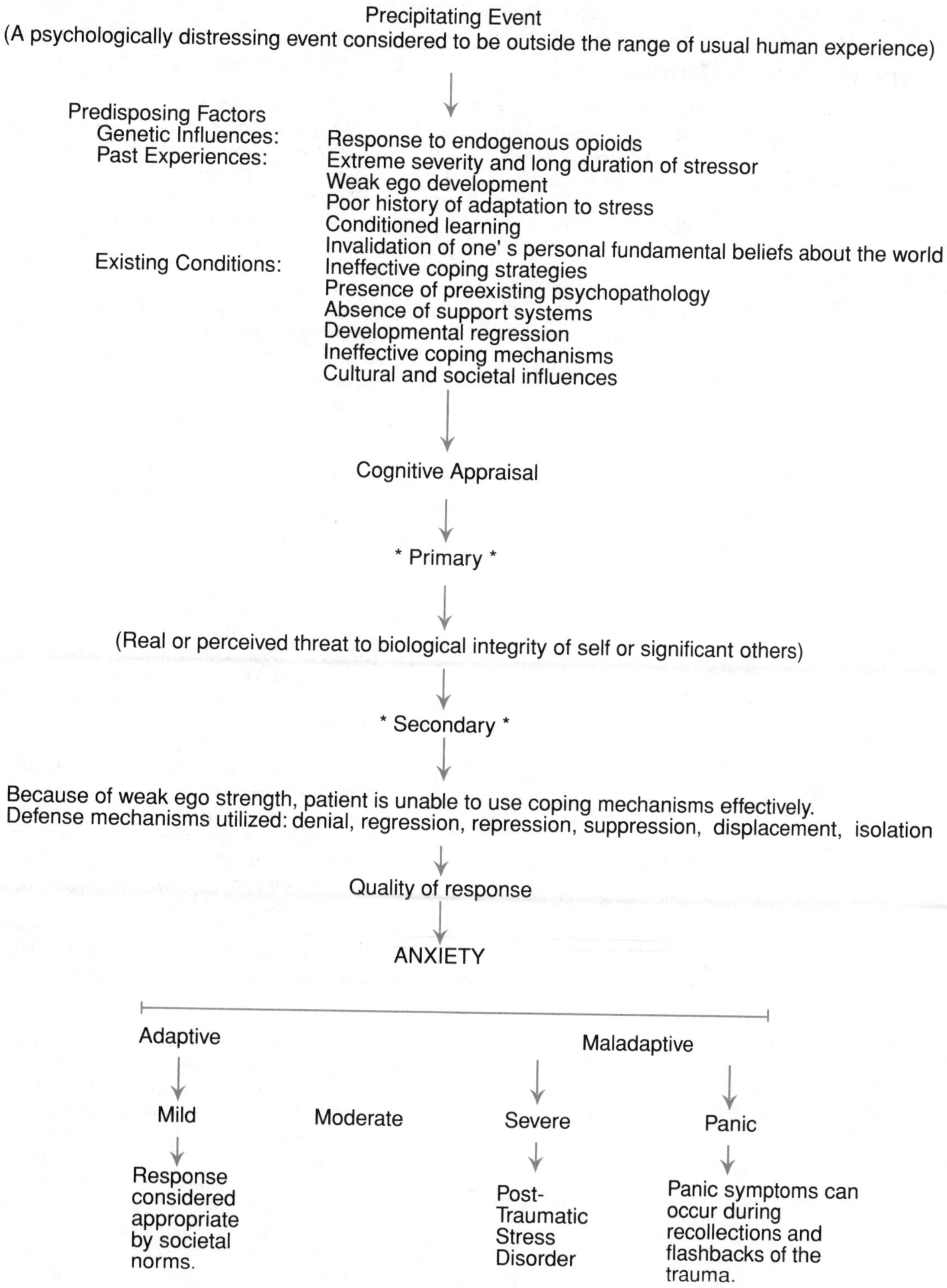

Precipitating Event
(A psychologically distressing event considered to be outside the range of usual human experience)

Predisposing Factors
Genetic Influences: Response to endogenous opioids
Past Experiences: Extreme severity and long duration of stressor
                         Weak ego development
                         Poor history of adaptation to stress
                         Conditioned learning
                         Invalidation of one's personal fundamental beliefs about the world
Existing Conditions: Ineffective coping strategies
                         Presence of preexisting psychopathology
                         Absence of support systems
                         Developmental regression
                         Ineffective coping mechanisms
                         Cultural and societal influences

Cognitive Appraisal

* Primary *

(Real or perceived threat to biological integrity of self or significant others)

* Secondary *

Because of weak ego strength, patient is unable to use coping mechanisms effectively.
Defense mechanisms utilized: denial, regression, repression, suppression, displacement, isolation

Quality of response

ANXIETY

Adaptive		Maladaptive	
Mild	Moderate	Severe	Panic
Response considered appropriate by societal norms.		Post-Traumatic Stress Disorder	Panic symptoms can occur during recollections and flashbacks of the trauma.

Figure 20.5 The dynamics of post-traumatic stress disorder using the transactional model of stress/adaptation.

Table 20.10   CARE PLAN FOR THE PATIENT WITH POST-TRAUMATIC STRESS DISORDER

Nursing Diagnoses	Objectives	Nursing Interventions
Post-trauma response related to distressing event considered to be outside the range of usual human experience, evidenced by flashbacks, intrusive recollections, nightmares, psychological numbness related to the event, dissociation, or amnesia.	The patient will integrate the traumatic experience into his or her persona, renew significant relationships, and establish meaningful goals for the future.	*In order to facilitate trust:* a. Assign the same staff as often as possible b. Use a nonthreatening, matter-of-fact, but friendly approach c. Respect patient's wishes regarding interaction with individuals of opposite sex at this time (especially important if the trauma was rape) d. Be consistent; keep all promises; convey acceptance; spend time with patient Stay with patient during periods of flashbacks and nightmares. Offer reassurance of safety and security, and that these symptoms are not uncommon following a trauma of the magnitude he or she has experienced. *Presence of a trusted individual may calm fears for personal safety and reassure patient that he or she is not "going crazy."* Obtain accurate history from significant others about the trauma and the patient's specific response. *Various types of traumas elicit different responses in patients (e.g., human-engendered traumas often generate a greater degree of humiliation and guilt in victims than trauma associated with natural disasters).* Encourage the patient to talk about the trauma at his or her own pace. Provide a nonthreatening, private environment, and include a significant other if the patient wishes. Acknowledge and validate patient's feelings as they are expressed. *This debriefing process is the first step in the progression toward resolution.* Discuss coping strategies used in response to the trauma, as well as those used during stressful situations in the past. Determine those that have been most helpful, and discuss alternative strategies for the future. Include available support systems, including religious and cultural influences. Identify maladaptive coping strategies (e.g., substance use, psychosomatic responses) and practice more adaptive coping strategies for possible future post-trauma responses. *Resolution of the post-trauma response is largely dependent on the effectiveness of the coping strategies employed.* Assist the individual to try to comprehend the trauma if possible. Discuss feelings of vulnerability and the individual's "place" in the world following the trauma. *Post-trauma response is largely a function of the shattering of basic beliefs the victim holds about self and world. Assimilation of the event into one's persona requires that some degree of meaning associated with the event be incorporated into the basic beliefs, which will effect how the individual eventually comes to reappraise self and world (Epstein, 1990).*

(continued)

Table 20.10 CONTINUED

Nursing Diagnoses	Objectives	Nursing Interventions
Dysfunctional grieving related to loss of self as perceived prior to the trauma or other actual/perceived losses incurred during/following the event, evidenced by irritability and explosiveness, self-destructiveness, substance abuse, verbalization of survival guilt or guilt about behavior required for survival.	Patient will demonstrate progress in dealing with stages of grief and will verbalize a sense of optimism and hope for the future.	Acknowledge feelings of guilt or self-blame that patient may express. *Guilt at having survived a trauma in which others died is common. The patient needs to discuss these feelings and recognize that he or she is not responsible for what happened but must take responsibility for own recovery.* Assess stage of grief in which the patient is fixed. Discuss normalcy of feelings and behaviors related to stages of grief. *Knowledge of grief stage is necessary for accurate intervention. Guilt may be generated if patient believes it is unacceptable to have these feelings. Knowing they are normal can provide a sense of relief.* Assess impact of the trauma on patient's ability to resume regular activities of daily living. Consider employment, marital relationship, sleep patterns. *Following a trauma, individuals are at high risk for physical injury due to disruption in ability to concentrate/problem solve and lack of sufficient sleep. Isolation and avoidance behaviors may interfere with interpersonal relatedness.* Assess for self-destructive ideas and behavior. *The trauma may result in feelings of hopelessness and worthlessness, leading to high risk for suicide.* Assess for maladaptive coping strategies, such as substance abuse, *that serve to delay the recovery process.* Identify available community resources to whom the individual may seek assistance if problems with dysfunctional grieving persist. *Support groups for victims of various types of traumas exist within most communities. Presence of support systems in the recovery environment has been identified as a major predictor in the successful recovery from trauma (Wilson & Krauss, 1985).*

11. Verbalizes desire to put the trauma in the past and progress with his or her life.

Evaluation Reassessment is conducted to determine whether the nursing actions have been successful in achieving the objectives of care. Evaluation of the nursing actions for the patient with PTSD may be facilitated by gathering information using the following types of questions.

Is the patient able to discuss the traumatic event without experiencing panic anxiety? Does the patient voluntarily discuss the traumatic event? Can the patient discuss changes that have occurred in his or her life due to the traumatic event? Does the patient experience "flashbacks?" Is the patient able to sleep without medication? Does the patient have nightmares? Has the patient learned new, adaptive coping strategies for assistance with recovery? Can the patient demonstrate successful use of these new coping strategies in times of stress? Can the patient verbalize stages of grief and the normal behaviors associated with each? Can he or she recognize own position in the grieving process? Is guilt being alleviated? Has the patient maintained or regained satisfactory relationships with significant others? Is he or she able to look to the future with optimism? Does the patient attend regular support group for victims of similar traumatic experiences? Does the patient have a plan of action for dealing with symptoms should they return?

Table 20.11 CRITICAL PATHWAY OF CARE FOR THE POST-TRAUMA PATIENT

Estimated Length of Stay: 14 days—Variations from designated pathway should be documented in progress notes

Nursing Diagnoses and Categories of Care	Time Dimension	Goals and/or Actions	Time Dimension	Goals and/or Actions	Time Dimension	Discharge Outcome
Post-trauma response	Day 1	Reassurance of patient safety.	Ongoing	Environment is made safe for patient.	Day 14	Patient is able to carry out activities of daily living. Fewer flashbacks, nightmares.
Referrals	Day 1	Psychiatrist Psychologist Social worker Clinical nurse specialist Music therapist Occupational therapist Recreational therapist Chaplain			Day 14	Discharge with follow-up appointments as required.
Diagnostic studies	Day 1 Day 2–5	Drug screen EKG; EEG MMPI Impact of event scale (IES)				
Medications	Day 1	Antidepressant medication, as ordered (tricyclics or MAOIs). Antianxiety medication, as ordered (benzodiazepines) May be given prn due to addictive quality. Clonidine or propranolol (for intrusive thoughts and hyperarousal). Sedative/hypnotics for sleep disturbances. May be given prn.	Day 1–14	Assess for effectiveness and side effects of medications. Administer addictive medications judiciously and taper dosage.	Day 14	Discharged with scripts as ordered by physician (e.g., antidepressants; clonidine; propranolol)

(continued)

Table 20.11 CONTINUED

Estimated Length of Stay: 14 days—Variations from designated pathway should be documented in progress notes

Nursing Diagnoses and Categories of Care	Time Dimension	Goals and/or Actions	Time Dimension	Goals and/or Actions	Time Dimension	Discharge Outcome
Additional assessments	Day 1 Day 1	VS every shift Assess: • Mental status • Mood swings • Anxiety level • Social interaction • Ability to carry out activities of daily living • Suicide ideation • Sleep disturbances • "Flashbacks" • Presence of guilt feelings	Day 2–14 Day 2–14	VS daily if stable Ongoing assessments	Day 14	Anxiety is maintained at manageable level. Mood is appropriate. Interacts with others. Carries out activities of daily living independently. Denies suicide ideation. Sleeps without medication. Is able to interrupt flashbacks with adaptive coping strategies. Has worked through feelings of guilt.
Diet	Day 1	Patient's choice or low tyramine if patient on MAOIs	Day 2–14	Same	Day 14	Patient eats well-balanced diet.
Patient education	Day 1	Orient to unit	Day 5–12 Day 12–13	Stages of grief Side effects of medications Coping strategies Low tyramine diet Community resources Support group Importance of not mixing drugs and alcohol Reinforce teaching	Day 14	Patient is discharged. Verbalizes understanding of information presented prior to discharge.

TREATMENT MODALITIES

Individual Psychotherapy

Most patients will experience a marked lessening of anxiety when given the opportunity to discuss their difficulties with a concerned and sympathetic therapist (Kaplan & Sadock, 1989). Gray (1978) states that the ultimate goal of individual psychotherapy with patients who have anxiety disorders is "to help the patient make responsible choices and to attain personal freedom." This he says is accomplished through four aspects of psychotherapy that are of particular importance:

1. *The therapeutic relationship.* An effective relationship ideally is based on mutual respect, confidence, and trust. Both therapist and patient should participate in the process with feelings of openness and frankness. Dependence on the therapist must be prevented, and treatment should be terminated when optimal benefit has been attained for the patient.

2. *Communication.* The ability of the patient to talk to the therapist and unburden himself or herself of guilt, conflict, anxiety, shame, and so forth affords the patient a feeling of relief and communion with another human being. The opportunity to reveal inner secrets that are a source of pain and suffering can free the individual to see and understand his or her behavior as never before. These shared insights open pathways for change.

3. *Education and reeducation.* Uncertainties and doubts are relieved from the mind through education. Knowledge has been shown to dissolve the fear that is fostered by ignorance. The therapist can use logical and rational explanations to increase the patient's understanding about various situations that create anxiety in his or her life.

4. *Change or transformation.* Gray (1978) suggests that this change in the patient's total being leads to his or her personal freedom to make conscious choices, to act according to these choices, and to accept the responsibility for the consequences of the action. The patient is able to choose the degree to which others can influence him or her. The anxiety response diminishes with this achievement of personal control.

Cognitive Therapy

The cognitive model relates how individuals respond in stressful situations to their subjective cognitive appraisal of the event (Beck & Emery, 1985). Anxiety is experienced when the cognitive appraisal is one of danger with which the individual perceives that he or she is unable to cope. Impaired cognition can contribute to anxiety disorders when the individual's appraisals are chronically negative. Automatic negative appraisals provoke self-doubts, negative evaluations, and negative predictions. Anxiety is maintained by this dysfunctional appraisal of a situation.

Cognitive therapy strives to assist the individual to reduce anxiety responses by altering cognitive distortions. Anxiety is described as being the result of exaggerated, *automatic* thinking.

Cognitive therapy for anxiety is brief and time-limited — usually from 5 to 20 sessions. Brief therapy discourages the patient's dependency on the therapist, which is prevalent in anxiety disorders, and encourages the patient's self-sufficiency.

A sound therapeutic relationship is a necessary condition for effective cognitive therapy. The patient must be able to talk openly about fears and feelings for the therapeutic process to occur. A major part of treatment consists of encouraging the patient to face frightening situations so as to be able to view them realistically, and talking about them is one way of achieving this. Treatment is a collaborative effort between patient and therapist.

Rather than offering suggestions and explanations, the therapist uses questions to encourage the patient to correct his or her anxiety-producing thoughts. The patient is encouraged to become aware of the thoughts, examine them for cognitive distortions, substitute more balanced thoughts, and eventually develop new patterns of thinking.

Cognitive therapy is very structured and orderly, which is important for the anxious patient who is often confused and lacks self-assurance. The focus is on solving present problems. Together the patient and therapist work to identify and correct maladaptive thoughts and behaviors that are maintaining a problem and blocking its solution.

Cognitive therapy is based on education. The premise is that one develops anxiety because he or she has learned inappropriate ways of handling life experiences. The belief is that with practice individuals can learn more effective ways of responding to these experiences. Homework assignments, which are a central feature of cognitive therapy, provide an experimental, problem-solving approach to overcoming long-held anxieties. Through fulfillment of these personal "experiments," the effectiveness of specific strategies and techniques is determined.

Behavior Therapy

Two common forms of behavior therapy include *systematic desensitization* and *implosion therapy* (flooding). They are commonly used to treat patients with phobic disorders and to modify stereotyped behavior of patients with PTSD (Embry, 1990). They have also been shown to be effective in a variety of other anxiety-producing situations (Wolpe, 1973).

SYSTEMATIC DESENSITIZATION

Systematic desensitization is a gradual exposing of the patient to the feared situation or object in imagination or in reality (Gray, 1978). The concept was introduced by Wolpe in 1958 and is based on behavioral conditioning principles. Emphasis is placed on *reciprocal inhibition* or counterconditioning.

Reciprocal inhibition is described as the restriction of anxiety prior to the effort of reducing avoidance behavior. The rationale behind this concept is that because relaxation is antagonistic to anxiety, individuals cannot be anxious and relaxed at the same time.

Systematic desensitization with reciprocal inhibition involves two main elements:

1. Training in relaxation techniques
2. Progressive exposure to a hierarchy of fear stimuli while in the relaxed state

The individual is instructed in the art of relaxation, using techniques most effective for him or her (e.g., progressive relaxation, mental imagery, tense and relax, meditation). When the individual has mastered the relaxation technique, exposure to the phobic stimulus is initiated. He or she is asked to present a hierarchical arrangement of situations pertaining to the phobic stimulus in order from most disturbing to least disturbing. While in a state of maximum relaxation, the patient may be asked to imagine the phobic stimulus. Initial exposure is focused on a concept of the phobic stimulus that produces the least amount of fear or anxiety. In subsequent sessions, the individual is gradually exposed to more fearful stimuli. Sessions may be executed in fantasy or in real life (*in vivo*) situations, or sometimes a combination of both.

CASE STUDY

John was afraid to ride on elevators. He had been known to climb 24 flights of stairs in an office building to avoid riding the elevator. John's own insurance office had plans for moving the company to a high-rise building soon, with offices on the 32nd floor. John sought assistance from a therapist for this problem. He was taught to achieve a sense of calmness and well-being through employment of a combination of mental imagery and progressive relaxation techniques. In the relaxed state, John was initially instructed to imagine the entry level of his office building, with a clear image of the bank of elevators. In subsequent sessions, and always in the relaxed state, John progressed to images of walking onto an elevator, having the elevator door close after he had entered, riding the elevator to the 32nd floor, and emerging from the elevator once the doors were opened.

Therapy for John also included *in vivo* sessions, in which he was exposed to the phobic stimulus in real-life situations (always after achieving a state of relaxation). This technique, combining imagined and *in vivo* procedures, proved very successful for John, and his employment in the high-rise complex was no longer in jeopardy due to claustrophobia.

IMPLOSION THERAPY (FLOODING)

Flooding is a therapeutic process in which the patient must imagine situations or participate in real-life situations that he or she finds extremely frightening for a prolonged period. Relaxation training is not a part of this technique. Plenty of time must be allowed for these sessions, since brief periods may be ineffective or even harmful. A session is terminated when the patient responds with considerably less anxiety than at the beginning of the session. Chambless and Goldstein (1979) describe flooding techniques in the following manner:

"The flooding technique requires that the therapist get as much information as possible concerning situations that trigger inappropriate anxiety. In a case of agoraphobia, a client reports that going out of the house leads to anxiety and that the anxiety is worse in public conveyances, elevators, and crowds. She fears she might be sent to an asylum and that no one will take care of her children, and so on. The client is asked to close her eyes and to imagine as vividly as possible what will be described without reflecting on it or evaluating its appropriateness. The therapist begins describing an anxiety-evoking situation in vivid detail starting with the client's preparing to go out alone. The flooding therapist is guided by the client's reactions: the more anxiety, the more appropriate the narrative. Modifications are made on the basis of new clues given by the client's reactions or statement. The same theme is repeated if it continues to arouse anxiety; it will be repeated as frequently as possible over as many sessions as necessary. Criteria for continuing are reports that anxiety is decreasing between sessions and that the client is instead entering formerly avoided situations."

Group/Family Therapy

Group therapy has been strongly advocated for patients with PTSD (Kaplan & Sadock, 1989). It has proved especially effective with survivors of combat trauma. Kolb (1986) stressed the importance of being able to share their experiences with empathic fellow veterans, to talk about problems in social adaptation, and to discuss options for managing their aggression toward others. Some groups are informal and leaderless, such as veterans' "rap" groups, and some are led by experienced group therapists who may have had some firsthand experience with the trauma. Some groups involve family members, thereby recognizing that the symptoms of PTSD may also severely affect them (Kaplan & Sadock, 1989).

Psychopharmacology

FOR PANIC AND GENERALIZED ANXIETY DISORDERS

Anxiolytics The benzodiazepine class of anti-anxiety drugs are the most commonly used group in the treatment of generalized anxiety disorders. Some researchers have suggested that they are not as effective in preventing panic attacks, and indeed evidence does show that low-to-moderate dosages of most benzodiazepines are inadequate in achieving relief (Kaplan & Sadock, 1989). However, recent investigations indicate that two high-potency benzodiazepines, alprazolam and clonazepam, have been found to be effective in the treatment of panic disorder (Beeber, 1989; Roy-Byrne & Katon, 1987). With long-term use, benzodiazepines produce physical dependence and tolerance. Withdrawal symptoms can be life threatening, so patients must be warned against abrupt discontinuation of the drug.

Antidepressants Several antidepressants have been shown to be effective as major antianxiety agents. The tricyclic imipramine has been used with success in patients experiencing panic disorder with agoraphobia. Clinically, it appears that most tricyclic antidepressants are equally effective with panic disorder (Schatzberg & Cole, 1986). Monamine oxidase (MAO) inhibitors, particularly phenelzine, and the antidepressant trazodone also exert antipanic effects. Imipramine appears to be the only antidepressant useful in the treatment of patients with generalized anxiety disorder (Kaplan & Sadock, 1989).

Antihypertensive Agents In recent years, a number of studies have called attention to the effectiveness of beta blockers (e.g., propranolol) and alpha$_2$ receptor agonists (e.g. clonidine) in the amelioration of anxiety symptoms (Schatzberg & Cole, 1986). Propranolol has potent effects on the somatic manifestations of anxiety (e.g., palpitations, tremors, etc.), with less dramatic effects on the psychological component of anxiety. It apparently has been used with some success in generalized anxiety disorder but is not particularly effective in blocking panic attacks (Gorman et al., 1983).

Clonidine has been found to be effective in blocking the acute anxiety effects in conditions such as opioid and nicotine withdrawal. However, it has had limited usefulness in the long-term treatment of panic and generalized anxiety disorders, particularly due to the development of tolerance to its antianxiety effects (Kaplan & Sadock, 1989).

FOR PHOBIC DISORDERS

Anxiolytics The benzodiazepines have been the most widely prescribed drug for the relief of phobic disorders, with mixed results. Alprazolam and clonazepam appear to be successful in reducing the symptoms of agoraphobia associated with panic disorder (Kaplan & Sadock, 1989).

Antidepressants The tricyclic imipramine and the MAO inhibitor phenelzine have been found to be effective in diminishing symptoms of agoraphobia and social phobias. However, with discontinuation of the medication, the phobic response often returns (Goodwin, 1983). Most simple phobias do not appear to respond to pharmacological intervention (Kaplan & Sadock, 1989).

Antihypertensives The beta blocker propranolol has been tried with success in patients experiencing anticipatory performance anxiety or "stage fright" (Goodwin, 1983). This type of phobic response produces symptoms such as sweaty palms, racing pulse, trembling hands, dry mouth, labored breathing, nausea, and memory loss. Propranolol appears to be quite effective in reducing these symptoms in some individuals.

FOR OBSESSIVE COMPULSIVE DISORDER

Antidepressants The tricyclic antidepressant clomipramine has proved to be effective in the treatment of obsessive compulsive disorder. In fact, clomipramine is the only drug currently approved by the Food and Drug Administration for use in this disorder (Jonas & Schaumburg, 1991). Other antidepressants with action similar to clomipramine have also been tried for treatment of obsessive compulsive disorder. Fluoxetine, which also blocks the reuptake of serotonin, has been shown to be effective in alleviating the obsessions and compulsions associated with the disorder (Jonas & Schaumburg, 1991).

FOR POST-TRAUMATIC STRESS DISORDER

Antidepressants Studies have shown that tricyclic antidepressants, and in particular amitriptyline and imipramine, have been effective in alleviating the depression, intrusive thoughts, sleep disorders, and nightmares associated with PTSD (Kaplan & Sadock, 1989). Efficacy of the MAO inhibitor phenelzine has also been demonstrated in reducing intrusive, depressive, and generalized anxiety symptoms with post-trauma patients (Friedman, 1990).

Anxiolytics Alprazolam has been prescribed for PTSD patients for its antidepressant and antipanic effects. Other benzodiazepines have also been widely used, despite the absence of controlled studies demonstrating their efficacy in PTSD (Friedman, 1990). Kaplan and Sadock (1989) state:

> "The benzodiazepines can interfere with the patient's ability to cope with severe emotions, can cause paradoxical rage, and can lead to abuse. Generally, therefore, they should not be used in PTSD."

Antihypertensives The beta blocker propranolol and alpha$_2$ receptor agonist clonidine have been successful in alleviating some of the symptoms associated with PTSD. In clinical trials, Kolb et al (1984) reported marked reductions in nightmares,

intrusive recollections, hypervigilance, insomnia, startle responses, and angry outbursts with the use of these drugs.

Other Drugs Carbamazepine and lithium carbonate have been shown to be effective in alleviating symptoms of intrusive recollections, flashbacks, nightmares, impulsivity, irritability, and violent behavior in PTSD patients (van der Kolk, 1988). Antipsychotics have been used with success in the treatment of refractory PTSD marked by paranoid behavior, aggressive psychotic symptoms, uncontrollable anger, self-destructive behavior, and frequent flashback episodes marked by frank auditory and visual hallucinations of traumatic episodes (Friedman, 1990). Further controlled trials are needed with these drugs to validate their efficacy in PTSD.

SUMMARY

Anxiety is a necessary force for survival and has been experienced by man throughout the ages. It was first described as a physiological disorder and identified by its physical symptoms, particularly the cardiac symptoms. The psychological implications for the symptoms were not recognized until the early 1990s.

Anxiety is considered a normal reaction to a realistic danger or threat to biologic integrity or self-concept. "Normality" of the anxiety experienced in response to a stressor is defined by societal and cultural standards.

Anxiety disorders are more common in women than in men by at least two to one. Studies of familial patterns suggest that a familial predisposition to anxiety disorders probably exists.

The *DSM-III-R* identifies four broad categories of anxiety disorders. They include panic and generalized anxiety disorders, phobic disorders, obsessive compulsive disorder, and PTSD. The etiology of these disorders is not entirely known. A number of elements, including psychosocial factors, biological influences, and learning experiences, enter into the development of these disorders.

Treatment of anxiety disorders include individual psychotherapy, cognitive therapy, behavior therapy, group and family therapy, and psychopharmacology. Common behavior therapies include systematic desensitization and implosion therapy (flooding). Nursing care is accomplished using the steps of the nursing process.

Nurses encounter patients experiencing anxiety in virtually all types of health-care settings. Nurses should be able to recognize the symptoms of anxiety and assist patients to understand that these symptoms are normal and acceptable.

Patients with anxiety disorders are generally seen in emergency departments or psychiatric facilities. Here nurses help patients to gain insight and increase self-awareness in relation to their illness. Intervention focuses on assisting patients to learn techniques with which they may interrupt the escalation of anxiety before it reaches unmanageable proportions. Maladaptive behavior patterns are replaced by new, more adaptive coping skills.

REVIEW QUESTIONS
Self-Examination/Learning Exercise

*Select the answer that is **most** appropriate for each of the following questions.*

Situation: Ms. T. has been diagnosed with agoraphobia.

1. Which behavior would be most characteristic of this disorder?
   a. Ms. T. experiences panic anxiety when she encounters snakes.
   b. Ms. T. refuses to fly in an airplane.
   c. Ms. T. will not eat in a public place.
   d. Ms. T. stays in her home for fear of being in a place from which she cannot escape.

2. The therapist who works with Ms. T. would likely choose which of the following therapies for her.
   a. 10 mg Valium qid.
   b. Group therapy with other agoraphobics
   c. Facing her fear in gradual step progression
   d. Hypnosis

3. Should the therapist choose to use implosion therapy, Ms. T. would be:
   a. taught relaxation exercises.
   b. subjected to graded intensities of the fear.
   c. instructed to stop the therapeutic session as soon as anxiety is experienced.
   d. presented with massive exposure to a variety of stimuli associated with the phobic object/situation.

Situation: Sandy is a 29-year-old woman who has been admitted to the psychiatric unit with a diagnosis of obsessive-compulsive disorder. She spends many hours during the day and night washing her hands.

4. The most likely reason Sandy washes her hands so much is:
   a. it relieves her anxiety.
   b. to reduce the probability of infection.
   c. it gives her a feeling of control over her life.
   d. it increases her self-concept.

5. The initial care plan for Sandy would include which of the following nursing interventions?
   a. Keep Sandy's bathroom locked so she cannot wash her hands all the time.
   b. Structure Sandy's schedule so that she has plenty of time for washing her hands.

    c. Put Sandy in isolation until she promises to stop washing her hands so much.

    d. Explain Sandy's behavior to her, since she is probably unaware that it is maladaptive.

6. On Sandy's fourth hospital day, she says to the nurse, "I'm feeling better now. I feel comfortable on this unit, and I'm not ill-at-ease with the staff or other patients anymore." In light of this change, which nursing intervention is most appropriate?

    a. Give attention to the ritualistic behaviors each time they occur and point out their inappropriateness.

    b. Ignore the ritualistic behaviors, and they will be eliminated for lack of reinforcement.

    c. Set limits on the amount of time Sandy may engage in the ritualistic behavior.

    d. Continue to allow Sandy all the time she wants to carry out the ritualistic behavior.

Situation: John is a 28-year-old high-school science teacher whose Army Reserve unit was called to fight in Operation Desert Storm. John did not want to fight. He admits that he joined the reserves to help pay off his college loans. In Saudi Arabia, he participated in combat and witnessed the wounding of several from his unit, as well as the death of his best friend. He has been experiencing flashbacks, intrusive recollections, and nightmares. His wife reports he is afraid to go to sleep, and his work is suffering. Sometimes he just sits as though he is in a trance. John is diagnosed with PTSD.

7. John says to the nurse, "I can't figure out why God took my buddy instead of me." From this statement, the nurse assesses which of the following in John?

    a. Repressed anger

    b. Survivor's guilt

    c. Intrusive thoughts

    d. Spiritual distress

8. John experiences a nightmare during his first night in the hospital. He explains to the nurse that he was dreaming about gunfire all around and people being killed. The nurse's most appropriate initial intervention is:

    a. administer alprazolam as ordered prn for anxiety.

    b. call the physician and report the incident.

    c. stay with John and reassure him of his safety.

    d. have John listen to a tape of relaxation exercises.

9. Which of the following therapy regimens would most appropriately be ordered for John?

    a. Imipramine and group therapy

    b. Diazepam and implosion therapy

    c. Alprazolam and behavior therapy

    d. Carbamazepine and cognitive therapy

10. Which of the following may be influential in the predisposition to PTSD?

    a. Unsatisfactory parent/child relationship

    b. Excess of the neurotransmitter serotonin

    c. Distorted, negative cognitions

    d. Severity of the stressor and availability of support systems

REFERENCES

American Psychiatric Association. (1987). *Diagnostic and statistical manual of mental disorders* (3rd ed, rev.). Washington, DC: American Psychiatric Association.

Beck, A. T. & Emery, G. (1985). *Anxiety disorders and phobias*. New York: Basic Books.

Beeber, L. S. (1989). Treatment of anxiety. *J Psychosoc Nurs, 27*: 42.

Chambless, D. L. & Goldstein, A. J. (1979). Behavioral psychotherapy. In R. J. Corsini (Ed.), *Current psychotherapies* (2nd ed.). Itasca, IL: FE Peacock Publishers.

Embry, C. K. (1990). Psychotherapeutic interventions in chronic post-traumatic stress disorder. In Wolf & Mosnaim (Eds.), *Post-traumatic stress disorder: Etiology, phenomenology, and treatment.* Washington, DC: American Psychiatric Press.

Emmelkamp, P. M. G. (1982). *Phobic and obsessive-compulsive disorders: Theory, research, and practice.* New York: Plenum Press.

Epstein, S. (1990). Beliefs and symptoms in maladaptive resolutions of the traumatic neurosis. In Ozer et al. (Eds.), *Perspectives on personality* (Vol. 3). London: Jessica Kingsley.

Erikson, E. (1968). *Youth, identity, and crisis.* New York: Norton.

Freud, S. (1959). On the grounds for detaching a particular syndrome from neurasthenia under the description 'anxiety neurosis.' In *The standard edition of the complete psychological works of Sigmund Freud* (Vol. 3). London: Hogarth Press.

Friedman, M. J. (1990). Interrelationships between biological mechanisms and pharmacotherapy of post-traumatic stress disorder. In Wolf & Mosnaim (Eds.), *Post-traumatic stress disorder: Etiology, phenomenology, and treatment.* Washington, DC: American Psychiatric Press.

Goodwin, D. W. (1983). *Phobia: The facts.* New York: Oxford University Press.

Gorman, J. M. et al (1983). Effect of acute beta adrenergic blockade on lactate-induced panic. *Arch Gen Psychiatry, 40*: 1079–1082.

Gray, M. (1978). *Neuroses: A comprehensive and critical view.* New York: Van Nostrand Reinhold Co.

Green, B. L., Wilson, J. P., & Lindy, J. D. (1985). Conceptualizing post-traumatic stress disorder: A psychosocial framework. In C. R. Figley (Ed.), *Trauma and its wake: The study and treatment of post-traumatic stress disorder.* New York: Brunner/Mazel.

Helzer, J., Robins, L., & McEvoy, L. (1987). Post-traumatic stress disorder in the general population. *N Engl J Med, 317*: 1630–1634.

Johnson, J. H. & Sarason, I. G. (1978). Life stress, depression and anxiety: Internal-external control as a moderator variable. *J Psychosom Res. 22*: 205–208.

Jonas, J. M. & Schaumburg, R. (1991). *Everything you need to know about Prozac.* New York: Bantam Books.

Kaplan, H. I. & Sadock, B. J. (1989). *Comprehensive textbook of psychiatry* (Vol. 1) (5th ed.). Baltimore: Williams & Wilkins.

Kardiner, A. (1941). *The traumatic neuroses of war.* New York: Hoeber.

Keable, D. (1989). *The management of anxiety: A manual for therapists.* New York: Churchill Livingstone.

Keane, T. M. et al. (1985). A behavioral approach to assessing and treating PTSD in Vietnam veterans. In C. R. Figley (Ed.), *Trauma and its wake.* New York: Brunner/Mazel.

Kolb, L. C., Burris, B. C., & Griffiths, S. (1984). Propranolol and clonidine in the treatment of the chronic post-traumatic stress disorders of war. In B. A. van der Kolk (Ed.), *Post-traumatic stress disorder: Psychological and biological sequelae.* Washington, DC: American Psychiatric Press.

Kolb, L. C. (1986). Treatment of chronic post-traumatic stress disorder. *Current Psychiatric Therapies, 23*: 119–126.

Kulka, R., Schlenger, W., & Fairbank, J. (1988). *National Vietnam veterans readjustment study (NVVRS) report: Description, current status, and initial PTSD prevalence estimates.* Washington, DC: Veterans Administration.

Nemiah, J. C. (1971). *Foundations of psychopathology.* New York: Oxford University Press.

Peterson, K. C., Prout, M. F., & Schwartz, R. A. (1991). *Post-traumatic stress disorder: A clinician's guide.* New York: Plenum Press.

Rachman, S. & Hodgson, R. J. (1980). *Obsessions and compulsions.* Englewood Cliffs, NJ: Prentice-Hall.

Roy-Byrne, P. P. & Katon, W. (1987, August). An update on treatment of the anxiety disorders. *Hospital and Community Psychiatry, 38*: 835–843.

Schatzberg, A. F. & Cole, J. O. (1986). *Manual of clinical psychopharmacology.* Washington, DC: American Psychiatric Press.

Teasdale, J. D. (1974). Learning models of obsessional-compulsive disorder. In H. R. Beech (Ed.), *Obsessional states.* London: Methuen.

Uhde, T. W. & Nemiah, J. C. (1989). Anxiety disorders. In H. I. Kaplan & B. J. Sadock (Eds.), *Comprehensive textbook of psychiatry* (Vol. 1) (ed. 5). Baltimore: Williams and Wilkins.

van der Kolk, B. A. (1988). The biological response to trauma. In F. Ochberg (Ed.), *Post-traumatic therapy and victims of violence.* New York: Brunner/Mazel.

Weissman, M. M. (1985). The epidemiology of anxiety disorders: Rates, risks, and familial patterns. In Tuma & Maser (Eds.), *Anxiety and the anxiety disorders.* Hillsdale, NJ: Lawrence Erlbaum Associates Publishers.

Wilson, J. P. & Krauss, G. E. (1985). Predicting post-traumatic stress disorders among Vietnam veterans. In W. E. Kelly (Ed.), *Post-traumatic stress disorder and the war veteran patient.* New York: Brunner/Mazel.

Wolpe, J. (1958). *Psychotherapy and reciprocal inhibition.* Stanford: Stanford University Press.

Wolpe, J. (1973). *The practice of behavior therapy.* New York: Pergamon Press.

BIBLIOGRAPHY

Blair, D. T. & Hildreth, N. A. (1991). PTSD and the Vietnam veteran: The battle for treatment. *J Psychosoc Nurs, 29*(10): 15–20.

Gerlock, A. A. (1991). Vietnam: Returning to the scene of the trauma. *J Psychosoc Nurs, 29*(2): 4–8.

Mowrer, O. H. (1960). *Learning theory and behavior.* New York: John Wiley & Sons.

Simoni, P. S. (1991). Obsessive-compulsive disorder: The effect of research on nursing care. *J Psychosoc Nurs, 29*(4): 19–23.

Townsend, M. C. (1990). *Drug guide for psychiatric nursing.* Philadelphia: FA Davis.

Townsend, M. C. (1991). *Nursing diagnoses in psychiatric nursing: A pocket guide for care plan construction* (2nd ed.). Philadelphia: FA Davis.

Tuma, A. H. & Maser, J. (Eds.). (1985). *Anxiety and the anxiety disorders.* Hillsdale, NJ: Lawrence Erlbaum Associates Publishers.

Whitley, G. G. (1991). Ritualistic behavior: Breaking the cycle. *J Psychosoc Nurs, 29*(10): 31–35.

Wolf, M. E. & Mosnaim, A. D. (Eds.). (1990). *Post-traumatic stress disorder: Etiology, phenomenology, and treatment.* Washington, DC: American Psychiatric Press.

21

SOMATOFORM DISORDERS

KEY TERMS
anosmia
aphonia
hypochondriasis
hysteria
la belle indifference
primary gain
pseudocyesis
secondary gain
somatization

OBJECTIVES

After reading this chapter, the student will be able to:

1. Define the term *hysteria*.
2. Discuss historical aspects and epidemiological statistics related to somatoform disorders.
3. Describe various types of somatoform disorders and identify symptomatology associated with each. Use this information in patient assessment.
4. Identify predisposing factors in the development of somatoform disorders.
5. Formulate nursing diagnoses and goals of care for patients with somatoform disorders.
6. Describe appropriate nursing interventions for behaviors associated with somatoform disorders.
7. Evaluate the nursing care of patients with somatoform disorders.
8. Discuss various modalities relevant to treatment of somatoform disorders.

INTRODUCTION

The somatoform disorders are characterized by physical symptoms suggesting medical disease, but no demonstrable organ pathology or pathophysiological mechanism can be found to account for them (Barsky, 1989). They are classified as mental disorders because pathophysiological processes are not demonstrable or understandable by existing laboratory procedures and are conceptualized most clearly by means of psychological constructs (American Psychiatric Association [APA], 1987). Somatization refers to all those mechanisms by which anxiety is translated into physical illness or bodily complaints.

A large proportion of patients in general medical outpatient clinics and private medical offices do not have organic disease requiring medical treatment (Purcell, 1988). Many of these patients may have somatoform disorders, but they do not perceive themselves as having a psychiatric problem and thus do not seek treatment from psychiatrists.

This chapter focuses on disorders that are characterized by anxiety that has been repressed and is being expressed in the form of physiological symptoms. Historical and epidemiological statistics are presented. Predisposing factors that have been implicated in the etiology of somatoform disorders provide a framework for studying the dynamics of somatization disorder, somatoform pain disorder, hypochondriasis, conversion disorder, and body dysmorphic disorder.

An explanation of the symptomatology is presented as background knowledge for assessing the patient with a somatoform disorder. Nursing care is described in the context of the nursing process. Various medical treatment modalities are explored.

HISTORICAL ASPECTS

The term *hysteria* describes a polysymptomatic disorder that usually begins in adolescence, rarely after the 20s, chiefly affects women, and is characterized by recurrent, multiple somatic complaints often described dramatically (Goodwin & Guze, 1989). The concept of hysteria is at least 4,000 years old and probably originated in Egypt. The name has been in use since the time of Hippocrates.

Witchcraft, demonology, and sorcery were associated with hysteria in the Middle Ages (Vieth, 1965). Mysterious symptoms and unusual behavior were frequently considered manifestations of supernatural, evil influences, with the patient being considered as either the evil spirit itself or the victim of the evil force.

In the 19th century, the French physician Paul Briquet attributed the disorder to dysfunction in the nervous system (Stoudemire, 1988). He conceptualized that the disorder was the result of stressful events that acted on the affective part of the brain in vulnerable individuals. Another French physician, Jean Martin Charcot, proposed an essentially physical theory for the disorder, attributing the symptoms to a hereditary degenerative process of the nervous system. Despite his feelings about a physical basis for hysteria, he became famous for his use of hypnosis in the treatment of the disorder (Goodwin & Guze, 1989).

Freud, whose interest in hysterical disorders had developed while he was working in Paris with Charcot, observed that under hypnosis, patients could recall past memories and emotional experiences that would relieve their symptoms. This led to his proposal that emotion that is not expressed can be "converted" into physical symptoms (Jones, 1980).

In the 1960s, a series of studies originated with a subgroup of hysteria patients who presented with multiple somatic symptoms, a chronic course, and excessive amounts of medical and surgical care. The disorder that delineated this homogeneous group came to be known as Briquet's syndrome, and is occasionally designated by this terminology even today (Barsky, 1989). Somatization disorder, as it is described in the *Diagnostic and Statistical Manual of Mental Disorders, ed. 3, revised (DSM-III-R)*, is a simplified version of Briquet's syndrome.

Of the somatoform disorders described in the *DSM-III-R*, only conversion disorder still carries the connotation of "hysteria." Its alternate diagnostic label is hysterical neurosis, conversion type (APA, 1987).

EPIDEMIOLOGICAL STATISTICS

Somatization disorder is rare in men. Its lifetime prevalence rate in women is between 0.2 percent and 2 percent (Smith et al, 1986). Tendencies toward somatization are apparently more common in those who are poorly educated, rural, religious fundamentalists, ethnic, and from lower socioeconomic classes (Stoudemire, 1988).

Prevalence rates of conversion disorders, derived out of general hospital populations, have been reported as 5 percent to 13 percent (Lazare, 1981). It occurs more frequently in women than in men and is more common in adolescents and young adults. A higher prevalence exists in lower socioeconomic groups, rural populations, and among those with less education (Barsky, 1989).

Hypochondriasis is present in 3 percent to 14 percent of patients in general medical practice (Barsky, 1989). The disorder is equally common among men and women, and the most common age at onset is between 20 and 30 years (APA, 1987).

Pain is likely the most frequent presenting complaint in medical practice today. Somatoform pain disorder is diagnosed more frequently in women. Its onset can occur at any age but is most frequently diagnosed in the 30s and 40s (APA, 1987). It is more common among people in blue-collar occupations (Barsky, 1989).

Body dysmorphic disorder is rare, although it may be more common than once believed (APA, 1987). As many as 2 percent of plastic surgery consultations have been reported from patients with this disorder (Stoudemire, 1988). Psychiatrists see only a small fraction of the cases. A profile of these patients reveals that they are usually in the late teens or 20s and unmarried. Follow-up studies have revealed the presence of severe neuroses and psychoses in a significant number of patients with body dysmorphic disorder (Connolly & Gibson, 1978).

APPLICATION OF THE NURSING PROCESS

Classifications of Somatoform Disorders: Background Assessment Data

SOMATIZATION DISORDER

Somatization disorder is a chronic syndrome of multiple somatic symptoms that cannot be explained medically and are associated with psychosocial distress and long-term seeking of assistance from health-care professionals (Barsky, 1989). Symptoms may be vague, dramatized, or exaggerated in their presentation. They may represent

virtually any organ system but commonly are expressed as neurological, gastrointestinal, psychosexual, or cardiopulmonary disorders (Kolb & Brodie, 1982). Anxiety and depression are frequently manifested, and suicidal attempts and threats are not uncommon.

The disorder usually runs a fluctuating course, with periods of remission and exacerbation. Patients often receive medical care from several physicians, sometimes simultaneously (APA, 1987). They have a tendency to seek relief through overmedicating with prescribed analgesics or antianxiety agents. Drug abuse and dependence are not uncommon complications of somatization disorder. When suicide results, it is usually in association with substance abuse (Purcell, 1988).

McCracken (1985) describes personality characteristics common to patients with somatization disorder. He suggests that there may be some overlapping of features associated with histrionic personality disorder, such as heightened emotionality, vague impressionistic thought, seductiveness, strong dependency needs, and a preoccupation with symptoms and oneself.

The *DSM-III-R* diagnostic criteria for somatization disorder are presented in Table 21.1.

Predisposing Factors to Somatization Disorder

Psychodynamic Theory This theory emphasizes a disturbance in the early mother-child relationship. McCracken (1985) describes the mother as one who, because of her own conflicts regarding sexuality and dependency, alternately clings to and rejects the child. Out of this conditional nurturing by the mother, the child fails to develop feelings of self-security. He or she defends against this insecurity by learning to gain affection and care through illness.

Theory of Family Dynamics In some families, there appears to be a marked deficiency in the abilities of the family members to openly express emotions, a failure to resolve conflicts verbally, and the denial of psychological problems in general (Stoudemire, 1988). In these "psychosomatic families," when the child becomes ill, a shift in focus is made from the open conflict to the child's illness, leaving unresolved the underlying issues that the family is unable to confront in an open manner. Thus, somatization by the child brings some stability to the family, as harmony replaces discord and the child's welfare becomes the common concern. The child in

Table 21.1 DIAGNOSTIC CRITERIA FOR SOMATIZATION DISORDER

A. A history of many physical complaints or a belief that one is sickly, beginning before the age of 30 and persisting for several years.

B. At least 13 symptoms from the list below. To count a symptom as significant, the following criteria must be met:

1. No organic pathology or pathophysiological mechanism (e.g., a physical disorder or the effects of injury, medication, drugs, or alcohol) to account for the symptom or, when there is related organic pathology, the complaint or resulting social or occupational impairment is grossly in excess of what would be expected from the physical findings.
2. Has not occurred only during a panic attack.
3. Has caused the person to take medicine (other than over-the-counter pain medication), see a doctor, or alter life-style.

Symptom list:

Gastrointestinal symptoms:
1. **Vomiting (other than during pregnancy)**
2. Abdominal pain (other than when menstruating)
3. Nausea (other than motion sickness)
4. Bloating (gassy)
5. Diarrhea
6. Intolerance of (gets sick from) several different foods

Pain symptoms:
7. **Pain in extremities**
8. Back pain
9. Joint pain
10. Pain during urination
11. Other pain (excluding headaches)

Cardiopulmonary symptoms:
12. **Shortness of breath when not exerting oneself**
13. Palpitations
14. Chest pain
15. Dizziness

Conversion or pseudoneurologic symptoms:
16. **Amnesia**
17. **Difficulty swallowing**
18. Loss of voice
19. Deafness
20. Double vision
21. Blurred vision
22. Blindness
23. Fainting or loss of consciousness
24. Seizure or convulsion
25. Trouble walking
26. Paralysis or muscle weakness
27. Urinary retention or difficulty urinating

Sexual symptoms for major part of the person's life after opportunities for sexual activity:
28. **Burning sensation in sexual organs or rectum (other than during intercourse)**
29. Sexual indifference
30. Pain during intercourse
31. Impotence

Female reproductive symptoms judged by the person to occur more frequently or severely than in most women:
32. **Painful menstruation**
33. Irregular menstrual periods
34. Excessive menstrual bleeding
35. Vomiting throughout pregnancy

Note: The presence of two or more items in boldface suggests a high likelihood of the disorder.
Source: From American Psychiatric Association (1987) with permission.

turn receives positive reinforcement for the illness (Minuchin et al, 1975).

Somatization may also have its roots in the family system due to parental teaching and parental example. The effectiveness of learning through role modeling has been well established and may be instrumental in teaching children to respond to anxious situations with somatization.

Cultural and Environmental Factors Some cultures and religions carry implicit sanctions against verbalizing or directly expressing emotional states (Stoudemire, 1988). Cross-cultural studies have shown that the somatization symptoms associated with depression are relatively similar, but the "cognitive" or emotional symptoms such as guilt are predominately seen in Western societies (Kleinman & Mechanic, 1980). In Middle Eastern and Oriental cultures, depression is almost exclusively manifested by somatic/vegetative symptoms. This unacceptability of emotional expression is reinforced in various cultures by the absence of vocabulary within the language to express psychological and emotional states (Leff, 1973).

Environmental influences may be significant in the predisposition to somatization disorder. Some studies have suggested that a tendency toward somatization appears to be more common in the poorly educated, rural, and lower socioeconomic classes (Stoudemire, 1988). This may be related to a lack of language sophistication required to express oneself psychologically or social restrictions against conceptualizing life difficulties in psychological terminology (Barsky, 1979; Mechanic, 1972).

Genetic Factors Although this disorder is presumed to be psychological in origin, and no conclusive evidence exists otherwise, studies that have shown a 10- to 20-fold increase in the incidence of the disorder in female first-degree relatives cannot be ignored (McCracken, 1985). These statistics may imply a possible inheritable predisposition. The deficiency of twin and adoption studies further impedes the ability to make assumptions regarding a genetic link to this disorder.

Transactional Model of Stress/Adaptation The etiology of somatization disorder is most likely influenced by multiple factors. In Figure 21.1, a graphic depiction of this theory of multiple causation is presented in the Transactional Model of Stress/Adaptation.

Nursing Diagnosis, Planning/Implementation Nursing diagnoses are formulated from the data gathered during the assessment phase and with background knowledge regarding predisposing factors to the disorder. Some common nursing diagnoses for patients with somatization disorder include:

Ineffective individual coping related to repressed anxiety and unmet dependency needs, evidenced by verbalization of numerous physical complaints in the absence of any pathophysiological evidence; total focus on the self and physical symptoms.

Knowledge deficit (psychological causes for physical symptoms) related to strong denial defense system, evidenced by history of doctor shopping for evidence of organic pathology to substantiate physical symptoms and statements such as, "I don't know why the doctor put me on the psychiatric unit. I have a physical problem."

In Table 21.2, these nursing diagnoses are presented in a plan of care for the patient with somatization disorder. Goals of care and appropriate nursing interventions are included for each. Rationales are provided in italics.

Outcome Criteria The following criteria may be used for measurement of outcomes in the care of the patient with somatization disorder.

The patient:

1. Is able to demonstrate adaptive coping strategies.
2. Is able to effectively use adaptive coping strategies during stressful situations without resorting to physical symptoms.
3. Is able to identify stressors that cause anxiety level to rise.
4. Verbalizes understanding of correlation between times of increased anxiety and onset of physical symptoms.
5. Demonstrates control over life situation by meeting needs in an assertive manner.

Evaluation Reassessment is conducted to determine if the nursing actions have been successful in achieving the objectives of care. Evaluation of the nursing actions for the patient with somatization disorder may be facilitated by gathering information using the following types of questions.

Can the patient recognize signs and symptoms of escalating anxiety? Can the patient intervene with adaptive coping strategies to interrupt the escalating anxiety before exacerbation of physical symptoms occurs? Is the patient able to verbalize an understanding of the correlation between physical symptoms and times of escalating anxiety? Does he or she have a plan for dealing with increased stress so that exacerbation of physical symptoms is prevented? Is the patient able to demonstrate assertiveness skills? Does the patient exercise control over life situation by participating in decision-making process? Is the patient able to name resources outside the hospital from whom he or she may seek assistance during times of extreme stress?

SOMATOFORM PAIN DISORDER

The predominant disturbance in somatoform pain disorder is severe and prolonged pain for which no adequate medical explanation exists (Barsky, 1989). This diagnosis is made when the pain pattern is not consistent with anatomical distribution of pain receptors, no organic etiology is detectable to explain the pain, and no pathophysiological mechanisms can be employed to fully account for the pain (APA, 1987). Even when organic

Precipitating Event
(Any event sufficiently stressful to threaten an already weak ego)

Predisposing Factors
  Genetic Influences: Possible familial predisposition
  Past Experiences: Weak ego development
    Feelings of insecurity
    Unmet dependency needs
    Positive reinforcement for somatization
    Role modeling
    Cultural/social sanctions against expressing emotions directly
  Existing Conditions: Developmental regression
    Absence of support systems
    Poor coping mechanisms

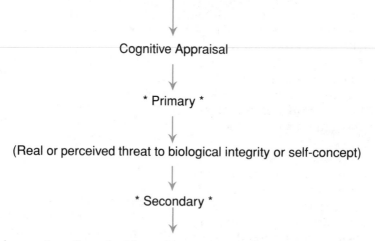

Cognitive Appraisal

* Primary *

(Real or perceived threat to biological integrity or self-concept)

* Secondary *

Because of weak ego strength, patient is unable to use coping mechanisms effectively.
Defense mechanisms utilized: denial, regression, repression, suppression

Quality of response

ANXIETY

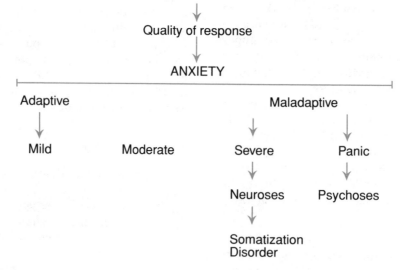

Adaptive   Maladaptive

Mild   Moderate   Severe   Panic

Neuroses   Psychoses

Somatization
Disorder

Figure 21.1 The dynamics of somatization disorder using the transactional model of stress/adaptation.

pathology is detected, the pain complaints are excessive of what would be expected from the underlying physical condition. Psychological implications in the etiology of the pain complaint may be evidenced by the correlation of a stressful situation with the onset of the symptom. Additional psycho-logical implications may be supported by: 1) the fact that appearance of the pain enables the patient to avoid some unpleasant activity and 2) the pain's promotion of emotional support or attention that the patient might not otherwise receive (Stoudemire, 1988).

Table 21.2 CARE PLAN FOR THE PATIENT WITH SOMATIZATION DISORDER

Nursing Diagnoses	Objectives	Nursing Interventions
Ineffective individual coping related to repressed anxiety and unmet dependency needs, evidenced by verbalization of numerous physical complaints in the absence of any pathophysiological evidence; total focus on the self and physical symptoms.	Patient will demonstrate ability to cope with stress by means other than preoccupation with physical symptoms.	Monitor physician's ongoing assessments, laboratory reports, and other data to maintain assurance that possibility of organic pathology is clearly ruled out. Review findings with patient. *Knowledge of this data is vital for the provision of adequate and appropriate care. Honest explanation may help patient understand psychologic implications.* Recognize and accept that the physical complaint is real to the patient, even though no organic etiology can be identified. *Denial of the patient's feelings is nontherapeutic and interferes with establishment of a trusting relationship.* Identify gains that the physical symptoms are providing for the patient: increased dependency, attention, distraction from other problems. *These are important assessment data to be used in assisting the patient with problem resolution.* Initially, fulfill patient's most urgent dependency needs, but gradually withdraw attention to physical symptoms. Minimize time given in response to physical complaints. *Anxiety and maladaptive behaviors will increase if dependency needs are ignored initially. Gradual lack of positive reinforcement will discourage repetition of maladaptive behaviors.* Explain to patient that any new physical complaints will be referred to the physician and give no further attention to them. Ensure physician's assessment of the complaint. *The possibility of organic pathology must always be considered. Failure to do so could jeopardize patient safety.* Encourage patient to verbalize fears and anxieties. Explain that attention will be withdrawn if rumination about physical complaints begins. Follow through. *Without consistency of limit setting, change will not occur.* Discuss possible alternative coping strategies patient may use in response to stress (e.g., relaxation exercises; physical activities; assertiveness skills). Give positive reinforcement for use of these alternatives. *Patient may need help with problem solving. Positive reinforcement encourages repetition.* Help patient identify ways to achieve recognition from others without resorting to physical symptoms. *Positive recognition from others enhances self-esteem and minimizes the need for attention through maladaptive behaviors.*

(*continued*)

Table 21.2 CONTINUED

Nursing Diagnoses	Objectives	Nursing Interventions
Knowledge deficit (psychological causes for physical symptoms) related to strong denial defense system, evidenced by history of doctor shopping for evidence of organic pathology to substantiate physical symptoms and statements such as, "I don't know why the doctor put me on the psychiatric unit. I have a physical problem."	Patient will verbalize psychological implications for physical symptoms.	Assess patient's level of knowledge regarding effects of psychologic problems on the body. Assess level of anxiety and readiness to learn. *An adequate data base is necessary for the development of an effective teaching plan. Learning does not occur beyond the moderate level of anxiety.* Discuss results of laboratory tests and physical examinations with patient. *Objective information about physical condition may help to break through the strong denial defense.* Have patient keep a diary of appearance, duration, and intensity of physical symptoms. A separate record of situations that the patient finds especially stressful should also be kept. *Comparison of these records may provide objective data from which to observe the relationship between physical symptoms and stress.* Help patient identify needs that are being met through the sick role. Formulate a more adaptive means for fulfilling these needs. Practice by role playing. *Change cannot occur until patient realizes that physical symptoms are used to fulfill unmet needs. Anxiety is relieved by role playing, as the patient is able to anticipate responses to stressful situations.* Evaluate teaching by having patient demonstrate adaptive methods of stress management: relaxation exercises, meditation, deep-breathing exercises, autogenics, and mental imagery.

Characteristic behaviors include frequent visits to physicians in an effort to obtain relief, excessive use of analgesics, requests for surgery, and assumption of the role of invalid (APA, 1987). Symptoms of depression are common and often are severe enough to warrant a diagnosis of major depression. Dependence on minor tranquilizers or narcotic analgesics is a typical complication of somatoform pain disorder.

In approximately one-half the cases of somatoform pain disorder, onset of the pain occurs immediately following a physical trauma (e.g., accident or surgery). *DSM-III-R* diagnostic criteria for this disorder are presented in Table 21.3.

Predisposing Factors to Somatoform Pain Disorder

Psychoanalytic Theory Engel (1959) associated psychogenic pain with unconscious guilt and masochism. He theorized that pain in these patients could often serve the purposes of punishment and atonement for unconscious guilt. He found that life

Table 21.3 DIAGNOSTIC CRITERIA FOR SOMATOFORM PAIN DISORDER

A. Preoccupation with pain for at least 6 months.
B. Either 1) or 2):
  1. Appropriate evaluation uncovers no organic pathology or pathophysiological mechanism (e.g., a physical disorder or the effects of injury) to account for the pain.
  2. When there is related organic pathology, the complaint of pain or resulting social or occupational impairment is grossly in excess of what would be expected from the physical findings.

Source: From American Psychiatric Association (1987) with permission.

histories of these patients were characterized by repeated episodes of real or perceived failures. Childhood was marked by physical abuse, the use of pain as punishment, and emotional distance from parents, resulting in repressed anger and feelings of helplessness. Children who have been severely punished feel guilty and unconsciously come to believe that they must indeed be bad. Such children may grow up with an unconscious need for suffering and pain to assuage this guilt (Barsky, 1989).

Behavioral Theory In behavioral terminology, psychogenic pain is explained as a response that is learned through operant and classical conditioning. In classical conditioning, a previously neutral stimulus may become a trigger for pain-related behaviors when it becomes associated in the mind of the individual with a painful stimulus. For example, the room where a painful event occurred may itself alone evoke pain-related behaviors because it has become associated with the painful event.

In operant conditioning, learning occurs when pain behaviors are positively or negatively reinforced. When pain behavior elicits attention, sympathy, and nurturing, this positive reinforcement increases the probability of the pain behavior continuing. Negative reinforcement results when the pain behavior prevents an undesirable response from occurring (e.g., provides relief from responsibilities for the patient).

Theory of Family Dynamics "Pain games" may be played in families burdened by conflict. Pain may be used by a family member to control and coerce others and for manipulating and gaining the advantage in interpersonal relationships. Pain may also serve as a *tertiary gain* for a family who maintains the identified patient in such a position that the real issue is disregarded and remains unresolved, even though some of the conflict is relieved.

Neurophysiological Theory This theory postulates that the cerebral cortex is involved in inhibiting the firing of afferent pain fibers (Barsky, 1989). Serotonin and the endorphins probably play a role in the central modulation of pain. The levels of serotonin and endorphins are believed to be decreased in patients with chronic, intractable pain. This deficiency seems to correlate with the augmentation of incoming sensory (pain) stimuli.

Transactional Model of Stress/Adaptation The etiology of somatoform pain disorder is most likely influenced by multiple factors. In Figure 21.2, a graphic depiction of this theory of multiple causation is presented in the Transactional Model of Stress/Adaptation.

Nursing Diagnosis, Planning/Implementation Nursing diagnoses are formulated from the data

gathered during the assessment phase and with background knowledge regarding predisposing factors to the disorder. Some common nursing diagnoses for patients with somatoform pain disorder include:

Chronic pain related to repressed anxiety and learned maladaptive coping skills evidenced by verbal complaints of pain, in the absence of pathophysiological evidence; excessive use of analgesics

Social isolation related to preoccupation with self and pain evidenced by seeking to be alone; refusal to participate in therapeutic activities.

In Table 21.4, these nursing diagnoses are presented in a plan of care for the patient with somatoform pain disorder. Goals of care and appropriate nursing interventions are included for each. Rationales are provided in italics.

Outcome Criteria The following criteria may be used for measurement of outcomes in the care of the patient with somatoform pain disorder.

The patient:
1. Is able to demonstrate adaptive coping strategies.
2. Verbalizes relief from pain.
3. Is able to effectively use adaptive coping strategies during stressful situations to prevent the onset of pain.
4. Is able to identify stressors that cause anxiety level to rise.
5. Verbalizes understanding of correlation between times of increased anxiety and onset of pain.
6. Demonstrates control over life situation by meeting needs in an assertive manner.
7. Interacts with others in an appropriate manner.
8. Demonstrates the ability to focus on the needs of others rather than totally focus on the self and pain.

Evaluation Reassessment is conducted to determine if the nursing actions have been successful in achieving the objectives of care. Evaluation of the nursing actions for the patient with somatoform pain disorder may be facilitated by gathering information using the following types of questions.

Can the patient recognize signs and symptoms of escalating anxiety? Can the patient intervene with

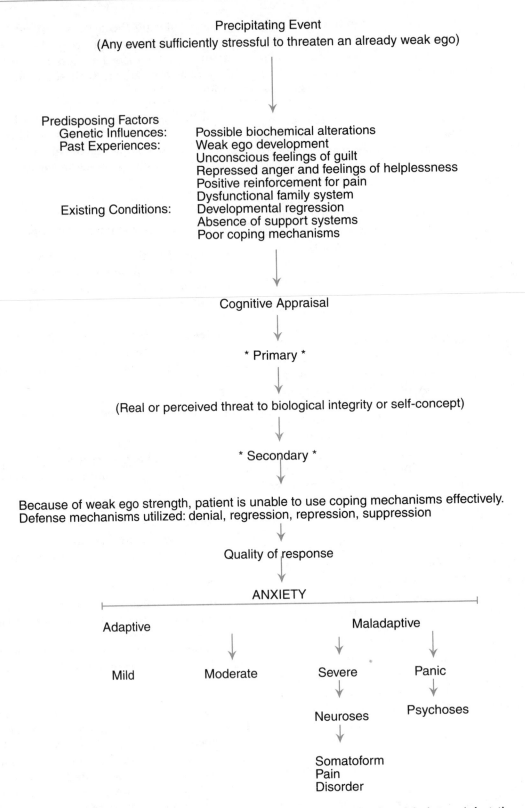

Figure 21.2 The dynamics of somatoform pain disorder using the transactional model of stress/adaptation.

adaptive coping strategies to interrupt the escalating anxiety before pain becomes unmanageable? Is the patient able to verbalize an understanding of the correlation between onset of pain and times of escalating anxiety? Does he or she have a plan for dealing with increased stress so that the pain response can be prevented? Is the patient able to demonstrate assertiveness skills. Does the patient exercise control over life situation by participating in decision-making process? Is the patient willingly and voluntarily interacting with others in an appropriate manner? Does he or she verbalize understanding of how pain behaviors interfere with the development of satisfactory interpersonal rela-

Table 21.4 CARE PLAN FOR THE PATIENT WITH SOMATOFORM PAIN DISORDER		
Nursing Diagnoses	**Objectives**	**Nursing Interventions**
Chronic pain related to repressed anxiety and learned maladaptive coping skills, evidenced by verbal complaints of pain, in the absence of pathophysiological evidence; excessive use of analgesics	Patient will verbalize relief from pain.	Monitor physician's ongoing assessments and laboratory reports *to ascertain that organic pathology is clearly ruled out.* Recognize and accept that the pain is indeed real to the patient, even though no organic etiology can be identified. *Denying the patient's feelings is nontherapeutic and hinders the development of a trusting relationship.* Observe and record the duration and intensity of the pain. Note factors that precipitate the onset of pain. *Identification of the precipitating stressor is important for assessment and care planning.* Provide pain medication as prescribed by physician. *Patient comfort and safety are nursing priorities.* Provide nursing comfort measures (e.g., backrub, warm bath, heating pad) with a matter-of-fact approach that does not reinforce the pain behavior. *May provide some relief from pain. Secondary gains from physical symptoms may prolong maladaptive behaviors.* Offer attention at times when patient is not focusing on pain. *Positive reinforcement encourages repetition of adaptive behaviors.* Identify activities that serve to distract patient from focus on self and pain. *These distractors serve in a therapeutic manner as a transition from focus on self/pain to focus on unresolved psychological issues.* Encourage verbalization of feelings. Explore meaning that pain holds for patient. Help patient connect symptoms of pain to times of increased anxiety and to identify specific situations that cause anxiety to rise. *Verbalization of feelings in a nonthreatening environment facilitates expression and resolution of disturbing emotional issues.* Encourage patient to identify alternative methods of coping with stress. *These may avert the use of pain as a maladaptive response to stress.* Explore ways to intervene as symptoms begin to intensify, *so that pain does not become disabling* (e.g., visual or auditory distractions, mental imagery, deep-breathing exercises, application of hot or cold compresses, relaxation exercises). Provide positive reinforcement for times when patient is not focusing on pain. *Positive reinforcement, in the form of the nurse's presence and attention, may encourage a continuation of these more adaptive behaviors.*

(continued)

Table 21.4 CONTINUED		
Nursing Diagnoses	**Objectives**	**Nursing Interventions**
Social isolation related to preoccupation with self and pain, evidenced by seeking to be alone; refusal to participate in therapeutic activities.	Patient will voluntarily spend time with other patients and staff members in group activities on the unit.	Spend time with the patient after setting limits on attention-seeking behaviors. Withdraw presence if ruminations about pain begin. *The nurse's presence conveys a sense of worthwhileness to the patient. Lack of reinforcement of maladaptive behaviors may help to decrease their repetition.* Increase amount of attention given during times when the patient is not focusing on pain. *This separates the person from the behavior. The patient experiences unconditional acceptance without a need for the pain behavior.* Describe to the patient how the focus on pain and self discourages others from wanting to spend time with him or her. *Patient may not realize how own behavior is perceived and may result in alienation from others.* Teach patient to recognize the difference between passive, assertive, and aggressive behaviors and the importance of respecting the human rights of others while protecting one's own basic human rights. *These assertive techniques enhance self-esteem and facilitate communication and mutual acceptance in interpersonal relationships.* Provide positive feedback for any attempts at social interaction in which the patient's focus is on others rather than on self or pain. *Positive feedback enhances self-esteem and encourages repetition of desirable behaviors.*

tionships? Does patient show concern for the needs of others and focus less on self/pain? Is the patient able to verbalize resources outside the hospital from whom he or she may seek assistance during times of extreme stress?

HYPOCHONDRIASIS

Hypochondriasis may be defined as unrealistic preoccupation with fear of having a serious illness (Stoudemire, 1988). The *DSM-III-R* suggest that this fear arises out of an unrealistic interpretation of physical signs and sensations. The fear becomes disabling and persists despite appropriate reassurance that no organic pathology can be detected. Occasionally medical disease may be present, but in the hypochondriacal individual, the symptoms are grossly disproportionate to the degree of pathology (Barsky, 1989).

The preoccupation may be with a specific organ or disease (e.g., cardiac disease), with bodily functions, such as peristolsis or heartbeat, or with minor physical alterations, such as a small sore or

an occasional cough (APA, 1987). They may become convinced that a rapid heart rate indicates they have heart disease or that the small sore is skin cancer. Hypochondriacs are profoundly preoccupied with their bodies and are totally aware of even the slightest change in feeling or sensation. However, their response to these small changes is usually unrealistic and exaggerated.

Individuals with hypochondriasis often have a long history of "doctor shopping," and are convinced that they are not receiving the proper care. Anxiety and depressed mood are common, and obsessive-compulsive traits frequently accompany the disorder.

Preoccupation with the fear of serious disease may interfere with social or occupational functioning. However, some individuals are able to function appropriately on the job, while limiting their physical complaints to nonwork time.

Hypochondriacs are so totally convinced that their symptoms are related to organic pathology that they adamantly reject, and are often irritated by, any implication that stress or psychosocial fac-

Table 21.5 DIAGNOSTIC CRITERIA FOR HYPOCHONDRIASIS

A. Preoccupation with the fear of having, or the belief that one has, a serious disease, based on the person's interpretation of physical signs or sensations as evidence of physical illness.

B. Appropriate physical evaluation does not support the diagnosis of any physical disorder that can account for the physical signs or sensations or the person's unwarranted interpretation of them, and the symptoms in A are not just symptoms of panic attacks.

C. The fear of having, or belief that one has, a disease persists despite medical reassurance.

D. Duration of the disturbance is at least 6 months.

E. The belief in A is not of delusional intensity, as in delusional disorder, somatic type (i.e., the person can acknowledge the possibility that his or her fear of having, or belief that he or she has, a serious disease is unfounded).

Source: From APA (1987) with permission.

tors play any role in their condition (Barsky, 1989). They are so apprehensive and fearful that they become alarmed at the slightest intimation of serious illness. Even reading about a disease or hearing that someone they know has been diagnosed with an illness precipitates alarm on their part.

The *DSM-III-R* diagnostic criteria for hypochondriasis are presented in Table 21.5.

Predisposing Factors to Hypochondriasis

Psychodynamic Theory Some psychodynamicists view hypochondriasis as an ego defense mechanism. Physical complaints are the expression of low self-esteem and feelings of worthlessness, as it is easier to feel something is wrong with the body than to feel something is wrong with the self (Barsky, 1989).

Another psychodynamic view explains hypochondriasis as the transformation of aggressive and hostile wishes toward others into physical complaints to others. Repressed anger, originating from past disappointments and unfulfilled needs for nurturing and caring, is expressed in the present by soliciting other people's help and concern and then thwarting and rejecting them as ineffective.

Still other psychodynamicists have viewed hypochondriasis as a defense against guilt (Kenyon,

1976). The individual views the self as "bad," based on real or imagined past misconduct, and views physical suffering as the deserved punishment required for atonement.

Cognitive Theory Studies show that noxious sensory input undergoes a cognitive screening process involving assessment and clarification, which may serve to amplify or reduce the sensations (Chapman, 1978). Cognitive theorists view hypochondriasis as arising out of perceptual and cognitive abnormalities. Barsky and Klerman (1983) cite three components of this theory:

1. These patients amplify normal bodily sensory input.
2. They incorrectly assess and misinterpret somatic symptoms of emotional arousal.
3. They are innately predisposed to thinking and perceiving in concrete rather than emotional or subjective terms.

Benign bodily sensations are misinterpreted and negative cognitive meanings are attached to them. Barsky and Klerman (1983) state:

> "Once formed, the incorrect attribution tends to persist because all future perceptions are interpreted to fit the cognitive set that the individual has a disease."

Sociocultural/Familial Factors Somatic complaints are often reinforced when the sick role serves to relieve the individual from the need to deal with a stressful situation, whether it be within society or within the family constellation. When the sick person is allowed to avoid stressful obligations, postpone unwelcome challenges, and is excused from troublesome duties, or becomes the prominent focus of attention because of the illness, positive reinforcement virtually guarantees repetition of the response. Barsky (1989) states:

> "Sick patients have special powers within their families—sickness and suffering allow them to avoid intimacy ("Not tonight, dear, I have a headache"), to control and manipulate others, and to express their hostility, since temper tantrums and irritability are excusable if one is sick."

Past Experience with Physical Illness Hypochondriacs seem to have an increased incidence of childhood medical illness and more extensive past medical histories (Barsky, 1989). This early exposure instills a knowledge of the terminology required to translate psychological distress into physical expression.

Personal experience, or the experience of close family members, with serious or life-threatening illness can predispose an individual to hypochondriasis. Once an individual has experienced a threat to biological integrity, he or she may develop a fear of recurrence. Increased bodily sensitivity develops, and the individual becomes strongly in tune to changes that may occur. The fear of recurring illness generates an exaggerated response leading to hypochondrical behaviors.

Genetic Influences Although little is known about the inheritance of hypochondriasis, some evidence indicates an increased prevalence of hypochondriasis among identical twins and other first-degree relatives (Barsky, 1989).

Transactional Model of Stress/Adaptation The etiology of hypochondriasis is most likely influenced by multiple factors. In Figure 21.3, a graphic depiction of this theory of multiple causation is presented in the Transactional Model of Stress/Adaptation.

Nursing Diagnosis, Planning/Implementation Nursing diagnoses are formulated from the data gathered during the assessment phase and with background knowledge regarding predisposing factors to the disorder. Some common nursing diagnoses for patients with hypochondriasis include:

Fear (of having serious disease) related to past experience of life-threatening illness, evidenced by preoccupation with and unrealistic interpretation of bodily signs and sensations.

Self-esteem disturbance related to unfulfilled childhood needs for nurturing and caring evidenced by transformation of internalized anger into physical complaints and hostility toward others.

In Table 21.6, these nursing diagnoses are presented in a plan of care for the patient with hypochondriasis. Goals of care and appropriate nursing interventions are included for each. Rationale are presented in italics.

Outcome Criteria The following criteria may be used for measurement of outcomes in the care of the patient with hypochondriasis.

The patient:
1. Is able to interpret bodily sensations rationally.

2. Verbalizes significance the irrational fear held for him or her.
3. Has decreased the number and frequency of physical complaints.
4. Has identified the correlation between increased anxiety and the exacerbation of physical symptoms.
5. Has identified life situations that precipitate anxiety.
6. Demonstrates more adaptive ways of coping with stress than with physical symptoms.
7. Demonstrates acceptance of self as a worthwhile person.
8. Expresses self-confidence in dealing with stressful life situations.
9. Makes life changes for improvement and accepts those situations that cannot be changed.
10. Sets realistic goals for the future.

Evaluation Reassessment is conducted to determine if the nursing actions have been successful in achieving the objectives of care. Evaluation of the nursing actions for the patient with hypochondriasis may be facilitated by gathering information using the following types of questions.

Does the patient demonstrate a decrease in ruminations about physical symptoms? Have fears of serious illness diminished? Is the patient able to correlate the exacerbation of physical symptoms to times of escalating anxiety? Is he or she able to use more adaptive coping mechanisms to interrupt the anxiety response? Can the patient demonstrate assertiveness and effective communication skills? Does the patient exercise control over life situation by participating in decision-making process? Does the patient set realistic goals for the future? Is the patient able to maximize his or her potential by making the most of personal strengths? Is the patient able to name resources outside the hospital from whom he or she may seek assistance during times of extreme stress?

CONVERSION DISORDER

Conversion disorder is a loss of or change in bodily functioning resulting from a psychological conflict, the bodily symptoms of which cannot be explained by any known medical disorder or pathophysiological mechanism (Barsky, 1989). Patients are unaware of the psychological basis and are thus not able to control their symptoms.

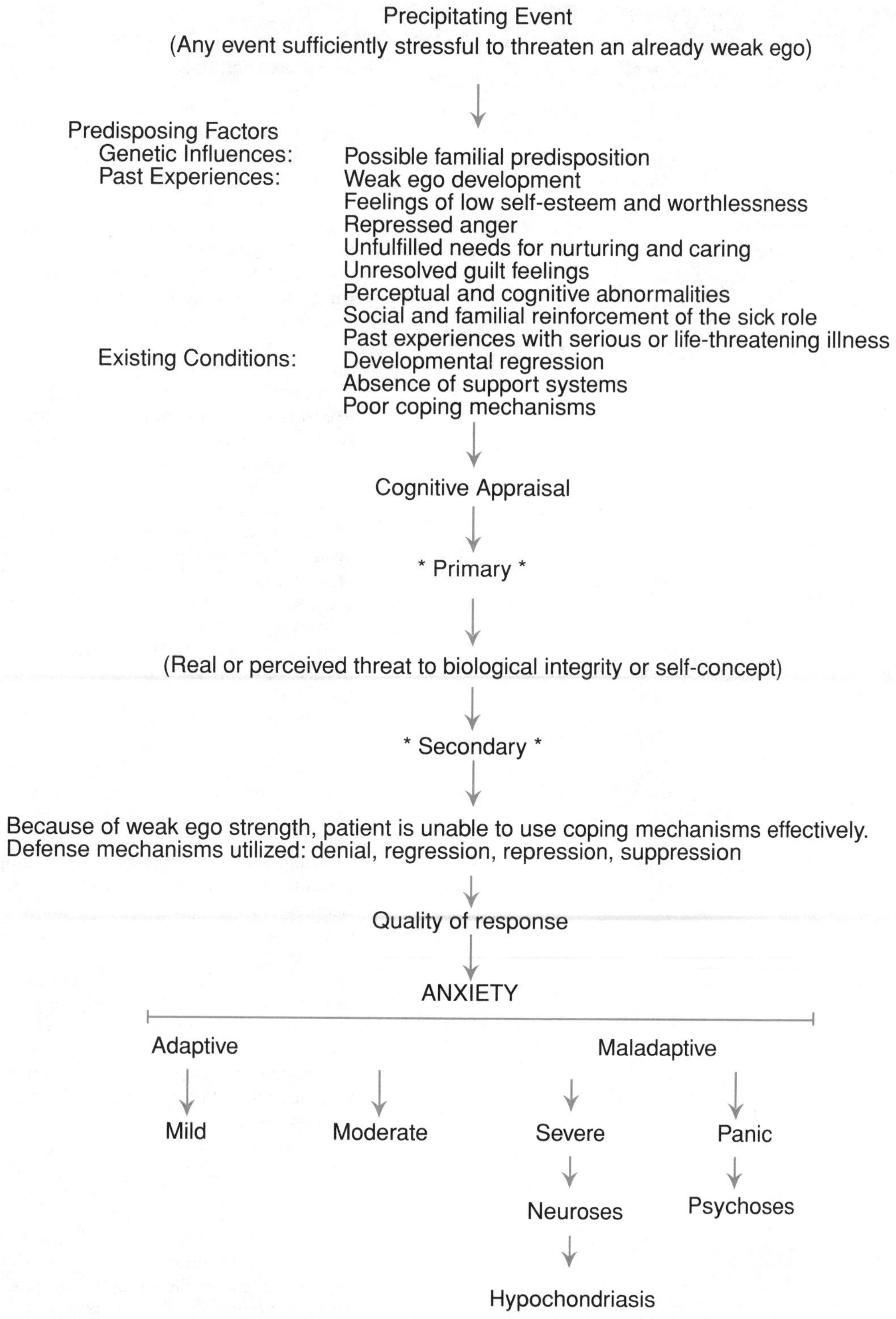

Precipitating Event
(Any event sufficiently stressful to threaten an already weak ego)

↓

Predisposing Factors
    Genetic Influences: Possible familial predisposition
    Past Experiences: Weak ego development
                     Feelings of low self-esteem and worthlessness
                     Repressed anger
                     Unfulfilled needs for nurturing and caring
                     Unresolved guilt feelings
                     Perceptual and cognitive abnormalities
                     Social and familial reinforcement of the sick role
                     Past experiences with serious or life-threatening illness
    Existing Conditions: Developmental regression
                     Absence of support systems
                     Poor coping mechanisms

↓

Cognitive Appraisal

↓

* Primary *

↓

(Real or perceived threat to biological integrity or self-concept)

↓

* Secondary *

↓

Because of weak ego strength, patient is unable to use coping mechanisms effectively.
Defense mechanisms utilized: denial, regression, repression, suppression

↓

Quality of response
↓

ANXIETY

Adaptive		Maladaptive	
↓	↓	↓	↓
Mild	Moderate	Severe	Panic
		↓	↓
		Neuroses	Psychoses
		↓	
		Hypochondriasis	

Figure 21.3 The dynamics of hypochondriasis using the transactional model of stress/adaptation.

Table 21.6 CARE PLAN FOR PATIENT WITH HYPOCHONDRIASIS

Nursing Diagnoses	Objectives	Nursing Interventions
Fear (of having a serious disease) related to past experience of life-threatening illness, evidenced by preoccupation with and unrealistic interpretation of bodily signs and sensations.	Patient will verbalize irrationality of fear and interpret bodily sensations correctly.	Monitor physician's ongoing assessments and laboratory reports *to ascertain that organic pathology is clearly ruled out.* Refer all new physical complaints to physician. *To assume that all physical complaints are hypochondriacal would place patient's safety in jeopardy.* Assess function patient's illness is fulfilling for him or her (e.g., unfulfilled needs for dependency, nurturing, caring, attention, and control). *This information may provide insight into reasons for maladaptive behavior and provide direction for planning patient care.* Identify times during which preoccupation with physical symptoms is worse. Determine extent of correlation of physical complaints with times of increased anxiety. *Patient is unaware of the psychosocial implications of the physical complaints. Knowledge of the relationship is the first step in the process for creating change.* Convey empathy. Let patient know that you understand how a specific symptom may conjure up fears of previous life-threatening illness. *Unconditional acceptance and empathy promote a therapeutic nurse/patient relationship.* Initially allow patient a limited amount of time (e.g., 10 minutes each hour) to discuss physical symptoms. *Because this has been his or her primary method of coping for so long, complete prohibition of this activity would likely raise patient's anxiety level significantly, further exacerbating the hypochondriacal behavior.* Help patient determine what techniques may be most useful for him or her to intervene when fear and anxiety are exacerbated (e.g., relaxation techniques; mental imagery; thought-stopping techniques; physical exercise). *All of these techniques are effective to reduce anxiety and may assist patient in the transition from focusing on fear of physical illness to the discussion of honest feelings.* Gradually increase the limit on amount of time spent each hour in discussing physical symptoms. If patient violates the limits, withdraw attention. *Lack of positive reinforcement may help to extinguish maladaptive behavior.* Encourage patient to discuss feelings associated with fear of serious illness. *Verbalization of feelings in a nonthreatening environment facilitates expression and resolution of disturbing emotional issues. When the patient is able to express feelings directly, there is less need to express them through physical symptoms.* Role play the patient's plan for dealing with the fear the next time it assumes control and before it becomes disabling through the exacerbation of physical symptoms. *Anxiety and fears are minimized when the patient has achieved a degree of comfort through practicing a plan for dealing with stressful situations in the future.*

(continued)

Table 21.6 CONTINUED

Nursing Diagnoses	Objectives	Nursing Interventions
Self-esteem disturbance related to unfulfilled childhood needs for nurturing and caring, evidenced by transformation of internalized anger into physical complaints and hostility toward others.	Patient will demonstrate acceptance of self as a person of worth, as evidenced by setting realistic goals, limiting physical complaints and hostility toward others, and verbalizing positive prospects for the future.	Convey acceptance, unconditional positive regard, and remain nonjudgmental at all times. *These interventions offer the patient respect and dignity, which add to feelings of self-worth.* Encourage patient to participate in decision making regarding care, as well as life situations. *This offers the patient some feeling of personal control, and decreases feelings of powerlessness.* Help patient to recognize and focus on strengths and accomplishments. Minimize attention given to past (real or perceived) failures. *Lack of attention may help to eliminate negative ruminations.* Encourage participation in group activities *from which patient may receive positive feedback and support from peers.* Ensure that patient is not becoming increasingly dependent. Withdraw attention at times when patient is focusing on physical symptoms. *Independent functioning increases feelings of self-worth. Lack of reinforcement may help to extinguish maladaptive behaviors.* Ensure that therapy groups offer patient simple methods of achievement. Offer recognition and positive feedback for actual accomplishments. *Successes and recognition increase self-esteem.* Teach assertiveness techniques and effective communication techniques. *Self-esteem is enhanced by the ability to interact with others in an effective manner.* Offer positive feedback when patient responds to stressful situation with coping strategies other than physical complaints. *Positive feedback enhances self-esteem and encourages repetition of desirable behaviors.*

The *DSM-III-R* identifies the most obvious and "classic" conversion symptoms as those that suggest neurologic disease. Examples include paralysis, aphonia, seizures, coordination disturbance, akinesia, dyskinesia, blindness, tunnel vision, anosmia, anesthesia, and paresthesia. Pseudocyesis is a conversion symptom and may represent both a wish for, and a fear of, pregnancy (APA, 1987).

Precipitation of conversion symptoms must be explained by psychological factors, and this may be evidenced by the presence of primary or secondary gain. When an individual achieves "primary gain," the conversion symptoms serve to prevent internal conflicts or painful issues or events from attaining awareness. Conversion symptoms promote "secondary gains" for the individual by enabling him or her to avoid difficult situations or to obtain support that might not otherwise be forthcoming.

The symptom usually occurs following a situation that produces extreme psychological stress for the individual. The symptom appears suddenly, and often the person expresses a relative lack of concern that is out of keeping with the severity of the impairment (APA, 1987). This lack of concern is identified as *la belle indifference* and is often a clue to the physician that the problem may be psychological rather than physical.

The prognosis of conversion seems to be highly variable. Some conversion symptoms resolve themselves over a period of days to months without treatment, while some may persist for years in spite of intense efforts at treatment (Purcell, 1988). The prognosis seems to have little to do with the specific symptom involved, and is seemingly dependent on the interplay of the individual's psychologic makeup, the social environment, and the

Table 21.7 DIAGNOSTIC CRITERIA FOR CONVERSION DISORDER

A. A loss of, or alteration in, physical functioning suggesting a physical disorder.

B. Psychological factors are judged to be etiologically related to the symptom because of a temporal relationship between a psychosocial stressor that is apparently related to a psychological conflict or need and initiation or exacerbation of the symptom.

C. The person is not conscious of intentionally producing the symptom.

D. The symptom is not a culturally sanctioned response pattern and cannot, after appropriate investigation, be explained by a known physical disorder.

E. The symptom is not limited to pain or to a disturbance in sexual functioning.

Source: From American Psychiatric Association (1987) with permission.

response to the symptom by people who are important to the patient.

The *DSM-III-R* diagnostic criteria for conversion disorder are presented in Table 21.7.

Predisposing Factors to Conversion Disorder

Psychoanalytic Theory This theory proposes that emotions associated with a traumatic event that the individual cannot express because of moral or ethical unacceptability are "converted" into physical symptoms. The unacceptable emotions are repressed and converted to a somatic hysterical symptom that is symbolic in some way of the original emotional trauma. An example might be the young soldier who, knowing that at daybreak he will be sent to the front lines to participate in battle, develops a paralysis of his arms and is unable to pick up his rifle.

Theory of Interpersonal Communication In this conceptual model, conversion symptoms are viewed as a type of nonverbal communication. When direct verbal communication becomes blocked in an interpersonal relationship, a message is conveyed through the employment of "somatic" language (Ford & Folks, 1985). With physical symptoms, the individual communicates that he or she (or the relationship) needs special treatment or consideration. Physical symptoms also may function as a nonverbal means of controlling or manipulating others (Barsky, 1989).

Neurophysiological Theory This theory suggests that some patients with conversion disorder have a disturbance in central nervous system arousal. Symptoms are thought to be derived from corticofugal inhibition of afferent stimulation at the level of the reticular activating system (Ludwig, 1972). This activity diminishes the awareness of bodily sensation and would explain the observed sensory deficits in some conversion disorder patients and their apparently low levels of anxiety and relative indifference to their impairment (Barsky, 1989).

Behavioral Theory Behavioral theorists believe that conversion symptoms are learned through positive reinforcement from cultural, social, and interpersonal influences (Stoudemire, 1988). The individual uses physical symptoms to communicate helplessness and in return gains attention and support from the environment. These secondary gains serve as reinforcement for the perpetuation of symptom formation during times of stress or conflict.

Transactional Model of Stress/Adaptation The etiology of conversion disorder is most likely influenced by multiple factors. In Figure 21.4, a graphic depiction of this theory of multiple causation is presented in the Transactional Model of Stress/Adaptation.

Nursing Diagnosis, Planning/Implementation Nursing diagnoses are formulated from the data gathered during the assessment phase and with background knowledge regarding predisposing factors to the disorder. Some common nursing diagnoses for patients with conversion disorder include:

Sensory-perceptual alteration related to repressed severe anxiety evidenced by loss or alteration in physical functioning without evidence of organic pathology; and "la belle indifference"

Self-care deficit related to loss or alteration in physical functioning evidenced by the need for assistance to carry out self-care activities, such as eating, dressing, hygiene, and toileting.

In Table 21.8, these nursing diagnoses are presented in a plan of care for the patient with conversion disorder. Goals of care and appropriate nursing interventions are included for each. Rationales are presented in italics.

Outcome Criteria The following criteria may be used for measurement of outcomes in the care of the patient with conversion disorder.

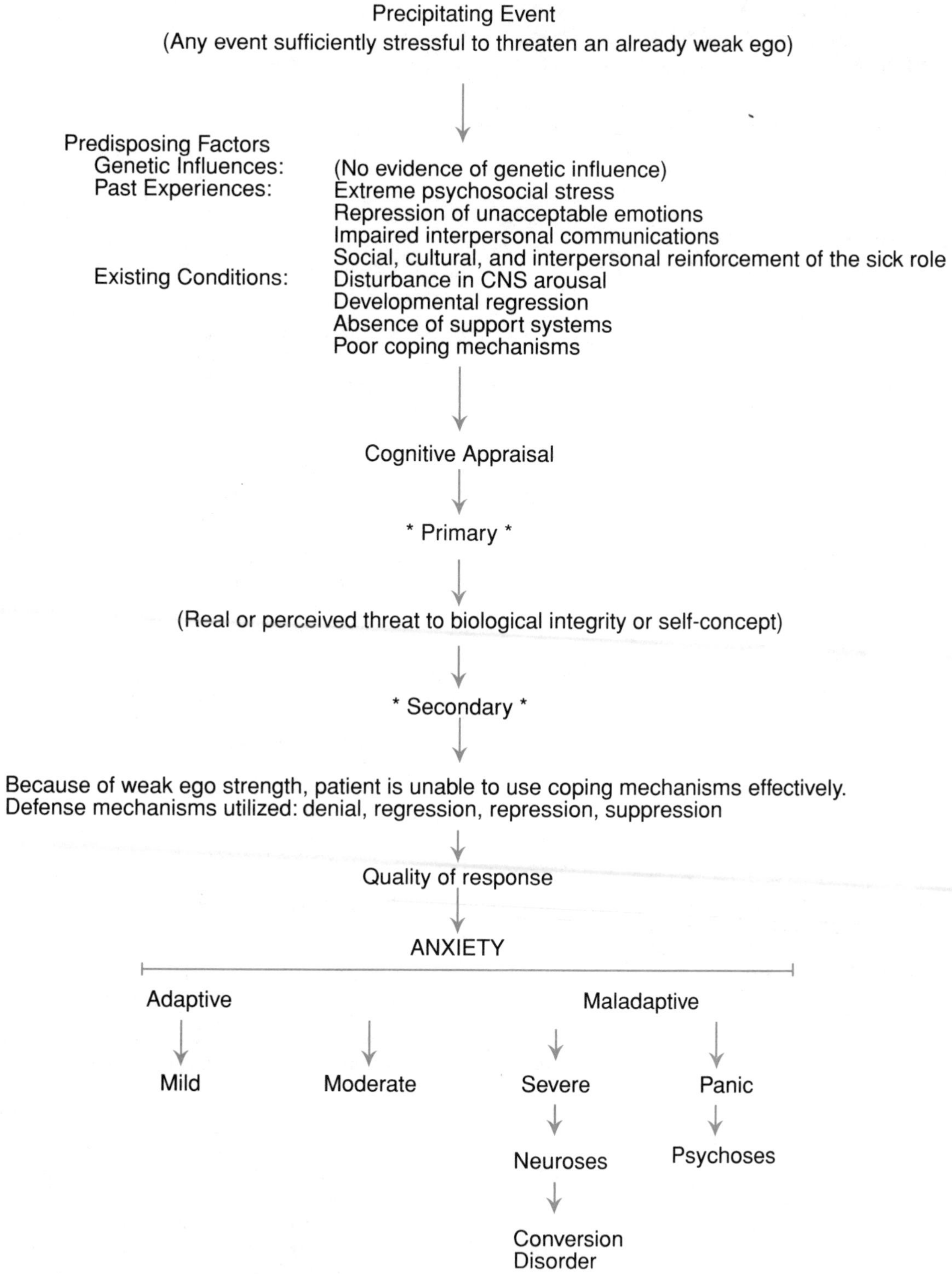

Precipitating Event
(Any event sufficiently stressful to threaten an already weak ego)

Predisposing Factors
  Genetic Influences: (No evidence of genetic influence)
  Past Experiences: Extreme psychosocial stress
                   Repression of unacceptable emotions
                   Impaired interpersonal communications
                   Social, cultural, and interpersonal reinforcement of the sick role
  Existing Conditions: Disturbance in CNS arousal
                   Developmental regression
                   Absence of support systems
                   Poor coping mechanisms

Cognitive Appraisal

* Primary *

(Real or perceived threat to biological integrity or self-concept)

* Secondary *

Because of weak ego strength, patient is unable to use coping mechanisms effectively.
Defense mechanisms utilized: denial, regression, repression, suppression

Quality of response

ANXIETY

Adaptive   Maladaptive

Mild   Moderate   Severe   Panic

Neuroses   Psychoses

Conversion
Disorder

Figure 21.4 The dynamics of conversion disorder using the transactional model of stress/adaptation.

Table 21.8 CARE PLAN FOR THE PATIENT WITH CONVERSION DISORDER

Nursing Diagnoses	Objectives	Nursing Interventions
Sensory-perceptual alteration related to repressed severe anxiety, evidenced by loss or alteration in physical functioning, without evidence of organic pathology; "la belle indifference."	Patient will demonstrate recovery of lost or altered function.	Monitor physician's ongoing assessments, laboratory reports, and other data to maintain assurance that possibility of organic pathology is clearly ruled out. *Failure to do so may jeopardize patient safety.* Identify primary or secondary gains that the physical symptom is providing for the patient (e.g., increased dependency, attention, protection from experiencing a stressful event). *These are considered to be etiological factors and will be used to assist in problem resolution.* Do not focus on the disability, and encourage patient to be as independent as possible. Intervene only when patient requires assistance. *Positive reinforcement would encourage continual use of the maladaptive response for secondary gains, such as dependency.* Do not allow the patient to use the disability as a manipulative tool to avoid participation in therapeutic activities. Withdraw attention if patient continues to focus on physical limitation. *Lack of reinforcement may help to extinguish the maladaptive response.* Encourage patient to verbalize fears and anxieties. Help identify physical symptoms as a coping mechanism that is used in times of extreme stress. *Patients with conversion disorder are usually unaware of the psychological implications of their illness.* Help patient identify coping mechanisms that he or she could use when faced with stressful situations, rather than retreating from reality with a physical disability. *Patient needs assistance with problem solving at this severe level of anxiety.* Give positive reinforcement for identification or demonstration of alternative, more adaptive coping strategies. *Positive reinforcement enhances self-esteem and encourages repetition of desirable behaviors.*
Self-care deficit related to loss or alteration in physical functioning, evidenced by the need for assistance to carry out self-care activities, such as eating, dressing, hygiene, and toileting.	Patient will be able to perform self-care activities independently.	Assess patient's level of disability. Note areas of strength and impairment. *This information will be used to plan care for the patient.* Encourage patient to perform self-care to his or her level of ability. Intervene when patient is unable to perform. *Successful performance of independent activities enhances self-esteem.* Maintain nonjudgmental attitude when providing assistance to the patient. The physical symptom is not within the patient's conscious control and is very real to him or her. *A judgmental attitude interferes with the nurse's ability to provide therapeutic care for the patient. In order to ensure patient comfort and safety:* a. Feed patient, if necessary, or provide assistance with containers, positioning, and so forth. b. Bathe patient, or assist with bath, as required. c. Assist with dressing, oral hygiene, combing hair, applying makeup. d. Provide bedpan, commode, or assistance to bathroom, as required.

(continued)

Table 21.8 CONTINUED		
Nursing Diagnoses	**Objectives**	**Nursing Interventions**
		Avoid fostering dependency by intervening when patient is capable of performing independently. Allow ample time to complete these activities to the best of patient's ability without assistance. Provide positive reinforcement for independent accomplishments. *Success and positive reinforcement enhance self-esteem and encourage repetition of desirable behaviors.* Help patient understand the purpose this disability is serving for him or her. Discuss honest feelings. *Self-disclosure and exploration of feelings with a trusted individual may help patient fulfill unmet needs and confront unresolved issues.*

The patient:

1. Is free of physical disability.
2. Is able to verbalize the correlation between the loss or alteration in function and extreme emotional stress.
3. Is able to identify the stressful situation that precipitates the physical disability.
4. Is able to verbalize the purpose the disability serves for him or her.
5. Is able to demonstrate more adaptive coping strategies for dealing with stress in the future.
6. Is able to perform all self-care activities without assistance.

Evaluation Reassessment is conducted to determine if the nursing actions have been successful in achieving the objectives of care. Evaluation of the nursing actions for the patient with conversion disorder may be facilitated by gathering information using the following types of questions.

Does the patient demonstrate full recovery from previous physical disability? Is the patient able to perform all self-care activities independently? Is he or she able to verbalize why the disability occurred? Can the patient verbalize the relationship between loss of function and stressful event? Does he or she recognize what unfulfilled need the loss of function was serving? Can the patient openly discuss feelings associated with the stressful event? Is he or she able to directly confront the conflict that was previously repressed and somaticized? Can the patient demonstrate more adaptive coping skills for dealing with stress/conflict? Does he or she

have a plan for coping with future stressful situations? Is the patient able to verbalize resources outside the hospital to whom he or she may turn when feeling the need for assistance?

BODY DYSMORPHIC DISORDER

This disorder was formerly called *dysmorphophobia*, and is characterized by the exaggerated belief that the body is deformed or defective in some specific way. The most common complaints involve facial flaws, such as wrinkles, spots on the skin; excessive facial hair; shape of the nose, mouth, jaw, or eyebrows; and swelling of the face (APA, 1987). Some patients may present with complaints involving other parts of the body, and in some instances, a true defect is present. However, the significance of the defect and the person's concern are unrealistically exaggerated.

Symptoms of depression and characteristics associated with obsessive-compulsive personality are common in individuals with body dysmorphic disorder. Social and occupational impairment may occur due to the excessive anxiety experienced by the individual in relation to the imagined defect. The person's medical history may reflect numerous visits to plastic surgeons and dermatologists in an unrelenting drive to correct the imagined defect. He or she may undergo unnecessary surgical procedures toward this effort.

This disorder has been closely associated with delusional thinking, although the *DSM-III-R* distin-

Table 21.9 DIAGNOSTIC CRITERIA FOR BODY DYSMORPHIC DISORDER

A. Preoccupation with some imagined defect in appearance in a normal-appearing person. If a slight physical anomaly is present, the person's concern is grossly excessive.

B. The belief in the defect is not of delusional intensity, as in delusional disorder, somatic type (i.e., the person can acknowledge the possibility that he or she may be exaggerating the extent of the defect or that there may be no defect at all).

C. Occurrence not exclusively during the course of anorexia nervosa or transsexualism.

Source: From American Psychiatric Association (1987) with permission.

guishes between it and delusional disorder, somatic subtype. Some follow-up studies have revealed the presence of severe personality disorders and schizophrenia in individuals with body dysmorphic disorder (Connolly & Gibson, 1978; Andreasen and Bardach, 1977). In Europe, where the syndrome has been more widely studied, it is considered to be a psychosis (Barsky, 1989).

The *DSM-III-R* diagnostic criteria for body dysmorphic disorder are presented in Table 21.9.

Predisposing Factors to Body Dysmorphic Disorder

The etiology of body dysmorphic disorder is unknown. In some patients, the belief is due to another more pervasive psychiatric disorder, such as schizophrenia, major mood disorder, or severe personality disorder (Barsky, 1989). In any case, the etiology of this disorder is presumed to be psychological (Purcell, 1988).

Body dysmorphic disorder has been classified as one of several *monosympotomatic hypochondriacal syndromes.* Each of these syndromes is characterized by a single hypochondriacal belief about one's body. Body dysmorphic disorder is one of the most common such syndromes. Others include delusions of parasitosis (i.e., the false belief that one is infested with some parasite or vermin), and delusions of bromosis (i.e., the false belief that one is emitting an offensive body odor).

Body dysmorphic disorder, or dysmorphophobia, has also been defined as the fear of some physical defect thought to be noticeable to others although the patient appears normal (Kolb & Brodie,

1982). These interpretations suggest that the disorder may be related to predisposing factors similar to those associated with hypochondriasis or phobias. Repression of morbid anxiety is undoubtedly an underlying factor, and it is very likely that multiple factors are involved in the predisposition to body dysmorphic disorder.

Nursing Diagnosis, Planning/Implementation
Nursing diagnoses are formulated from the data gathered during the assessment phase and with background knowledge regarding predisposing factors to the disorder. Nursing diagnoses for patients with body dysmorphic disorder may include:

Body image disturbance related to repressed severe anxiety evidenced by preoccupation with imagined defect; verbalizations that are out of proportion to any actual physical abnormality that may exist; and numerous visits to plastic surgeons or dermatologists seeking relief.

In Table 21.10, this nursing diagnosis is presented in a plan of care for the patient with body dysmorphic disorder. The goal of care and appropriate nursing interventions are included. Rationales are presented in italics.

Outcome Criteria The following criteria may be used for measurement of outcomes in the care of the patient with body dysmorphic disorder:

The patient:
1. Verbalizes a realistic perception of his or her appearance.
2. Expresses feelings of self-worth that reflect a positive body image and acceptance of personal appearance.
3. Is able to verbalize fears and anxieties that may contribute to altered body image.
4. Is able to verbalize adaptive strategies for dealing with fears and anxieties more effectively.
5. Expresses satisfaction with accomplishments unrelated to physical appearance.
6. Verbalizes intent to participate in a support group.

Evaluation Reassessment is conducted to determine if the nursing actions have been successful in achieving the objectives of care. Evaluation of the nursing actions for the patient with body dysmorphic disorder may be facilitated by gathering information using the following types of questions.

Table 21.10 CARE PLAN FOR THE PATIENT WITH BODY DYSMORPHIC DISORDER

Nursing Diagnosis	Objectives	Nursing Interventions
Body image disturbance related to repressed severe anxiety evidenced by preoccupation with imagined defect; verbalizations that are out of proportion to any actual physical abnormality that may exist; and numerous visits to plastic surgeons or dermatologists seeking relief.	Patient will verbalize realistic perception of body appearance.	Assess patient's perception of his or her body image. Keep in mind that this image is real to the patient. *Assessment information is necessary in developing an accurate plan of care. Denial of the patient's feelings impedes the development of a trusting, therapeutic relationship.* Help patient to see that his or her body image is distorted or that it is out of proportion in relation to the significance of an actual physical anomaly. *Recognition that a misperception exists is necessary before the patient can accept reality and reduce the significance of the imagined defect.* Encourage verbalization of fears and anxieties associated with identified stressful life situations. Discuss alternative adaptive coping strategies. *Verbalization of feelings with a trusted individual may help the patient come to terms with unresolved issues. Knowledge of alternative coping strategies may help the patient respond to stress more adaptively in the future.* Involve patient in activities that reinforce a positive sense of self not based on appearance. *When the patient is able to develop self-satisfaction based on accomplishments and unconditional acceptance, significance of the imagined defect or minor physical anomaly will diminish.* Make referrals to support groups of individuals with similar histories (e.g., Adult Children of Alcoholics (ACOA), Victims of Incest, Survivors of Suicide (SOS), Adults Abused as Children.) *Having a support group of understanding, empathic peers can help the patient accept the reality of the situation, correct distorted perceptions, and make adaptive life changes.*

Does the patient demonstrate a decrease in ruminations about the imagined defect? Is the patient able to maximize his or her potential by making the most of personal strengths? Has the patient verbalized a realistic perception of personal appearance? Does he or she demonstrate satisfactory acceptance of personal appearance? Does patient interact with others comfortably? Does patient focus attention on activities or personal accomplishments rather than personal appearance? Does patient demonstrate a positive self-worth not based on appearance? Has he or she expressed fears and anxieties that may have provided the foundation for preoccupation with imagined defect? Is patient able to demonstrate strategies for coping more adaptively with stress in the future? Is the patient able to verbalize resources from whom he or she may seek assistance during times of extreme stress (including regular attendance in a support group)?

TREATMENT MODALITIES

Patients with somatoform disorders are difficult to treat (Goodwin & Guze, 1989). The typical clinical picture of recurrent, multiple, vague symptoms combined with doctor shopping and frequent requests for time and attention may generate frustration and anger in the physician. Many patients with these disorders ignore referrals to psychiatrists, and those who do follow through rarely persist with the treatment. Thus, the majority of care for these patients continues to rest with other physicians, even though studies show that psychiatric consultation can reduce both extent and cost of medical care (Smith et al, 1986).

Individual Psychotherapy

The goal of psychotherapy is to help patients develop healthy and adaptive behaviors, encourage them to move beyond their somatization, and help them manage their lives more effectively (Barsky, 1989). The focus is on personal and social difficulties that the patient is experiencing in daily life and the achievement of practical solutions for these difficulties.

Treatment is initiated with a complete physical examination to rule out organic pathology. Once this has been ensured, the physician turns his or her attention to the patient's social and personal problems and away from the somatic complaints.

In the case of conversion disorder, the therapist will attempt to identify precipitating stressors and conflicts. He or she may be assisted in this effort by the use of hypnosis and narcoanalysis (amytal interview). These techniques consist of placing the patient in a relaxed state, and through questioning and suggestion, allowing him or her to reexperience the precipitating stress, fully reliving the repressed emotions, and thus freeing the patient of the psychological need for the symptom (McCracken, 1985).

Psychotherapy appears to be useful with very few hypochondriacal patients. Treatment consists of a complete medical examination by the primary physician to rule out organic pathology. Since most people with hypochondriasis are opposed to psychiatric treatment, the best approach seems to be a supportive and accepting relationship with a general medical practitioner who tolerates the patient's behavior without judgment and who is available during periods of distress and increased symptoms. This type of support can help to minimize incapacitating anxiety, doctor shopping, and further regression (McCracken, 1985).

Group Psychotherapy

Group therapy may be helpful for somatoform disorders because it provides a setting where patients can share their experiences of illness, learn to verbalize thoughts and feelings, and be confronted by group members and leaders when they reject responsibility for maladaptive behaviors (McCracken, 1985). It has been reported to be the treatment of choice for both somatization disorder and hypochondriasis, in part because it provides the social support and social interaction that these patients need (Barsky, 1989).

Behavior Therapy

Behavior therapy is more likely to be successful in instances when secondary gain is prominent. This may involve working with the patient's family or other significant others who may be perpetuating the physical symptoms by rewarding passivity and dependency and by being overly solicitous and helpful (Barsky, 1989). Behavioral therapy focuses on teaching these individuals to reward the patient's autonomy, self-sufficiency, and independence. This process becomes more difficult when the patient is very regressed and the sick role is well established.

Psychopharmacology

With somatoform pain disorder, the drugs of choice are aspirin and the nonsteroidal anti-inflammatory agents. They are most effective if used on a regularly scheduled basis rather than as needed. Opiates have a high addiction potential and should be reserved for patients suffering from pain that is clearly pathogenic (Barsky, 1989).

Some clinicians believe that antianxiety agents and antidepressants are helpful in instances when anxiety or depression is prominent. Careful monitoring of the use of antianxiety agents is important due to the high addiction potential.

Antidepressants have also been used to treat chronic pain. Amitryptilene (Elavil), imipramine (Tofranil), doxepin (Sinequan), and phenelzine (Nardil) are extensively used, and often provide pain relief at a dosage below that used to treat depression (Barsky, 1989). The analgesic action of antidepressant medications is not known.

Anticonvulsants such as phenytoin (Dilantin), carbamazepine (Tegretol), and clonazepam (Klonopin) have been reported to be effective in treating neuropathic and neuralgic pain, at least for short periods. Their efficacy in other somatoform pain disorders is less clear.

SUMMARY

Somatoform disorders, known historically as "hysteria," affect about 1 percent of the female population. There is a higher prevalence rate among the lower socioeconomic groups, rural populations, and the less educated. Somatoform disorders include somatization disorder, somatoform pain disorder, hypochondriasis, conversion disorder, and body dysmorphic disorder.

The person with somatization disorder has physical symptoms that may be vague, dramatized, or exaggerated in their presentation. No evidence of organic pathology can be identified. In somatoform pain disorder, the predominant symptom is pain, for which there is no medical explanation. Individuals with these disorders commonly have long histories of doctor shopping in search of validation of their symptoms.

Hypochondriasis is an unrealistic preoccupation with fear of having a serious illness. This disorder may follow a personal experience, or the experience of a close family member, with serious or life-threatening illness.

The individual with conversion disorder experiences a loss or alteration in bodily functioning, unsubstantiated by medical or pathophysiological explanation. Psychological factors are evident by the primary or secondary gains the individual achieves from experiencing the physiological manifestation. A relative lack of concern regarding the symptom is identified as *la belle indifference*.

Body dysmorphic disorder, formerly called *dysmorphophobia*, is the exaggerated belief that the body is deformed or defective in some way. It may be related to more serious psychiatric illness.

Various modalities have been implemented in the treatment of somatoform disorders, including individual psychotherapy, group psychotherapy, behavior therapy, and psychopharmacology. Nursing care is accomplished using the steps of the nursing process. Nurses can assist patients with somatoform disorders by helping them to replace maladaptive behavior patterns with new, more adaptive coping skills.

REVIEW QUESTIONS
Self-Examination/Learning Exercise

*Select the answer that is **most** appropriate for each of the following questions.*

Situation: Amy, age 24, was selected to represent the local children's home in the upcoming 26-mile marathon. If she wins, the children's home gets the new playground equipment they want so badly. If she loses, they will have to wait until another financial source can be located. Amy wants desperately to win for them. The morning of the race, she falls when she tries to get out of bed. She discovers her right leg is paralyzed.

1. Amy's mother takes her to the emergency room. Her physician is notified. It is likely that his initial intervention will be to:
   a. prescribe an antianxiety medication.
   b. rule out organic pathology.
   c. refer her to the rehabilitation clinic.
   d. refer her to a psychiatrist.

2. Amy shows a relative lack of concern for her sudden paralysis, even though her athletic abilities have always been a source of pride to her. This manifestation is known as:
   a. Tardive dyskinesia
   b. Secondary gain
   c. Malingering
   d. La belle indifference

3. Amy is admitted to the psychiatric unit with a diagnosis of conversion disorder. The primary nursing diagnosis for Amy would be:
   a. Self-care deficit related to inability to walk without assistance
   b. Severe anxiety related to fear of losing the race
   c. Ineffective individual coping related to severe anxiety
   d. Fear related to lack of confidence in her athletic ability

4. Which of the following nursing interventions would be most appropriate for Amy?
   a. Promote Amy's dependence, so that unfulfilled dependency needs can be met.
   b. Encourage her to discuss her feelings about the paralysis.
   c. Explain to her that the paralysis is not "real."
   d. Promote independence and withdraw attention when she continues to focus on the paralysis.

5. Conversion symptoms provide primary and secondary gains for the individuals experiencing them. Which of the following is an example of a primary gain for Amy?
   a. Allows her to receive additional personal attention
   b. Allows her to be totally dependent on others
   c. Allows her an acceptable excuse for not running in the race
   d. Allows her to feel more accepted and cared for by others

Situation: Lorraine is a frequent visitor to the outpatient clinic. She has been diagnosed with somatization disorder.

6. Which of the following symptom profiles would you expect when assessing Lorraine?
   a. Multiple somatic symptoms in several body systems
   b. Fear of having a serious disease
   c. Loss or alteration in sensorimotor functioning
   d. Belief that the body is deformed or defective in some way

7. Which of the following ego defense mechanisms describes the underlying dynamics of somatization disorder?
   a. Denial of depression
   b. Repression of anxiety
   c. Suppression of grief
   d. Displacement of anger

8. Nursing care for Lorraine would focus on helping her to:
   a. eliminate the stress in her life.
   b. discontinue her numerous physical complaints.
   c. take her medication only as prescribed.
   d. learn more adaptive coping strategies.

9. Lorraine states, "My doctor thinks I should see a psychiatrist. I can't imagine why he would make such a suggestion!" What is the basis for Lorraine's statement?
   a. She thinks her doctor wants to get rid of her as a patient.
   b. She doesn't understand the correlation of symptoms and stress.
   c. She thinks psychiatrists are only for "crazy" people.
   d. She thinks her doctor has made an error in diagnosis.

10. Lorraine tells the nurse about a pain in her side. She says she has not experienced it before. Which is the most appropriate response by the nurse?

    a. "I don't want to hear about another physical complaint. You know they are all in your head. It's time for group therapy now."

    b. "Let's sit down here together and you can tell me about this new pain you are experiencing. You'll just have to miss group therapy today."

    c. "I will report this pain to your physician. In the meantime, group therapy starts in 5 minutes. You must leave now to be on time."

    d. "I will call your physician and see if he will order a new pain medication for your side. The one you have now doesn't seem to provide relief. Why don't you get some rest for now."

REFERENCES

American Psychiatric Association. (1987). *Diagnostic and statistical manual of mental disorders* (3rd ed., rev.). Washington, DC: American Psychiatric Association.

Andreasen, N. C. & Bardach, J. (1977). Dysmorphophobia: Symptom or disease? *Am J Psychiatry, 134*: 673–676.

Barsky, A. J. (1979). Patients who amplify bodily sensations. *Ann Intern Med, 91*: 63–70.

Barsky, A. J. Somatoform disorders. (1989). In H. I. Kaplan & B. J. Sadock (Eds.), *Comprehensive textbook of psychiatry* (Vol. 1) (5th ed.). Baltimore: Williams & Wilkins.

Barsky, A. J. & Klerman, G. L. (1983). Overview: Hypochondriasis, bodily complaints, and somatic styles. *Am J Psychiatry, 140*: 273–283.

Chapman, C. R. (1978). Pain: The perception of noxious events. In R. A. Sternbach (Ed.), *The psychology of pain.* New York: Raven Press.

Connolly, F. H. & Gibson, M. (1978). Dysmorphophobia: A long-term study. *Br J Psychiatry, 132*: 568–570.

Engel, G. E. (1959). Psychogenic pain and the pain-prone patient. *Am J Med, 16*: 899–918.

Ford, C. V. & Folks, D. G. (1985). Conversion disorders: An overview. *Psychosom, 26*: 371–383.

Goodwin, D. W. & Guze, S. B. (1989). *Psychiatric diagnosis* (4th ed.). New York: Oxford University Press.

Jones, M. M. (1980). Conversion reaction: Anachronism or evolutionary form? A review of the neurologic, behavioral, and psychoanalytic literature. *Psychol Bull, 87*: 427–441.

Kenyon, F. E. (1976). Hypochondriacal states. *Br J Psychiatry, 129*: 1–14.

Kleinman, A. & Mechanic, D. (1980). Mental illness and psychosocial aspects of medical problems in China. In Kleinman et al. (Eds.), *Normal and abnormal behavior in chinese culture.* Boston: Reidel Publishing.

Kolb, L. C. & Brodie, H. K. H. (1982). *Modern clinical psychiatry* (10th ed.). Philadelphia: WB Saunders.

Lazare, A. (1981). Current concepts in psychiatry: Conversion symptoms. *N Engl J Med, 305*: 745–748.

Leff, J. (1973). Culture and the differentiation of emotional states. *Br J Psychiatry, 123*: 299–306.

Ludwig, A. M. (1972). Hysteria: A neurobiological theory. *Arch Gen Psychiatry, 27*: 771–777.

McCracken, J. T. (1985). Somatoform disorders. In J. I. Walker (Ed.), *Essentials of clinical psychiatry.* Philadelphia: JB Lippincott.

Mechanic, D. (1972). Social psychological factors affecting the presentation of bodily complaints. *N Engl J Med, 286*: 1132–1139.

Minuchin, S. et al. (1975). Family organization and family therapy. *Arch Gen Psychiatry, 32*: 1031–1038.

Purcell, S. D. (1988). Somatoform disorders. In H. H. Goldman (Ed.), *Review of general psychiatry* (2nd ed.). Norwalk, CT: Appleton & Lange.

Smith, G. R. et al. (1986). Psychiatric consultation in somatization disorder: A randomized controlled study. *N Engl J Med, 314*: 1407–1413.

Stoudemire, G. A. (1988). Somatoform disorders, factitious disorders, and malingering. In Talbott, Hales, & Yudofsky (Eds.), *Textbook of psychiatry.* Washington, DC: American Psychiatry Press.

Vieth, I. (1965). *Hysteria: The history of a disease.* Chicago: University of Chicago Press.

BIBLIOGRAPHY

Berger, D. M. (1985). Somatization, conversion, and hypochondriasis. In S. E. Greben, V. M. Rakoff, and G. Voineskos (Eds.), *A method of psychiatry* (ed. 2). Philadelphia: Lea & Febiger.

Townsend, M. C. (1991). *Nursing diagnoses in psychiatric nursing: A pocket guide for care plan construction.* (2nd ed.). Philadelphia: FA Davis.

Townsend, M. C. (1990). *Drug guide for psychiatric nursing.* Philadelphia: FA Davis.

22

DISSOCIATIVE DISORDERS

KEY TERMS
abreaction
amnesia
association
    directed
    free
continuous amnesia
depersonalization
derealization
fugue
generalized amnesia
hypnosis
integration
localized amnesia
selective amnesia

OBJECTIVES

After reading this chapter, the student will be able to:

1. Discuss historical aspects and epidemiological statistics related to dissociative disorders.
2. Describe various types of dissociative disorders and identify symptomatology associated with each. Use this information in patient assessment.
3. Identify predisposing factors in the development of dissociative disorders.
4. Formulate nursing diagnoses and goals of care for patients with dissociative disorders.
5. Describe appropriate nursing interventions for patients with dissociative disorders.
6. Evaluate nursing care of patients with dissociative disorders.
7. Discuss various modalities relevant to treatment of dissociative disorders.

INTRODUCTION

The *Diagnostic and Statistical Manual of Mental Disorders, ed. 3, revised (DSM-III-R)* describes the essential feature of dissociative disorders as a disturbance or alteration in the normally integrative functions of identity, memory, or consciousness (American Psychiatric Association [APA], 1987). Dissociative responses occur when anxiety becomes overwhelming and a disorganization of the personality ensues. Defense mechanisms that normally govern consciousness, identity, and memory break down, and behavior occurs with little or no participation on the part of the conscious personality (Kolk & Brodie, 1982). Four types of dissociative disorders are described by the *DSM-III-R:* psychogenic amnesia, psychogenic fugue, multiple personality, and depersonalization disorder.

This chapter focuses on disorders that are characterized by severe anxiety that has been repressed and is being expressed in the form of dissociative behavior. That is, certain mental contents are removed from consciousness to protect the ego from experiencing the painful anxiety. Historical and epidemiological statistics are presented. Predisposing factors that have been implicated in the etiology of dissociative disorders provide a framework for studying the dynamics of psychogenic amnesia, psychogenic fugue, multiple personality, and depersonalization disorder.

An explanation of the symptomatology is presented as background knowledge for assessing the patient with a dissociative disorder. Nursing care is described in the context of the nursing process. Various medical treatment modalities are explored.

HISTORICAL ASPECTS

There was a great deal of interest in the phenomena of dissociative processes during the 19th century. The concept of dissociation was first formulated during this period by the French physician and psychologist, Pierre Janet. He used it to explain the myriad bizarre symptoms of hysteria, which he characterized as "a form of mental disintegration characterized by a tendency toward the permanent and complete undoubling of consciousness" (Janet, 1907).

Freud (1962) viewed dissociation as a type of repression, an active defense mechanism used in the removal of threatening or unacceptable mental contents from conscious awareness. He also described the defense of splitting of the ego in the management of incompatible mental contents (Freud, 1964).

Professional interest in the dissociative disorders waned following the turn of the century but has recently been revived, with the study of multiple personality, in particular, achieving a level surpassing all previous periods. Despite the fact that Janet pioneered the study of dissociative processes in the 1890s, scientists still know remarkably little about the phenomena. Is dissociation a psychopathological process, or is it an ego-protective device? Is the dissociative process under voluntary control, or is it a totally unconscious effort? The wide scope of current studies concerning the dissociative syndromes promises to lead to a more accurate picture of their scope, etiology, and underlying mechanisms.

EPIDEMIOLOGICAL STATISTICS

Dissociative syndromes are statistically quite rare, but when they do occur, they may present very dramatic clinical pictures of severe disturbances in normal personality functioning (Purcell, 1988). Psychogenic amnesia is rare, though it occurs most frequently under conditions of war or during natural disasters (APA, 1987). Women are affected more often than men, with the most common age group being adolescence and young adulthood. It is rarely observed in the elderly.

Psychogenic fugue is also rare and occurs most often under conditions of war, natural disasters, or other intense psychosocial stress. Information regarding gender distribution and familial patterns of occurrence is not available.

Until recently, multiple personality disorder was considered to be a rare phenomenon. However, the modern discovery of hundreds of new cases of the disorder is forcing a reappraisal of its rarity, although there are not as yet sufficient data to permit a reliable determination of its incidence (Nemiah, 1989). The disorder occurs from three to nine times more frequently in women than in men, and onset almost invariably occurs in childhood (APA, 1987).

Clinical symptoms generally are not recognized until late adolescence or early adulthood (Purcell, 1988). The disorder seems to be more common in first-degree biological relatives of people with the disorder than in the general population.

The prevalence of severe episodes of depersonalization disorder is unknown, although single brief episodes of depersonalization may occur at some time in as many as 70 percent of young adults, particularly in the event of severe psychosocial stress (APA, 1987). Symptoms usually begin in adolescence or early adulthood. The disorder runs a chronic course and is characterized by periods of remission and exacerbation. The incidence of depersonalization disorder is high under conditions of sustained traumatization, such as in military combat or prisoner-of-war camps. It has also been reported in many individuals who endure near-death experiences (Kluft, 1988).

APPLICATION OF THE NURSING PROCESS

Classifications of Dissociative Disorders: Background Assessment Data

PSYCHOGENIC AMNESIA

Psychogenic amnesia is defined as a sudden inability to recall important personal information that is too extensive to be explained by ordinary forgetfulness and which is not due to an organic mental disorder, including states of drug intoxication and withdrawal (APA, 1987). Four types of disturbance in recall have been described. In the following example, the individual is involved in a traumatic automobile accident in which a loved one is killed.

1. *Localized amnesia.* The inability to recall all incidents associated with the traumatic event for a specific period following the event (usually a few hours to a few days). *Example:* Inability to recall events of the automobile accident and events occurring during a period following the accident (a few hours to a few days).
2. *Selective amnesia.* The inability to recall only certain incidents associated with a traumatic event for a specific period following the event. *Example:* Individual may not remember events leading to impact of the accident but

may remember being taken away in the ambulance.

3. *Generalized amnesia.* The inability to recall anything that has happened during the individual's entire lifetime, including personal identity. Generalized amnesia is a rare phenomenon.
4. *Continuous amnesia.* The inability to recall events occurring after a specific time up to and including the present. *Example:* The individual is unable to remember events associated with the automobile accident and anything that has occurred since. That is, the individual is unable to form new memories even though apparently alert and aware (Purcell, 1988).

The individual with amnesia usually appears alert and may give no indication to observers that anything is wrong, although at the onset of the episode there may be a brief period of disorganization (Berger, 1985). Patients suffering from amnesia are often brought to general hospital emergency departments by police who have found them wandering confusedly around the streets (Nemiah, 1989).

Onset of an amnestic episode usually follows severe psychosocial stress. Termination is typically abrupt and followed by complete recovery. Recurrences are unusual. *DSM-III-R* diagnostic criteria for psychogenic amnesia are presented in Table 22.1.

Predisposing Factors to Psychogenic Amnesia

Psychodynamic Theory Freud (1962) described amnesia as the result of repression of distressing mental contents from conscious awareness. He believed in the unconscious as a dynamic entity where repressed mental contents were stored and unavailable to conscious recall. Current psychody-

---

Table 22.1 DIAGNOSTIC CRITERIA FOR PSYCHOGENIC AMNESIA

A. The predominant disturbance is an episode of sudden inability to recall important personal information that is too extensive to be explained by ordinary forgetfulness.

B. The disturbance is not a result of multiple personality disorder or an organic mental disorder (e.g., blackouts during alcohol intoxication).

Source: American Psychiatric Association (1987) with permission.

namic explanations of dissociation are based on Freud's concepts. The repression of mental contents is perceived as a mechanism for protecting the patient from emotional pain that has arisen either from disturbing external circumstances or from anxiety-provoking internal sources (Nemiah, 1989).

Behavioral Theory   Psychogenic amnesia may also be explained by potential gains derived from the response. Reinforcement, in the form of primary and secondary gains for the individual, may contribute to the maladaptive functioning associated with this disorder. Primary gain from the amnesia would be protection from a painful emotional experience. Secondary gains may be derived from the gratifying responses of others that fulfill certain psychological needs and thus serve to maintain the amnesia after it is established (Purcell, 1988).

Biological Theory   Some efforts have been made to explain psychogenic amnesia on the basis of neurophysiological dysfunction, particularly in the ascending reticular activating system, thalamocortical projections, and other neurological pathways (Nemiah, 1989). However, most clinicians agree that current information attempting to explain the relationship between amnesia and neurophysiological processes is inadequate and lacking in credibility and usefulness.

Transactional Model of Stress/Adaptation   The etiology of psychogenic amnesia is most likely influenced by multiple factors. In Figure 22.1, a graphic depiction of this theory of multiple causation is presented in the Transactional Model of Stress/Adaptation.

Nursing Diagnosis, Planning/Implementation   Nursing diagnoses are formulated from the data gathered during the assessment phase and with background knowledge regarding predisposing factors to the disorder. The following nursing diagnoses may be used for the patient with psychogenic amnesia:

Altered thought processes related to severe psychological stress and repression of anxiety evidenced by loss of memory.

Powerlessness related to inability to cope effectively with severe anxiety evidenced by verbalizations of frustration over lack of control and dependence on others.

In Table 22.2, these nursing diagnoses are presented in a plan of care for the patient with psychogenic amnesia. Goals of care and appropriate nursing interventions are included for each. Rationales are presented in italics.

Outcome Criteria   The following criteria may be used for measurement of outcomes in the care of the patient with psychogenic amnesia.

The patient:
1. Is able to recall events associated with a traumatic event.
2. Is able to recall all events of past life.
3. Is able to demonstrate more adaptive coping strategies to avert amnestic behaviors in the face of severe anxiety.
4. Verbalizes control over certain life situations.
5. Verbalizes acceptance of certain life situations over which he or she has no control.
6. Sets realistic goals and expresses a sense of control over outcomes for the future.

Evaluation   Reassessment is conducted to determine if the nursing actions have been successful in achieving the objectives of care. Evaluation of the nursing actions for the patient with psychogenic amnesia may be facilitated by gathering information using the following types of questions.

Has the patient's memory been restored? Is he or she able to connect occurrence of psychological stress to loss of memory? Can the patient verbalize more adaptive methods of coping with stress? Can he or she demonstrate use of these more adaptive coping strategies? Is the patient able to carry out activities of daily living independently? Can the patient identify aspects of life situation over which control can be achieved? Does he or she verbalize acceptance of aspects of life situation over which control is not possible? Does the patient set realistic goals for the future? Does he or she express positive outcomes for the future? Is the patient able to verbalize the names of support groups of which he or she may become a member in an effort to deal successfully with stressful life situations? Does he or she express intention to become affiliated with one of these self-help groups?

PSYCHOGENIC FUGUE

The characteristic feature of psychogenic fugue is a sudden, unexpected travel away from home or

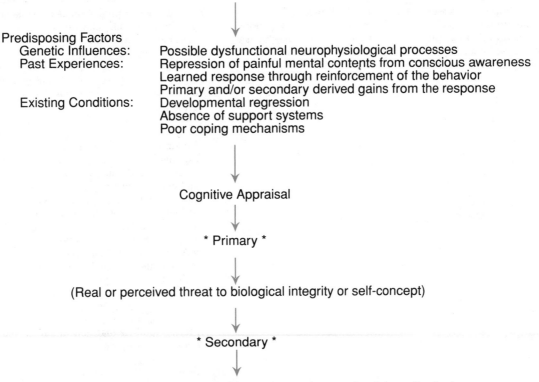

Precipitating Event
(Any event sufficiently stressful to threaten a fragile ego)

Predisposing Factors
 Genetic Influences: Possible dysfunctional neurophysiological processes
 Past Experiences: Repression of painful mental contents from conscious awareness
                         Learned response through reinforcement of the behavior
                         Primary and/or secondary derived gains from the response
 Existing Conditions: Developmental regression
                         Absence of support systems
                         Poor coping mechanisms

Cognitive Appraisal

* Primary *

(Real or perceived threat to biological integrity or self-concept)

* Secondary *

Because of weak ego strength, patient is unable to use coping mechanisms effectively.
Defense mechanisms utilized: denial, regression, repression, suppression

Quality of response

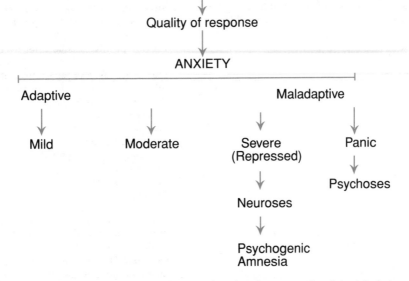

ANXIETY

Adaptive   Maladaptive

Mild   Moderate   Severe   Panic
                            (Repressed)
                                            Psychoses
                            Neuroses

                            Psychogenic
                            Amnesia

Figure 22.1   The dynamics of psychogenic amnesia using the transactional model of stress/adaptation.

Table 22.2 CARE PLAN FOR THE PATIENT WITH PSYCHOGENIC AMNESIA

Nursing Diagnoses	Objectives	Nursing Interventions
Altered thought processes related to severe psychological stress and repression of anxiety, evidenced by loss of memory.	Patient will recover deficits in memory and develop more adaptive coping mechanisms to deal with stress.	Obtain as much information as possible about the patient from family and significant others if possible. Consider likes, dislikes, important people, activities, music, pets. *A comprehensive baseline assessment is important for the development of an effective plan of care.* Do not flood patient with data regarding his or her past life. *Individuals who are exposed to painful information from which the amnesia is providing protection may decompensate even further into a psychotic state.* Instead, expose patient to stimuli that represent pleasant experiences from the past such as smells associated with enjoyable activities, beloved pets, and music known to have been pleasurable to the patient. As memory begins to return, engage patient in activities that may provide additional stimulation. *Recall may occur during activities that simulate life experiences.* Encourage patient to discuss situations that have been especially stressful and to explore the feelings associated with those times. *Verbalization of feelings in a nonthreatening environment may help patient come to terms with unresolved issues that may be contributing to the dissociative process.* Identify specific conflicts that remain unresolved, and assist patient to identify possible solutions. *Unless these underlying conflicts are resolved, any improvement in coping behaviors must be viewed as only temporary.* Provide instruction regarding more adaptive ways to respond to anxiety *so that dissociative behaviors are no longer needed.*
Powerlessness related to inability to cope effectively with severe anxiety, evidenced by verbalizations of frustration over lack of control and dependence on others.	Patient will be able to effectively problem solve ways to take control of life situation.	Allow patient to take as much responsibility as possible for own self-care practices. *Providing patient with choices will increase feelings of control.* Provide positive feedback for decisions made. Respect patient's right to make those decisions independently, and refrain from attempting to influence him or her toward those that may seem more logical. *Positive feedback encourages repetition of desirable behaviors.* Assist patient to set realistic goals for the future. *Unrealistic goals set the patient up for failure and reinforce feelings of powerlessness.* Help patient identify areas of life situation that he or she can control. *Patient's memory deficits may interfere with his or her ability to solve problems. Assistance is required to perceive the benefits and consequences of available alternatives accurately.* Help patient identify areas of life situation that are not within his or her ability to control. Encourage verbalization of feelings related to this inability *in an effort to deal with unresolved issues and accept what cannot be changed.* Identify ways in which patient can achieve. Encourage participation in these activities, and provide positive reinforcement for participation, as well as for achievement. *Positive*

(continued)

Table 22.2 CONTINUED

Nursing Diagnoses	Objectives	Nursing Interventions
		reinforcement enhances self-esteem and encourages repetition of desirable behaviors. Encourage **patient's participation in supportive self-help groups.** *In support groups, patient can learn ways to achieve greater control over life situation through direct feedback and by hearing about the experiences of others.*

customary workplace (APA, 1987). An individual in a fugue state is unable to recall personal identity, and assumption of a new identity is common. Nemiah (1989) states:

"During the fugue, they completely forget their past lives and associations. But unlike the patients with amnesia, they are unaware that they have forgotten anything. It is only when they suddenly come back to their former selves that they recall the time preceding the onset of the fugue, but now they are amnesic for the period covered by the fugue itself."

Individuals in a fugue state do not appear to be behaving in any way out of the ordinary. Contacts with other people are minimal. The assumed identity may be simple and incomplete or complex and elaborate. If a complex identity is established, the individual engages in intricate interpersonal and occupational activities and is often more socially gregarious and uninhibited than was the patient's previous style (Purcell, 1988).

Patients with psychogenic fugue often are picked up by the police when they are found wandering in a somewhat confused and frightened condition after emerging from the fugue in unfamiliar surroundings. They are usually presented to emergency departments of general hospitals. Upon assessment, they are able to provide details of earlier life situation but have no recall from the beginning of the fugue state. Information from other sources usually reveals that the occurrence of severe psychological stress or excessive alcohol use precipitated the fugue behavior.

Duration is usually brief, that is, hours to days or more rarely, months, and recovery is rapid and complete. Recurrences are rare. *DSM-III-R* diagnostic criteria for psychogenic fugue are presented in Table 22.3.

Table 22.3 DIAGNOSTIC CRITERIA FOR PSYCHOGENIC FUGUE

A. The predominant disturbance is sudden, unexpected travel away from home or one's customary place of work, with inability to recall one's past.

B. Assumption of a new identity (partial or complete).

C. The disturbance is not due to multiple personality disorder or to an organic mental disorder (e.g., partial complex seizures in temporal lobe epilepsy).

Source: American Psychiatric Association (1987) with permission.

Predisposing Factors to Psychogenic Fugue The theoretical models described as predisposing factors to psychogenic amnesia also have relevance for psychogenic fugue. Psychodynamic features, behavioral aspects, and possible biological factors are considered as having etiological implications for both disorders. In addition, dysfunctional family dynamics may be implicated in the predisposition to psychogenic fugue. The theory of family dynamics will be described here. Other theoretical models may be reviewed under the section on psychogenic amnesia.

Theory of Family Dynamics Fugue is sometimes related to a person's search for a lost parent (Berger, 1985). The unsatisfactory parent/child relationship, with subsequent internalization of loss, results in episodes of depression and suicidal ideation, common in patients who experience fugues. Unfulfilled separation anxiety, a defect in personality development, and unmet dependency needs are other associated features of psychogenic fugue that are related to dysfunctional family dynamics.

Transactional Model of Stress/Adaptation The etiology of psychogenic fugue is most likely influenced by multiple factors. In Figure 22.2, a

Precipitating Event
(Any event sufficiently stressful to threaten a fragile ego)

↓

Predisposing Factors
    Genetic Influences: Possible dysfunctional neurophysiological processes
    Past Experiences: Repression of painful mental contents from conscious awareness
                      Learned response through reinforcement of the behavior
                      Primary and/or secondary derived gains from the response
                      Dysfunctional family dynamics resulting in internalized loss
                      Unfulfilled separation anxiety and dependency needs
                      Defect in personality development
    Existing Conditions: Developmental regression
                      Absence of support systems
                      Poor coping mechanisms

↓

Cognitive Appraisal
↓
* Primary *
↓
(Real or perceived threat to biological integrity or self-concept)
↓
* Secondary *
↓
Because of weak ego strength, patient is unable to use coping mechanisms effectively.
Defense mechanisms utilized: denial, regression, repression, suppression
↓
Quality of response
↓
ANXIETY

Adaptive   Maladaptive

Mild   Moderate   Severe   Panic
                              (Repressed)
                                ↓   Psychoses
                              Neuroses
                              ↓
                              Psychogenic
                              Fugue

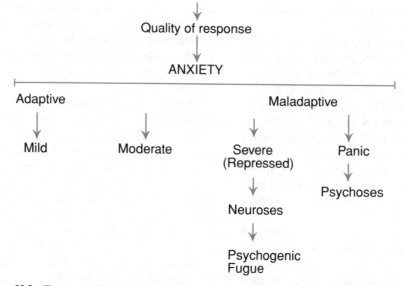

Figure 22.2 The dynamics of psychogenic fugue using the transactional model of stress/adaptation.

graphic depiction of this theory of multiple causation is presented in the Transactional Model of Stress/Adaptation.

Nursing Diagnosis, Planning/Implementation- Nursing diagnoses are formulated from the data gathered during the assessment phase and with background knowledge regarding predisposing factors to the disorder. Some common nursing diagnoses for patients with psychogenic fugue include:

High risk for violence directed toward others related to fear of unknown circumstances surrounding emergence from fugue state.

Ineffective individual coping related to dysfunctional family system and repressed severe anxiety evidenced by sudden travel away from home with inability to recall previous identity.

In Table 22.4, these nursing diagnoses are presented in a plan of care for the patient with psychogenic fugue. Goals of care and appropriate nursing interventions are included for each. Rationales are provided in italics.

Outcome Criteria The following criteria may be used for measurement of outcomes in the care of the patient with psychogenic fugue.

The patient:
1. Has not harmed self or others.
2. Is able to maintain anxiety at a level at which he or she feels no need for aggression.
3. Is able to discuss fears and anxieties with staff.
4. Is able to verbalize the extreme anxiety that precipitated the fugue state.
5. Is able to demonstrate more adaptive coping strategies in the face of extreme anxiety.
6. Is able to name resources from whom he or she may seek assistance in times of extreme anxiety.

Evaluation Reassessment is conducted to determine if the nursing actions have been successful in achieving the objectives of care. Evaluation of the nursing actions for the patient with psychogenic fugue may be facilitated by gathering information using the following types of questions.

Is the patient able to control anxiety without using violence? Is he or she able to demonstrate strategies for relieving anxiety without resorting to aggression? Does the patient discuss fears and anxieties with members of the staff. Has he or she confronted these fears and anxieties and dealt with them in an effort toward resolution? Can the patient verbalize and demonstrate adaptive coping strategies for dealing with extreme stress without resorting to dissociation? Does the patient recall the extreme stressor that precipitated the fugue state? Does he or she have a plan for dealing with the stressor should it reoccur in the future? Can he or she verbalize resources for seeking assistance in the face of extreme stress?

MULTIPLE PERSONALITY DISORDER

Multiple personality disorder (MPD) is a relatively rare phenomenon that is characterized by the existence of two or more personalities within a single individual (Purcell, 1988). Only one of the personalities is evident at any given moment, and one of them is dominant most of the time during the course of the disorder. Each personality is unique and comprised of a complex set of memories, behavior patterns, and social relationships that surface during the dominant interval. The transition from one personality to another is usually sudden, often dramatic, and usually precipitated by stress. O'Regan and Hurley (1985) state:

"Transition may be voluntary or involuntary, initiated either through conscious willing, in response to an unconscious emotion or a situation that triggers 'automatic' switching, or as a result of biochemical changes in the body."

Prior to therapy, the original personality usually has no knowledge of the other personalities, but when there are two or more subpersonalities, they are usually aware of each other's existence. Most often, the various subpersonalities have different names, but they may be unnamed and may be of a different sex, race, and age (Purcell, 1988). The various personalities are almost always quite disparate and may even appear to be the exact opposite of the original personality. For example, a normally shy, socially withdrawn, faithful husband may become a gregarious womanizer and heavy drinker with the emergence of another personality.

Various personalities may respond to a stressful situation in different ways. An example cited by the *DSM-III-R* suggests that a person may have one personality that responds to aggression with childlike fright and flight, another that responds with maso-

Table 22.4   CARE PLAN FOR THE PATIENT WITH PSYCHOGENIC FUGUE

Nursing Diagnoses	Objectives	Nursing Interventions
High risk for violence directed toward others related to fear of unknown circumstances surrounding emergence from fugue state.	Patient will not harm self or others.	Maintain low level of stimuli in patient's environment (low lighting, few people, simple decor, low noise level). *Anxiety level rises in stimulating environment. Individuals may be perceived as threatening by a fearful and agitated patient.* Observe patient's behavior frequently. *Close observation is necessary so that intervention can occur if required to ensure patient's (and others') safety.* Remove all dangerous objects from patient's environment, *so that in his or her agitated, confused state, patient may not use them to harm self or others.* Try to redirect violent behavior with physical outlets for the patient's anxiety (e.g., punching bag). *Physical exercise is a safe and effective way of relieving pent-up tension.* Staff should maintain and convey a calm attitude to patient. *Anxiety is contagious and can be transmitted from staff to patient.* Have sufficient staff available to indicate a show of strength to patient if it becomes necessary. *This shows the patient evidence of control over the situation and provides some physical security for staff.* Administer tranquilizing medications as ordered by physician. Monitor medication for its effectiveness and for any adverse side effects. *The avenue of the "least restrictive alternative" must be selected when planning intervention for a psychiatric patient.* If the patient is not calmed by "talking down" or by medication, use of mechanical restraints may be necessary. Be sure to have sufficient staff available to assist. Follow protocol established by the institution. Most states require that the physician reevaluate and issue a new order for restraints every 3 hours, except between midnight and 8:00 A.M. If the patient has previously refused medication, administer after restraints have been applied. Most states consider this intervention appropriate in emergency situations or in the event that a patient would likely harm self or others. Observe the patient in restraints every 15 minutes (or according to institutional policy). Ensure that circulation is not compromised (check temperature, color, pulse). Assist patient with needs related to nutrition, hydration, and elimination. Position patient so that comfort is facilitated and aspiration can be prevented. *Patient safety is a nursing priority.* As agitation decreases, assess patient's readiness for restraint removal or reduction. Remove one restraint at a time, while assessing patient's response. *This minimizes risk of injury to patient and staff.*

(continued)

Table 22.4 CONTINUED		
Nursing Diagnoses	**Objectives**	**Nursing Interventions**
Ineffective individual coping related to dysfunctional family system and repressed severe anxiety, evidenced by sudden travel away from home with inability to recall previous identity.	Patient will demonstrate more adaptive ways of coping in stressful situations than resorting to dissociation.	Reassure patient of safety and security through your presence. Dissociative behaviors may be frightening to the patient. *Presence of a trusted individual provides feeling of security and assurance of freedom from harm.* Identify stressor that precipitated severe anxiety. *This information is necessary to the development of an effective plan of patient care and problem resolution.* Explore feelings that patient experienced in response to the stressor. Help patient understand that the disequilibrium felt is acceptable in times of severe stress. *Patient's self-esteem is preserved by the knowledge that others may experience these behaviors under similar circumstances.* As anxiety level decreases and memory returns, use exploration and an accepting, nonthreatening environment to encourage patient to identify repressed traumatic experiences that contribute to chronic anxiety. *Patient must confront and deal with painful issues to achieve resolution.* Have patient identify methods of coping with stress in the past and determine whether the response was adaptive or maladaptive. *In times of extreme anxiety, patient is unable to evaluate appropriateness of response. This information is necessary for patient to develop a plan of action for the future.* Help patient define more adaptive coping strategies. Make suggestions of alternatives that might be tried. Examine benefits and consequences of each alternative. Assist patient in the selection of those that are most appropriate for him or her. *Depending on current level of anxiety, patient may require assistance with problem solving and decision making.* Provide positive reinforcement for patient's attempts to change. *Positive reinforcement enhances self-esteem and encourages repetition of desired behaviors.* Identify community resources to which the individual may go for support if past maladaptive coping patterns return.

chistic submission, and yet another that responds with counterattack (APA, 1987).

Generally, there is amnesia for the events that took place when another personality was in the dominant position. Often, however, one personality state is not bound by such amnesia and retains complete awareness of the existence, qualities, and activities of the other personalities (Nemiah, 1989). Subpersonalities that are amnestic for the other subpersonalities experience the periods when others are dominant as "lost time" or blackouts. They may "wake up" in unfamiliar situations with no idea where they are, how they got there, or who the people around them are. They may frequently be accused of lying when they deny remembering or being responsible for events or actions that occurred while another personality controlled the body.

Multiple personality disorder is not always incapacitating. Some MPD victims maintain responsible positions, complete graduate degrees, and are successful spouses and parents prior to diagnosis and while in treatment.

Eighty-nine percent of MPD victims have been misdiagnosed at least once (O'Regan & Hurley, 1985). Common misdiagnoses include depression, borderline and sociopathic personality disorders, schizophrenia, epilepsy, and bipolar disorder.

The *DSM-III-R* diagnostic criteria for multiple personality disorder are presented in Table 22.5.

Predisposing Factors to Multiple Personality Disorder Kluft (1984, 1987) developed the "four-factor" theory of the etiology of multiple personality disorder. The four factors he considers necessary for the development of multiplicity are:

1. A biological capacity for dissociation.
2. A history of trauma or abuse.
3. Specific psychological factors that influence the shaping of the various personalities as they take form at the time of the traumatic mobilization of the dissociative defense. These would be factors such as developmental stage, cultural, societal, and family influences.
4. A lack of adequate nurturing or opportunities to recover from the abuse.

These four factors may be explained by the following theories.

Biological Theories These theories include:

1. *Genetics.* Several studies have indicated that MPD is more common in first-degree biological relatives of people with the disorder than in the general population (APA, 1987). Braun (1985) concludes from his studies that at least one early caretaker of the individual who will develop MPD has exhibited severe psychopathology. Multiplicity is often seen in more

---

Table 22.5 DIAGNOSTIC CRITERIA FOR MULTIPLE PERSONALITY DISORDER

A. The existence within the person of two or more distinct personalities or personality states (each with its own relatively enduring pattern of perceiving, relating to, and thinking about the environment and self).

B. At least two of these personalities or personality states recurrently take full control of the person's behavior.

Source: American Psychiatric Association (1987) with permission.

---

than one generation of a family. While some psychiatrists believe this may reflect a genetic component of MPD—perhaps linked to the psychobiological capacity for dissociation—others correlate this dissociation process to the effects of the violent personalities of adult caregivers (O'Regan & Hurley, 1985).

2. *Organic.* The role of organic influences in the development of MPD remains unclear. Various studies (Allison, 1977; Horton and Miller, 1972; Schenk & Bear, 1981) have suggested a possible link to certain neurological alterations and MPD. These neurological conditions include temporal lobe epilepsy, severe migraine headaches, cerebral cortical damage, and visual alterations. Electroencephalographic abnormalities were observed in some patients with MPD.

The decided majority of individuals with these organic alterations evidence no signs of multiple personality. Based on the body of present knowledge, there is insufficient evidence to support the hypothesis of organic dysfunction as a determinant of MPD (Confer & Ables, 1983).

Psychological Influences A growing body of evidence points to the etiology of MPD as a set of traumatic experiences that overwhelms the individual's capacity to cope by any means other than dissociation. These experiences usually take the form of severe physical, sexual, or psychological abuse by a parent or significant other in the child's life (O'Regan & Hurley, 1985). Benjamin (1990) has stated, "MPD develops when people have been so overcome by early traumas that they have to put up mental partitions in order to function in everyday life." The most widely accepted etiological explanation for MPD is that it begins as a survival strategy that serves to help children cope with horrendous sexual, physical, or psychological abuse. In this traumatic environment, the child is reduced to experiencing the self as a passive victim unable to ward off cruel and unwanted stimuli (Confer & Ables, 1983). He or she creates a new being who is able to experience the overwhelming pain of the cruel reality, while the primary self is then able to escape awareness of the pain. Each new personality has as its nucleus a means of responding without anxiety and distress to various painful or dangerous stimuli.

Studies have revealed a great diversity in the nature and scope of the trauma that individuals with MPD have suffered (O'Regan & Hurley, 1985). *Sexual* abuse has included rape, incest, sodomy, and heterosexual and homosexual fellatio. Some individuals report being forced to witness the physical or sexual abuse of other children. Multiples have given examples of *psychological* abuse as being compelled to participate in murders, including cult activities involving ritual murders. *Physical* abuse has included burying, torture, beatings, excessive enemas and massive doses of cathartics, as well as total neglect. Kluft (1984) suggests that the number of a multiple's alternate personalities is related to the number of different types of abuse he or she suffered as a child. Individuals with many personalities have usually been severely abused well into adolescence.

Theory of Family Dynamics Studies by Braun (1986) indicate that individuals with MPD do not find the necessary healing support in their environment. Research has revealed a profile of the family of origin of the individual with MPD. The family of the multiple:

1. Upholds rigid religious or mystical beliefs.
2. Presents a united front to the community, yet internally is riddled with conflict.
3. Is isolated from the community and uncooperative regarding intervention or assistance.
4. Includes at least one caretaker who exhibits severe psychopathology.
5. Subjects the child to contradictory communications.
6. Is polarized by one overadequate parent (the abuser) and one underadequate parent (the enabler).

The individual who is not given the opportunity to heal following abuse and dissociation adopts this defense as a routine strategy for dealing with life problems.

Transactional Model of Stress/Adaptation The etiology of MPD is most likely influenced by multiple factors. In Figure 22.3, a graphic depiction of this theory of multiple causation is presented in the Transactional Model of Stress/Adaptation.

Nursing Diagnosis, Planning/Implementation Nursing diagnoses are formulated from the data gathered during the assessment phase and with background knowledge regarding predisposing factors to the disorder. Some common nursing diagnoses for patients with MPD include:

High risk for self-directed violence related to unresolved grief and self-blame associated with childhood abuse.

Personal identity disturbance related to childhood trauma/abuse evidenced by the presence of more than one personality within the individual.

In Table 22.6, these nursing diagnoses are presented in a plan of care for the patient with MPD. Goals of care and appropriate nursing interventions are included for each. Rationales are presented in italics.

Outcome Criteria The following criteria may be used for measurement of outcomes in the care of the patient with MPD.

The patient:
1. Has not harmed self or others.
2. Seeks out staff when aggressive feelings emerge.
3. Verbalizes understanding about the existence of multiple personalities.
4. Verbalizes understanding about the purpose the various personalities serve.
5. Verbalizes understanding that transition from one personality to another occurs in times of stress.
6. Verbalizes knowledge of various situations that precipitate stress.
7. Verbalizes understanding of and willingness to participate in integration therapy.

Evaluation Hospitalization of the patient with MPD usually only occurs in an acute situation (e.g., an attempted suicide, or an attempt to integrate a personality that the therapist is anticipating may precipitate violence and requires a more structured setting). In these cases, the nursing interventions would be directed toward the most critical issues.

Reassessment is ongoing and determines if the nursing actions have been successful in achieving the stated objectives of care. Evaluation of the nursing actions for the patient with MPD disorder may be facilitated by gathering information using the following types of questions.

Is the patient able to maintain control over hostile impulses? Has injury to the patient and others

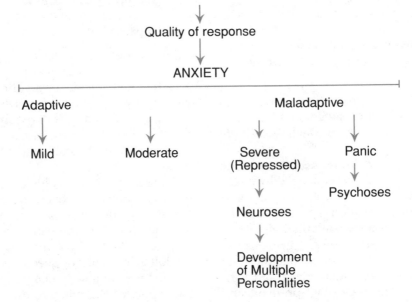

Precipitating Event
(Any event sufficiently stressful to threaten a fragile ego)

↓

Predisposing Factors
Genetic Influences: Possible hereditary factors
Past Experiences: Extreme sexual, psychological, and/or physical abuse
                      Repression of painful mental contents from conscious awareness
                      Splitting of the personality to protect the primary self
                      Dysfunctional family system with at least one parent exhibiting psychopathology
                      Lack of healing support from within the family system
Existing Conditions: Developmental regression
                      Absence of support systems
                      Poor coping mechanisms
                      Possible influences from neurological alterations, e.g., temporal lobe epilepsy,
                          severe migraine headaches, cerebral cortical damage, EEG abnormalities

↓

Cognitive Appraisal

↓

* Primary *

↓

(Real or perceived threat to biological integrity or self-concept)

↓

* Secondary *

↓

Because of weak ego strength, patient is unable to use coping mechanisms effectively.
Defense mechanisms utilized: denial, regression, repression, suppression

↓

Quality of response

↓

ANXIETY

Adaptive   Maladaptive

↓   ↓   ↓   ↓

Mild   Moderate   Severe   Panic
                          (Repressed)

                              ↓   ↓

                          Neuroses   Psychoses

                              ↓

                          Development
                          of Multiple
                          Personalities

Figure 22.3 The dynamics of multiple personality disorder using the transactional model of stress/adaptation.

Table 22.6 CARE PLAN FOR THE PATIENT WITH MULTIPLE PERSONALITY DISORDER

Nursing Diagnoses	Objectives	Nursing Interventions
High risk for self-directed violence related to unresolved grief and self-blame associated with childhood abuse.	Patient will not harm self.	Assess suicidal or harmful intent. Discuss consideration of a plan and availability of means. Assess sudden changes in behavior. *Impulse control may be impaired. Sudden changes may signal a switch to the "suicidal" personality.* Help patient identify stressful precipitating factors that initiate emergence of the "suicidal" personality. *Early detection allows time to manipulate the environment to reduce the possibility of injury.* Establish trust and secure a promise that patient seek out support when self-destructive impulses are present. *This allows the patient to assume some of the responsibility for his or her behavior, while still offering assistance if self-control is lacking.* Seek assistance from another, strong-willed personality *to help control the behavior of the "suicidal" personality.* Assist the patient in identifying alternative behaviors to self-destructive behaviors (e.g., verbal or written expression; physical activity). *These activities may provide a nondestructive alternative in the face of overwhelming aggressive impulse.* Place in isolation or provide physical restraint in a nonpunitive manner *to ensure patient safety when internal controls fail.* Assess physical and emotional status every 15 minutes while in restraints. *Patient safety and security are nursing priorities.* Administer antidepressant and antianxiety medications as ordered by physician. *Depression is common and the patient may become frustrated with the long-term treatment (sometimes in excess of 10 years). Anxiolytics may be required to reduce anxiety until internal controls are achieved.*
Personal identity disturbance related to childhood trauma/abuse evidenced by the presence of more than one personality within the individual.	Patient will verbalize understanding about the existence of multiple personalities within the self, the reason for their existence, and the importance of eventual integration of the personalities into one.	The nurse must develop a trusting relationship with the original personality and with each of the subpersonalities. *Trust is the basis of a therapeutic relationship. Each of the personalities views itself as a separate entity and must initially be treated as such.* Help patient understand the existence of the subpersonalities and the need each serves in the personal identity of the individual. *Patient may initially be unaware of the dissociative response. Knowledge of the needs each personality fulfills is the first step in the integration process.* Help patient identify stressful situations that precipitate transition from one personality to another. Carefully observe and record these transitions. *This knowledge is required to assist patient in responding more adaptively and to eliminate the need for transition to another personality.* Use nursing interventions necessary to deal with maladaptive behaviors associated with individual subpersonalities. For example, if one personality is suicidal, precautions must be taken to guard against patient's self-harm. If another personality has a tendency toward physical hostility,

(continued)

Table 22.6 CONTINUED		
Nursing Diagnoses	**Objectives**	**Nursing Interventions**
		precautions must be taken to protect others. *The safety of patient and others is a nursing priority.* Help subpersonalities to understand that their "being" will not be destroyed but rather integrated into a unified identity within the individual. *Because subpersonalities function as separate entities, the idea of total elimination generates fear and defensiveness.* Provide support during disclosure of painful experiences, and reassurance when patient becomes discouraged with lengthy treatment. *Positive reinforcement may encourage repetition of desirable behaviors.*

been avoided? Does the patient seek support from staff when aggressive feelings emerge? Is the patient able to discuss the presence of various personalities within the self? Is he or she able to verbalize why these personalities exist? Is the patient able to verbalize situations that precipitate transition from one personality to another? Does he or she ever switch from one personality to another voluntarily? Can the patient demonstrate alternative, more adaptive coping strategies? Does the patient verbalize understanding of the process of integration? Is he or she willing to undergo the lengthy therapy required for integration? Do the alternate personalities resist integration? Do the alternate personalities understand that integration does not mean extinction but instead a "coming together" of all the personalities into one identity? Does the patient have a plan for dealing with stress outside the therapy setting, particularly those situations that provoke feelings of violence to self or others? If so, has the plan been demonstrated (e.g., through role play?). Can the patient name resources outside the hospital from whom he or she may seek assistance during times of extreme stress?

DEPERSONALIZATION DISORDER

Depersonalization disorder is characterized by a temporary change in the quality of self-awareness, which often takes the form of feelings of unreality, changes in body image, feelings of detachment from the environment, or a sense of observing oneself from outside the body (Marciniak, 1985). *Depersonalization* (a disturbance in the perception of

oneself) is differentiated from *derealization*, which describes an alteration in the perception of the external environment. Both of these phenomena occur in a variety of psychiatric illnesses, such as schizophrenia, depression, anxiety states, and organic mental disorders, as well as depersonalization disorder. As stated earlier, the symptom of depersonalization is very common. Up to 70% of "healthy" adults may experience transient episodes of depersonalization (APA, 1987). The diagnosis of depersonalization disorder is not made, even if episodes are recurrent, unless the symptom causes social or occupational dysfunction (Purcell, 1988).

The *DSM-III-R* describes this disorder as "the occurrence of one or more episodes of depersonalization, not due to any other mental disorder, that causes marked distress." The individual feels detached from, or as an outside observer of, his or her body. There may be a mechanical or dreamlike feeling, or belief that the body's physical characteristics have changed. If derealization is present, objects in the environment are perceived as altered in size or shape. Other people in the environment may seem automated or mechanical.

These altered perceptions are experienced as disturbing and are often accompanied by anxiety, dizziness, fear of going insane, depression, obsessive thoughts, somatic complaints, and a disturbance in the subjective sense of time (APA, 1987). The disorder has been found to occur at least twice as often in women as in men and is a disorder of younger people, rarely occurring in individuals older than 40 years of age (Nemiah, 1989). The diagnostic criteria for depersonalization disorder are presented in Table 22.7.

Table 22.7 DIAGNOSTIC CRITERIA FOR DEPERSONALIZATION DISORDER

A. Persistent or recurrent experiences of depersonalization as indicated by either 1) or 2):
   1. An experience of feeling detached from, and as if one is an outside observer of, one's mental processes or body.
   2. An experience of feeling like an automaton or as if in a dream.
B. During the depersonalization experience, reality testing remains intact.
C. The depersonalization is sufficiently severe and persistent to cause marked distress.
D. The depersonalization experience is the predominant disturbance and is not a symptom of another disorder, such as schizophrenia, panic disorder, or agoraphobia without history of panic disorder but with limited symptom attacks or depersonalization, or temporal lobe epilepsy.

Source: American Psychiatric Association (1987) with permission.

Predisposing Factors to Depersonalization Disorder

Physiological Theories A variety of empirical observations have led some investigators to suggest that the phenomenon of depersonalization has a neurophysiological basis (Purcell, 1988). Patients with diseases of the central nervous system, such as brain tumors and epilepsy, have reported depersonalization episodes in association with their neurological impairment. Electrical stimulation of the cortex of the temporal lobes has produced the same effect. Some psychotomimetic drugs, such as LSD and mescaline, create distortions of perception and alterations in the sense of reality. A number of researchers have reported that individuals subjected to severe sensory deprivation sometimes experience the phenomenon of depersonalization.

Psychodynamic Theories Psychodynamic explanations place emphasis on psychological conflict and disturbances of ego structure in the predisposition to depersonalization disorder.

Perceiving the self as "not real" would serve as a defense mechanism and offer protection or escape from anxiety or some other unpleasant emotion resulting from internal psychological conflict (Purcell, 1988). For example, an individual who experiences extreme anxiety after a severe automobile accident perceives himself or herself (or the situation) as "not real" and therefore escapes the emotional pain associated with the incident.

Theories related to disturbances in ego structure focus on problems with personal identity and ego boundaries. Depersonalization occurs in response to psychological conflicts within the ego itself. The conflict results in a split in the ego between an observing self and an acting self, or a split between conflicting identifications (Nemiah, 1989). Proponents of this theory believe that explanation of depersonalization lies primarily in understanding the pathology of the structure and function of the ego.

Transactional Model of Stress/Adaptation The etiology of depersonalization disorder is most likely influenced by multiple factors. In Figure 22.4, a graphic depiction of this theory of multiple causation is presented in the Transactional Model of Stress/Adaptation.

Nursing Diagnosis, Planning/Implementation Nursing diagnoses are formulated from the data gathered during the assessment phase and with background knowledge regarding predisposing factors to the disorder. Some common nursing diagnoses for patients with depersonalization disorder include:

Sensory-perceptual alteration (visual and kinesthetic) related to repressed severe anxiety and underdeveloped ego evidenced by alteration in the perception or experience of the self or the environment.
Anxiety (severe to panic) related to fears of losing control or going insane evidenced by dizziness, somatic complaints, obsessive thoughts, and disturbances in the sense of time.

In Table 22.8, these nursing diagnoses are presented in a plan of care for the patient with depersonalization disorder. Goals of care and appropriate nursing interventions are included for each. Rationales are presented in italics.

Outcome Criteria The following criteria may be used for measurement of outcomes in the care of the patient with depersonalization disorder:

The patient:
1. Maintains a sense of reality during stressful situations.
2. Perceives self and environment accurately.
3. Verbalizes correlation between severe anxiety and symptoms of depersonalization.
4. Is able to maintain anxiety at a manageable level.
5. Verbalizes understanding of the role deper-

Precipitating Event
(Any event sufficiently stressful to threaten a fragile ego)

Predisposing Factors
  Genetic Influences: (No known hereditary factors)
  Past Experiences: Impairment in ego development
                           Development of inadequate ego defense mechanisms
  Existing Conditions: Use of psychotomimetic drugs
                           Personal identity disturbance
                           Ego too weak to deal with overwhelming stress
                           Developmental regression
                           Possible influences from neurological alterations, e.g., brain tumors, epilepsy,
                           Absence of support systems

Cognitive Appraisal

* Primary *

(Real or perceived threat to biological integrity or self-concept)

* Secondary *

Because of weak ego strength, patient is unable to use coping mechanisms effectively.
Defense mechanisms utilized: denial, regression, repression, suppression

Quality of response

ANXIETY

Adaptive   Maladaptive

Mild   Moderate   Severe   Panic
                          (Repressed)

                                          Psychoses

                           Neuroses

                  Depersonalization
                  Derealization

Figure 22.4   The dynamics of depersonalization disorder using the transactional model of stress/adaptation.

Table 22.8 CARE PLAN FOR THE PATIENT WITH DEPERSONALIZATION DISORDER

Nursing Diagnoses	Objectives	Nursing Interventions
Sensory-perceptual alteration (visual/kinesthetic) related to repressed severe anxiety and underdeveloped ego evidenced by alteration in the perception or experience of the self or the environment.	Patient will demonstrate the ability to perceive stimuli correctly and maintain a sense of reality during stressful situations.	Provide support and encouragement during times of depersonalization. Patients manifesting these symptoms may express fear and anxiety at experiencing such behaviors. They do not understand the response and may express a fear of going insane. *Support and encouragement from a trusted individual provide a feeling of security when fears and anxieties are manifested.* Explain the depersonalization behaviors and the purpose they usually serve for the patient. *This knowledge may help to minimize fears and anxieties associated with their occurrence.* Explain the relationship between severe anxiety and depersonalization behaviors. Help relate these behaviors to times of severe psychological stress that patient has experienced. *The patient may be unaware that the occurrence of depersonalization behaviors is related to severe anxiety.* Explore past experiences and possibly repressed painful situations, such as trauma or abuse. *Traumatic experiences may predispose individuals to dissociative disorders.* Discuss these painful experiences with the patient, and encourage him or her to deal with the feelings associated with these situations. Work to resolve the conflicts these repressed feelings have nurtured. *These interventions will serve to decrease the need for the dissociative response to anxiety.* Discuss ways the patient may more adaptively respond to stress, and role-play with him or her to practice using these new methods.
Anxiety (severe to panic) related to fears of losing control or going insane evidenced by dizziness, somatic complaints, obsessive thoughts, and disturbances in the sense of time.	Patient will verbalize understanding of purpose depersonalization behaviors fulfill, thereby decreasing fears and anxieties associated with experiencing them.	Maintain a calm, nonthreatening manner while working with the patient. *Anxiety is contagious and may be transferred from staff to patient or vice versa. Patient develops feeling of security in presence of calm staff person.* Reassure patient of his or her safety and security. This can be conveyed by the physical presence of the nurse. Do not leave the patient alone at this time. *The patient may fear for his or her life. The presence of a trusted individual provides the patient with a feeling of security and assurance of personal safety.* Use simple words and brief messages, spoken calmly and clearly. *In an intensely anxious situation, the patient is unable to comprehend anything but the most elemental communication.* Explain to the patient what is happening. Assure the patient that the experiencing of depersonalization behaviors does not mean that he or she is going crazy. *The feeling of a lack of control over behavior he or she does not understand will contribute to anxiety. Explanations should offer some relief.* When depersonalization behaviors have diminished and anxiety has been reduced, explore with the patient the stressful situation that may have precipitated the response. *The patient may be unaware that the occurrence of depersonalization behaviors is related to severe anxiety.* Discuss with

(continued)

Table 22.8 CONTINUED		
Nursing Diagnoses	**Objectives**	**Nursing Interventions**
		the patient ways in which he or she might respond to stressful situations that would be less likely to result in depersonalization behaviors. *This may have been the patient's way of dealing with stress for a long time. He or she may need help to identify alternative coping strategies.* Use role-play to practice new, more adaptive coping strategies. *Role-play allows the patient to practice and be better prepared to deal with the stressful situation should it reoccur. Being prepared provides a feeling of security and offers a sense of control to the patient.*

sonalization behaviors play in the management of anxiety.

6. Is able to verbalize more adaptive strategies for coping with stress.

Evaluation Reassessment is conducted to determine if the nursing actions have been successful in achieving the objectives of care. Evaluation of the nursing actions for the patient with depersonalization disorder may be facilitated by gathering information using the following types of questions.

Does the patient demonstrate the ability to perceive stimuli correctly? Does he or she maintain a sense of reality during stressful situations? Is the patient able to verbalize the purpose depersonalization behaviors serve? Is the patient able to verbalize a correlation between stressful situations and the onset of depersonalization behaviors? Can the patient demonstrate more adaptive coping strategies for dealing with stress without resorting to dissociation? Has the patient role-played these strategies in preparation for their use in real-life situations? Can the patient verbalize types of situations that precipitate extreme stress? Can the patient discuss more adaptive ways that he or she plans to deal with these times of extreme stress in the future? Is the patient able to name resources outside the hospital to whom he or she may turn when feeling the need for assistance?

TREATMENT MODALITIES

Psychogenic Amnesia

Many cases of psychogenic amnesia resolve spontaneously when the individual is removed from the stressful situation (Purcell, 1988). For other, more refractory conditions, intravenous administration of amobarbital is useful in the retrieval of lost memories. Most clinicians recommend supportive psychotherapy also to reinforce adjustment to the psychological impact of the retrieved memories and the emotions associated with them (Purcell, 1988).

In some instances, psychotherapy is used as the primary treatment. Techniques of persuasion and free or directed association are used to help the patient remember. In other cases, hypnosis may be required to mobilize the memories. Once the memories are obtained, the suggestion is made to patients that they will retain them in consciousness after awakening (Nemiah, 1989).

Psychogenic Fugue

Recovery from psychogenic fugue is usually rapid, spontaneous, and complete, and no specific treatment is required other than supportive care (Purcell, 1988). In some instances, manipulation of the environment or psychotherapeutic support may be helpful in diminishing stress or in helping the patient adapt to stress in the future.

When the fugue state is prolonged, techniques of gentle encouragement, persuasion, or directed association may be helpful, either alone or in combination with hypnosis or amobarbital interviews, which are also aimed at facilitating recall of the previous identity (Purcell, 1988).

Multiple Personality Disorder

The goal of therapy for the patient with MPD is to optimize the patient's function and potential. The achievement of integration is usually considered desirable, but in some cases a reasonable degree of conflict-free collaboration among the personalities is all that can be achieved (Kluft, 1988).

Some success has been achieved with intensive, long-term psychotherapy directed toward uncovering the underlying psychological conflicts, providing the patient with insight into these conflicts, and striving to synthesize the various identities into one integrated personality (Purcell, 1988). Patients are assisted to recall past traumas in detail. They must mentally reexperience the abuse that caused their illness. This process, called *abreaction*, or "remembering with feeling," is so painful that patients sometimes scream, sob, and flail about, just as they did during the real event (Gupta, 1990).

During therapy, each personality is actively explored and encouraged to become aware of the others across previously amnestic barriers. Traumatic memories, especially those related to childhood abuse, associated with the different personality manifestations are examined.

Braun (1986) and Kluft (1988) have identified the following principles of therapy for the person with MPD:

1. Use hypnosis to access personalities that do not emerge spontaneously.
2. Identify the relationships among subpersonalities and work with each personality equally.
3. Provide all personalities with information about their role in the dissociated system.
4. Encourage awareness, communication, empathy, and cooperation among personalities.
5. Use medications sparingly. Almost any medicine is fraught with "switch potential"—idiosyncratic responses to medication that vary across personalities.
6. Expect some degree of relapse following initial integration.
7. Do not assume that the course of treatment will be smooth. The course of treatment is often difficult and anxiety provoking to the patient and doctor alike, especially when aggressive or suicidal personalities are in the dominant role. In these instances, brief periods of hospitalization may be necessary as an interim supportive measure (Nemiah, 1989).

When integration is achieved, the individual becomes a total of all the feelings, experiences, memories, skills, and talents that were previously in the command of the various personalities. He or she learns how to function effectively without the necessity for creating new personalities to cope with life. This is possible only after years of intense psychotherapy, and even then, recovery is very often incomplete.

Depersonalization Disorder

Information about the treatment of depersonalization disorder is sparse and inconclusive. Various regimens have been tried, although none have proven widely successful. Pharmacotherapy with dextroamphetamines or amobarbital (Amytal) has been tried with inconclusive results (Purcell, 1988). Benzodiazepines provide symptomatic relief if anxiety is an important element of the clinical condition (Marciniak, 1985). For patients with evident intrapsychic conflict, use of analytically oriented insight psychotherapy may be useful, although many clinicians believe that a successful outcome requires a minimum of 5 years of therapy (Nemiah, 1989). Specific recommendations for the management of depersonalization disorder must await more extensive clinical investigation.

SUMMARY

A dissociative response has been described as a defense mechanism to protect the ego in the face of overwhelming anxiety. Dissociative responses result in an alteration in the normally integrative functions of identity, memory, or consciousness. Classification of dissociative disorders includes psychogenic amnesia, psychogenic fugue, multiple personality disorder, and depersonalization disorder.

In comparison to other primary psychiatric disorders, dissociative disorders are relatively rare. However, dissociative behaviors are not uncommonly observed in patients with other disorders.

The individual with psychogenic amnesia is unable to recall important personal information that is too extensive to be explained by ordinary forgetfulness. The memory deficit may be described as *localized*, *selective*, *generalized*, or *continuous*. Psychogenic fugue is characterized by a sudden, unexpected travel away from home with inability to recall the past, including personal identity. Duration of the fugue is usually brief, and once it is over the individual recovers memory of the past life, but is amnestic for the period covered by the fugue. The prominent feature of MPD is the existence of two or more personalities within a single individual. An individual may have many personalities, each of which serves a purpose for that individual of enduring painful stimuli that the original personality is too weak to face. Depersonalization disorder is characterized by an alteration in the perception of oneself (sometimes described as a feeling of having separated from the body and watching the activities of the self from a distance).

Nursing care of individuals with dissociative dis-

orders is accomplished using the steps of the nursing process. Background assessment data were presented, along with nursing diagnoses common to each disorder. Interventions appropriate to each nursing diagnosis and relevant outcome criteria for each were included. An overview of current medical treatment modalities was discussed.

Nurses in all areas of clinical practice should be aware of patient potential for dissociative responses and be able to recognize these behaviors should they occur. The initial health-care encounter of patients exhibiting dissociative behaviors often occurs in areas other than psychiatry.

REVIEW QUESTIONS
Self-Examination/Learning Exercise

*Select the answer that is **most** appropriate for each of the following questions.*

Situation: Ellen, age 32, was diagnosed as having MPD at age 28. Since that time, she has been in therapy with a psychiatrist, who has detected the presence of 12 personalities and identified a history of childhood abuse. Yesterday, Beth, the personality with suicidal ideations, swallowed a bottle of 20 diazepam (Valium). Ellen's roommate found her when she returned from work and called the emergency medical service. Ellen was stabilized in the emergency department and 48 hours later was transferred to the psychiatric unit.

1. The primary nursing diagnosis for Ellen would be:
   a. personal identity disturbance related to childhood abuse.
   b. sensory-perceptual alteration related to repressed anxiety.
   c. altered thought processes related to memory deficit.
   d. high risk for self-directed violence related to unresolved grief.

2. In establishing trust with Ellen, the nurse must:
   a. try to relate to Ellen as though she did not have multiple personalities.
   b. establish a relationship with each of the personalities separately.
   c. ignore behaviors that Ellen attributes to Beth.
   d. explain to Ellen that you will work with her only if she maintains the status of the primary personality.

3. The ultimate goal of therapy for Ellen is:
   a. integration of the personalities into one.
   b. for her to have the ability to switch from one personality to another voluntarily.
   c. for her to select which personality she wants to be her dominant self.
   d. for her to recognize that the various personalities exist.

4. The ultimate goal of therapy will most likely be achieved through:
   a. crisis intervention and directed association.
   b. psychotherapy and hypnosis.
   c. psychoanalysis and free association.
   d. insight psychotherapy and dextroamphetamines.

5. Which of the following is an appropriate nursing intervention for controlling the behavior of the "suicidal personality," Beth?
   a. When Beth emerges, put the patient in restraints.
   b. Keep Ellen in isolation during her hospitalization.
   c. Make a verbal contract with Ellen that Beth will do no harm.
   d. Elicit the help of another, strong-willed personality to help control Beth's behavior.

The following are general questions related to dissociative disorders:

6. Which of the following nursing interventions is most appropriate for the nurse working with the patient experiencing psychogenic amnesia?
   a. Use the technique of implosion therapy (flooding) to help the patient remember.
   b. Use hypnosis to help the patient remember.
   c. Expose the patient to stimuli that represent pleasant memories from the past.
   d. Expose the patient to stimuli that represent the painful stimuli for which the amnesia is providing the protection.

7. The nurse should understand that, when an individual awakens from a fugue state, he or she:
   a. will have no memory for what occurred during the fugue.
   b. will remember everything that occurred during the fugue.
   c. will have no memory of life before the fugue occurred.
   d. will have total recall of the time before and during the fugue.

8. Bob was driving his automobile that was involved in an accident in which his wife and child were killed. Unable to carry on with his life, he has sought emotional help. He says to the nurse, "I don't know how I managed to make all the funeral arrangements. At times it seemed as though I was an outside observer of everything that was happening." What is this phenomenon called?
   a. Derealization
   b. Abreaction
   c. Depersonalization
   d. Psychosis

9. Bob continues, "At other times, when I was with a group of people, it would appear as though everyone was moving in slow motion." What is this phenomenon called?
   a. Derealization
   b. Abreaction
   c. Depersonalization
   d. Psychosis

10. Which of the following examples of Bob's situation describes selective amnesia?
    a. Bob was unable to remember anything having to do with the accident until 3 days after the accident.
    b. Bob could not remember the accident but remembered hearing the ambulance siren and being admitted to the emergency room.
    c. Bob is unable to remember anything that has happened during his entire lifetime.
    d. Bob can remember nothing from the time of the accident to the present.

REFERENCES

Allison, R. B. (1984). A new treatment approach for multiple personalities. *Am J Clin Hypn, 17*(1): 15–32.

American Psychiatric Association. (1987). *Diagnostic and statistical manual of mental disorders* (3rd ed., rev.). Washington, DC: American Psychiatric Association.

Benjamin, R. (1990, March). In N. E. Gupta, Who Am I? *Ladies Home Journal, CVII*(3): 233.

Berger, D. M. (1985). Dissociative disorders. In S. E. Greben, Rakoff, V. M. and Voineskos, G. (Eds.), *A method of psychiatry* (2nd ed.). Philadelphia: Lea & Febiger.

Braun, B. G. (1985). The transgenerational incidence of dissociation and multiple personality disorder: A preliminary report. In R. P. Kluft (Ed.), *Childhood antecedents of multiple personality.* Washington, DC: American Psychiatric Press.

Braun, B. G. (1986). *Treatment of multiple personality disorder.* Washington, DC: American Psychiatric Press.

Confer, W. N. & Ables, B. S. (1983). *Multiple personality: Etiology, diagnosis, and treatment.* New York: Human Sciences Press.

Freud, S. (1962). The neuro-psychoses of defense (1894). In J. Strachey (Ed.), *Standard edition of the complete psychological works of Sigmund Freud, vol. 3.* London: Hogarth Press. (Original work published 1894)

Freud, S. (1964). Splitting of the ego in the process of defense. In J. Strachey (Ed.), *Standard edition of the complete psychological works of Sigmund Freud, vol. 22.* London: Hogarth Press. (Original work published 1940)

Gupta, N. E. (1990, March). Who Am I? *Ladies Home Journal CVII*(3): 161, 233–237.

Horton, P. C. & Miller, D. H. (1972). The etiology of multiple personality. *Comprehensive psychiatry. 13*(2): 151–159.

Janet, P. (1907). *The major symptoms of hysteria.* New York: Macmillan.

Kluft, R. P. (1984). Multiple personality in childhood. *Psychiatr Clin North Am, 7:* 121–134.

Kluft, R. P. (1987). Multiple personality disorder: An update. *Hosp Community Psychiatry, 38:* 363–373.

Kluft, R. P. (1988). The dissociative disorders. In Talbott, Hales, & Yudofsky (Eds.), *Textbook of psychiatry.* Washington, DC: American Psychiatric Press.

Kolb, L. C. & Brodie, H. K. H. (1982). *Modern clinical psychiatry* (10th ed.). Philadelphia: WB Saunders.

Marciniak, R. D. (1985). Other psychiatric disorders. In J. I. Walker (Ed.), *Essentials of clinical psychiatry.* Philadelphia: JB Lippincott.

Nemiah, J. C. (1989). Dissociative disorders (hysterical neuroses, dissociative type). In H. I. Kaplan & B. J. Sadock (Eds.), *Comprehensive textbook of psychiatry* (5th ed., Vol. I). Baltimore: Williams & Wilkins.

O'Regan, B. & Hurley, T. J. (1985). Multiple personality—Mirrors of a new model of mind? *Investigations, 1*(3/4): 1–23, Sausalito, CA: The Institute of Noetic Sciences.

Purcell, S. D. (1988). Dissociative disorders. In H. H. Goldman (Ed.), *Review of general psychiatry* (2nd ed.). Norwalk, CT: Appleton & Lange.

Schenk, L. & Bear, D. (1981). Multiple personality and related dissociative phenomena in patients with temporal lobe epilepsy. *Am J Psychiatry, 138:* 1311–1316.

BIBLIOGRAPHY

Townsend, M. C. (1991). *Nursing diagnoses in psychiatric nursing: A pocket guide for care plan construction* (2nd ed.). Philadelphia: FA Davis.

SEXUAL DISORDERS

KEY TERMS
anorgasmia
dyspareunia
exhibitionism
fetishism
frotteurism
gonorrhea
homosexuality
lesbianism
masochism
orgasm
paraphilia
pedophilia
premature ejaculation
retarded ejaculation
sadism
sensate focus
syphilis
transsexualism
transvestic fetishism
vaginismus
voyeurism

OBJECTIVES

After reading this chapter, the student will be able to:

1. Describe developmental processes associated with human sexuality.
2. Discuss historical and epidemiological aspects of paraphilias.
3. Identify various types of paraphilias.
4. Discuss predisposing factors associated with the etiology of paraphilias.
5. Describe the physiology of the human sexual response.
6. Discuss historical and epidemiological aspects of sexual dysfunction.
7. Identify various types of sexual dysfunction.
8. Discuss predisposing factors associated with the etiology of sexual dysfunction.
9. Conduct a sexual history.
10. Formulate nursing diagnoses and goals of care for patients with sexual disorders.
11. Describe appropriate nursing interventions for patients with sexual disorders.
12. Evaluate nursing care of patients with sexual disorders.
13. Identify various treatment modalities for patients with sexual disorders.
14. Discuss alternative sexual life-styles.
15. Identify various types of sexually transmitted diseases and discuss the consequences of each.

INTRODUCTION

Human beings are sexual beings. Sexuality is a basic need and an aspect of humanness that cannot be separated from life events (Hogan, 1980). It influences our thoughts, actions, and interactions and is involved in aspects of physical and mental health.

Society's attitude toward sexuality is changing. Patients are more open to seeking assistance in matters that pertain to sexuality. Although not all nurses need to be educated as sex therapists, they can readily integrate information on sexuality in the care they give by focusing on preventive, therapeutic, and educational interventions to help individuals attain, regain, or maintain sexual health.

This chapter focuses on disorders associated with sexual function. Primary consideration is given to the categories of paraphilias and sexual dysfunction, as classified in the *Diagnostic and Statistical Manual of Mental Disorders, ed 3, revised* (*DSM-III-R*) (American Psychiatric Association [APA], 1987). An overview of human sexual development throughout the life span is presented. Historical and epidemiological information associated with sexual disorders is included. Predisposing

factors that have been implicated in the etiology of sexual disorders provide a framework for studying the dynamics of paraphilias and disorders of sexual function. Various medical treatment modalities are explored. A discussion of alternative sexual life-styles is included. Various types of sexually transmitted diseases are described, and an explanation of the consequences of each is presented.

Symptomatology of each disorder is presented as background knowledge for assessing patients with sexual disorders. A tool for acquiring a sexual history is included. Nursing care is described in the context of the nursing process.

DEVELOPMENT OF HUMAN SEXUALITY

Birth Through Age 12

Although the sexual identity of an infant is determined prior to birth by chromosomal factors and physical appearance of the genitals, postnatal factors can greatly influence the way in which developing children perceive themselves sexually. Masculinity and femininity, as well as sex roles, are by and large culturally defined. For example, pink rooms or blue rooms, frilly, delicate dresses or tough, sturdy rompers initiate the differentiation of roles at birth.

It is not uncommon for infants to touch and explore their genitals. In fact, research on infantile sexuality indicates that both male and female infants are capable of sexual arousal and orgasm (Katchadourian & Lunde, 1975).

By age 2 or 2½, children know what gender they are (Hyde, 1986). They know that they are like the parent of the same gender and different from the parent of the opposite gender and from other children of the opposite gender. They become aware of differences in the genital region and differences in positions during urination (Martinson, 1973).

By age 4 or 5, children engage in heterosexual play. "Playing doctor" can be a popular game at this age. They form a concept of marriage to a member of the opposite gender.

Children increasingly gain experience with masturbation during childhood, although certainly not all children masturbate during this period. In a study of college students, 15 percent of the men and 20 percent of the women recalled that their first masturbation experiences occurred between ages 5 and 8 (Arafat & Cotton, 1974).

Late childhood and preadolescence may be characterized by homosexual play (Martinson, 1973). Generally, the activity involves no more than touching the other's genitals. Girls at this age become interested in menstruation, and both sexes are interested in learning about fertility, pregnancy, and birth. Interest in the opposite sex increases. Children of this age become self-conscious about their bodies and are concerned with physical attractiveness.

Children aged 10 to 12 are preoccupied with pubertal changes and the beginnings of romantic interest in the opposite gender. Prepubescent boys may engage in group sexual activities, such as genital exhibition or group masturbation. Homosexual sex play is not uncommon (Hogan, 1980). Prepubescent girls may engage in some genital exhibition but are usually not as preoccupied with the genitalia as boys of this age (Rosenbaum, 1976).

Adolescence

Adolescence represents an acceleration in terms of biological changes and psychosocial and sexual development. This time of turmoil is nurtured by awakening endocrine forces and a wide variety of psychosocial tasks demanding mastery (Kolodny

et al, 1979). Included in these tasks are issues relating to sexuality, such as how to deal with new or more powerful sexual feelings, whether to participate in various types of sexual behavior, how to recognize love, how to prevent unwanted pregnancy, and how to define age-appropriate sex roles.

Biologically, puberty begins for the female adolescent with breast enlargement, widening of the hips, and growth of pubic and ancillary hair. The onset of menstruation usually occurs between the ages of 11 and 13 years. In the male adolescent, growth of pubic hair and enlargement of the testicles begin at 12 to 16 years of age. Penile growth and the ability to ejaculate usually occur from the ages of 13 to 17. There is a marked growth of the body between ages 11 and 17, accompanied by the growth of body and facial hair, increased muscle mass, and a deeper voice (Hogan, 1980).

Sexuality is slower to develop in the female than in the male adolescent. Women show steady increases in sexual responsiveness that peak in their middle 20s or early 30s. Men reach the sexual acme of their lives during adolescence (Hogan, 1980). Masturbation is a common sexual activity among male adolescents. Studies indicate that nearly all males and almost two-thirds of females have masturbated to orgasm by the time they complete adolescence (Kinsey, Pomeroy, & Martin, 1948).

Many individuals have their first experience with sexual intercourse during the adolescent years. Although studies indicate a variety of statistics related to incidence of adolescent coitus, three notable trends have become evident during the past 2 decades. They are:

1. More adolescents are engaging in premarital intercourse.
2. The incidence of premarital intercourse for females has increased.
3. The average age of first intercourse is decreasing (Hyde, 1986).

The American culture has ambivalent feelings toward adolescent sexuality. Psychosexual development is desired, but parents want to avoid anything that may encourage teenage sex (Reiss, 1976).

Adulthood

This period of the life cycle begins at approximately 20 years of age and continues to age 65. Sexuality associated with ages 65 and older will be discussed in Chapter 27.

MARITAL SEX

Choosing a marital partner or developing a sexual relationship with another individual is one of the major tasks in the early years of this life-cycle stage. It is clear from the perspective of the 1980s that the institution of marriage has survived (Hyde, 1986). About 80 percent to 90 percent of all people in the United States marry, and of those who divorce, a high percentage remarry. Intimacy in marriage is one of the most common forms of sexual expressions for adults. The average American couple has coitus about two or three times per week when they are in their 20s, with the frequency gradually declining to about once per week for those aged 45 and older (Hyde, 1986). Many adults continue to masturbate even though they are married and have ready access to heterosexual sex. This behavior is perfectly normal, although it often evokes feelings of guilt and may be done secretly.

EXTRAMARITAL SEX

Approximately one-half of all married men have extramarital sex at some time in their lives compared with about one-quarter of all women (Hyde, 1986). Although the incidence of extramarital sex for men seems to be holding constant, the incidence for women is increasing and may be approaching the rate for men (Thompson, 1983).

Although attitudes toward premarital sex have changed substantially during the past several decades, attitudes toward extramarital sex have remained relatively stable. Between 80 percent and 98 percent of both women and men say they would object if their spouse engaged in sexual activity with someone else (Hyde, 1986).

SEX AND THE SINGLE PERSON

Attitudes about sexual intimacy among singles—never married, divorced, widowed—vary from individual to individual. Some are looking for any kind of relationship, casual or committed, to enrich their lives. Others vehemently deny any desire for marriage or sexual intimacy (Hogan, 1980).

Never-married singles may find their life-style exciting and enjoy its freedom, with no intention of ever marrying. Others may be desperately searching for a spouse, with the desperation increasing as the years wear on.

Most divorced women, but fewer widowed women, return to having an active sex life following separation from, or loss of, their spouse. Virtually all divorced and widowed men return to an active sex life (Hyde, 1986).

THE "MIDDLE" YEARS—46 to 65

With the advent of the middle years, a decrease in hormonal production initiates a number of changes in the sex organs, as well as the rest of the body. The average age of onset of menopause for women is around 50, although changes can be noted from about age 46 to 60 (Hogan, 1980). This decrease in the amount of estrogen can result in loss of vaginal lubrication, making intercourse painful. Other symptoms may include insomnia, "hot flashes," headaches, heart palpitations, and depression. Hormonal supplements may alleviate some of these symptoms.

With the decrease of androgen production during these years, men also experience sexual changes. The amount of ejaculate may decrease and ejaculation may be less forceful. The testes decrease in size, and erections may be less frequent and less rigid. By age 50, the refractory period increases, and men may require 8 to 24 hours after orgasm before another erection can be achieved (Masters & Johnson, 1966).

Biological drives decrease, and interest in sexual activity may decrease during these "middle" years. Although men need longer stimulation to reach orgasm and intensity of pleasure may decrease, women stabilize at the same level of sexual activity as at the previous stage in the life cycle (Hogan, 1980). Both sexes should continue sexual activity, since long sexual abstinence decreases sexual functioning (Masters & Johnson, 1966).

SEXUAL DISORDERS

Paraphilias

The term *paraphilia* is used to identify repetitive or preferred sexual fantasies or behaviors that involve any of the following:

1. The preference for use of a nonhuman object.
2. Repetitive sexual activity with humans involving real or simulated suffering or humiliation.
3. Repetitive sexual activity with nonconsenting partners (Abel, 1989).

The *DSM-III-R* specifies that these sexual fantasies or behaviors must persist for at least 6 months. It also requires that the individual repeatedly act on these urges or be markedly distressed by them (APA, 1987).

HISTORICAL ASPECTS

Historically, it seems, some restrictions on human sexual expression have always existed. Sexual prohibitions provide possible containment for sexuality's potentially disruptive power (Abel, 1989). Under the code of Orthodox Judaism, masturbation was punishable by death. Ancient Catholicism considered it a carnal sin. In the late 19th century, this activity was viewed as a major cause of insanity.

Pedophilia, the sexual exploitation of children, was condemned in ancient cultures, as it continues to be today. Incest remains the one taboo that crosses cultural barriers. It was punishable by death in Babylonia, Judea, and ancient China, and offenders were handed the death penalty as late as 1650 in England (Abel, 1989).

Oral-genital, anal, homosexual, and animal sexual contacts were viewed by the early Christian church as unnatural and, in fact, as greater transgressions than extramarital sexual activity because they did not lead to biological reproduction (Abel, 1989). Today, of these church-condemned, non-procreative behaviors, only sex with animals (zoophilia) retains its classification as a paraphilia in the *DSM-III-R*.

EPIDEMIOLOGICAL STATISTICS

Relatively limited data exist on the prevalence or course of the paraphilias. Most information that is available has been obtained from studies of incarcerated sex offenders. Another source of information has been from outpatient psychiatric services for paraphiliacs outside the criminal justice system.

Because few paraphiliacs experience personal distress from their behavior, most individuals come for treatment due to pressure from their partners or the authorities (Becker & Kavoussi, 1988). Data suggest that the majority of paraphiliacs seeking outpatient treatment do so for pedophilia (45 percent), exhibitionism (25 percent), or voyeurism (12 percent).

The majority of individuals with paraphilias are men, and more than 50 percent of these individuals develop the onset of their paraphilic arousal prior to age 18 (Becker & Kavoussi, 1988). The behavior peaks between ages 15 and 25 and gradually declines, so that by age 50, the occurrence of paraphilic acts is very low, except for those paraphilic behaviors that occur in isolation or with a cooperative partner. Some individuals with these disorders experience multiple paraphilias (Abel et al, 1985).

TYPES OF PARAPHILIAS

The following types of paraphilias are identified by the *DSM-III-R*:

Exhibitionism Exhibitionism is characterized by recurrent, intense sexual urges and sexually arousing fantasies, of at least 6 months' duration, involving the exposure of one's genitals to a stranger (APA, 1987). Masturbation may occur during the exhibitionism. The condition apparently only occurs in men, and the victims are women in 99 percent of the cases (Abel, 1989).

The exhibitionist's urges to expose himself intensify when he has excessive free time or is under significant stress (Abel, 1989). Most exhibitionists have rewarding sexual relationships with adult partners but concomitantly expose themselves to other women.

Fetishism Fetishism involves recurrent, intense sexual urges and sexually arousing fantasies, of at least 6 months' duration, involving the use of non-living objects (APA, 1987). Common fetish objects include bras, women's underpants, stockings, shoes, boots, or other wearing apparel. The fetish object is generally used during masturbation or incorporated into sexual activity with another person to produce sexual excitation.

When the fetish involves cross-dressing, the disorder is called *transvestic fetishism*. The individual is a heterosexual man who keeps a collection of women's clothes that he intermittently uses to cross-dress when alone. While cross-dressed, he usually masturbates and imagines other men being attracted to him as a woman in his female attire (APA, 1987).

Requirement of the fetish object for sexual arousal may become so intense in some individuals that to be without it may result in impotence. Onset of the disorder usually occurs during adolescence.

The disorder is chronic, and the complication arises when the individual becomes progressively more intensely aroused to sexual behaviors that exclude a sexual partner. Distancing between the paraphiliac and his partner may result to the point that the partner eventually terminates the relationship.

In addition to their fetishism, significant numbers of fetishists are concomitantly or have previously been involved in exhibitionism, frotteurism, pedophilia, rape, or voyeurism (Abel, 1989).

Frotteurism Frotteurism is defined as the recurrent preoccupation with intense sexual urges or fantasies of at least 6 months' duration involving touching or rubbing against a nonconsenting person (APA, 1987). Sexual excitement is derived from the actual touching or rubbing, not from the coercive nature of the act.

The individual usually chooses to commit the act in crowded places, such as on buses or subways during rush hour. In this way, he can provide rationalization for his behavior should someone complain, and more easily escape arrest. The frotteur waits in a crowd until he identifies a victim, follows her and allows the rush of the crowd to push him against her. He fantasizes a relationship with his victim while rubbing his genitals against her thighs and buttocks, or touching her genitalia or breasts with his hands. He often escapes detection due to the victim's initial shock and denial that such an act has been committed in this public place.

Significant numbers of frotteurs are concomitantly or have previously been involved in exhibitionism, pedophilia, sadism, rape, or voyeurism (Abel, 1989).

Pedophilia The *DSM-III-R* describes the essential feature of this disorder as recurrent sexual urges and sexually arousing fantasies, of at least 6 months' duration, involving sexual activity with a prepubescent child. The age of the molester is 16 or older, and is at least 5 years older than the child. This category of paraphilia is the most common of sexual assaults (Abel, 1989).

The majority of child molestations involve genital fondling or oral sex. Vaginal or anal penetration of the child is most common in cases of incest (Abel, 1989). Others may limit their activity to undressing the child and looking, exposing themselves, masturbating in the presence of the child, or gentle touching and fondling of the child (APA, 1987).

Onset usually occurs during adolescence, and the disorder often runs a chronic course, particularly with male pedophiles who demonstrate a preference for male children. A significant number of pedophiles are concomitantly or have previously been involved in exhibitionism, voyeurism, or rape (Abel, 1989).

Sexual Masochism The identifying feature of this disorder is recurrent, intense sexual urges and sexually arousing fantasies, of at least 6 months' duration, involving the act (real, not simulated) of being humiliated, beaten, bound, or otherwise made to suffer (APA, 1987). These masochistic activities may be fantasized (e.g., being raped), solitary (e.g., self-inflicted pain), or with a partner (e.g., being restrained, spanked, or beaten by the partner). Some masochistic activities have resulted in death, in particular those that involve sexual arousal by oxygen deprivation.

The disorder is usually chronic and can progress to the point at which the individual is unable to achieve sexual satisfaction without masochistic fantasies or activities. A significant number of masochists are concomitantly or have previously been involved in exhibitionism, pedophilia, rape, or transvestism (Abel, 1989).

Sexual Sadism The *DSM-III-R* identifies the essential feature of this disorder as recurrent, intense, sexual urges and sexually arousing fantasies, of at least 6 months' duration, involving acts (real, not simulated) in which the psychological or physical suffering (including humiliation) of the victim is sexually exciting (APA, 1987). The sadistic activities may be fantasized or acted upon with a consenting or nonconsenting partner. In all instances, sexual excitation occurs in response to the suffering of the victim. Examples of sadistic acts include restraint, beating, burning, rape, cutting, torture, and even killing.

The course of the disorder is usually chronic, with the severity of the sadistic acts often increasing over time. Activities with nonconsenting partners are usually terminated by legal apprehension. A significant number of sadists are concomitantly or have previously been involved in exhibitionism, frotteurism, pedophilia, rape, or voyeurism (Abel, 1989).

Voyeurism This disorder is identified by recurrent, intense sexual urges and sexually arousing fantasies, of at least 6 months' duration, involving the act of observing unsuspecting people, usually strangers, who are either naked, in the process of disrobing, or engaging in sexual activity (APA, 1987). Sexual excitement is achieved through the act of looking, and no contact with the person is attempted. Masturbation usually accompanies the window peeping but may occur later as the individual fantasizes about the voyeuristic act.

Onset of voyeuristic behavior usually occurs before age 15, and the disorder often runs a chronic course. Most individuals who engage in voyeurism enjoy satisfying sexual relationships with an adult partner. Few apprehensions occur because most targets of voyeurism are unaware that they are being observed. In addition to their voyeurism, a significant number of voyeurs are concomitantly or have previously been involved in exhibitionism, frotteurism, pedophilia, rape, or sadism (Abel, 1989).

PREDISPOSING FACTORS TO PARAPHILIAS

Biological Factors Various studies have implicated several organic factors in the etiology of paraphilias. Destruction of parts of the limbic system in animals has been shown to cause hypersexual behavior (Becker & Kavoussi, 1988). Temporal lobe diseases, such as psychomotor seizures or temporal lobe tumors, have been implicated in some paraphiliacs. Abnormal levels of androgens also may contribute to inappropriate sexual arousal. The results of these studies are inconclusive at this time. The majority were conducted with violent sex offenders and cannot accurately be generalized specifically to paraphiliacs (Bradford & McLean, 1984).

Psychoanalytic Theory The psychoanalytic approach defines a paraphiliac as one who has failed the normal developmental process toward heterosexual adjustment (Abel, 1989). This occurs when the individual fails to resolve the oedipal crisis and either identifies with the parent of the opposite gender or selects an inappropriate object for libido cathexis. Becker and Kavoussi (1988) offer the following explanation:

> "Severe castration anxiety during the oedipal phase of development leads to the substitution of a symbolic object (inanimate or an anatomic part) for the mother, as in fetishism and transvestism. Similarly, anxiety over arousal to the mother can lead to the choice of 'safe,' inappropriate sexual partners, as in pedophilia and zoophilia, or 'safe' sexual behaviors in which there is no sexual contact, as in exhibitionism and voyeurism."

Behavioral Theory The behavioral model hypothesizes that whether or not an individual engages in paraphiliac behavior depends on the type of reinforcement he receives following the behavior. Abel (1989) suggests that the initial act may be committed for various reasons. Some examples include recalled memories of experiences from an individual's early life (especially the first shared sexual experience), modeling behavior of others who have carried out paraphilic acts, mimicking sexual behavior depicted in the media, and sometimes recalling emotional events from the past, such as one's own molestation.

Once the initial act has been committed, a conscious evaluation of the behavior occurs and a choice is made of whether or not to repeat it. Fear of punishment or perceived harm or injury to the victim, or a lack of pleasure following the experience may all lead to nonrecurrence of the paraphilic act. However, when negative consequences do not occur, when the act itself is highly pleasurable, or when the paraphilic person immediately escapes and thereby avoids seeing any negative consequences experienced by the victim, the activity is more likely to be repeated (Abel, 1989).

Transactional Model of Stress/Adaptation In some individuals, paraphilic arousal occurs during periods of stress and conflict. The etiology of paraphilias most likely is influenced by multiple factors. In Figure 23.1, a graphic depiction of this theory of multiple causation is presented in the Transactional Model of Stress/Adaptation.

TREATMENT MODALITIES

Biological Treatment Biological treatment of paraphilias has focused on blocking or decreasing

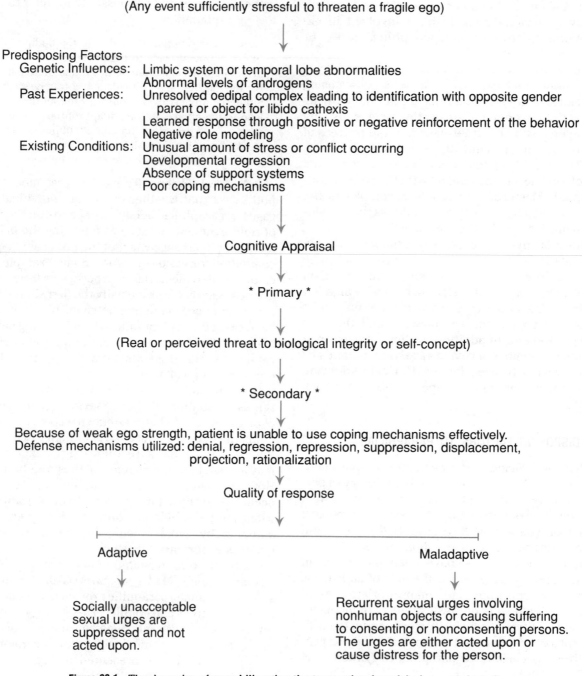

Precipitating Event
(Any event sufficiently stressful to threaten a fragile ego)

Predisposing Factors
    Genetic Influences: Limbic system or temporal lobe abnormalities
                           Abnormal levels of androgens
    Past Experiences: Unresolved oedipal complex leading to identification with opposite gender
                               parent or object for libido cathexis
                           Learned response through positive or negative reinforcement of the behavior
                           Negative role modeling
    Existing Conditions: Unusual amount of stress or conflict occurring
                           Developmental regression
                           Absence of support systems
                           Poor coping mechanisms

Cognitive Appraisal

* Primary *

(Real or perceived threat to biological integrity or self-concept)

* Secondary *

Because of weak ego strength, patient is unable to use coping mechanisms effectively.
Defense mechanisms utilized: denial, regression, repression, suppression, displacement,
projection, rationalization

Quality of response

Adaptive   Maladaptive

Socially unacceptable   Recurrent sexual urges involving
sexual urges are   nonhuman objects or causing suffering
suppressed and not   to consenting or nonconsenting persons.
acted upon.   The urges are either acted upon or
                               cause distress for the person.

Figure 23.1   The dynamics of paraphilia using the transactional model of stress/adaptation.

the level of circulating androgens. The most extensively used of the antiandrogenic medications are the progestin derivatives that block testosterone synthesis (Becker & Kavoussi, 1988). They do not influence the direction of sexual drive toward appropriate adult partners. Instead they act to decrease libido and thus break the individual's pattern of compulsive deviant sexual behavior (Becker & Kavoussi, 1988). They are not meant to be the sole source of treatment and work best when given in conjunction with the paraphiliac's participation in individual or group psychotherapy.

Psychoanalytic Therapy Psychoanalytic approaches have been tried in the treatment of paraphilias. In this type of therapy, the therapist assists the patient to identify unresolved conflicts and traumas from early childhood. The therapy focuses on helping the individual resolve these early conflicts, thus relieving the anxiety that prevents him or her from forming appropriate sexual relationships. In turn, the individual has no further need for paraphilic fantasies.

Behavioral Therapy Aversion techniques have been used to modify undesirable behavior. Aversion therapy methods in the treatment of paraphilias have included the use of electric shock and chemical induction of nausea and vomiting, usually in combination with exposure to photographs depicting the undesired behavior (Kolodny et al, 1979).

Other behavioral approaches to decreasing inappropriate sexual arousal have included covert sensitization and satiation. With covert sensitization, the individual combines inappropriate sexual fantasies with aversive, anxiety-provoking scenes under the guidance of the therapist (Becker & Kavoussi, 1988). Satiation is a technique in which the postorgasmic individual repeatedly fantasizes deviant behaviors to the point of saturation with the deviant stimuli, consequently making the fantasies and behavior boring (Marshall & Barbaree, 1978).

ROLE OF THE NURSE

Treatment of the paraphiliac is often very frustrating for both the patient and the therapist. Most paraphiliacs deny that they have a problem and seek psychiatric care only after their inappropriate behavior comes to the attention of others. In secondary prevention, the focus is to diagnose and treat the problem as early as possible, so that difficulties are minimized. These individuals should be referred to specialists who are accustomed to working with this very special population.

Nursing may best become involved in the primary prevention process. The focus of primary prevention in sexual disorders is to intervene in home life or other facets of childhood in an effort to prevent problems from developing. An additional concern of primary prevention is to assist in the development of adaptive coping strategies to deal with stressful life situations.

Bancroft (1978) has suggested that there are three components of sexual development. A disturbance in one or more of these components in development might lead to a variety of sexual deviations. These three components include:

1. Gender identity — the sense of maleness or femaleness developed in early childhood.
2. Sexual responsiveness — arousal to appropriate stimuli.
3. Formation of relationships with others.

Different developmental components seem to be disturbed in the various sexual deviations. For example, gender identity may be disturbed in transvestism or transsexualism. The second component, sexual responsiveness to appropriate stimuli, is disturbed in the case of the fetishist. In the case of the exhibitionist or the frotteur, the ability to form relationships is disturbed.

Nurses can participate in the regular evaluation of these developmental components to assure that as children mature, their development in each of these three components is healthy, thereby preventing deviant sexual behaviors. Nurses who work in pediatrics, psychiatry, public health, ambulatory clinics, schools, and any other facility requiring contact with children must be knowledgeable about human sexual development. Accurate assessment and early intervention by these nurses can contribute a great deal toward primary prevention of sexual disorders.

Sexual Dysfunctions

THE SEXUAL RESPONSE CYCLE

An understanding of anatomy and physiology is a prerequisite to considerations of pathology and treatment. The sexual response cycle is fundamentally the same for men and women. Although most physiologists describe four phases in the cycle, the *DSM-III-R* identifies an additional stage (appetitive) that is distinctly psychological in nature.

Phase I: Appetitive   This phase is distinct from any identified solely through physiology and reflects the psychiatrist's fundamental concern with motivations, drives, and personality (Sadock, 1989). This phase is characterized by sexual fantasies and the desire for sexual activity.

Phase II: Excitement   Excitation occurs as a result of sexual stimulation, which may be either physical or psychological in origin (Kolodny et al, 1979).

The Female Response   The initial response to sexual stimulation in women is vaginal lubrication. Vasocongestion results in enlargement of the labia and clitoris. There is an elongation and ballooning of the vagina, and its color turns a deep purple. Nipples of the breast become erect.

The Male Response   Men's first physiological response to sexual stimulation is penile erection, which occurs as a direct result of vasocongestive changes within the spongelike tissue of the penis (Kolodny et al, 1979). This is followed by a tightening and lifting of the scrotal sac and an enlargement and elevation of the testes.

Phase III: Plateau   This phase is a continuation of the processes of vasoconstriction and myotonia begun in the excitement phase. Both men and women experience a significant increase in the heart and respiration rates, and in blood pressure.

The Female Response   In women, the most notable change during the plateau phase is a swelling of the tissues surrounding the outer third of the vagina. The size of the vaginal entrance actually becomes smaller, and there may be a noticeable increase in gripping of the penis. This change is called the orgasmic platform (Hyde, 1986).

The Male Response   The plateau phase in men is characterized by a slight swelling and deepening of the reddish purple color of the glans penis. The testes may be 50 percent larger than in the unaroused state. A few drops of fluid, probably secreted by the Cowper's glands, may appear at the tip of the penis. Although this fluid is not the ejaculate, it may contain active sperm (Hyde, 1986).

Phase IV: Orgasm   Orgasm is identified as a peaking of sexual pleasure, with release of sexual tension and rhythmic contraction of the perineal muscles and pelvic reproductive organs (APA, 1987). The pulse increases to more than twice its usual rate. Respirations may rise to three times the usual rate, and blood pressure increases by 30 to 100 mm Hg systolic and 20 to 50 mg Hg diastolic (usually higher in men than in women) (Hogan, 1980).

The Female Response   Orgasm in women is marked by simultaneous rhythmic contractions of the uterus, the orgasmic platform, and the rectal sphincter (Kolodny et al, 1979).

The Male Response   The male orgasm begins with a series of contractions aimed at collecting seminal fluid from the prostate gland, the seminal vesicles, and the vas deferens. The sphincter of the neck of the urinary bladder closes tightly, and the collected fluid is propelled anteriorly by rhythmic contractions of the prostate, the perineal muscles, and the shaft of the penis.

Phase V: Resolution   If orgasm has occurred, this phase is characterized by disgorgement of blood from the genitalia (detumescence), creating a sense of general relaxation, well-being, and muscular relaxation. If orgasm does not occur, resolution may take 2 to 6 hours and be associated with irritability and discomfort (Sadock, 1989).

The Female Response   Women have the potential to be multiorgasmic — that is, to have a series of identifiable orgasmic responses without dropping below the plateau phase of arousal (Kolodny et al, 1979). Muscles and organs return to the prearousal state within a few minutes. However, unlike men, women experience no refractory period and may be able to respond to additional stimulation almost immediately (APA, 1987).

The Male Response   Following orgasm, detumescence results in rapid loss of the erection and a return of the scrotum and testes to their prearousal state. Following the resolution period, men have a refractory period that may last from several minutes to many hours. During that time, they cannot be stimulated to further orgasm (Sadock, 1989). For most men, this interval lengthens with age and is typically longer with each repeated ejaculation within a time span of several hours (Kolodny et al, 1979).

HISTORICAL AND EPIDEMIOLOGICAL ASPECTS RELATED TO SEXUAL DYSFUNCTION

Concurrent with the cultural changes occurring during the sexual revolution of the 1960s and 1970s came an increase in scientific research into sexual physiology and sexual dysfunctions. Masters and

Johnson (1966; 1970) pioneered this work with their studies on human sexual response and the treatment of sexual dysfunctions. Sadock (1989) states:

"Historically, problems of sexual conflict and sexual dysfunction have always been the province of psychiatry. Problems of dysfunction are particularly distressing to patients and have often been resistant to treatment. The current approach to sexual dysfunctions reflects the cultural and scientific developments of recent years, the development of specific techniques for the treatment of these problems, the historical interest of psychiatry in this area, and the recognition of its importance in psychiatric practice."

Sexual dysfunction consists of an impairment or disturbance in any of the phases of the sexual response cycle. No one knows exactly how many people experience sexual dysfunctions. Knowledge exists only about those who seek some kind of treatment for the problem, and they may be few in number compared with those who have a dysfunction but suffer quietly and never seek therapy (Hyde, 1986).

A number of studies have revealed a variety of statistics. Frank et al (1978), in a survey of 100 well-educated, reportedly happily married couples, reported the information presented in Table 23.1. Masters and Johnson (1970) reported that 50 percent of all American couples suffer from some type of sexual dysfunction. A study by Robins et al (1984) estimated that 24 percent of the U.S. population will experience a sexual dysfunction at some time in their lives. Finally, Nathan (1986) conducted an analysis of the results of 22 surveys within the general population in an effort to estimate prevalence rates for the various sexual dysfunctions. The results of this study are presented in Table 23.2.

Table 23.1 SURVEY OF SEXUAL DYSFUNCTION

Sexual Dysfunctions	Men (n=100)	Women (n=100)
Erectile or ejaculatory dysfunctions	40%	
Arousal or orgasmic dysfunctions		63%
Other sexual difficulties (e.g., lack of interest or inability to relax)	50%	77%

Source: Frank et al (1978).

Table 23.2 ESTIMATES OF PREVALENCE* RATES FOR SEXUAL DYSFUNCTIONS—AN ANALYSIS OF THE LITERATURE

Disorder	Men	Women
Sexual desire disorders		
Hypoactive sexual desire disorder	1%–15%	1%–35%
Sexual arousal disorders		
Male erectile disorder	10%–20%	
Orgasm disorders		
Inhibited female orgasm		5%–30%
Inhibited male orgasm	5%	
Premature ejaculation	35%	

*This "prevalence" rate refers to an estimate of the number of people who have a disorder at any given time.
Source: Nathan (1986).

TYPES OF SEXUAL DYSFUNCTION

Sexual Desire Disorders

Hypoactive Sexual Desire Disorder   This disorder is defined by the *DSM-III-R* (APA, 1987) as a persistent or recurrent deficiency or absence of sexual fantasies and desire for sexual activity. The judgment of deficiency or absence is made by the clinician, taking into account factors that affect sexual functioning, such as age, sex, and the context of the person's life.

An individual's absolute level of sexual desire may not be the problem, but rather the problem may be a discrepancy between the partners' levels (Hyde, 1986). The conflict may occur if one partner wants sex more often than the other. Care must be taken not to label one partner as pathological when the problem actually lies in the discrepancy of sexual desire.

An estimated 20% of the total population has hypoactive sexual desire disorder (Sadock, 1989). The complaint is more common among women than men.

Sexual Aversion Disorder   This disorder is characterized by a persistent or recurrent extreme aversion to, and avoidance of, all or almost all genital sexual contact with a sexual partner. Whereas individuals displaying hypoactive desire are often neutral or indifferent toward sexual interaction, sexual aversion implies disgust, anxiety, or even panic responses to genital contact (Leiblum & Rosen, 1988).

Sexual Arousal Disorders

Female Sexual Arousal Disorder This disorder is identified in the *DSM-III-R* by one of the following criteria:

1. Persistent or recurrent partial or complete failure to attain or maintain the lubrication-swelling response of sexual excitement until completion of the sexual activity.
2. Persistent or recurrent lack of a subjective sense of sexual excitement and pleasure in a woman during sexual activity.

Male Sexual Arousal Disorder This disorder is also called erectile dysfunction or impotence. Either of the following criteria may be present to make this diagnosis (APA, 1987):

1. Persistent or recurrent partial or complete failure in a man to attain or maintain erection until completion of the sexual activity.
2. Persistent or recurrent lack of a subjective sense of sexual excitement and pleasure in a man during sexual activity.

Primary erectile dysfunction refers to cases in which the man has never been able to have intercourse; *secondary erectile dysfunction* refers to cases in which the man has difficulty getting or maintaining an erection but has been able to have vaginal or anal intercourse at least once (Hyde, 1986).

Orgasm Disorders

Inhibited Female Orgasm (Anorgasmia) This disorder is defined as the recurrent and persistent inhibition of the female orgasm, as manifested by the absence or delay of orgasm following a period of sexual excitement judged adequate in intensity and duration to produce such a response (APA, 1987). Women who are able to achieve orgasm through noncoital clitoral stimulation but are not able to experience it during coitus in the absence of manual clitoral stimulation are not necessarily categorized as anorgasmic (Sadock, 1989).

A woman is considered to have *primary orgasmic dysfunction* when she has never experienced orgasm by any kind of stimulation. *Secondary orgasmic dysfunction* exists if the woman has experienced at least one orgasm, regardless of the means of stimulation, but no longer does so.

Inhibited Male Orgasm (Retarded Ejaculation) With this disorder, the man is unable to ejaculate, even though he has a firm erection and has had more than adequate stimulation (Hyde, 1986). The severity of the problem may range from only occasional problems ejaculating (secondary disorder) to a history of never having experienced an orgasm (primary disorder). In the most common version, the man is incapable of ejaculating during coitus but may be able to ejaculate as a result of other types of stimulation.

Premature Ejaculation The *DSM-III-R* describes this disorder as persistent or recurrent ejaculation with minimal sexual stimulation or before, upon, or shortly after penetration and before the person wishes it. Diagnosis should take into account factors that affect duration of the excitement phase, such as age, novelty of the sexual partner or situation, and frequency of sexual activity (APA, 1987).

An estimated 30 percent of the male population has this dysfunction, and about 40 percent of men treated for sexual disorders have premature ejaculation as the chief complaint (Sadock, 1989). It is particularly common among young men who have a very high sex drive and have not yet learned to control ejaculation (Hyde, 1986).

Sexual Pain Disorders

Dyspareunia This disorder is defined as recurrent or persistent genital pain in either a man or women before, during, or after sexual intercourse, that is not associated with vaginismus or with lack of lubrication (APA, 1987). In women, the pain may be felt in the vagina, around the vaginal entrance and clitoris, or deep in the pelvis. In men, the pain is felt in the penis. Dyspareunia makes intercourse very unpleasant and may even lead to abstention from sexual activity (Hyde, 1986).

Prevalence studies of dyspareunia have provided estimates ranging from 8 percent to 33 percent in women and 1 percent in men (Wincze & Carey, 1991). Dyspareunia in men is often associated with urinary tract infection, with pain being experienced during urination as well as during ejaculation.

Vaginismus Vaginismus is an involuntary constriction of the outer one-third of the vagina that prevents penile insertion and intercourse (Sadock, 1989). On the basis of data obtained from infertility studies, Barnes (1981) suggests that vaginismus occurs in 5 out of every 1,000 women, a rate of 0.5 percent. It most often afflicts highly educated women and those in the higher socioeconomic groups (Sadock, 1989).

PREDISPOSING FACTORS TO SEXUAL DYSFUNCTIONS

Biological Factors

Sexual Desire Disorders A recent study has found markedly decreased levels of serum testosterone in men complaining of hypoactive sexual desire disorder (Sadock, 1989). There is also suggestive evidence of a relationship between serum testosterone and increased female libido (Segraves, 1988). Evidence of diminished libido has been observed in both men and women with elevated levels of serum prolactin (Segraves, 1988). Various medications have also been implicated in the etiology of hypoactive sexual desire disorder. Some examples include antihypertensives, antipsychotics, antidepressants, anxiolytics, and anticonvulsants. Alcohol and cocaine have also been associated with impaired desire, especially after chronic use (Abel, 1985).

Sexual Arousal Disorders Postmenopausal women require a longer period of stimulation for lubrication to occur, and there is generally less vaginal transudate after menopause (Sadock, 1989). Various medications, particularly those with antihistaminic and anticholinergic properties, may also contribute to decreased ability for arousal in women. Arteriosclerosis may be the most common cause of male erectile disorder as a result of arterial insufficiency (Wagner & Metz, 1981). Various neurological disorders can contribute to erectile dysfunctions as well. The most common neurologically based cause may be diabetes, which places men at high risk for neuropathy (Wincze & Carey, 1991). Others include temporal lobe epilepsy and multiple sclerosis. Trauma (e.g., spinal cord injury or pelvic cancer surgery) can also result in erectile dysfunction. Several medications have been implicated in the etiology of this disorder, including antihypertensives, antipsychotics, antidepressants, and anxiolytics. Chronic use of alcohol has also been shown to be a contributing factor.

Orgasm Disorders Results of research on the increased ability to achieve orgasm in posthysterectomy women by administering an estrogen-androgen hormone combination have been mixed (Wincze & Carey, 1991). Although the hormone replacement did influence sexual desire and arousal, effects on orgasmic ability remains unclear. In a study on female orgasmic response by Malatesta et al. (1982), acute alcohol intoxication was found to be associated with difficulty achieving orgasm, as well as a decreased subjective intensity of orgasm. Some medical conditions (e.g., hypothyroidism, diabetes mellitus, and hyperprolactinemia), as well as medications (e.g., antihypertensives, antidepressants), can affect a woman's ability to have orgasms (Sadock, 1989).

Biological factors associated with inhibited male orgasm include surgery of the genitourinary tract (e.g., prostatectomy), various neurological disorders (e.g., Parkinson's disease), and other diseases (e.g., diabetes mellitus). Various medications have been implicated, including antihypertensives, anticholinergics, and antipsychotics. Transient cases of the disorder may occur with excessive alcohol intake (Sadock, 1989).

Premature ejaculation is almost always caused by psychological rather than physical factors (Kaplan, 1974). However, particularly in cases of secondary dysfunction, in which a man at one time had ejaculatory control but later lost it, physical factors may occasionally be involved (Hyde, 1986). Examples include a local infection, such as prostatitis, or a degenerative neural disorder, such as multiple sclerosis.

Sexual Pain Disorders Various organic factors can cause painful intercourse in women (Marmor, 1976a). They include:

1. Disorders of the vaginal entrance: intact hymen or irritated remnants of the hymen, episiotomy scar, infection of the Bartholin's glands
2. Irritation or damage to the clitoris.
3. Disorders of the vagina: infections, allergies (e.g., to spermicides), senile vaginitis, surgical scarring (e.g., hysterectomy)
4. Pelvic disorders: infections, endometriosis, tumors, cysts

Painful intercourse in men may also be caused by various organic factors. For example, infection caused by poor hygiene under the foreskin of an uncircumsized man can cause pain. Phimosis, a condition in which the foreskin cannot be pulled back, can also cause painful intercourse (Hyde, 1986). An allergic reaction to various vaginal spermicides or irritation caused by vaginal infections may be a contributing factor. Finally, various prostate problems may cause pain on ejaculation (Hyde, 1986).

Psychosocial Factors

Sexual Desire Disorders LoPiccolo and Friedman (1988) have identified a number of individual and relationship causes of hypoactive sexual desire disorder. Individual causes include religious orthodoxy, obsessive-compulsive personality, conflicts with gender identity or sexual preference, sexual phobias, fear of losing control over sexual urges, secret sexual deviations, fear of pregnancy, "widower's syndrome" (inadequate grieving following the death of a spouse), depression, and aging-related concerns (e.g., changes in physical appearance). Among the relationship causes are lack of physical attraction to one's partner, poor sexual skills in the partner, conflict in the marriage, and fear of closeness (for fear of personal vulnerability or rejection).

Sadock (1989) describes the possible etiology of sexual aversion disorder as follows:

"The disorder may result from a traumatic sexual assault, such as rape or childhood abuse, from repeated painful experiences with coitus, and from early developmental conflicts that have left the patient with unconscious connections between the sexual impulse and overwhelming feelings of shame and guilt. The disorder may also be a reaction to a perceived psychological assault by one's partner and to relationship difficulties."

Sexual Arousal Disorders Tollison and Adams (1979) list the following psychological factors as possible impediments to female arousal: doubt, guilt, fear, anxiety, shame, conflict, embarrassment, tension, disgust, irritation, resentment, grief, hostility toward partner, and puritanical/moralistic upbringing. Clinical experience suggests that history of sexual abuse may also be an important etiological factor (Becker, 1989).

The etiology of male erectile disorder may be related to an inability to express the sexual impulse because of fear, anxiety, anger, or moral prohibition (Sadock, 1989). Developmental factors that hinder the ability to be intimate, that lead to a feeling of inadequacy or distrust, or that develop a sense of being unloving or unlovable may also result in impotence. Relationship factors that may af-

fect erectile functioning include lack of attraction to one's partner, anger toward one's partner, or being in a relationship that is not characterized by trust (Wincze & Carey, 1991). Unfortunately, regardless of the etiology of the impotence, once it occurs, the man may become increasingly anxious about his next sexual encounter. This anticipatory anxiety about achieving and maintaining an erection may then perpetuate the problem.

Orgasm Disorders Numerous psychological factors are associated with inhibited female orgasm. They include fears of becoming pregnant or rejection by the sexual partner, hostility toward men, and feelings of guilt regarding sexual impulses (Sadock, 1989). Negative cultural conditioning ("nice girls don't enjoy sex") may also influence the adult female's sexual response. Various developmental factors also have relevance to orgasmic dysfunction. Examples include childhood exposure to rigid religious orthodoxy, negative family attitudes toward nudity and sex, and traumatic sexual experiences during childhood or adolescence, such as incest or rape (Kolodny et al, 1979).

Psychological factors are also associated with inhibited male orgasm. In the primary disorder (never experienced prior orgasm), the man often comes from a rigid, puritanical background. He perceives sex as sinful and the genitals as dirty, and he may have conscious or unconscious incest wishes and guilt (Sadock, 1989). In the case of secondary disorder (previously experienced orgasms, but they stopped), interpersonal difficulties are usually implicated. There may be some ambivalence about commitment, fear of pregnancy, or unexpressed hostility.

Kaplan (1974) focused on the main cause of premature ejaculation as being the man's lack of awareness of the premonitory sensations before ejaculation. The ability to control ejaculation occurs as a gradual maturing process with a sexual partner in which foreplay becomes more give-and-take "pleasuring," rather than strictly goal-oriented. The man becomes aware of the sensations and learns to delay the point of ejaculatory inevitability. Relationship problems, such as a stressful marriage, unexpressed anger, anxiety over intimacy, and lack of comfort in the sexual relationship may also contribute to this disorder (McCarthy, 1989).

Sexual Pain Disorders Vaginismus may occur in response to having experienced dyspareunia (painful intercourse) for various organic reasons stated in the "Biological Factors" section. This previous experience results in involuntary constriction within the vagina in response to anticipatory pain, making intercourse impossible. No organic process can be implicated as the cause of vaginismus itself (Kolodny et al, 1979). A variety of psychosocial factors have been implicated, including negative childhood conditioning of sex as dirty, sinful, and shameful. Early traumatic sexual experiences (e.g., rape or incest) may also cause vaginismus. Other factors that may be important in the etiology of vaginismus include homosexual orientation, traumatic experience with an early pelvic examination, pregnancy phobia, venereal disease phobia, or cancer phobia (Kolodny et al, 1979).

Transactional Model of Stress/Adaptation The etiology of sexual dysfunction is most likely influenced by multiple factors. In Figure 23.2, a graphic depiction of this theory of multiple causation is presented in the Transactional Model of Stress/Adaptation.

APPLICATION OF THE NURSING PROCESS

Assessment Most assessment tools for taking a general nursing history contain some questions devoted to sexuality. It is a subject about which many nurses feel uncomfortable obtaining information. However, accurate data must be collected if problems are to be identified and resolutions attempted. Hogan (1980) states, "Sexual health is an integral part of both emotional and physical health. The nursing history is incomplete if it does not include items directed toward sexuality."

Indeed, most nurses will not be required to obtain a sexual history as in depth as the one presented in this chapter. However, certain patients require a more extensive sexual history than that which is included in the general nursing history. These include patients who have medical or surgical conditions that may affect their sexuality; patients with infertility problems, sexually transmitted disease, or complaints of sexual inadequacy; patients who are pregnant or present with gynecological problems; those seeking information on abortion or family planning; and individuals in premarital, marital, and psychiatric counseling (Hogan, 1980).

The best approach for taking a sexual history is a nondirective one. That is, it is best to use the sexual history outline as a guideline but allow the interview to progress in a less restrictive manner than the outline permits (with one question immediately following the other). The order of the questions should be adjusted according to the patient's needs as they are identified during the interview. A nondirective approach allows time for the patient to interject information related to feelings or concerns about his or her sexuality.

The language used should be understandable to the patient. If he or she uses terminology that is unfamiliar, ask for clarification. Take level of education and cultural influences into consideration.

The nurse's attitude must convey warmth, openness, honesty, and objectivity. Personal feelings, attitudes, and values should be clarified and should not interfere with acceptance of the patient. The nurse must remain nonjudgmental. This is conveyed by listening in an interested but matter-of-fact manner, without overreacting or underreacting to any information the patient may present.

The content outline for a sexual history presented in Table 23.3 is not intended to be used as a rigid questionnaire but as guidelines from which the nurse may select appropriate topics for gathering information about the patient's sexuality. The outline should be individualized according to patient needs.

Nursing Diagnosis, Planning/Implementation Nursing diagnoses are formulated from the data gathered during the assessment phase and with background knowledge regarding predisposing factors to the disorder. The following nursing diagnoses may be used for the patient with sexual disorders:

Sexual dysfunction related to depression and conflict in marriage, evidenced by loss of sexual desire.

Altered sexuality patterns related to conflicts with sexual orientation or variant preferences, evidenced by expressed dissatisfaction with sexual behaviors (e.g., voyeurism, transvestism).

In Table 23.4, these nursing diagnoses are presented in a plan of care for the patient with sexual disorders. Goals of care and appropriate nursing interventions are included for each. Rationales are presented in italics.

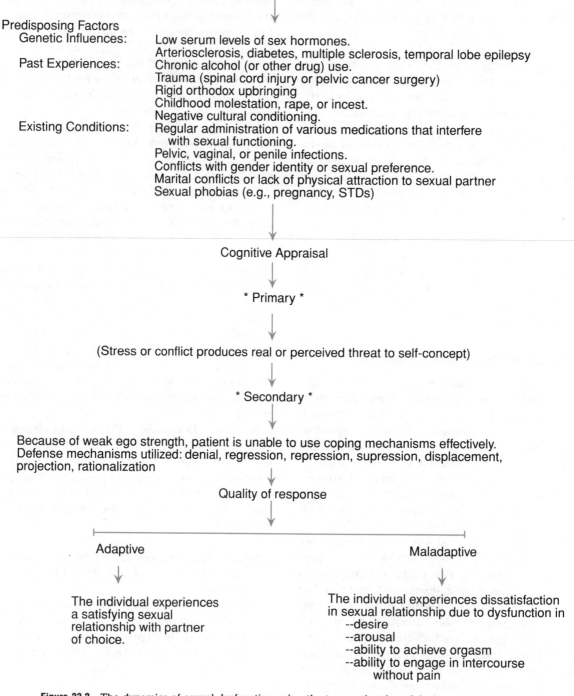

Figure 23.2 The dynamics of sexual dysfunction using the transactional model of stress/adaptation.

Table 23.3 SEXUAL HISTORY: CONTENT OUTLINE

I. Identify data
  A. Patient
    1. Age
    2. Gender
    3. Marital status
  B. Parents
    1. Ages
    2. Dates of death and ages at death
    3. Birthplace
    4. Marital status
    5. Religion
    6. Education
    7. Occupation
    8. Congeniality
    9. Demonstration of affection
    10. Feelings toward parents
  C. Siblings (same information as above)
  D. Marital partner (same information as above)
  E. Children
    1. Ages
    2. Gender
    3. Strengths
    4. Identified problems
II. Childhood sexuality
  A. Family attitudes about sex
    1. Parents' openness about sex
    2. Parents' attitudes about nudity
  B. Learning about sex
    1. Asking parents about sex
    2. Information volunteered by parents
    3. At what age and how did patient learn about: pregnancy, birth, intercourse, masturbation, nocturnal emissions, menstruation, homosexuality, sexually transmitted diseases (STDs)
  C. Childhood sex activity
    1. First sight of nude body:
      a. Same gender
      b. Opposite gender
    2. First genital self-stimulation:
      a. Age
      b. Feelings
      c. Consequences
    3. First sexual exploration at play with another child:
      a. Age (of self and other child)
      b. Gender of other child
      c. Nature of the activity
      d. Feelings and consequences

    4. Sexual activity with older persons:
      a. Age (of self and other person)
      b. Gender of other person
      c. Nature of the activity
      d. Patient willingness to participate
      e. Feelings and consequences
  D. Did you ever see your parents (or others) having intercourse? Describe your feelings.
  E. Childhood sexual theories or myths:
    1. Thoughts about conception and birth.
    2. Roles of male/female genitals and other body parts in sexuality
III. Onset of adolescence
  A. In girls:
    1. Information about menstruation:
      a. How received; from whom
      b. Age received
      c. Feelings
    2. Age:
      a. Of first period
      b. When breasts began to develop
      c. At appearance of ancillary and pubic hair
    3. Menstruation:
      a. Regularity; discomfort; duration
      b. Feelings about first period
  B. In boys:
    1. Information about puberty:
      a. How received; from whom
      b. Age received
      c. Feelings
    2. Age:
      a. Of appearance of ancillary and pubic hair
      b. Change of voice
      c. First orgasm (with or without ejaculation); emotional reaction
IV. Orgastic experiences
  A. Nocturnal emissions (male) or orgasms (female) during sleep
    1. Frequency
  B. Masturbation
    1. Age begun; ever punished?
    2. Frequency; methods used
    3. Marital partner's knowledge
    4. Practiced with others? Spouse?
    5. Emotional reactions
    6. Accompanying fantasies
  C. Necking and petting ("making out")
    1. Age when begun

(*continued*)

Table 23.3 CONTINUED

2. Frequency
3. Number of partners
4. Types of activity

D. Premarital intercourse
1. Frequency
2. Relationship with and number of partners
3. Contraceptives used
4. Feelings

E. Orgasmic frequency
1. Past
2. Present

V. Feelings about self as masculine/feminine
A. The male patient:
1. Does he feel masculine?
2. Accepted by peers?
3. Sexually adequate?
4. Feelings/concerns about body:
   a. Size
   b. Appearance
   c. Function

B. The female patient:
1. Does she feel feminine?
2. Accepted by peers?
3. Sexually adequate?
4. Feelings/concerns about body:
   a. Size
   b. Appearance
   c. Function

VI. Sexual fantasies and dreams
A. Nature of sex dreams
B. Nature of fantasies
1. During masturbation
2. During intercourse

VII. Dating
A. Age and feelings about:
1. First date
2. First kissing
3. First petting or "making out"
4. First going steady

VIII. Engagement
A. Age
B. Sex activity during engagement period:
1. With fiancee
2. With others

IX. Marriage
A. Date of marriage
B. Age at marriage: Spouse:
C. Spouse's occupation

D. Previous marriages: Spouse:
E. Reason for termination of previous marriages:
   Patient: Spouse:
F. Children from previous marriages:
   Patient: Spouse:
G. Wedding trip (honeymoon):
1. Where? How long?
2. Pleasant or unpleasant?
3. Sexual considerations?

H. Sex in marriage:
1. General satisfaction/dissatisfaction
2. Thoughts about spouse's general satisfaction/dissatisfaction

I. Pregnancies
1. Number: Ages of couple:
2. Results (normal birth, cesarean delivery, miscarriage, abortion)
3. Planned or unplanned
4. Effects on sexual adjustment
5. Sex of child wanted or unwanted

X. Extramarital sex
A. Emotional attachments
1. Number; frequency; feelings
B. Sexual intercourse
1. Number; frequency; feelings
C. Postmarital masturbation
1. Frequency; feelings
D. Postmarital homosexuality
1. Frequency; feelings
E. Multiple sex ("swinging")
1. Frequency; feelings

XI. Sex after widowhood, separation, or divorce:
A. Outlet
1. Orgasms in sleep
2. Masturbation
3. Petting
4. Intercourse
5. Homosexuality
6. Other
B. Frequency; feelings

XII. Sexual variations and disorders:
A. Homosexuality
1. First experience; describe circumstances
2. Frequency since adolescence
B. Sexual contact with animals
1. First experience; describe nature of contact
2. Frequency and recent contact
3. Feelings

(continued)

Table 23.3 CONTINUED

C. Voyeurism
1. Describe types of observation experienced
2. Feelings

D. Exhibitionism
1. To whom? When?
2. Feelings

E. Fetishes; transvestism
1. Nature of fetish
2. Nature of transvestite activity
3. Feelings

F. Sadomasochism
1. Nature of activity
2. Sexual response
3. Frequency; recency
4. Consequences

G. Seduction and rape
1. Has patient seduced/raped another?
2. Has patient ever been seduced/raped?

H. Incest
1. Nature of the sexual activity.
2. With whom?
3. When occurred? Frequency; recency
4. Consequences

I. Prostitution
1. Has patient ever accepted/paid money for sex?
2. Type of sexual activity engaged in.
3. Feelings about prostitution.

XIII. Certain effects of sex activities
A. STDs
1. Age at learning about STDs
2. Type of STD contracted
3. Age and treatment received

B. Illegitimate pregnancy
1. At what age(s)
2. Outcome of the pregnancy(ies)
3. Feelings

C. Abortion
1. Why performed?
2. At what age(s)?
3. How often?
4. Before or after marriage?
5. Circumstances: who, where, how?
6. Feelings about abortion: at the time; in retrospect; anniversary reaction.

XIV. Use of erotic material
A. Personal response to erotic material
1. Sexual pleasure—arousal
2. Mild pleasure
3. Disinterest; disgust

B. Use in connection with sexual activity
1. Type and frequency of use
2. To accompany what type of sexual activity

Source: Adapted from an outline prepared by the Group for Advancement of Psychiatry, based on the Sexual Performance Evaluation Questionnaire of the Marriage Council of Philadelphia with permission.

Outcome Criteria   The following criteria may be used for measurement of outcomes in the care of the patient with sexual disorders.

The patient:

1. Is able to correlate stressful situations that decrease sexual desire.
2. Is able to communicate with partner about sexual situation without discomfort.
3. Is able to verbalize ways to enhance sexual desire.
4. Verbalizes resumption of sexual activity at level satisfactory to self and partner.
5. Is able to correlate variant behaviors with times of stress.
6. Is able to verbalize fears about abnormality and inappropriateness of sexual behaviors.
7. Expresses desire to change variant sexual behavior.
8. Participates in and cooperates with extended plan of behavior modification.
9. Expresses satisfaction with own sexuality pattern.

Evaluation   Reassessment may be necessary to determine if selected interventions have been successful in assisting the patient to overcome problems with sexual functioning. Evaluation may be facilitated by gathering information using the following types of questions.

Has the patient identified life situations that promote feelings of depression and decreased sexual desire? Is he or she able to verbalize ways to deal with this stress? Can the patient satisfactorily com-

Table 23.4   CARE PLAN FOR THE PATIENT WITH A SEXUAL DISORDER

Nursing Diagnoses	Objectives	Nursing Interventions
Sexual dysfunction related to depression and conflict in marriage, evidenced by loss of sexual desire.	Patient identifies stressors that contribute to loss of sexual desire. Patient resumes sexual activity at level satisfactory to self and partner.	Assess patient's sexual history and previous level of satisfaction in sexual relationship. *This establishes a data base from which to work, and provides a foundation for goal setting.* Assess patient's perception of the problem. *Patient's idea of what constitutes a problem may differ from the nurse's. It is the patient's perception on which the goals of care must be established.* Help patient determine time dimension associated with the onset of the problem and discuss what was happening in life situation at that time. *Stress in all areas of life will affect sexual functioning. Patient may be unaware of correlation between stress and sexual dysfunction.* Assess patient's level of energy. *Fatigue decreases patient's desire and enthusiasm for participation in sexual activity.* Review medication regimen; observe for side effects. *Many medications can affect libido. Evaluation of drug and individual response is important to ascertain whether drug is responsible for the problem.* Provide information regarding sexuality and sexual functioning. *Increasing knowledge and correcting misconceptions can decrease feelings of powerlessness and anxiety and facilitate problem resolution.* Refer for additional counseling/sex therapy if required. *Patient and partner may need additional or more in-depth assistance if problems in sexual relationship are severe or remain unresolved.*
Altered sexuality patterns related to conflicts with sexual orientation or variant preferences, evidenced by expressed dissatisfaction with sexual behaviors (e.g., voyeurism; transvestism).	Patient will express satisfaction with own sexuality pattern.	Take sexual history, noting patient's expression of areas of dissatisfaction with sexual pattern. *Knowledge of what patient perceives as the problem is essential for providing the type of assistance he or she may need.* Assess areas of stress in patient's life and examine relationship with sexual partner. *Sexual variant behaviors are often associated with added stress in the patient's life.* Note cultural, social, ethnic, racial, and religious factors that may contribute to conflicts regarding variant sexual practices. *Patient may be unaware of the influence these factors exert in creating feelings of shame and guilt.* Be accepting and nonjudgmental. *Sexuality is a very personal and sensitive subject. The patient is more likely to share this information if he or she does not fear being judged by the nurse.* Assist therapist in plan of behavior modification to help patient decrease variant behaviors. *Individuals with paraphilias are treated by specialists who have experience in modifying variant sexual behaviors. Nurses can intervene by providing assistance with implementation of the plan for behavior modification.* Teach patient that sexuality is a normal human response and is not synonymous with any one sexual act; that it involves complex interrelationships among one's self-concept, body

(continued)

Table 23.4 CONTINUED		
Nursing Diagnoses	**Objectives**	**Nursing Interventions**
		image, personal history, family and cultural influences; and all interactions with others (VandeVusse & Simandl, 1992). *If patient feels abnormal or very unlike everyone else, the self-concept is likely to be very low — even worthless. Helping him or her to see that even though the behavior is variant, feelings and motivations are common, may help to increase feelings of self-worth and desire to change behavior.*

municate with sexual partner about the problem? Have the patient and sexual partner identified ways to enhance sexual desire and the achievement of sexual satisfaction for both? Are they seeking assistance with marital conflict? Do both partners agree on what the major problem is? Do they have the motivation to attempt change? Do they verbalize an increase in sexual satisfaction?

Is the patient able to correlate an increase in variant sexual behavior to times of severe stress? Has the patient been able to identify those stressful situations and verbalize alternative ways to deal with them? Does the patient express a desire to change variant sexual behavior and a willingness to cooperate with extended therapy to do so? Does the patient express an understanding about the normality of sexual feelings, aside from the inappropriateness of his or her behavior? Are expressions of increased self-worth evident?

TREATMENT MODALITIES

Sexual Desire Disorders

Hypoactive Sexual Desire Disorder   This disorder has been treated in the past with the administration of testosterone in both men and women. The masculinizing side effects makes this approach unacceptable to women, and there is no conclusive evidence that it is useful in increasing libido in men, even when normal levels have been measured as low (Bancroft, 1984).

Becker and Kavoussi (1988) describe the most effective treatment as a combination of cognitive therapy to deal with maladaptive beliefs; psychodynamic therapy to explore intrapsychic conflicts;

behavioral treatment, such as exercises to enhance sexual pleasuring and communication; and marital therapy to deal with the individual's use of sex to control the relationship.

Low sexual desire is not uncommonly the result of partner incompatibility. If this is the case, the therapist may choose to shift to helping a couple identify and deal with the incompatibility separate from the sexual issue (Wincze & Carey, 1991).

Sexual Aversion Disorder   Systematic desensitization (see Chapter 20) is often the treatment of choice for this disorder to reduce the patient's fear and avoidance of sex (Becker & Kavoussi, 1988). Gradual exposure, under relaxed conditions, to imagined and actual sexual situations serves to decrease the amount of anxiety generated by these experiences. Successful treatment of sexual phobias has also been reported by Kaplan (1979) using tricyclic or monoamine oxidase inhibitor medications and psychosexual therapy aimed at developing insight into unconscious conflicts.

Sexual Arousal Disorders

Female Sexual Arousal Disorder   The goal of treatment is to reduce the anxiety that is associated with sexual activity. Masters and Johnson (1970) have reported successful results using their behaviorally oriented *sensate focus exercises* to treat this disorder. The objective is to reduce the goal-oriented demands of intercourse on both the man and the woman, thus reducing performance pressures and anxiety associated with possible failure. Kolodny et al (1979) describe sensate focus exercises in the following manner:

"The couple are instructed to take turns touching one another's bodies—avoiding the breasts and genitals—to establish a sense of tactile awareness by noticing textures, contours, temperatures, and contrasts (while doing the touching) or to be aware of the sensations of being touched by their partner. They are carefully instructed that sexual excitation is not the purpose of this exercise (although it may occur); instead, their attention should focus on their own physical sensations and should minimize cognitive processes. The couple gradually moves through various levels of sensate focus that progress from nongenital touching to touching that includes the breasts and genitals; touching that is done in a simultaneous, mutual format rather than by one person at a time; and touching that extends to and allows eventually for the possibility of intercourse."

Male Erectile Disorder   Sensate focus has been used effectively for male erectile disorder as well. Clinicians widely agree that even in cases where significant organic factors have been identified, psychological factors may also be present and must be considered in treatment (Wincze & Carey, 1991).

Group therapy, hypnotherapy, and systematic desensitization have also been used successfully in reducing the anxiety that may contribute to erectile difficulties. Psychodynamic interventions may be helpful in alleviating intrapsychic conflicts contributing to performance anxiety (Becker & Kavoussi, 1988).

Various medications, including testosterone, yohimbine, and penile injections of phenoxybenzamine and papaverine, have been tried in men with erectile dysfunction, with inconclusive results (Brindley, 1986; Morales et al, 1982).

When erectile dysfunction occurs because of irreversible organic causes, penile prostheses may be implanted. Two basic types are currently available: a bendable silicon implant and an inflatable device. The bendable variety requires a relatively simple surgical technique for insertion but results in a perpetual state of semierection for the patient (Kolodny et al, 1979). The inflatable penile prosthesis produces an erection only when it is desired, and the appearance of the penis in both the flaccid and erect states is completely normal. Potential candidates for penile implantation should undergo careful psychological and physical screening. Although penile implants do not enable the patient to recover the ability to ejaculate or to have an orgasm, men with prosthetic devices have generally reported satisfaction with their subsequent sexual functioning (Sadock, 1989).

Orgasm Disorders

Inhibited Female Orgasm   Anxiety may be a contributing factor to the lack of orgasmic ability in women. For this reason, sensate focus is often advised in an effort to provide a framework for reducing anxiety, increasing awareness of physical sensations, and transferring communications skills from the verbal to the nonverbal domain (Kolodny et al, 1979). LoPiccolo and Stock (1986) describe a program of directed masturbation training for the individual with primary anorgasmia (never having had an orgasm). The systematic program involves discussion of feelings, special exercises, and gradual self-exploration of the body, and moves toward focused genital stimulation in combination with sexual fantasies. Treatment for secondary anorgasmia (had orgasms, then stopped) focuses on the couple and their relationship. Therapy with both partners is essential to successful treatment of this disorder.

Inhibited Male Orgasm   Treatment for this disorder is very similar to that described for the anorgasmic woman. A combination of sensate focus and masturbatory training has been used with a high degree of success in the Masters and Johnson (1970) clinic. Treatment for inhibited male orgasm almost always includes the sexual partner.

Premature Ejaculation   Masters and Johnson (1970) developed a highly successful technique for the treatment of premature ejaculation. Sensate focus is used, with progression to genital stimulation. When the man reaches the point of imminent ejaculation, the woman is instructed to apply the "squeeze" technique—applying pressure at the base of the glans penis with her thumb and first two fingers. Pressure is held for 5 seconds and then released. This technique is continued until the man is no longer on the verge of ejaculating. This technique is practiced during subsequent periods of sexual stimulation. Kolodny et al (1979) state, "For unknown neurophysiologic reasons, this maneuver reduces the urgency of ejaculatory tension and, used with consistency, reconditions the pattern of ejaculatory timing to improve control surprisingly well."

Sexual Pain Disorders

Dyspareunia Treatment for the pain of intercourse begins with a thorough physical and gynecological examination. When organic pathology has been eliminated, the patient's fears and anxieties underlying sexual functioning are investigated (Becker & Kavoussi, 1988). Systematic desensitization has been used successfully to decrease fears and anxieties associated with painful intercourse.

Vaginismus Treatment of this disorder begins with education of the woman and her sexual partner regarding the anatomy and physiology of the disorder—that is, what exactly is occurring during the vaginismus reflex and possible etiologies. The involuntary nature of the disorder is stressed in an effort to alleviate the perception on the part of the sexual partner that this occurrence is an act of willful withholding by the woman (Kolodny et al, 1979).

The second phase of treatment involves systematic desensitization. The patient is taught a series of tensing and relaxing exercises aimed at relaxation of the pelvic musculature. Relaxation of the pelvic muscles is followed by a procedure involving the systematic insertion of dilators of graduated sizes until the woman is able to accept the penis into the vagina without discomfort. This physical therapy, combined with treatment of any identified relationship problems, has been used by the Masters and Johnson (1970) clinic with a high degree of success.

ALTERNATIVE SEXUAL LIFE-STYLES

Homosexuality

Homosexual activity occurs under some circumstances in probably all known human cultures and all mammalian species for which it has been studied (Gadpaille, 1989). The term *homosexuality* is derived from the Greek root *homo* meaning "same" and refers to sexual preference for individuals of the same gender. It may be applied in a general way to homosexuals of both genders but is often used to specifically denote male homosexuality. The term *lesbianism*, used to identify female homosexuality, is traced to the Greek poet Sappho who lived on the island of Lesbos and is famous for the love poems she wrote to other women. Most homosexuals prefer the term "gay" to describe their life-style, as it is less derogatory in its lack of emphasis on the sexual aspects of the life-style (Hyde, 1986). A heterosexual is then referred to as straight.

The psychiatric community in general does not consider consensual homosexuality to be a mental disturbance (Becker & Kavoussi, 1988). The concept of homosexuality as a disturbance in sexual orientation no longer appears in the *DSM-III-R* (APA, 1987). Instead the *DSM-III-R* is concerned only with the individual who experiences "persistent and marked distress about his or her sexual orientation."

Many members of the American culture disapprove of the homosexual life-style. In a survey by Davis and Smith (1984), 73 percent of those surveyed responded that they believed sexual relations between two adults of the same sex was always wrong. Some experts believe that many Americans' attitudes toward homosexuals can best be described as homophobic (Fyfe, 1983). Homophobia is defined as a pathological fear of homosexuals and is usually indicative of a deep-seated insecurity about one's own gender identity (Hogan, 1980). Homophobic behaviors include extreme prejudice against, abhorrence of, and discomfort with homosexuals. These behaviors are usually rationalized by religious, moral, legal, or pseudoscientific considerations (Marmor, 1976b).

Relationship patterns are as varied among homosexuals as they are among heterosexuals (Gadpaille, 1989). Some homosexuals may remain with one partner for an extended period, even for a lifetime, while others prefer not to make a commitment, and "play the field" instead.

No one knows for sure why people are homosexual or heterosexual. Various theories have been proposed regarding the issue, but no single etiological factor has emerged in a consistent manner. Many contributing factors likely influence the development of sexual orientation.

PREDISPOSING FACTORS

Biological Theories As early as 1952, Kallman argued that there is a genetic predisposition to homosexuality. He based this theory on a study in which he found 100 percent concordance for homosexuality among all the identical-twin pairs he studied. However, subsequent investigators have failed to duplicate his findings, and although there appear to be at least familial factors in some instances of male homosexuality, definitive findings related to genetic influences have not yet been validated (Gadpaille, 1989).

A number of studies have been conducted to determine whether or not there is a hormonal influence in the etiology of homosexuality. Researchers have speculated that levels of testosterone may be lower and levels of estrogen higher in homosexual men than in heterosexual men. Results have been inconsistent. Some studies did find higher testosterone levels and lower estrogen levels among lesbians than among a control group of heterosexual women (Hyde, 1986). Results are inadequate to support a hormonal influence.

It has also been suggested that exposure to inappropriate hormones during the critical fetal period of sexual differentiation may contribute to homosexual orientation (Ehrhardt et al, 1985). This hypothesis lacks definitive evidence, and conclusions regarding its validity remain tentative.

Psychosocial Theories Freud (1930) believed that all humans are inherently bisexual, with the capacity for both heterosexual and homosexual behavior. He theorized all individuals go through a homoerotic phase as children. Thus, if homosexuality occurs later in life it is due to arrest of normal psychosexual development. He also believed homosexuality could occur as a result of pathological family relationships in which the child adopts a negative oedipal position, that is, there is sexualized attachment to the parent of the same gender and identification with the parent of the opposite gender.

Bieber et al (1962) found a dysfunctional family pattern as an etiological influence in the development of male homosexuality. The mother was described as dominant, overprotective, possessive, and seductive in her interactions with her son. The father was found to be passive, distant, and covertly or overtly hostile, and was openly devalued and dominated by the mother. Her behavior succeeds in undermining the father's availability as an acceptable object of gender identification for the boy, while hindering the child's capacity for trust in members of the opposite sex.

A study by Wolff (1971) revealed characteristics about the families of lesbians. Mothers of lesbians were found to be rejecting or indifferent while the fathers were found to be distant or absent. Wolff concluded from these findings that because the girl does not receive adequate love from her mother, she continues throughout her life to search for that missing love in other women. The distant or absent father results in her lack of ability to form satisfactory relationships with men.

SPECIAL CONCERNS

People with homosexual preferences have problems that are not all that different from their heterosexual counterparts. Considerations of attractiveness, finding a partner, and concerns about sexual adequacy are common to both. Sexually transmitted diseases (STDs) are epidemic among sexually active individuals of all sexual persuasions. Of particular concern is acquired immunodeficiency syndrome (AIDS), which was seen as a gay disease for the first few years of the epidemic (see Chapter 28). AIDS is a fatal viral illness that in the western world until recently was indeed mainly transmitted during male homosexual activity (Bancroft, 1989). Although it is now well known that AIDS is also spread through contaminated blood products and the sharing of needles by intravenous drug users, as well as heterosexual contact, there are still those individuals who believe AIDS is God's way of punishing homosexuals. These types of societal attitudes are described by many homosexuals as being their greatest burden.

Some individuals live in fear of the discovery of their sexual orientation — fear of being rejected by parents and significant others. They experience a great deal of cognitive dissonance related to the disparity between their overt behavior and their inner feelings. Social sanctions still exist in some areas for homosexuals in regard to employment, housing, and public accommodations. Gay rights are protected by the Human Rights Commission. However, evidence of discrimination is still widespread.

Nurses must examine their personal attitudes and feelings about homosexuality. They must be able to recognize when negative feelings are compromising the care they give. Increasing numbers of homosexuals are being honest about their lifestyles. Health-care workers must ensure that these individuals receive the care with dignity that is the right of all human beings. Nurses who have come to terms with their own feelings about homosexuality are able to separate the person from the behavior. Acceptance of the alternative life-style is not an essential component of nursing. Unconditional acceptance of the individual is.

Transsexualism

Transsexualism is a disorder of gender identity or gender dysphoria (unhappiness or dissatisfaction with one's gender) of the most extreme variety. An individual, despite having the anatomical characteristics of a given gender, has the self-perception of being of the opposite gender (Becker & Kavoussi, 1988). The disorder is rare, with an estimated prevalence of 1 in 30,000 for men and 1 in 100,000 for women (APA, 1987).

The *DSM-III-R* diagnostic criteria for transsexualism states that the individual (who has reached puberty) must have had a persistent preoccupation for at least 2 years with changing his or her primary and secondary sex characteristics to those of the opposite gender.

Individuals with this disorder do not feel comfortable wearing the clothes of their assigned gender and often engage in cross-dressing. They may find their own genitals repugnant and repeatedly submit requests to the health-care system for hormonal and surgical gender reassignment. Depression and anxiety are common and are often attributed by the individual to his or her inability to live in the desired gender role.

PREDISPOSING FACTORS

Biological Theories Several studies have been conducted to determine if sex hormone levels are abnormal in individuals with gender dysphoria (Starka et al, 1975; Sipova et al, 1977; Jones et al, 1973). The results of these studies were varied.

As with homosexuality, there has been some speculation that gender-disordered individuals may be exposed to inappropriate hormones during the prenatal period, which can result in a genetic woman having male genitals, or a genetic man having female genitals (Ehrhardt et al, 1985). Evidence that prenatal exposure to these hormones predisposes to transsexualism, however, remains inconclusive.

Psychosocial Theories A good deal of emphasis has been placed on the importance of social learning in gender identity development. The *DSM-III-R* states, "Extensive, pervasive childhood femininity in a boy or childhood masculinity in a girl increases the liklihood of transsexualism" (APA, 1987). Green (1976; 1985) found a number of factors thought to influence femininity in boys:

1. Parental indifference to feminine behavior in a boy.
2. Parental encouragement of feminine behavior in a boy.
3. Repeated cross-dressing of a young boy by a woman.
4. Maternal overprotection of a son and prohibition of "rough, boyish" play.
5. Excessive maternal attention and physical contact, resulting in lack of separation and individuation of the boy from his mother.
6. Absence of or rejection by the father.
7. Physical beauty of a boy, influencing adults to treat him in a feminine manner.
8. Lack of male playmates during early years of socialization.

Factors that influence masculinity in girls are not so clear cut. These characteristics are considerably more common and are also regarded as more socially acceptable, hence less attention is given to their significance. In a study of "tomboy" girls, Green et al (1982) found a preference for male sex-typed toys, male-gender peer group, participation in sports, male roles taken in playing house, as well as the stated wish to be a boy. Pauly (1974) found that a disturbed parental relationship was also commonly reported by a substantial majority of adult female transsexuals. The dynamics often included a weak or depressive mother or an aggressive, excessively masculine and often alcoholic father. Encouragement by both parents of masculinity in the daughter appears to be common.

SPECIAL CONCERNS

Treatment of the transsexual is a complex process. The true transsexual intensely desires to have the genitalia and physical appearance of the assigned gender changed to conform with his or her gender identity. This change requires a great deal more than surgical alteration of physical features.

In most cases, the individual must undergo extensive psychological testing and counseling, as well as live in the role of the desired gender for up to 2 years prior to surgery.

Hormonal treatment is initiated during this period. Male patients receive estrogens, which results in a redistribution of body fat in a more "feminine" pattern, enlargement of the breasts, a softening of the skin, and reduction in body hair. Females receive testosterone, which also causes a redistribution of body fat, growth of facial and body hair, enlargement of the clitoris, and deepening of the voice (Becker & Kavoussi, 1988). Amenorrhea usually occurs within 4 months (Levine, 1989).

Surgical treatment for the male-to-female transsexual involves removal of the penis and testes and creation of an artificial vagina. Care is taken to preserve sensory nerves in the area so that the individual may continue to experience sexual stimulation.

Surgical treatment for the female-to-male transsexual is more complex and generally less successful (Hyde, 1986). A mastectomy and sometimes a hysterectomy are performed. A penis and scrotum are constructed from tissues in the genital and abdominal area, and the vaginal orifice is closed. A penile implant is used to attain erection.

Both men and women continue to receive maintenance hormone therapy following surgery. Satisfaction with the results are high, and most consider the pain and discomfort worthwhile. Levine (1989) states, "Most systematic studies of patients who have had surgery indicate that approximately 85 percent are pleased that they underwent their operations and feel that their bodies and their minds are finally whole."

Nursing care of the post–sex-reassignment surgical patient is similar to that of most other post-surgical patients. Particular attention is given to maintaining comfort, preventing infection, preserving integrity of the surgical site, maintaining elimination, and meeting nutritional needs (Hogan, 1980). Psychosocial needs may have to do with body image, and fears and insecurities about relating to others and being accepted in the new gender role. This can begin with nursing in a healing atmosphere that is both nonthreatening and nonjudgmental.

Bisexuality

A bisexual person is not exclusively heterosexual or homosexual but engages in sexual activity with members of both genders. Bisexuals are also sometimes referred to as ambisexual.

Bisexuality is more common than exclusive homosexuality. Statistics suggest that approximately 75 percent of all men are exclusively heterosexual and only 2 percent are exclusively homosexual, leaving a relatively large percentage who have engaged in sexual activity with both men and women (Hyde, 1986).

MacDonald (1982) describes a diversity of sexual preferences among bisexuals. Some prefer men and women equally, while others have a preference for one gender but are accepting of sex with the other gender. Some bisexuals may alternate between homosexual and heterosexual activity for long periods, while others may have both a male and a female lover at the same time. Some individuals maintain their bisexual orientation throughout their lives, while others may become exclusively homosexual or heterosexual.

PREDISPOSING FACTORS

Little research exists on the etiology of bisexuality. Freud (1930) believed that all humans are inherently bisexual; that is, he believed that all individuals have the capacity for both heterosexual and homosexual interactions.

Most research on the development of homosexuality rests on the assumption that it is somehow determined by pathological conditions in childhood (Hyde, 1986). Many heterosexual individuals, however, have their first homosexual encounter later in life. It is unlikely that an initial homosexual encounter that occurs in the 30s or 40s was determined by a pathological condition that occurred when the child was 3 or 4 years old. Some encounters, too, are based solely on the situation, such as the heterosexual man who engages in homosexual behavior while in prison, then returns to heterosexuality following his release. This behavior most likely was determined by the circumstances rather than some pathological process that occurred 20 years before.

Riddle (1978) suggests that gender identity (determining whether one is male or female) seems to be established during the preschool years. Sexual identity (determining whether one is heterosexual or homosexual or both) most likely continues to evolve throughout one's lifetime.

SEXUALLY TRANSMITTED DISEASES

The term *sexually transmitted diseases (STDs)* refers to a large group of disease syndromes that can be transmitted sexually irrespective of whether the disease has genital pathological manifestations (Thompson et al, 1986). They may be transmitted from one person to another through heterosexual or homosexual anal, oral, or genital contact.

Sexually transmitted diseases are at epidemic levels in the United States. Individuals are beginning a longer, active sex life at an earlier age. More women are sexually active than ever before. The social changes that may have contributed to the increase in STDs are sometimes referred to as the three P's: permissiveness, promiscuity, and the pill (Darrow, 1975). The widespread knowledge that antibiotics were available to "cure" infections and the pill was available to prevent pregnancy resulted in significant increases in promiscuity and the subsequent exposure to and spread of STDs.

The nurse's first responsibility in STD control is to educate patients who may develop or have a sexually transmitted infection (Lamb et al, 1987). Nurses must be knowledgeable about which diseases are most prevalent, how they are transmitted, signs and symptoms, available treatment, and consequences of avoiding treatment (Table 23.5). They must teach this information to patients in the hospitals and clinics, and take an active role in programs of education in the community. Early education is the target for decreasing the spread of STDs.

Sexually transmitted diseases have a particularly emotive significance because they can be transmitted between sexual partners. As a consequence, such diseases have strong connotations of illicit or immoral sex and carry considerable social stigma as well as potentially horrifying medical consequences (Bancroft, 1989). Feelings of guilt can be overwhelming. Patients who have STDs need strong support to overcome not only the physical difficulties, but also the social and emotional aspects associated with having this type of illness.

Prevention of STDs is the ideal goal, but early detection and appropriate treatment continue to be considered a realistic objective. Nurses are in an excellent position to provide the education required for prevention, as well as the physical treatment, and social and emotional support to assist patients with STDs regain and maintain optimal wellness.

SUMMARY

This chapter has provided information related to the development of sexuality throughout the life cycle. Normal sexual response patterns were described in an effort to provide background information for the recognition and treatment of sexual disorders.

The *DSM-III-R* identifies two major categories of sexual disorders: paraphilias and sexual dysfunctions. Paraphilias define a group of behaviors that involve sexual activity with nonhuman objects or with nonconsenting partners or that involve suffering to others. Types of paraphilias include exhibitionism, fetishism, frotteurism, pedophilia, sexual masochism or sadism, and voyeurism.

Sexual dysfunctions are disturbances that occur in any of the phases of the normal human sexual response cycle. They include sexual desire disorders, sexual arousal disorders, orgasm disorders, and sexual pain disorders.

Predisposing factors and symptomatology for each of these sexual disorders was presented as background assessment data. A content outline for obtaining a sexual history was included. The delivery of nursing care was described in the context of the nursing process.

A description of the most current medical treatment modalities for each of the sexual disorders was presented. Alternative sexual life-styles, including homosexuality, transsexualism, and bisexuality, were discussed. Finally, information on the transmission, signs and symptoms, treatment, and potential complications of the most prevalent STDs

Table 23.5 SEXUALLY TRANSMITTED DISEASES

Disease	Organism of Transmission	Method of Transmission	Signs and Symptoms	Available Treatment	Potential Complications
Gonorrhea	*Neisseria gonorrhoeae* (bacterium)	Vaginal sex; anal sex; genital-oral sex; via hand moistened with infected secretions and placed in contact with mucous membranes such as the eyes.	Males; urethritis; dysuria, purulent discharge from urethra; proctitis; pharyngitis. Females: initially asymptomatic. Progress to infection of cervix, urethra, and fallopian tubes.	Tetracycline; penecillin G; amoxicillin; ampicillin; spectinomycin	Males: Sterility from orchitis or epididymitis. Females: Chronic pelvic inflammatory disease; infertility; ectopic pregnancy; blindness from gonococcal conjunctivitis
Syphilis	*Treponema pallidum* (spirochete)	Vaginal sex; anal sex; genital-oral sex; via contact of infected secretions with intact mucous membranes or abraded skin.	Primary stage: painless chancre on penis, vulva, vagina, mouth, anus, or other point of contact with mucous membranes or abraded skin. Secondary stage: rash, headache, anorexia, weight loss, fever, sore throat, body aches, anemia.	Long-acting penecillin G; tetracycline; erythromycin	Latent stage: lasts many years; no symptoms but can be passed on to fetus. Tertiary stage: blindness, heart disease, insanity, ulcerated lesions on skin, mucous membranes, or internal organs.
Chlamydial infection	*Chlamydia trachomatis* (intracellular bacterium)	Vaginal sex; anal sex; via hand moistened with infected secretions and placed in contact with mucous membranes	Females: cervicitis (either asymptomatic or may have discharge, dysuria, soreness, bleeding) Males: urethral discharge and dysuria.	Tetracycline; erythromycin	Scarring in the fallopian tubes; ectopic pregnancy; infertility.
Genital herpes	Herpes simplex virus, type 1 or type 2	Vaginal sex; anal sex; genital-oral sex; skin-to-skin contact with infected areas; to newborn through vaginal delivery.	Blistery lesions in the genital area causing pain, itching, burning. Also vaginal or urethral discharge, fever, headache, malaise, and myalgias.	Acyclovir applied directly to the area provides symptomatic relief. No cure.	Recurrences are possible. Potential complications include: meningitis, encephalitis, urethral strictures. Possible risk of cervical cancer.

(continued)

Table 23.5 CONTINUED					
Disease	**Organism of Transmission**	**Method of Transmission**	**Signs and Symptoms**	**Available Treatment**	**Potential Complications**
Genital warts	Condyloma acuminatum (human papilloma virus)	Vaginal sex; anal sex; skin-to-skin contact with infected areas.	Cauliflowerlike warts that appear on penis or scrotum in men, labia, vaginal walls or cervix in women. Mild itching may occur.	Application of fluorouracil (5-FU); cryotherapy; electrocautery; surgical removal.	Recurrences are possible. Possible increased risk of cervical cancer.
Hepatitis B	Hepatitis B Virus	Vaginal sex; anal sex; genital-oral sex; contact with infectious blood or blood products; contact of infectious secretions with mucous membranes or abrased skin.	Malaise, anorexia, nausea/ vomiting, fever, headache, mild pain in right upper quadrant of abdomen, jaundice.	No cure. Treatment involves supportive care; bedrest for extended period. Medications have not generally been found to be useful.	Complications include chronic hepatitis; cirrhosis; liver cancer.
Acquired immune deficiency syndrome (AIDS)	Human immuno-deficiency virus (HIV)	Exchange of body fluids via: Anal sex; vaginal sex; genital-oral sex; shared use of needles during drug use. Skin-to-skin contact when there are open sores on the skin. Transfusion with contaminated blood.	May be asymptomatic for as long as 10 years following infection with HIV. Early signs of AIDS include severe weight loss, diarrhea, fever, night sweats or the presence of a persistent opportunistic infection (e.g. herpes or candidiasis)	No cure. Zidovudine (AZT or Retrovir) used to slow growth of the virus. Other medications given for symptomatic relief.	Regardless of treatment, the outcome of AIDS is eventually fatal.

was suggested as material for use in programs of education intended to decrease the spread of STDs.

Human sexuality influences all aspects of physical and mental health. Patients are becoming more open to discussing matters pertaining to sexuality, and it is therefore important for nurses to integrate information on sexuality into the care they give. This can be done by focusing on preventive, therapeutic, and educational interventions to help individuals attain, regain, or maintain sexual health.

REVIEW QUESTIONS
Self-Examination/Learning Exercise

*Select the answer that is **most** appropriate for each of the following questions.*

1. Janice, age 24, and her husband are seeking treatment at the sex therapy clinic. They have been married for 3 weeks and have never had sexual intercourse together. Pain and vaginal tightness prevent penile entry. Sexual history reveals Janice was raped when she was 15 years old. The physician would most likely assign which of the following diagnoses to Janice?
   a. Dyspareunia
   b. Vaginismus
   c. Anorgasmia
   d. Sexual aversion disorder

2. The most appropriate nursing diagnosis for Janice would be:
   a. pain related to vaginal constriction.
   b. altered sexuality patterns related to inability to have vaginal intercourse.
   c. sexual dysfunction related to history of sexual trauma.
   d. dysfunctional grieving related to loss of self-esteem because of rape.

3. The first phase of treatment may be initiated by the nurse. It would include which of the following?
   a. Sensate focus exercises
   b. Tense and relaxation exercises
   c. Systematic desensitization
   d. Education about the disorder

4. The second phase of treatment includes which of the following?
   a. Gradual dilation of the vagina
   b. Sensate focus exercises
   c. Hypnotherapy
   d. Administration of minor tranquilizers

5. Statistically, the outcome of therapy for Janice and her husband is likely to:
   a. be unsuccessful.
   b. be very successful.
   c. be of very long duration.
   d. result in their getting a divorce.

Match each of the paraphilias listed on the left with its correct behavioral description from the column on the right.

_____ 6. Exhibitionism

_____ 7. Transvestic fetishism

a. Tom watches his neighbor through her window each night as she undresses for bed. Later he fantasizes about having sex with her.

b. Frank drives his car up to a strange woman, stops, and asks her for directions. As she is explaining, he reveals his erect penis to her.

_____ 8. Voyeurism

_____ 9. Frotteurism

_____ 10. Pedophilia

c. Tim, age 17, babysits for his 11-year-old neighbor, Jeff. Six months ago, Tim began fondling Jeff's genitals. They now engage in mutual masturbation each time they are together.

d. John is 32 years old. He buys women's clothing at the thrift shop. Sometimes he dresses as a woman and goes to a singles' bar. He becomes sexually excited as he fantasizes about men being attracted to him as a woman.

e. Fred rides a crowded subway every day. He stands beside a woman he views as very attractive. Just as the subway is about to stop, he places his hand on her breast and rubs his genitals against her buttock. As the door opens, he dashes out and away. Later he fantasizes she is in love with him.

REFERENCES

Abel, E. L. (1985). *Psychoactive drugs and sex.* New York: Plenum.

Abel, G. G. (1989). Paraphilias. In H. I. Kaplan & B. J. Sadock (Eds.), *Comprehensive textbook of psychiatry* (Vol. I) (5th ed.). Baltimore: Williams & Wilkins.

Abel, G. G., Mittelman, M. S., & Becker, J. V. (1985). Sexual offenders: Results of assessment and recommendations for treatment. In H. H. Ben-Aron, S. I. Hucker, & C. D. Webster (Eds.), *Clinical criminology.* Toronto: MM Graphics.

American Psychiatric Association (1987). *Diagnostic and statistical manual of mental disorders.* (3rd ed., rev.). Washington, DC: American Psychiatric Association.

Arafat, I. S. & Cotton, W. L. (1974). Masturbation practices of males and females. *Journal of Sex Research, 10*: 293–307.

Bancroft, J. (1978). The prevention of sexual offenses. In C. B. Qualls et al. (Eds.), *The prevention of sexual disorders.* New York: Plenum.

Bancroft, J. (1984). Testosterone therapy for low sexual interest and erectile dysfunctions in men. *Br J Psychiatry 144*: 146–151.

Bancroft, J. (1989). *Human sexuality and its problems* (2nd ed.). New York: Churchill Livingstone.

Barnes, J. (1981). Non-consummation of marriage. *Ir Med J, 74*: 19–21.

Becker, J. V. (1989). Impact of sexual abuse on sexual functioning. In S. R. Leiblum & R. C. Rosen (Eds.), *Principles and practice of sex therapy: Update for the 1990s* (2nd ed.). New York: Guilford Press.

Becker, J. V. & Kavoussi, R. J. (1988). Sexual disorders. In J. A. Talbott, R. E. Hales, & S. C. Yudofsky (Eds.), *Textbook of psychiatry.* Washington, DC: The American Psychiatric Press.

Bieber, I. et al. (1962). *Homosexuality.* New York: Basic Books.

Bradford, J. M. & McLean, D. (1984). Sexual offenders, violence, and testosterone: A clinical study. *Can J Psychiatry, 29*: 335–343.

Brindley, G. S. (1986). Maintenance treatment of erectile impotence by cavernosal unstriated muscle relaxant injection. *Br J Psychiatry, 49*: 210–215.

Darrow, W. W. (1975). Changes in sexual behavior and venereal diseases. *Clin Obstet Gynecol, 18*: 255–267.

Davis, J. A. & Smith, T. (1984). *General social surveys, 1972–1984: Cumulative data.* New Haven: Yale University, Roper Center for Public Opinion Research.

Ehrhardt, A. A. et al. (1985). Sexual orientation after prenatal exposure to exogenous estrogen. *Arch Sex Behav, 14*: 57–78.

Frank, E., Anderson, C., & Rubinstein, D. (1978). Frequency of sexual dysfunctions in normal couples. *N Engl J Med, 299*: 111–115.

Freud, S. (1930). *Three contributions to the theory of sex* (4th ed.). New York: Nervous and Mental Disease Publishing.

Fyfe, B. (1983). Homophobia, or homosexual bias reconsidered. *Arch Sex Behav, 12*: 549–554.

Gadpaille, W. J. (1989). Homosexuality. In H. I. Kaplan & B. J. Sadock (Eds.), *Comprehensive textbook of psychiatry* (Vol. 1) (5th ed.). Baltimore: Williams & Wilkins.

Green, R. (1976). One hundred and ten feminine and masculine boys: Behavioral contrasts and demographic similarities. *Arch Sex Behav, 5*: 425–446.

Green, R. (1985). Gender identity in childhood and later sexual orientation: Follow up of 78 males. *Am J Psychiatry, 142*: 339–341.

Green, R. et al. (1982). Ninety-nine 'tomboys' and 'non-tomboys': Behavioral contrasts and demographic similarities. *Arch Sex Behav, 11*: 247–266.

Hogan, R. M. (1980). *Human sexuality: A nursing perspective*. New York: Appleton-Century-Crofts.

Hyde, J. S. (1986). *Understanding human sexuality* (3rd ed.). New York: McGraw-Hill.

Jones, J. R. & Samimy, J. (1973). Plasma testosterone levels and female transsexualism. *Arch Sex Behav, 2*: 251–256.

Kallman, F. J. (1952). Comparative twin study on the genetic aspects of male homosexuality. *J Nerv Ment Dis, 115*: 283.

Kaplan, H. S. (1974). *The new sex therapy*. New York: Brunner/Mazel.

Kaplan, H. S. (1979). *Disorders of sexual desire and other new concepts and techniques in sex therapy*. New York: Brunner/Mazel.

Katchadourian, H. A. & Lunde, D. T. (1975). *Fundamentals of human sexuality*. (2nd ed.). New York: Holt.

Kinsey, A. C., Pomeroy, W. B., & Martin, C. E. (1948). *Sexual behavior in the human male*. Philadelphia: WB Saunders.

Kolodny, R. C., Masters, W. H., & Johnson, V. E. (1979). *Textbook of sexual medicine*. Boston: Little, Brown and Company.

Lamb, M, Olshansky, E. F., Power, D., & Woods, N. F. (1987). Interventions for persons with problems of the reproductive system. In W. J. Phipps, Long, B. C., & Woods, N. F. (Eds.), *Medical surgical nursing: Concepts and clinical practice* (3rd ed.). St. Louis: C.V. Mosby.

Leiblum, S. R. & Rosen, R. C. (Eds.). (1988). *Sexual desire disorders*. New York: The Guilford Press.

Levine, S. B. (1989). Gender identity disorders of childhood, adolescence, and adulthood. In H. I. Kaplan & B. J. Sadock (Eds.), *Comprehensive textbook of psychiatry* (Vol. 1) (5th ed.). Baltimore: Williams & Wilkins.

LoPiccolo, J. & Friedman, J. M. (1988). Broad-spectrum treatment of low sexual desire: Integration of cognitive, behavioral, and systemic therapy. In S. R. Leiblum & R. C. Rosen (Eds.), *Sexual desire disorders*. New York: Guilford Press.

LoPiccolo, J. & Stock, W. E. (1986). Treatment of sexual dysfunction. *J Consult Clin Psychol, 54*: 158–167.

MacDonald, A. P. (1982). Research on sexual orientation: A bridge that touches both shores but doesn't meet in the middle. *Journal of Sex Education and Therapy, 8*: 9–13.

Malatesta, V. J. et al. (1982). Acute alcohol intoxication and female orgasmic response. *Journal of Sex Research, 18*: 1–17.

Marmor, J. (1976a). Frigidity, dyspareunia, and vaginismus. In B. J. Sadock et al. (Eds.), *The sexual experience*. Baltimore: Williams & Wilkins.

Marmor, J. (1976b). Homosexuality and sexual orientation disturbances. In B. J. Sadock et al. (Eds.), *The sexual experience*. Baltimore: Williams & Wilkins.

Marshall, W. L. & Barbaree, H. E. (1978). The reduction of deviant arousal: Satiation treatment for sexual aggressors. *Criminal Justice and Behavior, 5*: 294–303.

Martinson, F. M. (1973). *Infant and child sexuality: A sociological perspective*. St. Peter, MN: Book Mark.

Masters, W. H. & Johnson, V. E. (1966). *Human sexual response*. Boston: Little, Brown, and Company.

Masters, W. H. & Johnson, V. E. (1970). *Human sexual inadequacy*. Boston: Little, Brown, and Company.

McCarthy, B. W. (1989). Cognitive-Behavioral strategies and techniques in the treatment of early ejaculation. In S. R. Leiblum & R. C. Rosen (Eds.), *Principles and practice of sex therapy: Update for the 1990s* (2nd ed.). New York: The Guilford Press.

Morales, A. et al. (1982). Nonhormonal pharmacologic treatment of organic impotence. *J Urol, 128*: 45–47.

Nathan, S. G. (1986). The epidemiology of the *DSM-III* psychosexual dysfunctions. *J Sex Marital Ther, 12*: 267–281.

Pauly, I. B. (1974). Female transsexualism. *Arch Sex Behav, 3*: 487–526.

Reiss, I. L. (1976). Adolescent sexuality. In W. W. Oaks, G. A. Melchiode, & I. Ficher (Eds.). *Sex and the life cycle.* New York: Grune and Stratton.

Riddle, D. I. (1978). Relating to children: Gays as role models. *Journal of Social Issues, 34*: 38–58.

Robins, L. N. et al. (1984). Lifetime prevalence of specific psychiatric disorders in three sites. *Arch Gen Psychiatry, 41*: 949–958.

Rosenbaum, M. B. (1976). Female sexuality, or why can't a woman be more like a woman. In W. W. Oaks, G. H. Melchiode, & I. Ficher (Eds.), *Sex and the life cycle.* New York: Grune and Stratton.

Sadock, V. A. (1989). Normal human sexuality and sexual disorders. In H. I. Kaplan & B. J. Sadock (Eds.), *Comprehensive textbook of psychiatry* (Vol. 1) (5 ed.). Baltimore: Williams & Wilkins.

Sadock, Kaplan, & Freedman (Eds.). (1986). *The sexual experience.* Baltimore: Williams & Wilkins.

Segraves, R. T. (1988). Hormones and libido. In S. R. Leiblum & R. C. Rosen, *Sexual desire disorders.* New York: The Guilford Press.

Sipova, I. & Starka, L. (1977). Plasma testosterone values in transsexual women. *Arch Sex Behav, 6*: 477–481.

Starka, L. et al. (1975). Plasma testosterone in male transsexuals and homosexuals. *Journal of Sex Research, 11*: 134–138.

Thompson, A. P. (1983). Extramarital sex: A review of the research literature. *Journal of Sex Research, 19*: 1–22.

Thompson, J. M., McFarland, G. K., Hirsch, J. E., Tucker, S. M., & Bowers, A. C. (1986). *Clinical nursing.* St. Louis: CV Mosby.

Tollison, C. D. & Adams, H. E. (1979). *Sexual disorders: Treatment, theory.* New York: Gardner Press.

VandeVusse, L. & Simandl, G. (1992). Sexuality patterns, altered. In K. V. Gettrust & P. D. Brabec (Eds.), *Nursing diagnosis in clinical practice: Guides for care planning.* Albany, NY: Delmar Publishers.

Wagner, G. & Metz, P. (1981). Arteriosclerosis and erectile failure. In G. Wagner & R. Green (Eds.), *Impotence: Physiological, psychological, surgical diagnosis and treatment.* New York: Plenum.

Wincze, J. P. & Carey, M. P. (1991). *Sexual dysfunction: A guide for assessment and treatment.* New York: The Guilford Press.

Wolff, C. (1971). *Love between women.* New York: Harper & Row.

BIBLIOGRAPHY

Doenges, M. E., Townsend, M. C., & Moorhouse, M. F. (1989). *Psychiatric care plans.* Philadelphia: FA Davis.

Kaplan, H. I. & Sadock, B. J. (1989). *Comprehensive textbook of psychiatry* (Vol. 1) (5th ed.). Baltimore: Williams & Wilkins.

Kinsey, A. C., Pomeroy, W. B., Martin, C. E., & Gebhard, P. H. (1953). *Sexual behavior in the human female.* Philadelphia: WB Saunders.

Leiblum, S. R. & Rosen, R. C. (Eds.). (1989). *Principles and practice of sex therapy* (2nd ed.). New York: The Guilford Press.

Lion, E. M. (Ed.). (1982). *Human sexuality in nursing process.* New York: John Wiley & Sons.

Talbott, J. A., Hales, R. E., & Yudofsky, S. C. (1988). *Textbook of psychiatry,* Washington, DC: The American Psychiatric Press.

Townsend, M. C. (1991). *Nursing diagnoses in psychiatric nursing: A pocket guide for care plan construction* (2nd ed.). Philadelphia: FA Davis.

ADJUSTMENT AND IMPULSE CONTROL DISORDERS

Intermittent Explosive Disorder
Kleptomania
Pathological Gambling
Pyromania
Trichotillomania
SUMMARY

OBJECTIVES
After reading this chapter, the student will be able to:
1. Discuss historical aspects and epidemiological statistics related to adjustment and impulse control disorders.
2. Describe various types of adjustment and impulse control disorders and identify symptomatology associated with each. Use this information in patient assessment.
3. Identify predisposing factors in the development of adjustment and impulse control disorders.
4. Formulate nursing diagnoses and goals of care for patients with adjustment and impulse control disorders.
5. Describe appropriate nursing interventions for behaviors associated with adjustment and impulse control disorders.
6. Evaluate nursing care of patients with adjustment and impulse control disorders.
7. Discuss various modalities relevant to treatment of adjustment and impulse control disorders.

INTRODUCTION

Adjustment disorder and impulse control disorders represent two separate diagnostic categories in the *Diagnostic and Statistical Manual of Mental Disorders, ed. 3, revised* (*DSM-III-R*) (American Psychiatric Association [APA], 1987). They do, however, share some similar characteristics. Adjustment disorders are precipitated by "an identifiable psychosocial stressor," and impulse disorders are often modulated directly by the severity of psychosocial stressors (Wise, 1988). Conversely, adjustment disorders are quite common, and impulse control disorders are relatively rare.

This chapter focuses on disorders that occur in response to stressful situations with which the individual has the inability to cope. The behavior may include:

1. Impairment in an individual's usual social and occupational functioning.
2. Compulsive acts that may be harmful to the person or others.

Historical and epidemiological statistics are presented. Predisposing factors that have been implicated in the etiology of adjustment and impulse control disorders provide a framework for studying the dynamics of these pathological conditions.

An explanation of the symptomatology is presented as background knowledge for assessing the patient with an adjustment or impulse control disorder. Nursing care is described in the context of the nursing process. Various medical treatment modalities are explored.

HISTORICAL AND EPIDEMIOLOGICAL FACTORS

Historically, patients with symptoms identified by adjustment or impulse control disorders were classified as having personality disturbances. Problems with these diagnostic categories began following World War II, when as a result of the lack of a standardized diagnostic system, psychiatrics began to experience difficulties communicating diagnoses for behaviors attributed by many to the exposure to combat stress.

The concept of impulse disorders dates back to the 19th century and was identified by the term *instinctive monomania* (Gibbens & Prince, 1962). The original monomanias included alcoholism, fire setting, homicide, and kleptomania.

Adjustment disorders are probably quite common, although there are no reliable studies on the epidemiology of these disorders (Wise, 1988). The diagnosis has likely often been assigned without regard to the existing criteria. In a study by Andreasen and Wasek (1980), 5 percent of inpatients received this diagnosis, and they state, "the percentage of new outpatients receiving this diagnosis was almost certainly substantially higher." A 1986 study by Hales and associates, who reviewed the records of more than 1,000 medical and surgical inpatients who had subsequently been referred to the psychiatric service of a large general hospital, found that adjustment disorder comprised the most frequent diagnosis given (almost 19 percent).

The *DSM-III-R* (APA, 1987) identifies five specific categories of impulse control disorders: intermittent explosive disorder, kleptomania, pathological gambling, pyromania, and trichotillomania. Apparently these disorders are quite rare. Various sources place the prevalence range at from less than 1 percent to 5 percent of the adult population, with kleptomania being at the higher end of the range. Intermittent explosive disorder, pathological gambling, and pyromania are more common among men, while kleptomania and trichotillomania are diagnosed more often in women (APA, 1987).

APPLICATION OF THE NURSING PROCESS

Adjustment Disorders

CLASSIFICATIONS OF ADJUSTMENT DISORDER: BACKGROUND ASSESSMENT DATA

An adjustment disorder is characterized by a maladaptive reaction to an identifiable psychosocial stressor or stressors that occurs within 3 months after onset of the stressor and has persisted for no longer than 6 months (APA, 1987). The individual shows impairment in social and occupa-

tional functioning or exhibits symptoms that are in excess of a normal and expectable reaction to the stressor. The symptoms are expected to remit soon after the stressor is relieved, or if the stressor persists, when a new level of adaptation is achieved. The *DSM-III-R* diagnostic criteria for adjustment disorder are presented in Table 24.1.

The stressor itself can be almost anything, but an individual's response to any particular stressor cannot be predicted. If an individual is highly predisposed or vulnerable to maladaptive response, a severe form of the disorder may follow what most people would consider only a mild or moderate stressor. On the other hand, a less vulnerable individual may develop only a mild form of the disorder in response to what others might consider a severe stressor.

A number of clinical presentations are associated with adjustment disorders. The following categories are identified by the *DSM-III-R* and are distinguished by the predominant features of the maladaptive response.

Adjustment Disorder with Anxious Mood   This category denotes a maladaptive response to a psychosocial stressor in which the predominant manifestation is anxiety. For example, the symptoms may reveal nervousness, worry, and jitteriness.

Table 24.1   DIAGNOSTIC CRITERIA FOR ADJUSTMENT DISORDER

A. A reaction to an identifiable psychosocial stressor (or multiple stressors) that occurs within 3 months of onset of the stressor(s).

B. The maladaptive nature of the reaction is indicated by either of the following:
1. Impairment in occupational (including school) functioning or in usual social activities or relationships with others
2. Symptoms that are in excess of a normal and expectable reaction to the stressor(s)

C. The disturbance is not merely one instance of a pattern of overreaction to stress or an exacerbation of another mental disorder.

D. The maladaptive reaction has persisted for no longer than 6 months.

E. The disturbance does not meet the criteria for any specific mental disorder and does not represent uncomplicated bereavement.

Source: American Psychiatric Association (1987) with permission.

The pervasiveness of anxiety as a symptom in psychiatric illness may contribute to the nebulosity and subsequent infrequent use of this category of adjustment disorder (Popkin, 1989). The clinician must make a differential diagnosis with anxiety disorders.

Adjustment Disorder with Depressed Mood This category is the most commonly diagnosed adjustment disorder. The clinical presentation is one of predominant mood disturbance, although less pronounced than that of major depression. The symptoms, such as depressed mood, tearfulness, and feelings of hopelessness, exceed what is an expected or normative response to an identified psychosocial stressor.

Adjustment Disorder with Disturbance of Conduct This category is characterized by conduct in which there is violation of the rights of others or of major age-appropriate societal norms and rules. Examples include truancy, vandalism, reckless driving, fighting, and defaulting on legal responsibilities. Differential diagnosis must be made from conduct disorder or antisocial personality disorder.

Adjustment Disorder with Mixed Disturbance of Emotions and Conduct The predominant features of this category include mood disturbances (e.g., depression) and emotional disturbances (e.g., anxiety) as well as conduct in which there is violation of the rights of others or of major age-appropriate societal norms and rules (e.g., truancy, vandalism, fighting).

Adjustment Disorder with Mixed Emotional Features This category designates a subtype of adjustment disorder that is characterized by a combination of depression and anxiety or other emotions. In making a diagnosis, the clinician must differentiate from depressive and anxiety disorders.

Adjustment Disorder with Physical Complaints This category identifies patients who respond to major life stressors with repression and external expression of somatic symptoms. It differs from somatoform disorders in that the latter must have presented symptoms for at least 6 months. Common symptoms include fatigue, backache, headache, or other aches and pains.

Adjustment Disorder with Withdrawal The predominant manifestation of this category is social withdrawal without significantly depressed or anxious mood. This behavior is presumed to be in response to a major psychosocial stressor.

Adjustment Disorder with Work (or Academic) Inhibition This category identifies the individual who prior to experiencing a major psychosocial stressor had been capable of performing adequately in either an occupational or academic role. Following the stressor, the individual manifests inability to perform usual job or academic tasks. Symptoms of anxiety and depression are also common to this disorder.

PREDISPOSING FACTORS TO ADJUSTMENT DISORDERS

Biological Theory The presence of chronic disorders, such as organic mental disorder or mental retardation, is thought to limit the general adaptive capacity of an individual (DeWitt, 1984). In these individuals, the normal process of adaptation to stressful life experiences is impaired, causing increased vulnerability to adjustment disorders.

Psychosocial Theories Some proponents of psychoanalytic theory view adjustment disorder as a maladaptive response to stress that is caused by early childhood trauma, increased dependency, and retarded ego development. Other psychoanalysists put considerable weight on the constitutional factor or birth characteristics that contribute to the manner in which individuals respond to stress. In adjustment disorder, a specific meaningful stress has found the point of vulnerability in a person of otherwise adequate ego strength (Popkin, 1989).

DeWitt (1984) describes the predisposition to adjustment disorder as an inability to complete the grieving process in response to a painful life change. She describes the presumed cause of this inability to adapt as *psychic overload*, "a level of intrapsychic strain that exceeds the individual's ability to cope and may therefore disrupt normal functioning and cause psychologic or somatic symptoms." Some individuals remain in denial, acting as though the event never occurred. In others, intrusive symptoms may predominate. In all instances, however, it is the persistence of unwanted emotions and images, and the feeling of being powerless to stop them, that precludes the dysfunctional response.

Transactional Model of Stress/Adaptation Why are some individuals able to confront stressful situations adaptively and even gain strength from the experience, while others not only fail to cope adaptively, but may even encounter psychopathological dysfunction? The Transactional Model of Stress/Adaptation takes into consideration the interaction between the individual and the environment.

The type of stressor that one experiences may influence one's adaptation. Sudden-shock stressors occur without warning, and continuous stressors are those that an individual is exposed to over an extended period. Although many studies have been directed to individuals' responses to sudden-shock stressors, Andreasen and Wasek (1980) found that continuous stressors were more commonly cited than sudden-shock stressors as precipitants to maladaptive functioning.

DeWitt (1984) cites situational context as a contributing factor to an individual's stress response. Situational factors include personal and general economic conditions; occupational and recreational opportunities; the availability of social supports, such as family, friends, and neighbors; and the availability of cultural or religious support groups.

Intrapersonal factors have also been implicated in the predisposition to adjustment disorder. Intrapersonal considerations include constitutional vulnerability. Chess and Thomas (1984) suggested that a child with a difficult temperament (defined as one who cries loudly and often; adapts to changes slowly; and has irregular patterns of hunger, sleep, and elimination) is at greater risk of developing a behavior disorder. Freud (1964) theorized that traumatic childhood experiences created points of fixation to which the individual, during times of stress, would be likely to regress. This might also apply to other unresolved conflicts or developmental issues. Other intrapersonal factors that might influence one's ability to adjust to a painful life change include social skills, coping strategies, the presence of psychiatric illness, degree of flexibility, and level of intelligence.

The etiology of adjustment disorder is most likely influenced by multiple factors. A graphic depiction of this theory of multiple causation is presented in Figure 24.1.

NURSING DIAGNOSIS, PLANNING/IMPLEMENTATION

Nursing diagnoses are formulated from the data gathered during the assessment phase and with background knowledge regarding predisposing factors to the disorder. The following nursing diagnoses may be used for the patient with adjustment disorder:

> Dysfunctional grieving related to real or perceived loss of any concept of value to the individual, evidenced by interference with life functioning, developmental regression, or somatic complaints.
>
> Impaired adjustment related to change in health status requiring modification in life-style (e.g., chronic illness, physical disability), evidenced by inability to problem solve or set realistic goals for the future.
>
> NOTE: According to the North American Nursing Diagnosis Association definition, this diagnosis would only be appropriate for the person with adjustment disorder if the precipitating stressor was a change in health status.

In Table 24.2, these nursing diagnoses are presented in a plan of care for the patient with adjustment disorder. Goals of care and appropriate nursing interventions are included for each. Rationales are presented in italics.

Outcome Criteria   The following criteria may be used for measurement of outcomes in the care of the patient with adjustment disorder.

The patient:
1. Is able to verbalize acceptable behaviors associated with each stage of the grief process.
2. Demonstrates a reinvestment in the environment.
3. Is able to accomplish activities of daily living independently.
4. Demonstrates ability for adequate occupational and social functioning.
5. Verbalizes awareness of change in health status and the effect it will have on life-style.
6. Is able to problem solve and set realistic goals for the future.
7. Demonstrates the ability to cope effectively with change in life-style.

EVALUATION

Reassessment is conducted to determine if the nursing actions have been successful in achieving the objectives of care. Evaluation of the nursing actions for the patient with adjustment disorder may be facilitated by gathering information using the following types of questions.

Does the patient verbalize understanding of the grief process and his or her position in the process?

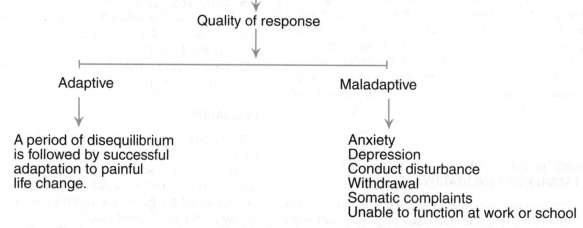

Precipitating Event
(Event that occurs without warning or stress that occurs over an extended period of time)

↓

Predisposing Factors
Genetic Influences: Mental retardation
                         Organic mental disorder
                         Temperamental characteristics at birth that promote vulnerability
Past Experiences: Traumatic childhood experiences
                         Unresolved grief
Existing Conditions: Retarded ego development
                         Unstable economic condition
                         Lack of occupational/recreational opportunities
                         Lack of social, cultural, or religious support groups
                         Inadequate social skills and coping strategies
                         Presence of psychiatric illness

↓

Cognitive Appraisal

↓

* Primary *

↓

(Real or perceived threat to biological integrity or self-concept)

↓

* Secondary *

↓

Because of weak ego strength, patient is unable to use coping mechanisms effectively.
Defense mechanisms utilized: denial, regression, rationalization, repression, suppression

↓

Quality of response

↓

Adaptive	Maladaptive
↓	↓
A period of disequilibrium is followed by successful adaptation to painful life change.	Anxiety Depression Conduct disturbance Withdrawal Somatic complaints Unable to function at work or school

Figure 24.1 The dynamics of adjustment disorder using the transactional model of stress/adaptation.

Table 24.2   CARE PLAN FOR THE PATIENT WITH ADJUSTMENT DISORDER

Nursing Diagnoses	Objectives	Nursing Interventions
Dysfunctional grieving related to real or perceived loss of any concept of value to the individual, evidenced by interference with life functioning, developmental regression, or somatic complaints.	Patient will be able to function adequately at age-appropriate level with evidence of progression toward resolution of grief.	Determine stage of grief in which patient is fixed. Identify behaviors associated with this stage. *Accurate baseline assessment data are necessary to plan effective care for the grieving patient.* Develop trusting relationship with the patient. Show empathy and caring. Be honest and keep all promises. *Trust is the basis for a therapeutic relationship.* Convey an accepting attitude so that the patient is not afraid to express feelings openly. *An accepting attitude conveys to the patient that you believe he or she is a worthwhile person. Trust is enhanced.* Allow patient to express anger. Do not become defensive if initial expression of anger is displaced on the nurse. Assist patient to explore angry feelings so that they may be directed toward the intended object or person. *Verbalization of feelings in a nonthreatening environment may help patient come to terms with unresolved issues.* Assist patient to discharge pent-up anger through participation in large motor activities (e.g., brisk walks, jogging, volleyball, punching bag, exercise bike). *Physical exercise provides a safe and effective method for discharging pent-up tension.* Explain to the patient the normal stages of grief and the behaviors associated with each stage. Help patient to understand that feelings such as guilt and anger toward the lost concept are appropriate and acceptable during the grief process. *Knowledge of the availability of the feelings associated with normal grieving may help to relieve some of the guilt that these responses generate.* Encourage patient to review relationship with lost concept. With support and sensitivity, point out reality of the situation in areas where misrepresentations are expressed. *Patient must give up idealized perception and be able to accept both positive and negative aspects about the painful life change before the grief process is complete.* Communicate to patient that crying is acceptable. Use of touch is generally therapeutic, although specific knowledge about the patient is important before using it *as touch is considered inappropriate in some cultures.* Assist patient in solving problems as he or she attempts to determine methods for more adaptive coping with the stressor. Provide positive feedback for strategies identified and decisions made. *Positive reinforcement enhances self-esteem and encourages repetition of desirable behaviors.* Encourage patient to reach out for spiritual support during this time in whatever form is desirable. Assess patient's spiritual needs and assist as necessary in their fulfillment. *Spiritual support can enhance successful adaptation to painful life experiences.*
Impaired adjustment related to change in health status requiring modification in life-style, evidenced by inability to problem solve or set realistic goals for the future.	Patient will willingly demonstrate competence to function independently to his or her optimal level of ability, considering change in health status.	Encourage patient to talk about life-style prior to the change in health status. Discuss coping mechanisms that were used at stressful times in the past. *Identify the patient's strengths so that they may be used to facilitate adaptation to the change in health status.* Encourage patient to discuss the health change and particularly to express anger associated with it. *Anger is a normal stage in the grieving process and if not released in an appropriate manner, may be turned inward on the self, leading to pathological depression.*

(continued)

Table 24.2 CONTINUED		
Nursing Diagnoses	**Objectives**	**Nursing Interventions**
		Encourage patient to express fears associated with the change or alteration in life-style that the change has created. *Change often creates a feeling of disequilibrium, and the individual may respond with fears that are irrational or unfounded. He or she may benefit from feedback that corrects misperceptions about how life will be with the change in health status.* Provide assistance with activities of daily living as required, but encourage independence to the limit that patient's ability will allow. Give positive feedback for activities accomplished independently. *Independent accomplishments and positive feedback enhance self-esteem and encourage repetition of desired behaviors. Successes also provide hope that adaptive functioning is possible and decrease feelings of powerlessness.* Help patient with decision making regarding incorporation of change into life-style. Identify problems the change is likely to create. Discuss alternative solutions, weighing potential benefits and consequences of each alternative. Support patient's decision in the selection of an alternative. *The high degree of anxiety that usually accompanies a major life-style change often interferes with an individual's ability to solve problems and to make appropriate decisions. Patient may need assistance with this process in an effort to progress toward successful adaptation.* Use role play *to decrease anxiety* as patient anticipates stressful situations that might occur in relation to the health status change. *Role play decreases anxiety and provides a feeling of security by preparing the patient with a plan of action to respond in an appropriate manner when a stressful situation occurs.* Ensure that patient and family are fully knowledgeable regarding the physiology of the change in health status and its necessity for optimal wellness. Encourage them to ask questions, and provide printed material explaining the change to which they may refer following discharge. Ensure that patient can identify resources within the community from which he or she may seek assistance in adapting to the change in health status. *Increased knowledge enhances successful adaptation.*

Does he or she recognize own adaptive and maladaptive behaviors associated with the grief response? Can the patient accomplish activities of daily living independently? If assistance is required, can he or she verbalize resources from whom help may be sought? Does the patient demonstrate evidence of progression along the grief response? Does the patient demonstrate ability to perform occupational and social activities adequately? Does the patient discuss the change in health status and modification of life-style it will effect? Does the patient demonstrate acceptance of the modification? Is the patient able to participate in decision making and problem solving for his or her future? Does the patient set realistic goals for the future? Does the patient demonstrate new adaptive coping strategies for dealing with the change in life-style? Is the patient able to verbalize available resources to whom he or she may go for support or assistance should it be necessary?

Impulse Control Disorders

CLASSIFICATIONS OF IMPULSE CONTROL DISORDERS: BACKGROUND ASSESSMENT DATA

The *DSM-III-R* (APA, 1987) describes the essential features of impulse control disorders as follows:

1. Failure to resist an impulse, drive, or temptation to perform some act that is harmful to the person or others. There may or may not be conscious resistance to the impulse. The act may or may not be premeditated or planned.
2. An increasing sense of tension or arousal before committing the act.
3. An experience of either pleasure, gratification, or release at the time of committing the act. The act is ego-syntonic, that is, it gratifies a conscious wish of the individual's at the moment. Immediately following the act, there may or may not be genuine regret, self-reproach, or guilt.

Impulse control disorders are characterized by a need or desire that must be satisfied immediately regardless of the consequences (Booth, 1984). The individuals seldom know why they do what they do or why it is pleasurable. These behaviors have been likened to sexual excitement and orgasmic release; some authors have noted that many of the behaviors have adverse or even destructive consequences for the person.

Booth (1984) states:

"People with impulse control disorders usually function well enough in other areas of their lives. Many are stable individuals with no serious disorders of thought or cognition. Although other behavior disorders are occasionally associated with some impulse control disorders, the problem for many of these individuals consists solely in a socially unacceptable discharge of tension that is momentarily gratifying but which causes misery and remorse later."

The *DSM-III-R* (APA, 1987) describes five specific categories of impulse control disorders: intermittent explosive disorder, kleptomania, pathological gambling, pyromania, and trichotillomania.

INTERMITTENT EXPLOSIVE DISORDER

This disorder is characterized by a loss of control of a violent or aggressive impulse that culminates in serious assaultive acts or destruction of property (APA, 1987). The individual is not normally an aggressive person between episodes, and the degree of aggressiveness expressed during the episodes is significantly out of proportion to any precipitating psychosocial stressor.

The symptoms appear suddenly, without any apparent provocation, and the violence is usually the result of an irresistible impulse to lash out. Some patients report sensorium changes, such as confusion during episodes or amnesia for events that occurred during episodes (Booth, 1984). Symptoms terminate abruptly, commonly lasting only minutes or at most a few hours, and are followed by feelings of genuine remorse and self-reproach about the inability to control, and the consequences of, the aggressive behavior.

Symptoms of the disorder most often begin in adolescence or young adulthood and gradually disappear as the individual approaches middle age. Patients often have histories of learning disabilities, hyperkinesis, and proneness to accidents in childhood (Booth, 1984). The disorder, which is relatively rare, occurs more often in men than in women (APA, 1987). The *DSM-III-R* diagnostic criteria for intermittent explosive disorder are presented in Table 24.3.

Table 24.3 DIAGNOSTIC CRITERIA FOR INTERMITTENT EXPLOSIVE DISORDER

A. Several discrete episodes of loss of control of aggressive impulses resulting in serious assaultive acts or destruction of property.

B. The degree of aggressiveness expressed during the episodes is grossly out of proportion to any precipitating psychosocial stressors.

C. There are no signs of generalized impulsiveness or aggressiveness between the episodes.

D. The episodes of loss of control do not occur during the course of a psychotic disorder, organic personality syndrome, antisocial or borderline personality disorder, conduct disorder, or intoxication with a psychoactive substance.

Source: American Psychiatric Association (1987) with permission.

Predisposing Factors to Intermittent Explosive Disorder

Biological Influences

1. **Genetic.** The disorder is apparently more common in first-degree biological relatives of people with the disorder than in the general population (APA, 1987).
2. **Physiological.** Any central nervous system insult may predispose to the general clinical syndrome (Booth, 1984). Although they were not included in the revised edition (APA, 1987), the *DSM-III* (APA, 1980) listed possible predisposing factors as perinatal trauma, infantile seizures, head trauma, and encephalitis. Individuals who show high-amplitude, paroxysmal, slow activation on the electroencephalogram are more likely to have aggressive outbursts than are those with either classic "seizure disorder" or normal patterns on electroencephalograms (Booth, 1984).

Psychosocial Influences

1. **Family Dynamics.** Individuals with intermittent explosive disorder often have very strong identifications with assaultive parental figures. The typical history includes a chaotic and violent early family milieu with heavy drinking by one or both parents, parental brutality, child abuse, and the emotional or physical unavailability of a father figure (Booth, 1984). The individual often has childhood memories of parental inconsistencies and unpredictability.

KLEPTOMANIA

The *DSM-III-R* describes kleptomania as "a recurrent failure to resist impulses to steal objects not needed for personal use or their monetary value." The stolen objects are either given away, discarded, returned surreptitiously, or kept and hidden. The individual usually has enough money to pay for the stolen objects (APA, 1987).

The kleptomaniac steals purely for the sake of stealing and for the sense of relief and gratification that follows an episode. The impulsive stealing is in response to increasing tension, and even though the individual almost always knows that the act is wrong, he or she cannot resist the force of mount-

Table 24.4 DIAGNOSTIC CRITERIA FOR KLEPTOMANIA

A. Recurrent failure to resist impulses to steal objects not needed for personal use or their monetary value.

B. Increasing sense of tension immediately before committing the theft.

C. Pleasure or relief at the time of committing the theft.

D. The stealing is not committed to express anger or vengeance.

E. The stealing is not due to conduct disorder or antisocial personality disorder.

Source: American Psychiatric Association (1987) with permission.

ing tension and the pursuit of pleasure and relief that follows (Booth, 1984). Seldom is attention given to the possibility or consequences of being apprehended.

The individual, who usually steals without assistance or collaboration from others, may feel shame or remorse following the incident. Others never experience guilt or regret for their behavior. Symptoms of depression and anxiety have been associated with the disorder.

Onset of the disorder is usually in adolescence. It tends to be chronic, with periods of waxing and waning throughout the course of the disorder. Although an exceedingly rare condition, it appears to be more common among women than men. Fewer than 5 percent of arrested shoplifters give a history that is consistent with kleptomania (Popkin, 1989).

The *DSM-III-R* diagnostic criteria for kleptomania are presented in Table 24.4.

Predisposing Factors to Kleptomania

Biological Influences As with other disorders of impulse control, brain disease and mental retardation are known on occasion to be associated with profitless stealing (Kaplan & Sadock, 1985). Disinhibition and poor impulse control have been associated with cortical atrophy in the frontal region and enlargement of the lateral ventricles of the brain (Popkin, 1989).

Psychosocial Influences Abraham (1953) observed that many kleptomaniacs experienced feelings of being neglected, injured, or unwanted. They reported childhood memories of abandonment (real or imagined) and a sense of lovelessness and deprivation. Booth (1984) states:

"Most dynamic theories of the causes of kleptomania center either on stealing as an attempt to obtain nourishment, esteem, and love or as a sexual equivalent—a quest for a penis in a woman or as a defense against castration anxiety in men. Some theories have been developed in which both mechanisms play a role."

PATHOLOGICAL GAMBLING

This disorder is defined by the *DSM-III-R* as "a chronic and progressive failure to resist impulses to gamble, and gambling behavior that compromises, disrupts, or damages personal, family, or vocational pursuits" (APA, 1987). The preoccupation with and impulse to gamble intensifies when the individual is under stress. Many impulsive gamblers describe a physical sensation of restlessness and anticipation that can only be relieved by placing a bet. Booth (1984) states:

"During a game or a race, the tension is amplified. Whether the pathologic gambler wins or loses, there is typically an immediate urge to place another bet until all the money is gone or until the impulse is temporarily quelled by a run of winning chances, which confers a heightened sense of self-esteem or security."

As the need to gamble increases, the individual is forced to obtain money by whatever means is available. This may include borrowing money from illegal sources or pawning personal items (or items that belong to others). As gambling debts accrue, or out of a need to continue gambling, the individual may desperately resort to forgery, theft, or even embezzlement. Family relationships are disrupted, and impairment in occupational functioning may occur due to absences from work in order to gamble.

Gambling behavior usually begins in adolescence; however, compulsive behaviors rarely occur before young adulthood. The disorder generally runs a chronic course, with periods of waxing and waning, largely dependent on periods of psychosocial stress.

The prevalence of pathological gambling in the United States is estimated at 2 percent to 3 percent of the adult population (APA, 1987). It is more common among men than women.

Various personality traits have been attributed to pathological gamblers. These individuals have

Table 24.5 **DIAGNOSTIC CRITERIA FOR PATHOLOGICAL GAMBLING**

Maladaptive gambling behavior, as indicated by at least four of the following:

1. Frequent preoccupation with gambling or with obtaining money to gamble.
2. Frequent gambling of larger amounts of money or over a longer period than intended.
3. A need to increase the size or frequency of bets to achieve the desired excitement.
4. Restlessness or irritability if unable to gamble.
5. Repeated loss of money by gambling and returning another day to win back losses ("chasing").
6. Repeated efforts to reduce or stop gambling.
7. Frequent gambling when expected to meet social or occupational obligations.
8. Sacrifice of some important social, occupation, or recreational activity in order to gamble.
9. Continuation of gambling despite inability to pay mounting debts or despite other significant social, occupational, or legal problems that the person knows to be exacerbated by gambling.

Source: American Psychiatric Association (1987) with permission.

been described as jovial, extroverted, brash, and energetic (Booth, 1984). Many gamblers exhibit characteristics associated with narcissism and grandiosity and often have difficulties with intimacy, empathy, and trust.

The *DSM-III-R* diagnostic criteria for pathological gambling are presented in Table 24.5.

Predisposing Factors to Pathological Gambling

Biological Influences

1. *Genetics.* The fathers of men with the disorder and the mothers of women with the disorder are more likely to have the disorder than is the population at large (Kaplan & Sadock, 1985).
2. *Physiological.* Various neurophysiological dysfunctions have been associated with pathological gambling behaviors. They include epilepsy, subcortical lesions, and minimal brain dysfunction (Booth, 1984).

Psychosocial Influences The *DSM-III-R* lists the following factors as possible contributors to pathological gambling: inappropriate parental discipline (absence, inconsistency, or harshness); exposure to gambling activities as an adolescent; a high family value placed on material and financial symbols; and a lack of family emphasis on saving, planning, and budgeting.

According to Kaplan and Sadock (1985), some psychodynamicists view the pathological gambler as continuing to struggle with the oedipal complex. In this case, the gambling may represent a challenge of the father figure for acceptance or rejection; a battle with the father figure for supremacy; an expression of extreme submissiveness; an attempt to bribe so that forbidden pleasures might be enjoyed; or an attempt to woo the father.

Other writers have attempted to explain compulsive gambling in terms of psychosexual maturation (Booth, 1984). The gambling is compared to masturbation; both of these activities derive motive force from a buildup of tension that is released through repetitive actions or the anticipation of them. The gambler's inherent need to lose may be based on guilt resulting from an unconscious aggression toward a mother who blocked the child's search for gratification in genital manipulation (Bergler, 1957).

PYROMANIA

Pyromania is the inability to resist the impulse to set fires (Booth, 1984). The act of starting the fire is preceded by tension or affective arousal. The individual experiences intense pleasure, gratification, or relief when setting the fires or witnessing or participating in their aftermath (APA, 1987). The sole motive for setting the fire is self-gratification — not revenge or to collect on insurance or for sabotage. Pyromaniacs may take precautions to avoid apprehension; however, many are totally indifferent to the consequences of their behavior.

The onset of symptoms usually begins in childhood. Many pyromaniacs report early fascination with fire and excitement associated with firefighting equipment and activities. The disorder is relatively rare and is much more common in men than in women. Characteristics associated with pyromaniacs include low intelligence, learning disabilities, hyperkinesis and enuresis in childhood, poor impulse control in other areas (e.g., heavy drinking is common), explosive temper, recklessness, and fascination with high speed (Booth, 1984).

The *DSM-III-R* diagnostic criteria for pyromania are presented in Table 24.6.

Table 24.6 DIAGNOSTIC CRITERIA FOR PYROMANIA

A. Deliberate and purposeful fire setting on more than one occasion.

B. Tension or affective arousal before the act.

C. Fascination with, interest in, curiosity about, or attraction to fire and its situational context or associated characteristics (e.g., paraphernalia, uses, consequences, exposure to fires).

D. Intense pleasure, gratification, or relief when setting fires, or when witnessing or participating in their aftermath.

E. The fire setting is not done for monetary gain, as an expression of sociopolitical ideology, to conceal criminal activity, to express anger or vengeance, to improve one's living circumstances, or in response to a delusion or hallucination.

Source: American Psychiatric Association (1987) with permission.

Predisposing Factors to Pyromania

Biological Influences Various physiological influences have been associated with fire setting. They include mental retardation, dementia, epilepsy, minimal brain dysfunction, and learning disabilities (Booth, 1984; Popkin, 1989). A biochemical influence has been suggested based on evidence of significantly low cerebrospinal fluid monoamine metabolite levels in a study of male arsonists (Virkkunen et al, 1987).

Psychosocial Influences Booth (1984) describes three major psychoanalytic issues that have been associated with impulsive fire setting: 1) an association between fire setting and sexual gratification, 2) concerns about inferiority, impotence, and annihilation, and 3) unconscious anger toward a parent figure. This is consistent with Freud's (1964) view of fire as a symbol of sexuality. He suggested that the warmth radiated by fire can be compared to the sensation that accompanies a state of sexual excitation. Several authors have described patients who have masturbated after setting fires and describe the gratification they experience as "orgasmic." Other psychoanalytic writers have suggested that fire may symbolize activities deriving from various levels of libidinal and aggressive development. They view the act of fire setting as a means of relieving accumulated rage over the frustration caused by a sense of social, physical, and sexual inferiority (Kaplan & Sadock, 1985).

TRICHOTILLOMANIA

The *DSM-III-R* defines this disorder "as the recurrent failure to resist impulses to pull out one's own hair" (APA, 1987). The impulse is preceded by an increasing sense of tension, and the individual experiences a sense of release or gratification from pulling out the hair. Hair loss usually occurs in the scalp region but can also involve hair from the eyebrows, eyelashes, beard, armpits, and pubic area. These areas of hair loss are more likely found on the opposite side of the body from the dominant hand (Wise, 1988). Pain is seldom reported to accompany the hair pulling, although tingling and pruritus in the area are not uncommon.

The disorder usually begins in childhood and may be accompanied by nail biting, head banging, scratching, biting, or other acts of self-mutilation (APA, 1987). This phenomenon is relatively rare, but occurs more often in women than in men.

The *DSM-III-R* diagnostic criteria for trichotillomania are presented in Table 24.7.

Predisposing Factors to Trichotillomania

Biological Influences A family history of alopecia has been demonstrated in one study of children with trichotillomania (APA, 1987). Trichotillomania can also be present as a major symptom in mental retardation (Krishnan et al, 1985).

Psychosocial Influences The *DSM-III-R* links the onset of symptoms to stressful situations in more than one quarter of cases (APA, 1987). Other factors include disturbances in mother-child relationships, fear of abandonment, and recent object loss.

The psychodynamic view associates trichotillomania with early emotional deprivation (Popkin, 1989). The mother is often described as rejecting, sadistic, and condemning; the father, as weak and passive. In some rudimentary and distorted way,

Table 24.7 DIAGNOSTIC CRITERIA FOR TRICHOTILLOMANIA

A. Recurrent failure to resist impulses to pull out one's own hair, resulting in noticeable hair loss.

B. Increasing sense of tension immediately before pulling out the hair.

C. Gratification or a sense of relief when pulling out the hair.

D. No association with a preexisting inflammation of the skin and not a response to a delusion or hallucination.

Source: American Psychiatric Association (1987) with permission.

hair pulling satisfies the need for tenderness and physical contact, and the fear of abandonment subsides.

Transactional Model of Stress/Adaptation The etiology of impulse control disorders is most likely influenced by multiple factors. In Figure 24.2, a graphic depiction of this theory of multiple causation is presented in the Transactional Model of Stress/Adaptation.

NURSING DIAGNOSIS, PLANNING/IMPLEMENTATION

Nursing diagnoses are formulated from the data gathered during the assessment phase and with background knowledge regarding predisposing factors to the disorder. The following nursing diagnoses may be used for the patient with impulse control disorder.

High risk for violence directed toward others related to dysfunctional family system, evidenced by episodes of violent, aggressive, or assaultive behavior.

Ineffective individual coping related to possible hereditary factors, physiological alterations, dysfunctional family, or unresolved developmental issues, evidenced by inability to control impulse to gamble, steal, set fires, or pull out own hair.

In Table 24.8, these nursing diagnoses are presented in a plan of care for the patient with impulse control disorder. Goals of care and appropriate nursing interventions are included for each. Rationales are presented in italics.

Outcome Criteria The following criteria may be used for measurement of outcomes in the care of the patient with impulse control disorder.

The patient:
1. Has not caused harm to self or others.
2. Is able to inhibit the impulse for violence and aggression.
3. Is able to verbalize the symptoms of increasing tension.
4. Is able to verbalize strategies to avoid becoming violent.
5. Is able to verbalize actual object at which anger is directed.
6. Is continuing to work on increasing frustration tolerance.

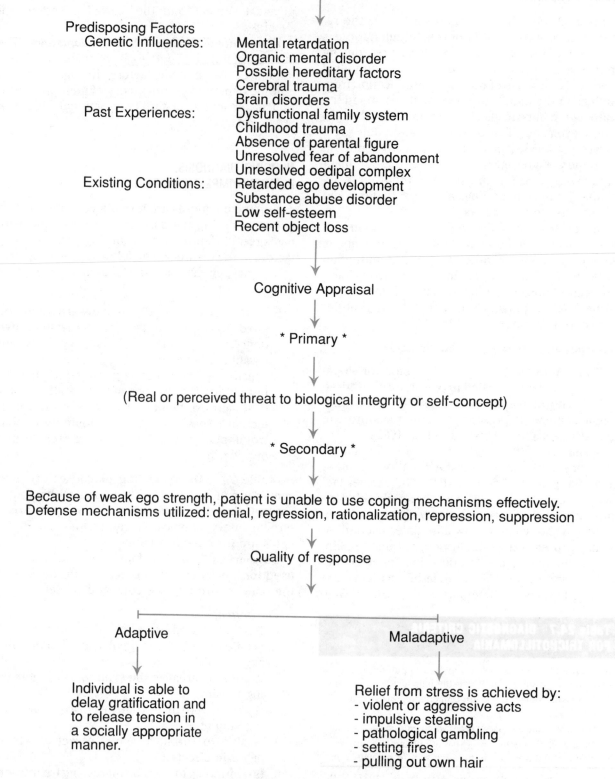

Figure 24.2 The dynamics of impulse control disorder using the transactional model of stress/adaptation.

Table 24.8 CARE PLAN FOR THE PATIENT WITH IMPULSE CONTROL DISORDER

Nursing Diagnoses	Objectives	Nursing Interventions
High risk for violence directed toward others related to dysfunctional family system, evidenced by episodes of violent, aggressive, or assaultive behavior.	Patient will not harm others or the property of others.	Convey an accepting attitude toward this patient. Feelings of rejection are undoubtedly familiar to him or her. Work on development of trust. Be honest, keep all promises, and convey the message that it is not him or her but the behavior that is unacceptable. *An attitude of acceptance promotes feelings of self-worth. Trust is the basis of a therapeutic relationship.* Maintain low level of stimuli in patient's environment (low lighting, few people, simple decor, low noise level). *A stimulating environment may increase agitation and promote aggressive behavior. Make the patient's environment as safe as possible* by removing all potentially dangerous objects. Help patient identify the true object of his or her hostility. *Because of weak ego development, patient may be unable to use ego defense mechanisms correctly. Helping him or her recognize this in a nonthreatening manner may help reveal unresolved issues so that they may be confronted.* Staff should maintain and convey a calm attitude. *Anxiety is contagious and can be transferred from staff to patient. A calm attitude provides patient with a feeling of safety and security.* Help patient recognize the signs that tension is increasing and ways in which violence can be averted. *Activities that require physical exertion are helpful in relieving pent-up tension.* Explain to patient that should explosive behavior occur, staff will intervene in whatever way is required (e.g., tranquilizing medication, restraints, isolation) to protect patient and others. *This conveys to the patient evidence of control over the situation and provides a feeling of safety and security.*
Ineffective individual coping related to possible hereditary factors, physiological alterations, dysfunctional family, or unresolved developmental issues, evidenced by inability to control impulse to gamble, steal, set fires, or pull out own hair.	Patient will be able to delay gratification and use adaptive coping strategies in response to stress.	Help patient gain insight into his or her own behaviors. Often these individuals rationalize to such an extent that they deny that what they have done is wrong. *Patient must come to understand that certain behaviors will not be tolerated within the society and that severe consequences will be imposed upon those individuals who refuse to comply. Patient must WANT to become a productive member of society before he or she can be helped.* Talk about past behaviors with patient. Discuss behaviors that are acceptable by societal norms and those that are not. Help patient identify ways in which he or she has exploited others. Encourage patient to explore how he or she would feel if the circumstances were reversed. *An attempt may be made to enlighten the patient to the sensitivity of others by promoting self-awareness in an effort to assist the patient gain insight into his or her own behavior.* Throughout relationship with patient, maintain attitude of "It is not you, but your behavior, that is unacceptable." *An attitude of acceptance promotes feelings of dignity and self-worth.* Work with patient to increase the ability

(*continued*)

Table 24.8 CONTINUED		
Nursing Diagnoses	**Objectives**	**Nursing Interventions**
		to delay gratification. **Reward desirable behaviors and provide immediate positive feedback.** *Rewards and positive feedback enhance self-esteem and encourage repetition of desirable behaviors.* **Help patient identify and practice more adaptive strategies for coping with stressful life situations.** *The impulse to perform the maladaptive behavior may be so great that the patient is unable to see any other alternatives to relieve stress.*

7. Is able to verbalize more adaptive strategies for coping with stressful situations.
8. Is able to demonstrate ability to delay gratification.
9. Verbalizes understanding that behavior is unacceptable and accepts responsibility for own behavior.

EVALUATION

Reassessment is conducted to determine if the nursing actions have been successful in achieving the objectives of care. Evaluation of the nursing actions for the patient with impulse control disorder may be facilitated by gathering information using the following types of questions.

Has violence, aggression, or assaultive behavior been avoided? Have the patient and others escaped harm? Does the patient verbalize understanding of the unacceptability of his or her behavior? Is he or she able to verbalize and demonstrate more adaptive strategies for coping with stress? Is the patient able to demonstrate the ability to delay gratification? Can he or she verbalize the symptoms of tension that precede unacceptable behavior? Can the patient demonstrate ways to intervene when tension rises that inhibit the compulsion for maladaptive behavior? Can the patient verbalize the types of stress that create the tension? Can he or she verbalize a plan to deal with the stress in the future without resorting to behaviors that are socially unacceptable?

TREATMENT MODALITIES

Adjustment Disorders

Various treatments are used for patients with adjustment disorder. The major goals of therapy for these individuals are:

1. To relieve symptoms.
2. To achieve a level of adaptation that at least equals the level of functioning before the stressful event.
3. To undergo positive change whenever possible (DeWitt, 1984).

INDIVIDUAL PSYCHOTHERAPY

Individual psychotherapy is the most common treatment for adjustment disorder. Horowitz and Kaltreider (1980) describe an approach to individual psychotherapy in which the patient's problems are seen to result from the meanings assigned by the individual to the stressful event and expressed by activation of unresolved conflicts, latent self-images, and developmental inadequacies. Treatment works to remove these blocks to adaptation so that normal developmental progression can resume. Techniques are used to clarify links between the current stressor and past experiences, and to assist with the development of more adaptive coping strategies.

FAMILY THERAPY

Focus of treatment is shifted from the individual to the system of relationships in which the individual is involved. The maladaptive response of the identified patient is viewed as symptomatic of a dysfunctional family system. All family members are included in the therapy, and treatment serves to improve the functioning within the family network. Emphasis is placed on communication, family rules, and interaction patterns among the family members.

BEHAVIORAL THERAPY

The goal of behavioral therapy is to replace ineffective response patterns with more adaptive ones. The situations that promote ineffective responses are identified, and carefully designed reinforcement schedules, along with role modeling, coaching, and didactic presentations, are used to alter the maladaptive response patterns (DeWitt, 1984). This type of treatment is very effective when implemented in an inpatient setting where the patient's behavior and its consequences are more readily controlled.

SELF-HELP GROUPS

Group experiences with or without a professional facilitator provide a context in which members may consider and compare their responses to similar life experiences (DeWitt, 1984). Members benefit from learning that they are not alone in their painful experiences. Hope is derived from knowing that others have survived and even grown from similar experiences. Members of the group exchange advice, share coping strategies, and provide support and encouragement for each other.

PSYCHOPHARMACOLOGY

Adjustment disorder is not commonly treated with medications. Reasons for this include 1) concerns that their effect is temporary and only masks the real problem, interfering with the possibility of finding a more permanent solution and 2) because psychoactive drugs carry the potential for physiological and psychological dependence.

When the patient with adjustment disorder has symptoms of anxiety or depression, the physician may prescribe antianxiety or antidepressant medication. These medications are considered only adjuncts to psychotherapy and should not be given as the primary therapy. In these instances, they are given to alleviate symptoms so that the individual may more effectively cope while attempting to adapt to the stressful situation.

Impulse Control Disorders

INTERMITTENT EXPLOSIVE DISORDER

Individual psychotherapy with intermittent explosive disorder has not been successful. Group therapy, with its elements of group loyalty, peer pressure, expectation, and confrontation, has been more useful (Booth, 1984). Family therapy may be helpful when the patient is an adolescent or young adult (Kaplan & Sadock, 1985).

Largely, treatment of patients with intermittent explosive disorder has been with psychopharmacologic agents. A variety of agents have been tried, including lithium, carbamazepine, phenytoin, benzodiazepines, and propranolol (Popkin, 1989). Recent data suggest a relationship between aggressive behavior and abnormal serotonin metabolism. Clinical management of the disorder with medications that block reuptake of serotonin warrants further investigation.

Neurosurgical procedures have been used in the treatment of intractable explosive behavior. Evidence of the effectiveness of this type of treatment is lacking.

KLEPTOMANIA

Insight-oriented psychodynamic psychotherapy has been the most successful method of treatment of kleptomania (Booth, 1984). It has been most helpful with those individuals who experience guilt and shame and are thus motivated to change their behavior.

Various methods of behavior therapy have also been reported as useful (Popkin, 1989). Systematic desensitization, aversive conditioning, and alteration of interactional strategies have been helpful in some instances.

PATHOLOGICAL GAMBLING

Because most pathological gamblers deny that they have a problem, treatment is very difficult. In fact, most gamblers only seek treatment due to legal difficulties, family pressures, or other psychiatric complaints (Kaplan & Sadock, 1985).

Behavioral therapy has been used with pathological gamblers. McConaghy et al (1983) reported that imaginal desensitization has been more successful than aversive therapy.

Lithium carbonate has been shown to be successful in the treatment of some pathological gamblers (Moskowitz, 1980). This medication likely is most effective in relieving associated mood disturbances.

Possibly the most effective treatment of pathological gambling is participation by the individual in Gamblers Anonymous (GA). This organization of inspirational group therapy is modeled after Alcoholics Anonymous. The only requirement for GA membership is an expressed desire to stop gambling (Wise, 1988). Treatment is based on peer pressure, public confession, and the availability of other reformed gamblers to help individuals resist the urge to gamble (Booth, 1984). Gam-Anon (for family and spouses of compulsive gamblers) and Gam-a-Teen (for adolescent children of compulsive gamblers) are also important sources for treatment.

PYROMANIA

Mavromatis and Lion (1977) have stated, "Treatment for firesetters has been traditionally problematic due to the frequent refusal to take responsibility for the act, the use of denial, the existence of alcoholism, and the lack of insight."

Aversive therapy and behavior therapy techniques have been used with moderate results. Group therapy and family therapy have been quite successful with children (Booth, 1984).

TRICHOTILLOMANIA

Behavior modification has been employed in the treatment of trichotillomania. Various techniques have been tried, including covert desensitization and habit reversal practices. When the techniques are managed by a therapist, a system of rewards and punishment is applied in an effort to modify the hair-pulling behaviors.

Psychodynamic intervention has been used in children with trichotillomania. Inquiry is made into areas of parent-child relationships or other areas of potential conflict that may provide some enlightenment about the problem (Wise, 1988).

Various psychopharmacologic agents, including chlorpromazine, amitriptyline, and lithium carbonate, have been tried in the treatment of trichotillomania. Isolated case results of successful treatment have been reported.

SUMMARY

This chapter has focused on disorders that occur in response to stressful situations with which the individual has the inability to cope. The behavior may include:

1. Impairment in an individual's usual social and occupational functioning.
2. Compulsive acts that may be harmful to the person or others.

Adjustment disorders are relatively common. In fact, some studies indicate they are the most commonly ascribed psychiatric diagnosis. Clinical symptoms include inability to function socially or occupationally in response to a psychosocial stressor. The disorder is distinguished by the predominant features of the maladaptive response. These include anxiety, depression, disturbance of conduct, disturbance of emotions and conduct, mixed emotional features, physical complaints, withdrawal, and inhibition of work or academics.

Of the two types of stressors discussed, (i.e., sudden-shock and continuous), it has been found that more individuals respond with maladaptive behaviors to continuous stressors to which they are exposed over an extended period. Treatment modalities for adjustment disorders include individual psychotherapy, family therapy, behavioral therapy, self-help groups, and psychopharmacology.

Impulse control disorders are quite rare but involve compulsive acts that may be harmful to the individual or to others. Individuals with impulse control disorders experience increased tension, followed by the inability to resist committing a specific act, after which the individual feels a sense of release and gratification.

Impulse control disorders include:

1. *Intermittent explosive disorder*—violent or aggressive behavior that culminates in serious assaultive acts or the destruction of property.
2. *Kleptomania*—inability to resist the impulse to steal.
3. *Pathological gambling*—inability to resist the impulse to gamble.
4. *Pyromania*—inability to resist the impulse to set fires.
5. *Trichotillomania*—inability to resist the impulse to pull out one's own hair.

Nursing care of individuals with adjustment and impulse control disorders is accomplished using the steps of the nursing process. Background assessment data were presented, along with nursing diagnoses common to each disorder. Interventions appropriate to each nursing diagnosis and relevant outcome criteria for each were included. An overview of current medical treatment modalities was discussed.

REVIEW QUESTIONS
Self-Examination/Learning Exercise

*Select the answer that is **most** appropriate for each of the following questions.*

Situation: Linda has been admitted to the psychiatric unit with a diagnosis of adjustment disorder with depressed mood. She recently left her husband after 10 years of a very stormy marriage. She did not want to leave but decided that the move was best for herself, as well as her two children (who are living with her). Linda was very dependent on her husband and is having difficulty living an independent life-style.

1. The primary nursing diagnosis for Linda would be:
   a. impaired adjustment related to breakup of marriage.
   b. dysfunctional grieving related to breakup of marriage.
   c. high risk for self-directed violence related to depressed mood.
   d. social isolation related to depressed mood.

2. Linda says to the nurse, "I feel so bad. I thought I would feel better once I left, but I feel worse!" Which is the *best* response by the nurse?
   a. "Cheer up, Linda. You have a lot to be happy about."
   b. "You are grieving for the marriage you did not have. It's natural for you to feel badly."
   c. "Try not to dwell on how you feel. If you don't think about it, you'll feel better."
   d. "You did the right thing, Linda. Knowing that should make you feel better."

3. The physician orders amitriptyline (Elavil) for Linda. This medication is intended to:
   a. increase energy and elevate mood.
   b. stimulate the central nervous system.
   c. prevent psychotic symptoms.
   d. produce a calming effect.

4. Which of the following is true regarding adjustment disorder?
   a. Linda will require long-term psychotherapy to achieve relief.
   b. Linda likely inherited a genetic tendency for the disorder.

    c. Linda's symptoms will likely remit once she has accepted the change in her life.

    d. Linda probably would not have experienced adjustment disorder if she had a higher level of intelligence.

5. The category of adjustment disorder with depressed mood identifies the individual who:

    a. violates the rights of others to feel better.

    b. expresses symptoms that reveal a high level of anxiety.

    c. exhibits severe social isolation and withdrawal.

    d. is experiencing a dysfunctional grieving process.

Match the behavior on the right to the appropriate diagnosis on the left.

6. Kleptomania   _____ a. Tony has been fascinated by fire for as long as he can remember. He played with matches as a child. As an adult, he has set numerous fires, always feeling exhilarated and even sexually stimulated afterward.

7. Intermittent explosive disorder   _____ b. Janet recently received a great deal of money and property in a divorce settlement. Shortly after the divorce, she experienced an impulse to enter a large department store and steal some inexpensive costume jewelry. Although she had been apprehended twice for shoplifting, she was indifferent to being discovered at this time.

8. Pathological gambling   _____ c. Frankie, a 16-year-old boy, had had temper tantrums since age 2. As he matured, the "tantrums" intensified, with explosions of rage, usually without identifiable provocation. He had attempted to molest his 12-year-old sister and went after his father with a butcher knife. He has an abnormal electroencephalogram.

9. Pyromania   _____ d. Callie, a 10-year-old girl, has been pulling her hair out of the crown of her head for several years. She has been referred to psychiatry from the dermatology clinic. Her mother reports the hair pulling usually occurs at night when Callie is tired. Further history reveals Callie's father left her mother when Callie was 4 years old and has never been heard from since. Callie tells the psychiatrist he left because she was a bad girl.

10. Trichotillomania   _____ e. Harold has borrowed a great deal of money from an illegal source in an

effort to pay back a gambling debt. He has continued to gamble so that he can pay back the loan with his winnings. Last night, the loan sharks threatened harm if he did not pay soon. He withdraws all the money from his joint account with his wife and heads for the race track.

REFERENCES

Abraham, K. (1953). Manifestations of the female castration complex. In D. Bryan & A. Strachey (Eds.), *Selected papers on psychoanalysis.* New York: Basic Books.

American Psychiatric Association. (1980). *Diagnostic and statistical manual of mental disorders* (3rd ed.). Washington, DC: American Psychiatric Association.

American Psychiatric Association. (1987). *Diagnostic and statistical manual of mental disorders* (3rd ed., rev.). Washington, DC: American Psychiatric Association.

Andreasen, N. C. & Wasek, P. (1980). Adjustment disorders in adolescents and adults. *Arch Gen Psychiatry, 37,* 1166–1170.

Bergler, E. (1957). *The psychology of gambling.* New York: International Universities Press.

Booth, G. K. (1984). Disorders of impulse control. In H. H. Goldman (Ed.), *Review of general psychiatry.* Los Altos, CA: Lange Medical Publications.

Chess, S. & Thomas, A. (1984). *Origins and evolution of behavior disorders.* New York: Brunner/Mazel.

DeWitt, K. N. (1984). Adjustment disorder. In H. H. Goldman (Ed.), *Review of general psychiatry.* Los Altos, CA: Lange Medical Publications.

Freud, S. (1964). New introductory lectures on psycho-analysis and other works. In *The Standard Edition of the Complete Psychological Works of Sigmund Freud* (Vol. 22). London: Hogarth Press.

Gibbens, T. C. N. & Prince, J. (1962). *Shoplifting.* London: Institute for the Study and Treatment of Delinquency.

Hales, R. E. et al. (1986). Psychiatric consultation in a military general hospital. *Gen Hosp Psychiatry, 8,* 173–182.

Horowitz, M. J. & Kaltreider, N. (1980). Psychotherapy of stress response syndromes. In T. Karasu & L. Bellak (Eds.), *Specialized techniques in individual psychotherapy.* New York: Brunner/Mazel.

Kaplan, H. I. & Sadock, B. J. (1985). *Modern synopsis of comprehensive textbook of psychiatry* (4th ed.). Baltimore: Williams & Wilkins.

Krishnan, K. R. R. et al. (1985). Trichotillomania—A review. *Comp Psychiatry, 26,* 123–138.

Mavromatis, M. & Lion, J. R. (1977). A primer on pyromania. *Dis Nerv Syst, 38,* 954–955.

McConaghy, N. et al. (1983). Controlled comparison of aversive therapy and imaginal desensitization in compulsive gambling. *Br J Psychiatry, 142,* 366–372.

Moskowitz, J. A. (1980). Lithium and lady luck. *NY State J Med, 80,* 785–788.

Popkin, M. K. (1989). Adjustment disorder and impulse control disorder. In H. I. Kaplan & B. J. Sadock (Eds.), *Comprehensive textbook of psychiatry* (Vol. 2) (5th ed.). Baltimore: Williams & Wilkins.

Virkkunen, M. et al. (1987). Cerebrospinal fluid monoamine metabolite levels in male arsonists. *Arch Gen Psychiatry, 44,* 241–247.

Wise, M. G. (1988). Adjustment disorders and impulse disorders not otherwise classified. In J. A. Talbott, R. E. Hales, & S. C. Yudofsky (Eds.), *Textbook of psychiatry,* Washington, DC: American Psychiatric Press.

BIBLIOGRAPHY

Eaton, M. T., Peterson, M. H., & Davis, J. A. (1981). *Psychiatry* (5th ed.). New York: Medical Examination Publishing.

Lanza, M. L. (1983). Origins of aggression. *J Psychosoc Nurs, 21*(6), 11–16.

Roper, J. M., Coutts, A., Sather, J., & Taylor, R. (1985). Restraint and seclusion. *J Psychosoc Nurs, 23*(6), 18–23.

Stilling, L. (1992). The pros and cons of physical restraints and behavior controls. *J Psychosoc Nurs, 30*(3), 18–20.

Townsend, M. C. (1991). *Nursing diagnoses in psychiatric nursing: A pocket guide for care plan construction* (2nd ed.). Philadelphia: FA Davis.

25

PSYCHOLOGICAL FACTORS AFFECTING PHYSICAL CONDITION

Rheumatoid Arthritis
Ulcerative Colitis
SUMMARY

OBJECTIVES

After reading this chapter, the student will be able to:

1. Differentiate between somatoform and psychophysiological disorders.
2. Identify various types of psychophysiological disorders.
3. Discuss historical and epidemiological statistics related to various psychophysiological disorders.
4. Describe symptomatology associated with various psychophysiological disorders and use this data in patient assessment.
5. Identify various predisposing factors to psychophysiological disorders.
6. Formulate nursing diagnoses and goals of care for patients with various psychophysiological disorders.
7. Describe appropriate nursing interventions for behaviors associated with various psychophysiological disorders.
8. Evaluate nursing care of patients with psychophysiological disorders.
9. Discuss various modalities relevant to treatment of psychophysiological disorders.

INTRODUCTION

Psychophysiological responses are those in which it has been determined that psychological factors contribute to the initiation or exacerbation of the physical condition. They differ from somatoform disorders in that there is evidence of either demonstrable organic pathology or a known pathophysiological process involved. No such organic involvement can be identified in somatoform disorders. The *Diagnostic and Statistical Manual of Mental Disorders, ed. 3, revised (DSM-III-R)* (American Psychiatric Association [APA], 1987) diagnostic criteria for psychological factors affecting physical condition are presented in Table 25.1.

Virtually any organic disorder can be considered psychophysiological in nature. Kaplan (1989) states that "all disease is influenced by psychologi-

Table 25.1 DIAGNOSTIC CRITERIA FOR PSYCHOLOGICAL FACTORS AFFECTING PHYSICAL CONDITION

A. Psychologically meaningful environmental stimuli are temporally related to the initiation or exacerbation of a specific physical condition or disorder.

B. The physical condition involves either demonstrable organic pathology (e.g., rheumatoid arthritis) or a known pathophysiological process (e.g., migraine headache).

C. The condition does not meet the criteria for a somatoform disorder.

Source: American Psychiatric Association (1987) with permission.

cal factors." A list of some (though certainly not all) psychophysiological disorders is presented in Table 25.2.

Table 25.2 EXAMPLES OF PSYCHOPHYSIOLOGICAL DISORDERS

Acne	Immune disease (e.g.,
Amenorrhea	multiple sclerosis,
Angina pectoris	systemic lupus
Asthma	erythematosus)
Cancer	Impotence
Cardiospasm	Irritable bowel syndrome
Coronary heart disease	Migraine headache
Duodenal ulcer	Nausea and vomiting
Dysmenorrhea	Neurodermatitis
Enuresis	Obesity
Essential hypertension	Pylorospasm
Gastric ulcer	Regional enteritis
Herpes	Rheumatoid arthritis
Hyperglycemia	Sacroiliac pain
Hyperthyroidism	Skin disease (e.g., psoriasis)
Hypoglycemia	Tension headache
	Tuberculosis
	Ulcerative colitis

Sources: APA (1987), Kaplan (1989), and Pelletier (1977).

The following psychophysiological disorders are discussed in this chapter:

asthma
cancer
coronary heart disease
peptic ulcer
hypertension
migraine headache
obesity
rheumatoid arthritis
ulcerative colitis

Historical and epidemiological statistics are presented. Predisposing factors that have been implicated in the etiology of each psychophysiological disorder provide a framework for study. An explanation of the symptomatology is presented as background knowledge for assessing the patient with a psychophysiological disorder. Nursing care is described in the context of the nursing process. Various medical treatment modalities are explored.

HISTORICAL ASPECTS

For more than a century, physicians have agreed that in some disorders there is an interaction between emotional and physical factors. Kaplan and Sadock (1985) describe four general types of reaction to stress:

1. *The normal,* in which there is increased alertness and a mobilization of defenses for action.
2. *The psychophysiological,* in which the defenses fail and the response is translated into somatic symptoms.
3. *The neurotic,* in which the anxiety is so great that the defense becomes ineffective and neurotic symptoms develop.
4. *The psychotic,* in which loss of control results in misperception of the environment.

This explanation of stress response corresponds to the concept of anxiety described by Peplau (1963) and the type of responses associated with each level (see Chapter 2). Along the continuum of anxiety, psychophysiological disorders occur at the moderate-to-severe level.

Selye (1976) studied the physiological response of a biological system to change imposed upon it. He found that regardless of the stressor, the biological entity responded with a syndrome of symptoms that he called the *general adaptation syndrome.* (This syndrome of symptoms is described in Chapter 1.) In this aroused state, the individual garners the strength to face the stress and mobilize the defenses to resolve it. However, if the defenses fail and the stressor is not quickly resolved, the body remains in this aroused state indefinitely, becoming susceptible to psychophysiological illness.

Historically, mind and body have been viewed as two distinct entities, each subject to different laws of causality. Indeed, in many instances, particularly in highly specialized areas of medicine, the biological and psychological components of disease remain separate. However, medical research shows that a change is occurring. Research associated with biological functioning is being expanded to include also the psychological and social determinants of health and disease (Bakal, 1979). This psychobiological approach to illness reflects a more holistic perspective and one that promotes concern for helping patients achieve optimal functioning.

APPLICATION OF THE NURSING PROCESS

Types of Psychophysiological Disorders

ASTHMA

Definition and Epidemiological Statistics
Asthma is a syndrome of airflow limitation characterized by increased responsiveness of the tra-

cheobronchial tree to various stimuli and manifested by airway smooth muscle contraction, hypersecretion of mucus, and inflammation (Anderson, 1991). It affects approximately 7 million adults and children in the United States (Brucia et al, 1987). The onset is commonly in childhood, and the incidence is higher in boys until the teen years. During adolescence and thereafter, the incidence is higher in women than men (Vachon, 1989).

Signs and Symptoms Asthma is characterized by episodes of bronchial constriction resulting in dyspnea, wheezing, productive cough, restlessness, and eosinophilia. Expiration is prolonged and breathing reflects use of accessory muscles. Tachypnea and nasal flaring are common. The individual is usually diaphoretic and quite apprehensive, with total attention focused on his or her breathing.

Predisposing Factors

Biological Influences Hereditary factors may play a role in the etiology of asthma. When both parents have the disease, it is known to occur in more than half the offspring, dropping to around 20 percent when only one parent is affected (Vachon, 1989). Twin studies show a concordance of about 50 percent.

Allergies play a major role in precipitating the attacks associated with asthma. Anderson (1991) lists the following specific agents known to stimulate bronchoconstriction: aspirin and all nonsteroidal anti-inflammatory drugs, chemicals, dust, grains, food additives, and beta-blocking agents (e.g., propranolol). Other nonspecific factors known to stimulate bronchoconstriction include exercise, cold air, environmental pollutants and irritants (e.g., infection, cigarette smoke), pharmacological agents (e.g., histamine, cholinergic agonists), and reflux esophagitis.

Psychosocial Influences Asthma has long been recognized as a "typical" psychophysiological response with evidence of symptoms being induced by emotional stress. The psychodynamic personality profile of the asthmatic person reflects excessive unresolved dependence on the mother (Alexander et al, 1968). This characteristic arises out of a fear of rejection, possibly based in part on the parent's attempt to instill independence in the child before he or she was ready. Separation from the parent was viewed as possible abandonment.

These unfulfilled needs may contribute to the precipitation of asthmatic attacks in later life when an individual experiences a disappointment in an interpersonal relationship that he or she perceives as loss or rejection, or is faced with a stressful situation in which he or she feels very insecure.

CANCER

Definition and Epidemiological Statistics Cancer is a malignant neoplasm in which the basic structure and activity of the cells have become deranged, usually due to changes in the DNA. These mutated cells grow wildly and rapidly, and lose their similarity to the original cells. The malignant cells spread to other areas by invading surrounding tissues and by entering the blood and lymphatic system. If left untreated, the malignant neoplasms usually result in death.

Cancer is the second leading cause of death in the United States today. However, 5-year survival rates have increased as a result of early diagnosis and treatment and the improvement of treatment modalities for most cancers. The largest number of deaths from cancer in both men and women is attributed to cancer of the lung (American Cancer Society [ACS], 1989).

In the black population, the mortality rates tend to be higher and the survival rates are lower than in the white population. Cancer has been called a "disease of the aging," as the likelihood of developing cancer increases with age.

Signs and Symptoms The ACS has identified seven significant changes that may occur as early warning signs of cancer. They include:

1. A change in bowel or bladder habits.
2. A sore that does not heal.
3. Unusual bleeding or discharge.
4. A thickening or lump in the breast or elsewhere.
5. Indigestion or difficulty in swallowing.
6. An obvious change in a wart or mole.
7. A nagging cough or hoarseness.

Specific effects are determined by site. Malignant tumors can also create effects at sites distant to the primary site. Late-stage cancer symptoms may include anemias, infections, thrombocytopenia, cachexia, weakness, weight loss, dyspnea, ascites, and pleural effusion (Hogan & Xistris, 1987).

Predisposing Factors

Biological Influences Certain cancers, such as those of the stomach, breast, colon, rectum, uterus, and lung, tend to occur in a familial pattern. Whether this indicates an inherited susceptibility or common exposure to an etiological factor is unknown (ACS, 1981).

Continuous irritation may predispose individuals to certain types of cancer. For example, chronic exposure to the sun may predispose to melanoma, and prolonged alcohol consumption is thought to be related to the development of esophageal cancer (ACS, 1981).

Exposure to occupational or environmental carcinogens may lead to specific cancers. Examples include cigarette smoke, aniline dye, radium, asphalt, arsenic, chromate, uranium, and asbestos. Various drugs have been implicated in the onset of cancer. They include immunosuppressive agents, diethylstilbestrol, oral contraceptives, cytotoxic agents, and radioisotopes.

Certain viruses have been isolated and identified as the causative factor of cancer in some animals. However, the role that viruses play in the etiology of cancer in humans has not been definitely established.

Psychosocial Influences Dreher (1988) reports on specific characteristics that have been associated with individuals who develop cancer. The term *type C personality* has been coined to describe these characteristics. Cancer has sometimes been called the "nice guy's disease." Dreher (1988) describes cancer-prone individuals in the following way: "They're always trying to please other people and constantly putting their own needs last. They rarely show anger and seldom share their problems with friends and family. They are some of the nicest people you'll ever meet."

Researchers who have studied these characteristics identify the following profile for the type C personality:

- Extreme suppression of anger and hostility (experiences these emotions, but doesn't express them)
- Exhibits a calm, placid exterior
- Feelings of depression and despair are common
- Low self-esteem; low self-worth
- Puts others' needs before own

- Has a tendency toward self-pity (the martyr)
- Sets unrealistic standards and is inflexible in the enforcement of these standards
- Holds resentment toward others for perceived "wrongs," although others are never aware of these feelings

LeShan (1977), who conducted psychotherapy for more than 30 years with cancer patients, says:

> "The single most significant factor in the weakening of the cancer defense mechanism is the loss of hope in ever achieving any meaning, zest or validity in life. It's the feeling that we can't ever really be ourselves—fully and richly as human beings—in being, relating or creating."

LeShan calls this the "loss of self." In his studies, he found that, as children, cancer patients were not allowed to express themselves in an honest manner but were forced to yield to the roles and expectations placed on them by others. They come to believe that they can either be themselves (and therefore unloved and alone), or they can be what others want and thus be loved and accepted. It is viewed as a hopeless situation from which the individual can never achieve any real self-gratification. LeShan (1966) described the profile of the family of origin of cancer patients as follows:

- Lack of close relationship with one or both parents
- Loss of parent through death in a large number of cases
- Child feels neglected, physically or emotionally
- Child feels loneliness and despair, and blames self for situation
- Comes to believe that life situation is hopeless, with little or no opportunity for self-gratification
- Continual efforts to conform to others' expectations to win their love and approval

Several studies have been conducted in an effort to determine if there is a link between psychosocial stress and the onset of cancer symptoms (Gallagher & Gallo, 1975; Riley, 1975). Results indicate a positive correlation between the effects of stress and the induction and growth of neoplastic tumors in extensive work with experimental animals and in more limited studies with humans. Biopsychosocial events appear to reduce immunological competence at a critical time and may allow a mutant cell to thrive and grow (Pelletier, 1977).

CORONARY HEART DISEASE

Definition and Epidemiological Statistics Coronary heart disease (CHD) is defined as myocardial impairment due to an imbalance between coronary blood flow and myocardial oxygen requirements caused by changes in the coronary circulation (Woods et al, 1991). It is the leading cause of death in the United States. Five million people have CHD. It is more prevalent in men than in women, although the number of women with CHD is increasing, probably as a result of greater social and economic pressures on women and changes in their life-styles. The incidence of CHD is higher in older individuals and in the affluent (Kavanagh, 1987).

Signs and Symptoms Artherosclerosis, or changes in the lining of the coronary arteries that affect lumen size, is the basic underlying problem associated with CHD. Size of the lumen is decreased as a result of an accumulation of cells, lipids, and connective tissue that adheres to the intima of the artery. This results in decreased oxygenated blood flow to the myocardium and possible myocardial ischemia. Myocardial ischemia may be asymptomatic, or the individual may experience discomfort in the chest.

Angina pectoris can occur spontaneously or in relation to increased myocardial oxygen demand. Common descriptions of pain associated with angina include sensations of strangling, aching, squeezing, pressing, expanding, choking, burning, constriction, indigestion, tightness, and heaviness (Woods et al, 1991). The discomfort of angina usually lasts from 2 to 5 minutes, sometimes as long as 15 minutes, and rarely as long as 30 minutes.

Pain associated with myocardial infarction (MI) is similar to that experienced in angina but lasts longer than 15 to 30 minutes. Symptoms may also include indigestion, nausea and vomiting, diaphoresis, syncope, palpitations, or dyspnea. In approximately 15 percent to 25 percent of cases, patients experiencing MI will not experience chest discomfort (Woods et al, 1991).

Predisposing Factors

Biological Influences A number of risk factors have been identified as predisposing factors to the development of CHD. A family history of CHD increases an individual's risk of developing atherosclerosis. It is not known whether there is a direct genetic link or if the risk is related more to environmental life-style patterns.

High serum lipoprotein levels, particularly cholesterol and triglycerides, are considered to be a major risk factor for CHD. Individuals with hypertension (blood pressures greater than 140/90 mm Hg) or diabetes mellitus are also at higher risk for the disease.

Various life-style habits have been implicated. The association between cigarette smoking and CHD has now been clearly established. Three compounds in cigarette smoke (tar, nicotine, and carbon monoxide) have been implicated as causative agents in CHD (Woods et al, 1991).

Obesity, defined as body mass index (weight/height^2) that is greater than 20 percent above the ideal value, has been associated with increased risk of developing CHD (Woods et al, 1991). It is unclear whether the increased risk is associated with the obesity itself or to other factors that frequently accompany obesity, such as high blood pressure or diabetes.

Sedentary life-style has also been implicated. Physical exercise may offer some protection from the complications of CHD, may help to maintain blood pressure at a lower level, and may be associated with a decrease in serum lipoproteins (Thompson et al, 1986; Woods et al, 1991).

Psychosocial Influences Friedman and Rosenman (1974) have completed the most comprehensive work to date in the area of personality and CHD. They developed a detailed profile of the CHD-prone individual, which they identified as type A personality. They also studied personality characteristics of individuals who experienced stress in a different manner and seemed less prone to CHD. This personality profile was entitled type B.

Friedman and Rosenman identified two character traits that when occurring together automatically classify an individual as type A personality. These two traits are excessive competitive drive and a chronic, continual sense of time urgency. Additional type A characteristics include:

- Easily aroused hostility; usually kept under control, but flares up unexpectedly, often when others would consider it unwarranted.
- Very aggressive, very ambitious, concentrates almost exclusively on his or her career.
- Has no time for hobbies, and if does find self

with leisure time, feels guilty if just relaxes; feels is wasting time.

- Seldom feels satisfied with accomplishments; always feels must do *more*.
- Measures achievements in numbers produced and dollars earned.
- The struggle to achieve is continual and there is never enough time; time becomes the type A's enemy.
- Appears to be very extroverted and social; often dominates conversation; outgoing personality often conceals a deep-seated insecurity about own worth.
- A driving ambition and need to win leads the type A personality to undertake all activities with the same competitive drive. Even recreational activities become aggressive when the individual puts undue pressure on himself or herself to compete.

Type B personalities are not the opposite of type As, only different. Type Bs are no less successful than type As. They may perform every bit as well on their jobs — maybe better. Type Bs do not feel the constant sense of time urgency the type As feel. They can function under time pressure when it is required, but it is not a pervasive part of their lives as it is with type As. The type B's ambition will probably be based on goals that have been well thought out. There is not the constant need for competition and comparison with peers. Self-worth often comes from goals other than material and social success. Type Bs recognize and accept both strengths and limitations. They view leisure time as a time to relax, and they do so without feeling guilty. They take the time to consider alternatives and to think things through before deciding or acting. These characteristics often result in more creative output by type Bs. Type As are prone to making more errors due to their impulsivity — to acting before thinking things through.

A 1975 study by Rosenman and colleagues reported the results of an 8½-year follow-up study for predicting CHD in men between the ages of 39 and 59. In this study, the incidence of CHD was significantly associated with parental history, diabetes, education, smoking, blood pressure, and serum-cholesterol levels. The study also concluded that type A behavior was a strong factor and that "this association could not be explained by association of behavior pattern with any single predictive risk factor or any combination of them" (Rosenman et al., 1975). Type A behavior risk factor could not be "explained away" by the other risk factors and was clearly a contributing factor in itself.

PEPTIC ULCER

Definition and Epidemiological Statistics Peptic ulcers are an erosion of the mucosal wall in the esophagus, stomach, duodenum, or jejunum. Deeper lesions may penetrate the mucosal layer and extend into the muscular layers of the intestinal wall (Simmons & Heitkemper, 1991).

One in every 10 men and one in every 40 women might expect to experience signs and symptoms of peptic ulcer disease during their lifetime (Lipsitt, 1989). Prevalence of the disease within the population is estimated at 6 percent to 15 percent. It is more common in men than women by about 3 or 4 to 1. Hospitalization, surgery, and mortality related to peptic ulcer disease places an economic burden on this country in the billions of dollars annually.

Signs and Symptoms Pain is the characteristic clinical manifestation of peptic ulcer disease. It is usually experienced in the upper abdomen near the midline and may radiate to the back, sternum, or lower abdomen. Pain is usually worse when the stomach is empty and gastric secretions are high. Food or antacid medication often relieves pain.

Predisposing Factors

Biological Influences There appears to be a hereditary predisposition to peptic ulcer disease, in that a person with a family member with ulcer disease has a three times greater risk of developing an ulcer as compared to the general population (Simmons & Heitkemper, 1991). The ulcer itself occurs as a result of an imbalance in the secretion of hydrochloric acid and the mucosal resistance factors. Any factor that stimulates higher-than-normal hydrochloric acid secretion can promote the development of peptic ulcers.

Several environmental factors have been associated with peptic ulcer disease. Cigarette smoking and regular use of aspirin have been strongly implicated. Other agents, such as alcohol, steroids, and nonsteroidal anti-inflammatory drugs, are ulcerogenic in that they can cause damage to the gastric mucosal barrier.

Psychosocial Influences Studies as early as the 1940s have observed increased gastric secretion and motility in the presence of conscious anxiety, resentment, and frustration (Lipsitt, 1989). The link between ulcers and stress has been related by some psychodynamic investigators to an unfulfilled dependency need in ulcer-prone individuals. It has been hypothesized that babies with an inherited trait for high acid secretion levels express high oral drives that are often experienced by the mother as frustrating in the earliest mother-child relationship. The mother's inability to meet the child's dependency needs promotes hypersecretion of gastric acid, with a subsequent breakdown of mucosal cells (Lipsitt, 1989). This hypothesis was tested by Weiner et al (1957) in a study in which they were able to accurately predict which army recruits with "intense oral cravings and conflicts" would develop duodenal ulcers in the presence of gastric acid hypersecretion caused by the stress of military training.

ESSENTIAL HYPERTENSION

Definition and Epidemiological Statistics Essential hypertension is the persistent elevation of blood pressure for which there is no apparent cause or associated underlying disease (Cunningham, 1991). It is a major cause of cerebrovascular accident (stroke), cardiac disease, and renal failure.

Thirty-eight percent of the population have a blood pressure of 140/90 mm Hg or higher, and these individuals have twice the risk of cardiovascular disease than those with lower blood pressure (Hackett et al, 1989). Because hypertension is often asymptomatic, the National Heart, Lung, and Blood Institute estimates that 50 percent of persons with hypertension do not know they have it (Walsh & Woloszyn, 1987). The disorder is more common in men than in women and is twice as prevalent in the black population as it is in the white population.

Signs and Symptoms Most commonly, hypertension produces no symptoms, particularly in the early stages. When symptoms do occur, they may include headache, vertigo, flushed face, spontaneous nosebleed, or blurred vision. Chronic, progressive hypertension may reveal signs and symptoms associated with specific organ system damage. For example, dyspnea, chest pain, or cardiac hypertrophy may indicate cardiovascular damage, confusion and paresthesia may be suggestive of cerebrovascular damage, and elevated serum creatinine or blood urea nitrogen levels may signal kidney damage.

Predisposing Factors

Biological Influences Individuals who have a positive family history of hypertension are at greater risk of developing the disorder than those who do not. Other environmental conditions that may contribute to hypertension are obesity and cigarette smoking.

Various physiological influences have been hypothesized. These include an imbalance of circulating vasoconstrictors (e.g., angiotensin) and vasodilators (e.g., prostaglandins), increased sympathetic nervous system activity resulting in increased vasoconstriction, and impairment in sodium and water excretion (Cunningham, 1991).

Psychosocial Influences Hackett et al (1989) offer the following psychodynamic explanation of the individual with essential hypertension:

> "The person at risk for hypertension appears compliant and congenial, longing for approval. Although superficially easy going, that person is inwardly suppressing anger and suspicion. This dilemma derives from childhood experiences with parents toward whom anger could not be expressed without real or imagined loss of love and security. The desire to please, in tandem with an antagonistic battle-ready stance, is felt to be characteristic of essential hypertensive persons."

MIGRAINE HEADACHE

Definition and Epidemiological Statistics Migraine headache is a vascular event in which pain arises from the scalp, its blood vessels, and muscles; from the dura mater and its venous sinuses; and from the blood vessels at the base of the brain (Schenk, 1987). Pain most commonly originates in the muscles of the face, neck, and head; the blood vessels; and the dura mater. The blood vessels dilate and become congested with blood. Pain results from the exertion of pressure on nerves that lie in or around these congested blood vessels.

Migraine headaches can occur at any age. They often begin in childhood, adolescence, or early adulthood, and lessen in frequency and intensity around age 50. They are more common in women than in men, and often are associated with various phases of the menstrual cycle.

Approximately 5 percent of the general population suffer from migraine headaches. There appears to be a strong hereditary component involved, as a definite familial pattern has been recognized and can often be traced over generations.

Signs and Symptoms The "classic" migraine headache occurs in two distinctive phases. In the prodromal phase, which may begin from minutes to days before the actual pain of the headache, the individual may experience visual disturbances, weakness and numbness on one side of the body, mental confusion, irritability, fatigue, sweating, and dizziness. The headache phase usually consists of pain on one side of the head. As it intensifies, the pain may spread to the other side as well. The ache is frequently dull, deep, and throbbing, and often begins in the forehead, ear, jaw, or in or around an eye or temple (Saper & Magee, 1981). Nausea, vomiting, mental cloudiness, total body aching, abdominal pain, chills, and cold hands and feet commonly accompany the headache. The actual attack usually lasts from 1 hour to more than a day. Following it, sore muscles, total body exhaustion, and a continued mild mental cloudiness may persist for days.

The most common form of migraine headache is a variation of the classic version. Many of the symptoms are similar, but in common migraine the distinctive phases of the classic migraine do not occur. Photophobia (sensitivity to light) and hyperacusis (sensitivity to sound) may be present in both types.

Predisposing Factors

Biological Influences A number of biologic influences have been identified as triggers for headache-prone individuals. Periods of hormonal change have been implicated, such as menstruation, ovulation, menopause, and at the beginning or just following pregnancy.

Heredity appears to play an important role in the etiology of migraine headaches. It is common to find individuals from several generations within the same family who experience the disorder. Occasionally members of one or two generations are spared, but a history of headaches in aunts, uncles, cousins, or grandparents is frequent (Saper & Magee, 1981).

Some foods, beverages, and drugs can precipitate migraine in certain individuals. These substances include caffeine, chocolate, aged cheese, vinegar, organ meats, alcoholic beverages, sour cream, yogurt, aspartame, citrus fruits, bananas, raisins, avocados, onions, smoked meats, monosodium glutamate, and products preserved with nitrites. Drugs that lower blood pressure, in particular reserpine and hydralazine, have been known to trigger migraine headaches.

Some people experience attacks only during or after physical exertion. This may be caused by either the chemical or blood vessel changes that occur during physical exertion or by the depletion of certain biological substances following the exercise.

Various other factors that have been implicated in the development of migraine headaches include cigarette smoking, bright lights, changes in the weather, high elevations, oral contraceptives, altered sleep patterns, and skipping meals.

Psychosocial Influences Certain characteristics have been identified as "the migraine personality." Saper and Magee (1981) identify the migraine sufferer as perfectionistic, overly conscientious, and somewhat inflexible. They may be meticulously neat and tidy, compulsive, and often very hard workers. They are usually quite intelligent, exacting, and place a very high premium on success, setting high (sometimes unrealistic) expectations on the self and others. Delegation of responsibility is difficult, as the individual feels no one can perform as well as he or she. Classically, there is repressed or suppressed anger. The individual experiences hostility and anger, but is unable to express these feelings openly.

Emotions play a critical role in the precipitation of migraine headaches. An individual who is experiencing emotional stress may develop a migraine headache. This may be in response to the secondary gains one receives from the sick role. Migraine headaches may provide a means of escape for dealing with the stressful situation. Other individuals experience migraine attacks only *after* the emotionally distressing event has passed or lessened. This has been called "let down" headache and can be one of the influential factors in provoking the weekend or holiday migraine, when the anxiety has been relieved, and the individual finally relaxes (Saper & Magee, 1981).

OBESITY

Definition and Epidemiological Statistics Obesity has been defined as a body mass index (weight/height^2) that is greater than 20 percent above the ideal value (Woods et al, 1991). Approximately one out of five persons older than the age of 19 years is obese (Heitkemper & Brubacher, 1991). Obesity is more common in black women than in white women and more common in white men than in black men. The prevalence among lower socioeconomic classes is six times that in upper socioeconomic classes, and there is a somewhat greater prevalence of obesity among Jews, followed by Roman Catholics, and then Protestants (Lomax, 1989). Approximately 0.1 percent of the population are categorized as "morbidly" obese, which is defined as 100 percent over ideal weight (Lomax, 1989; Heitkemper & Brubacher, 1991).

Signs and Symptoms The following formula is used to determine degree of obesity in an individual:

$$\text{Body mass index} = \frac{\text{Weight (kg)}}{\text{Height (m)}^2}$$

The body mass index range for normal weight is 20 to 25 for men and 19 to 24 for women. The individual is considered to be in the obese range once the body mass index range reaches 30. At this level, weight alone can contribute to increases in morbidity and mortality.

Obese people often present with hyperlipidemia, particularly elevated triglyceride and cholesterol levels. They commonly have hyperglycemia and are at risk for developing diabetes mellitus. Osteoarthritis may be evident due to trauma to weight-bearing joints. There is increased work load on the heart and lungs, often leading to symptoms of angina or respiratory insufficiency (Long & Neville, 1987).

Predisposing Factors

Biological Influences Genetics have been implicated in the development of obesity in that 80 percent of children born of two overweight parents will also be overweight (Ackerman, 1983). Studies of twins reared by normal and overweight parents have supported this implication of heredity as a factor (Long & Neville, 1987).

Lesions in the appetite and satiety centers in the hypothalamus may contribute to overeating and lead to obesity. Hypothyroidism is a problem that interferes with basal metabolism and may lead to weight gain. Weight gain can also occur in response to the decreased insulin production of diabetes mellitus and the increased cortisone production of Cushing's disease.

On an elementary level, obesity can be viewed as an ingestion of a greater number of calories than are expended. Weight gain occurs when caloric intake exceeds caloric output in terms of basal metabolism and physical activity. Many overweight individuals lead sedentary life-styles, making it very difficult to burn off calories.

Psychosocial Influences The psychoanalytic view of obesity proposes that obese individuals have unresolved dependency needs and are fixed in the oral stage of psychosexual development (Norman, 1984). The symptoms of obesity are viewed as depressive equivalents, attempts to regain "lost" or frustrated nurturance and care.

Lomax (1989) describes an oral character structure, the traits of which include excessive optimism or pessimism, greed, demandingness, dependency, and impatience. Together, these traits form a characteristic personality configuration that is etiologically significant and is found in strong association with obesity.

RHEUMATOID ARTHRITIS

Definition and Epidemiological Statistics Rheumatoid arthritis is a chronic systemic disease characterized by inflammation of the connective tissues throughout the body (Thompson et al, 1986). It commonly affects the tissues in and around joints, leading to joint destruction and deformity.

Rheumatoid arthritis affects 0.5 percent to 1 percent of the population of the United States between the ages of 20 and 80 years (Ananth, 1989). Average age of onset of symptoms is 35 (Pelletier, 1977). It is more prevalent in women than in men by about 3 to 1. The disease is characterized by periods of remission and exacerbation.

Signs and Symptoms Onset of the disease is usually insidious, with joint inflammation preceding the systemic symptoms of fatigue, malaise, anorexia, weight loss, low-grade fever, myalgias, and parasthesias (Cicero, 1991). About 8 percent to 10 percent of patients have an acute onset, with symptoms appearing in the course of a day. Individuals with acute onset have a good prognosis and often permanent remission, whereas an insidious onset with extra-articular involvement has the poorest prognosis (Harris, 1983). Joint involvement is usually characterized by swelling, pain, redness, warmth, and tenderness. Joints of the hands and feet are often affected early. As the disease progresses, any freely movable joint may be involved.

About one out of every five rheumatoid arthritis patients develops systemic manifestations, which can occur in virtually any body system. Cardiac, pulmonary, and renal involvement are the most serious consequences of rheumatoid arthritis (Cicero, 1991).

Predisposing Factors

Biological Influences Heredity appears to be an influential factor in the predisposition to rheumatoid arthritis. The serum protein rheumatoid factor is found in at least half of rheumatoid arthritics and frequently in their close relatives (Pelletier, 1977). It is an inherited characteristic that increases one's vulnerability to the disease. Although the rheumatoid factor is present in patients with other diseases, it is rare in the population at large.

An additional theory postulates that rheumatoid arthritis may be the result of a dysfunctional immune mechanism initiated by an infectious process, although the causative agent is yet to be identified. In such an instance, antibodies that form in keeping with a normal reaction to infection, become directed instead against the self in an autoimmune response that results in tissue damage.

Psychosocial Influences Rheumatoid arthritis patients are postulated to be self-sacrificing, masochistic, conforming, self-conscious, inhibited, and perfectionistic as a result of their inability to express feeling of anger and hostility (Ananth, 1989). Female rheumatoid arthritis patients are described as nervous, tense, worried, moody, depressed, and typically had mothers whom they felt rejected them and fathers who were unduly strict (Pelletier, 1977).

Evidence has accumulated during the past 4 decades suggesting that emotionally traumatic life events, such as the loss of a key person by death or separation, often precede the first symptoms of rheumatoid arthritis and precipitate its onset in between 22 percent and 100 percent of patients (Ananth, 1989). Thus, emotional decompensation in predisposed individuals may result in the onset or exacerbation of rheumatoid arthritis.

ULCERATIVE COLITIS

Definition and Epidemiological Statistics Ulcerative colitis is a chronic mucosal inflammatory disease of the colon and rectum (Thompson et al, 1986). The incidence of the disease in the U.S. is approximately 5 to 7 per 100,000 population (Heitkemper & Martin, 1991). It can occur at any age but is most prevalent between 15 and 30 years. The incidence of ulcerative colitis is more common among Jewish than non-Jewish populations and among whites than nonwhites (Lipsitt, 1989).

Signs and Symptoms The mucosa of the colon and rectum become inflamed, with diffuse areas of bleeding. Diarrhea is the predominant symptom of ulcerative colitis. There may be as many as 15 to 20 liquid stools a day containing blood, mucus, and pus (Long et al, 1987). Abdominal cramping may or may not precede the bowel movement. Generalized manifestations include fever, anorexia, weight loss, nausea, and vomiting (Heitkemper & Martin, 1991). During exacerbation of the illness, anemia and elevated white cell count are common.

As the disease progresses, the inflammation advances up the colon and the bleeding points enlarge and become ulcerated. The ulcers may bleed or perforate, forming scar tissue as they heal. The scar tissue causes the colon to thicken and become rigid, and normal elasticity and absorptive capability are diminished. Changes in the mucosa may result in the formation of pseudopolyps that can become cancerous.

Predisposing Factors

Biological Influences A genetic factor may be involved in the development, as individuals who have a family member with ulcerative colitis are at greater risk than the general population.

The possibility that ulcerative colitis may be an autoimmune disease has generated a great deal of research interest. High rates of anticolon antibodies are found in relatives of ulcerative colitis patients. This autoimmune precondition for inflammatory bowel disease may support Engel's (1955) statement that the disease may result from "unidentified changes that alter relationships in the colon so that it responds to its own flora as pathogens."

Psychosocial Influences Lipsitt (1989) states, "The precise role of psychosomatic factors in the pathogenesis of inflammatory bowel disease remains uncertain, although descriptions of patients as obsessive-compulsive, dependent, emotionally immature, and especially vulnerable to separations and loss have borne the test of time and clinical observation."

Engel (1955) described colitis patients as having an obsessive-compulsive behavior pattern involving excessive neatness, indecision, conformity, overintellectualism, rigid morality, anxiety, and depression. He found similarities in the personality profiles of colitis patients and those of rheumatoid arthritis patients. Neither could express hostility or anger directly, and both seemed immature and dependent. Colitis patients generally had mothers who were controlling and had a propensity to assume the role of martyr, much like the mothers of rheumatoid arthritis patients.

Onset or exacerbation of ulcerative colitis has been associated with stressful life events or psychological trauma. The altered immune status that accompanies psychological stress may be an influencing factor in predisposed individuals.

Transactional Model of Stress/Adaptation   The etiology of psychophysiological disorders is most likely influenced by multiple factors. In Figure 25.1, a graphic depiction of this theory of multiple causation is presented in the Transactional Model of Stress/Adaptation.

Nursing Diagnosis, Planning/Implementation

Nursing diagnoses are formulated from the data gathered during the assessment phase and with background knowledge regarding predisposing factors to the disorder. Some common nursing diagnoses for patients with specific psychophysiological disorders include:

Asthma
- Ineffective airway clearance
- Activity intolerance
- Anxiety (severe)

Cancer
- Fear
- Anticipatory grieving
- Body image disturbance

Coronary Heart Disease
- Pain
- Fear
- Activity intolerance

Peptic Ulcer Disease
- Pain
- Impaired tissue integrity

Hypertension
- High risk for altered tissue perfusion
- High risk for sexual dysfunction

Migraine Headache
- Pain
- Altered role performance

Obesity
- Altered nutrition: More than body requirements
- Body image disturbance
- Self-esteem disturbance

Rheumatoid Arthritis
- Pain
- Self-care deficit
- Activity intolerance

Ulcerative Colitis
- Pain
- Diarrhea
- High risk for altered nutrition: Less than body requirements

Some nursing diagnoses common to the general category of psychological factors affecting physical condition include:

Ineffective individual coping related to repressed anxiety and inadequate coping methods, evidenced by initiation or exacerbation of physical illness.

Knowledge deficit related to psychological factors affecting physical condition, evidenced by statements such as "I don't know why the doctor put me on the psychiatric unit. I have a physical problem."

Self-esteem disturbance related to unmet dependency needs, evidenced by self-negating verbalizations and demanding sick-role behaviors.

Altered role performance related to physical illness accompanied by real or perceived disabling symptoms, evidenced by changes in usual patterns of responsibility.

In Table 25.3, selected nursing diagnoses common to the general category are presented in a plan of care. Goals of care and appropriate nursing interventions are included for each. Rationales are presented in italics.

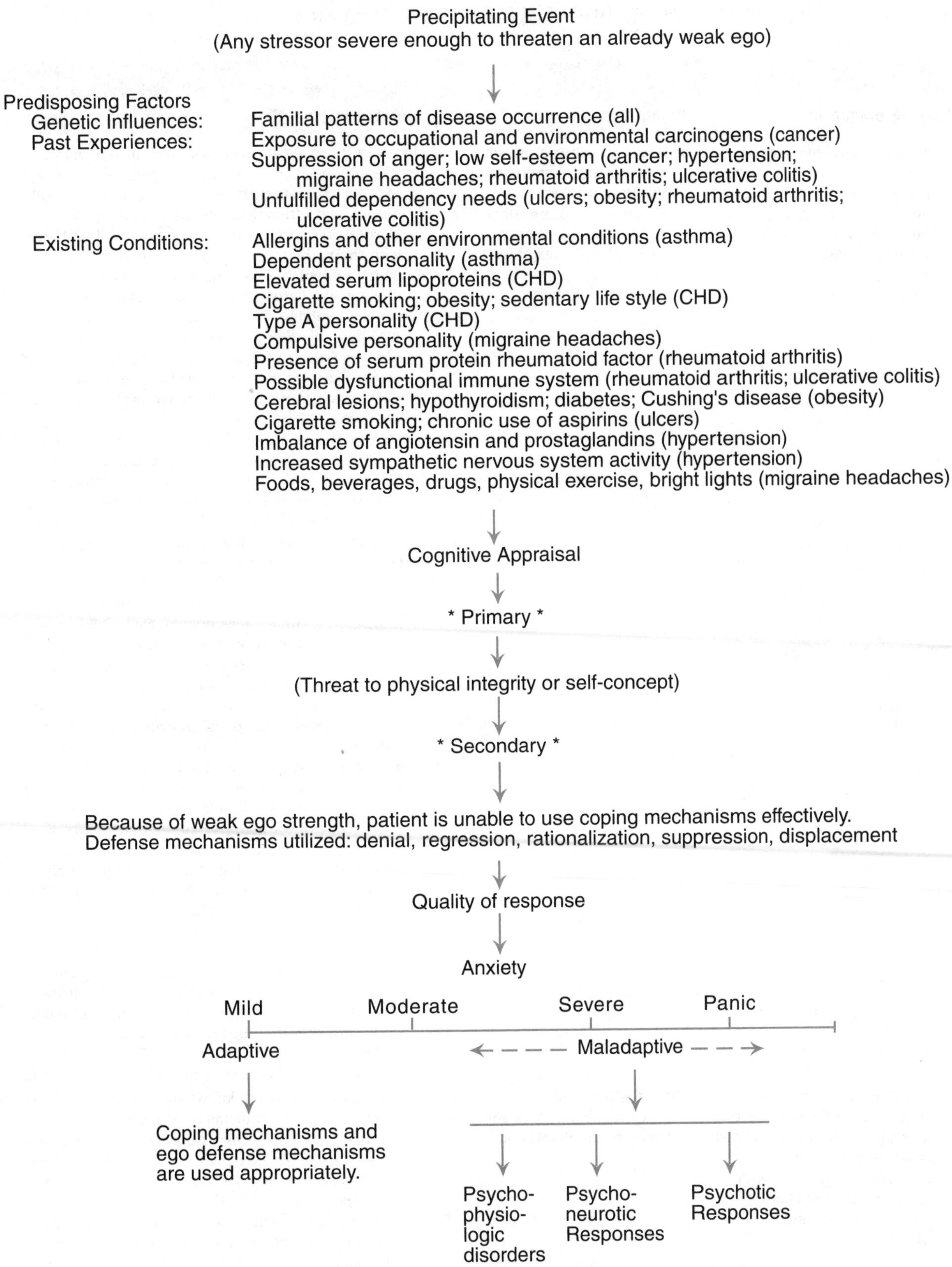

Precipitating Event
(Any stressor severe enough to threaten an already weak ego)

↓

Predisposing Factors
  Genetic Influences: Familial patterns of disease occurrence (all)
  Past Experiences: Exposure to occupational and environmental carcinogens (cancer)
                          Suppression of anger; low self-esteem (cancer; hypertension;
                              migraine headaches; rheumatoid arthritis; ulcerative colitis)
                          Unfulfilled dependency needs (ulcers; obesity; rheumatoid arthritis;
                              ulcerative colitis)
  Existing Conditions: Allergins and other environmental conditions (asthma)
                          Dependent personality (asthma)
                          Elevated serum lipoproteins (CHD)
                          Cigarette smoking; obesity; sedentary life style (CHD)
                          Type A personality (CHD)
                          Compulsive personality (migraine headaches)
                          Presence of serum protein rheumatoid factor (rheumatoid arthritis)
                          Possible dysfunctional immune system (rheumatoid arthritis; ulcerative colitis)
                          Cerebral lesions; hypothyroidism; diabetes; Cushing's disease (obesity)
                          Cigarette smoking; chronic use of aspirins (ulcers)
                          Imbalance of angiotensin and prostaglandins (hypertension)
                          Increased sympathetic nervous system activity (hypertension)
                          Foods, beverages, drugs, physical exercise, bright lights (migraine headaches)

↓

Cognitive Appraisal

↓

* Primary *

↓

(Threat to physical integrity or self-concept)

↓

* Secondary *

↓

Because of weak ego strength, patient is unable to use coping mechanisms effectively.
Defense mechanisms utilized: denial, regression, rationalization, suppression, displacement

↓

Quality of response

↓

Anxiety

Mild   Moderate   Severe   Panic

Adaptive   ← – – – Maladaptive – – →

↓   ↓

Coping mechanisms and   ↓   ↓   ↓
ego defense mechanisms
are used appropriately.   Psycho-   Psycho-   Psychotic
                           physio-   neurotic   Responses
                           logic   Responses
                           disorders

Figure 25.1 The dynamics of psychophysiologic disorders using the transactional model of stress/adaptation.

Table 25.3 CARE PLAN FOR THE PATIENT WITH A PSYCHOPHYSIOLOGICAL DISORDER		
Nursing Diagnoses	**Objectives**	**Nursing Interventions**
Ineffective individual coping related to repressed anxiety and inadequate coping methods, evidenced by initiation or exacerbation of physical illness.	Patient will achieve physical wellness and demonstrate the ability to prevent exacerbation of physical symptoms as a coping mechanism in response to stress.	Perform thorough physical assessment *to determine specific care required for patient's physical condition.* Monitor laboratory values, vital signs, intake and output, and other assessments necessary *to maintain an accurate ongoing appraisal.* Together with the patient, identify goals of care and ways in which patient believes he or she can best achieve those goals. Patient may need assistance with problem solving. *Personal involvement in his or her own care provides a feeling of control and increases chances for positive outcomes.* Encourage patient to discuss current life situations that he or she perceives as stressful and the feelings associated with each. *Verbalization of true feelings in a nonthreatening environment may help patient come to terms with unresolved issues.* During patient's discussion, note times during which a sense of powerlessness or loss of control over life situations emerges. Focus on these times and discuss ways in which the patient may maintain a feeling of control. *A sense of self-worth develops and is maintained when an individual feels power over his or her own life situations.* As patient becomes able to discuss feelings more openly, assist him or her in a nonthreatening manner to relate certain feelings to the appearance of physical symptoms. *Patient may be unaware of the relationship between physical symptoms and emotional problems.* Discuss stressful times when physical symptoms did not appear and the adaptive coping strategies that were used during those situations. *Therapy is facilitated by considering areas of strength and using them to the patient's benefit.* Provide positive reinforcement for adaptive coping mechanisms identified or used. Suggest alternative coping strategies but allow patient to determine which can most appropriately be incorporated into his or her life-style. *Positive reinforcement enhances self-esteem and encourages repetition of desired behaviors. Patient may require assistance with problem solving but must be allowed and encouraged to make decisions independently.* Help patient to identify a resource within the community (friend, significant other, group) to use as a support system for the expression of feelings *in an effort to prevent maladaptive coping through physical illness.*
Knowledge deficit related to psychological factors affecting physical condition, evidenced by statements such as "I don't know why the doctor put me on the psychiatric unit. I have a physical problem."	Patient will be able to verbalize psychological factors affecting his or her physical condition.	Assess patient's level of knowledge regarding effects of psychological problems on the body. *An adequate data base is necessary for the development of an effective teaching plan.* Assess patient's level of anxiety and readiness to learn. *Learning does not occur beyond the moderate level of anxiety.* Discuss physical examinations and laboratory tests that have been conducted. Explain purpose and results of each. *Patient has the right to know about and accept or refuse any medical treatment.* Explore

(continued)

Table 25.3 CONTINUED

Nursing Diagnoses	Objectives	Nursing Interventions
		feelings and fears held by patient. Go slowly. These feelings may have been suppressed/repressed for so long that their disclosure may be a very painful experience. Be supportive. *Expression of feelings in the presence of a trusted individual and in a nonthreatening environment may encourage the individual to confront unresolved feelings.* Have patient keep a diary of appearance, duration, and intensity of physical symptoms. A separate record of situations that the patient finds especially stressful should also be kept. *Comparison of these records may provide objective data from which to observe the relationship between physical symptoms and stress.* Help patient identify needs that are being met through the sick role. Together, formulate more adaptive means for fulfilling these needs. Practice by role playing. *Repetition through practice serves to reduce discomfort in the actual situation.* Provide instruction in assertiveness techniques, especially the ability to recognize the differences among passive, assertive, and aggressive behaviors and the importance of respecting the rights of others while protecting one's own basic rights. *These skills will preserve patient's self-esteem while also improving his or her ability to form satisfactory interpersonal relationships.* Discuss adaptive methods of stress management, such as relaxation techniques, physical exercise, meditation, breathing exercises, and autogenics. *Use of these adaptive techniques may decrease appearance of physical symptoms in response to stress.*

OUTCOME CRITERIA

The following criteria may be used for measurement of outcomes in the care of the patient with a psychophysiological disorder.

The patient:
1. Denies pain or other physical complaint.
2. Demonstrates the ability to perform more adaptive coping strategies in the face of stressful situations.
3. Verbalizes stressful situations that have led to physical symptoms in the past.
4. Verbalizes a plan to cope with stressful situations without resorting to physical symptoms.
5. Is able to perform activities of daily living independently.

Evaluation

Reassessment is conducted to determine if the nursing actions have been successful in achieving the objectives of care. Evaluation of the nursing actions for the patient with a psychophysiological disorder may be facilitated by gathering information using the following types of questions.

Does the patient complain of pain or any other physical symptom? Is the physical symptom interfering with role responsibilities? Does the patient verbalize that the physical symptom has been relieved? Is he or she able to carry out activities of daily living independently? Is the patient able to verbalize alternative coping strategies for dealing with stress? Is he or she able to demonstrate the ability to use these more adaptive coping strategies in the face of stress? Does the patient recognize which types of stressful situations exacerbate physical symptoms? Is he or she able to correlate the appearance of the physical symptoms with the stressful situation? Is the patient able to verbalize unfulfilled needs for which the sick role is compensating? Can he or she verbalize alternative ways to fulfill these needs? Can the patient name resources to whom he or she may go when feeling the need for assistance in times of stress?

TREATMENT MODALITIES

Asthma

The goals of medical treatment for patients with asthma are prevention of acute attacks and relief of the symptoms (Anderson, 1991). Medications are used for both of these purposes. The route of choice is generally inhalation from a metered-dose inhaler, and the most commonly prescribed medications are bronchodilators and corticosteroids. Bronchodilators increase the airway diameter, and corticosteroids reduce the inflammatory response.

The most commonly used bronchodilators are the beta-adrenergic agonists (e.g., terbutaline, albuterol). Theophylline and other methylxanthines are also used, but because they are usually given orally, they produce greater side effects than medications administered by inhaler.

Corticosteriods, such as prednisone and beclomethasone, may be given by inhaler in doses less than 15 mg/day; higher doses usually require oral administration (Anderson, 1991). Other medications prescribed for asthma include anticholinergics, which inhibit neural reflex effects that contribute to bronchoconstriction, and cromolyn sodium, which occupies a position on the mast cell and prevents release of the chemicals that stimulate bronchospasm and promote inflammation.

Some patients with asthma may be candidates for psychotherapy, either a short-term intervention or the longer-term approach. While having the internist or family physician maintain care of the physical component of the patient's illness, the psychotherapist focuses on attitudes and emotions, fears of confiding and rejection, and struggles between attachment and independence (Vachon, 1989). The psychological aspects are kept separate from the physical aspects of the illness so that the therapeutic relationship is not destroyed if the patient suffers an asthmatic attack during psychotherapy. Exacerbations during the treatment offer both the therapist and the patient an opportunity to become aware of the psychological context in which they occur. They then may be able to understand the emotional factors involved and, hopefully, to modify them.

Cancer

Surgery is perhaps the oldest method used to control or cure cancer. Surgical procedures can be used to diagnose malignancy (e.g., biopsy), to cure malignancies (e.g., mastectomy, hysterectomy), for rehabilitation measures (e.g., breast reconstruction), and for various other purposes of improving quality of life for cancer patients when a cure is impossible (e.g., palliative and supportive measures).

Radiation therapy is the use of high-energy ionizing emissions from a radioactive source to eradicate malignant tumors with as little damage to normal tissues as possible (Wheeler, 1991). It can be used singly or in combination with other forms of treatment to achieve maximum tumor control. It is also used as a palliative measure to control the pain of bone metastasis in patients with advanced neoplastic disease.

Chemotherapy is the administration of antineoplastic drugs, in a systemic or regional manner, to cure or control a malignancy (Wheeler, 1991). These drugs have the potential of curing certain cancers. In instances when a cure is not possible, they may be given for palliative measures, to control symptoms, or to extend the patient's useful life. They are often given in combination with other therapies, such as surgery or radiation therapy. Most chemotherapeutic agents have significant adverse effects (e.g., bone marrow depression, severe nausea and vomiting, alopecia), which should be measured against the potential benefits when outlining a course of treatment for a cancer patient.

In consideration of the psychosomatic dimensions of cancer, Simonton and Simonton (1975) report positive results with autogenic relaxation and mental imagery in the role of adjunct therapy for patients with malignant disease. Once relaxation has been achieved, the individual is taught to visualize the malignancy within his or her body.

Then the person visualizes a killer attack (from his or her own fantasy) on the malignant cells, followed by a visualization of the army of white cells transporting the dead cancer cells out of the body. The Simontons have had convincing results with this technique, particularly in patients who maintain a positive attitude about therapy. They strongly emphasize a high correlation between positive response to treatment and positive attitudes, both to the disease and to life in a more general sense. They also emphasize that the application of relaxation and visualization techniques is an *adjunct* to traditional treatment, not an *alternative*.

Psychotherapy may serve to help those possibly cancer-prone individuals with type C personality characteristics. The individual must begin by searching for and finding the "lost self." He or she must learn to express the feelings and emotions that have been suppressed. Overcoming some of the characteristics associated with type C personality may have the potential of diminishing the risk of developing cancer, as well as facilitating recovery from the disease.

Coronary Heart Disease

Thompson et al (1986) discuss the following therapies in the treatment of CHD:

Surgical intervention with coronary artery bypass grafting (CABG) is indicated for patients with significant obstruction of the major coronary arteries. It provides symptomatic relief in 80 percent of cases.

Percutaneous transluminal coronary angioplasty (PTCA) is a technique that does not alter the general disease process but is an alternative approach to CABG. PTCA attempts to restore patency of the arterial lumen by compressing atheromatous plaques.

Chemotherapeutic agents used in the treatment of CHD include:

1. Vasodilators — to increase coronary tissue perfusion (e.g., nitroglycerin, isosorbide)
2. Beta-adrenergic blocking agents — to treat angina and hypertension (e.g., propranolol, atenolol)
3. Calcium antagonists — to treat angina and hypertension (e.g., verapamil, nifedipine, diltiazem)
4. Antihyperlipidemic agents — to lower serum cholesterol and triglyceride levels (e.g., clofibrate, gemfibrozil, pravachol)

Various techniques have been tried in an attempt to modify the type A behavior pattern associated with CHD. Progressive relaxation, autohypnosis, meditation, biofeedback, and group therapy have been used with mixed results. Friedman and Rosenman (1974) have devised a therapeutic program designed to reduce type A behavior. Combining education of the patient with individualized behavior modification therapy, they were able to reduce type A behavior in 44 percent of the experimental subjects. The recurrence rate of nonfatal myocardial infarction was one half that of the control subjects who received the educational program but did not participate in the behavioral modification therapy.

Peptic Ulcer

The focus of treatment for peptic ulcer disease is to alleviate symptoms, promote healing, and prevent complications and recurrence (Simmons & Heitkemper, 1991).

Pharmacological interventions include:

1. Antacids — to neutralize gastric (HCl) acid (e.g., calcium carbonate, magnesium/aluminum salts)
2. Antisecretory agents — to inhibit secretion of HCl in the stomach
   a. Histamine H_2 antagonists (e.g., cimetidine, ranitidine)
   b. Anticholinergics (e.g., atropine, belladona, propantheline)
3. Cytoprotective agents — to coat ulcerated mucosal tissue and inhibit pepsin activity (e.g., sucralfate)

The selection of foods in dietary intervention is determined by patient tolerance. The traditional bland diet with emphasis on dairy products has become controversial. Spicy foods cause dyspepsia in some individuals. A reduction or elimination of caffeine and alcohol is recommended. Smoking and the intake of aspirin should be avoided.

Surgical intervention may be necessary if medical management does not result in symptomatic relief, when serious, life-threatening complications occur, or when there is possible malignancy (Simmons & Heitkemper, 1991). The most common types of surgical intervention include gastrectomy (removal of a portion of the stomach), vagotomy (severing the vagus nerve to reduce vagally stimulated HCl acid), and pyloroplasty (repairing or reopening of the pylorus to enhance gastric emptying).

Psychotherapy with ulcer patients whose personality characteristics, ego strength, and coping mechanisms favor increased vulnerability to stress has been described as beneficial (Lipsitt, 1989). Troublesome conflicts that have been associated with peptic ulcer disease, such as passivity, dependency, aggression, anger, and frustration, need to be evaluated and properly addressed in treatment, respecting the patient's defensive structure and need for support and reassurance. Various studies have been conducted with peptic ulcer patients (Lipsitt, 1989). The experimental groups received medication along with psychotherapy, while the control groups received medication alone. Results were significant for the experimental groups, who showed consistent and continuing improvement, while recurrence and complications were common among members of the control groups. Lipsitt (1989) states:

"Cumulative evidence to date of the efficacy of psychotherapy [in the treatment of peptic ulcer disease] is that psychotherapy, even for brief periods of time, offers more lasting benefits in social adjustment and symptom reduction than symptomatic medical treatment alone, measured by recurrences and complications."

Essential Hypertension

The treatment of patients with hypertension is directed toward lowering blood pressure in an attempt to halt or reverse progressive organ damage. Some individuals are able to lower the blood pressure by alterations in life-style. If the individual is unable or unwilling to do so, pharmacological therapy is recommended. Many individuals are treated with a combination of both approaches.

DIETARY MODIFICATIONS

The two most effective nonpharmacological modalities for the reduction of elevated blood pressure are weight reduction and sodium restriction (Langford et al., 1985). It may also be necessary for the individual who is on diuretic therapy to ensure that there is a sufficient intake of potassium, either through diet or with supplements. It is also important for the individual with high blood pressure to decrease intake of caffeine, alcohol, and saturated fats.

ENVIRONMENTAL FACTORS

The individual should not smoke.

PHYSICAL EXERCISE

Increased physical activity (e.g., aerobic-type exercise for 30 minutes two to three times a week) has been shown to lower blood pressure in hypertensive individuals (Hagberg et al., 1983).

PHARMACOTHERAPY

Physicians usually take a "stepped-care" approach to prescribing antihypertensive medications. If weight control, dietary restrictions, and physical exercise are not sufficient to maintain a lowered pressure, the first step of pharmacological intervention is usually with a low dose of a diuretic, beta-blocker, calcium channel blocker, or angiotensin-converting enzyme inhibitor. If these medications are not successful in lowering the pressure, either the dosage is increased or a second drug of a different classification is substituted or added. This continues until the desired blood pressure is achieved, side effects become intolerable, or the maximum amount of each drug has been reached (Walsh & Woloszyn, 1987).

RELAXATION TECHNIQUES

Relaxation techniques, such as meditation, yoga, hypnosis, and biofeedback, have been shown to reduce blood pressure in some individuals. They are especially useful for individuals with higher initial pressures and as adjunctive therapy to pharmacological treatment. Supportive psychotherapy, during which the individual is encouraged to express honest feelings, particularly anger, may also be helpful.

Migraine Headache

There currently is little that can consistently and effectively relieve a migraine attack once it has begun. Some physicians administer injections of narcotics, such as meperidine or codeine, which block the pain and allow the individual to sleep until the attack subsides. The newest drug to be introduced that has been effective in aborting a migraine is the serotonin receptor agonist sumatriptin. This drug induces cerebral vasoconstriction, and studies in England have shown it to be effective in preventing as well as interrupting migraine attacks.

Other treatments during a migraine attack that may provide some relief include: cold compresses to the head and neck; bedrest in a quiet, darkened room; application of pressure to the temples; and perhaps application of heat to neck and shoulder muscles that have contracted in response to headache pain.

Some medications are prescribed to be taken at the first sign of onset of a migraine attack. If taken in the prodromal phase at the very first sign, ergotamine tartrate may prevent the vasodilation that creates the pain of migraine. It is ineffective once the attack has begun. Ergotamine is available in combination with other drugs, such as caffeine, sedatives, and antiemetics, and is marketed in various forms, including tablets, suppositories, inhalants, and sublinguals. Ergotamine can safely be given only once or twice a week at the most, so it is not appropriate for individuals who have headaches more often than this. It can be very harmful because of its vasoconstrictive properties and the potential for preventing adequate tissue perfusion.

Most medications are used for prophylactic treatment of migraine headaches. A variety of classifications of drugs have been used for this purpose and have shown varying degrees of effectiveness with individual patients. The most commonly used classes include the beta-blockers (e.g., propranolol), antidepressants (e.g., amitriptyline, fluoxetine), and calcium-channel blockers (e.g., verapamil). Other agents that are sometimes used include antihistamines (e.g., methysergide, cyproheptadine), antihypertensives (e.g., clonidine), psychotropics (e.g., chlorpromazine), and lithium carbonate.

Saper and Magee (1981) suggest the following nonpharmacological interventions to help prevent migraine attacks:

1. Discontinue or avoid any circumstances, events, foods, over-the-counter medications, or beverages that could have been involved in precipitation of an attack.

2. If headaches seem related to the use of oral contraceptives or other prescription medications, discuss with physician. No medication should be discontinued without first consulting with physician.

3. Learn relaxation techniques. Ensure that at least half an hour is set aside for relaxation exercises to reduce stress. Use of these exercises may help prevent poststress headaches.

4. Regularly participate in enjoyable hobbies and relaxing activities.

5. Regular physical exercise is advisable, unless it has been known to provoke migraine attacks.

6. It is best to obtain the same amount of sleep each night. Don't oversleep or do without sleep.

7. Biofeedback, behavior modification, yoga, or meditation appear to be worthwhile in some cases of migraine.

8. Migraine may be related to repressed/suppressed anger, hostility, and guilt. Honest expression of these feelings may serve to remove some of the emotional predisposition to the disorder. Psychotherapy may be necessary in some instances, both to help relieve unresolved anger and to help modify some of the characteristics associated with "migraine personality."

9. Some individuals report relief from migraines after they quit smoking. The products of combustion may play a role in dilating arteries.

Obesity

Treatment of obese people is determined by degree of obesity and motivation for change. Lomax (1989) suggests a variety of treatments based on these two factors.

BEHAVIORAL THERAPY

Essential to this type of treatment is the patient's self-awareness regarding eating behaviors. This is accomplished by keeping a food diary for 1 to 2 weeks before starting the treatment program, recording what was eaten, how much, when, where, with whom, and feelings at the time. High-calorie foods in the home should be replaced with low-calorie foods. Eating should not take place while doing anything else (e.g., watching TV, reading) that would distract from the consciousness of food intake. An exercise program should be undertaken, starting very modestly and increasing to more vigorous efforts. A system of rewards should be initiated and awarded promptly for changes in eating and exercise behavior (not for weight loss).

SELF-HELP GROUPS

Support groups such as Overeaters Anonymous, Weight Watchers, and Take Off Pounds Sensibly (TOPS) rely on group process and motivational support, which seem to strengthen the program of behavior modification. Some of the groups provide inspirational lecturers. They have experienced a moderate degree of success in helping some individuals lose weight. However, the attrition rate is high, and the individual must be motivated to avoid returning to old patterns of eating once the structured program is concluded and the target weight has been achieved.

PHARMACOLOGICAL TREATMENT

Some physicians may prescribe anorexigenic drugs as a diet aid for individuals attempting to lose weight. Common medications for this purpose include diethylpropion (Tenuate), fenfluramine (Pondimin), mazindol (Sanorex), and phendimetrazine (Anorex). All are indicated for the short-term management of obesity and do carry a potential for abuse and dependence. The use of appetite suppressants alone is not currently recommended, since weight lost as a result of their use is usually rapidly regained (Norman, 1984).

SURGICAL INTERVENTIONS

Surgical procedures, such as intestinal bypass operations and gastric stapling, have been effective in producing weight loss in some individuals. However, the risk of surgery and anesthesia are greater in obese individuals. Postoperative complications, such as malabsorption syndromes, are possible following bypass procedures. Therefore, these interventions should be limited to the treatment of mas-

sive and morbid obesity that has not responded to conservative management (Norman, 1984). Wiring the jaws shut to prevent the intake of solid food has also helped some individuals lose weight.

PSYCHOTHERAPY

Psychotherapy has been shown to be effective in helping a small number of individuals lose weight. The decrease of body image disturbance through psychotherapy is substantial, and these individuals have a history of maintaining their weight loss well. Treatment focuses on the person's capacity to recognize needs and make decisions about them, rather than on abnormal eating patterns. Feelings are explored, and alternatives to food as a means of diminishing anxiety, worry, and frustration are identified. Some clinicians suggest that psychotherapy may be a helpful adjunct to surgical intervention (Lomax, 1989).

Rheumatoid Arthritis

The goals of therapy for rheumatoid arthritis are to relieve discomfort and achieve remission. Treatment depends on the extent of the disability, psychosocial variables, and the results of laboratory examinations.

PHARMACOLOGICAL TREATMENT

Aspirin is the cornerstone of drug therapy for the patient with rheumatoid arthritis. In large doses, it has potent anti-inflammatory action, as well as analgesic and antipyretic actions. Up to 5 g/day is prescribed for the patient with rheumatoid arthritis.

Nonsteroidal anti-inflammatory agents (e.g., ibuprofen, fenoprofen, naproxen, sulindac) are used with patients for whom salicylate therapy is ineffective or inappropriate. Persistent articular inflammation may be treated with antirheumatic agents (e.g., gold, penicillamine, hydroxychloroquine sulfate). Corticosteroids (e.g., prednisone, prednisolone, hydrocortisone) provide dramatic results in alleviating pain and inflammation but are not often used because of numerous adverse effects. Antineoplastic agents (e.g., azathioprine, cyclophosphamide, methotrexate, sulfasalazine) have afforded some relief to patients with particularly severe and resistant forms of the disease (Cicero, 1991).

SURGICAL TREATMENT

Various surgical treatments are available for patients with rheumatoid arthritis (Thompson et al, 1986). Synovectomy is performed to relieve pain and maintain muscle and joint balance. Joint fusion may provide stability to a joint and decrease deformity. Spinal fusion may be necessary to treat subluxation. Total joint replacements are considered for patients with severe deformities, significant functional disabilities, or poorly controlled pain (Cicero, 1991).

PSYCHOLOGICAL TREATMENT

Psychotherapy and prompt recognition and treatment of psychiatric morbidity help patients cope and adapt (Ananth, 1989). A patient's initial reaction to the diagnosis of rheumatoid arthritis will depend on the degree of incapacity at the time and the immediate threat to his or her life-style. Denial of the illness is a common initial response. Over time, a number of adaptive processes, including resignation, episodic anger, sadness, and anxiety, may occur (Ananth, 1989). Patients may blame themselves or believe that the disease is the result of past behaviors. Depression may need to be treated separately. Patients should be encouraged to function as independently as possible. Emphasis should be deflected from a focus on cure to one on control of the disease and prevention of disability.

Ulcerative Colitis

The goals of care for the patient with ulcerative colitis are to relieve discomfort and to promote and maintain remission of the disease. This is accomplished through nutritional therapy, pharmacological treatment, surgical intervention if necessary, and psychological support.

NUTRITIONAL THERAPY

There are no general restrictions on diet. Patients should avoid foods that they identify as irritating. Usually a low-residue diet is initiated and advanced as tolerated, with one food added at a time (Thompson et al, 1986). Milk may be a problem for some patients. When the disease is severe or extensive, and absorption problems have resulted in dehydration and cachexia, total parenteral nutrition may be necessary. Tube feedings may be initiated if severe anorexia is present (Long et al, 1987).

PHARMACOLOGICAL TREATMENT

Sulfasalazine is the most commonly prescribed medication for inflammatory bowel disease (Heitkemper & Martin, 1991). It appears to have both anti-inflammatory and antimicrobial properties. Severe forms of the disease are treated with corticosteroids (e.g., hydrocortisone, prednisone, prednisolone). Corticosteroids provide relief through suppression of inflammation but have no effect on cure of ulcerative colitis. To provide symptomatic relief, antidiarrheals (e.g., loperamide, diphenoxylate) and antispasmodics (e.g., propantheline) may be prescribed.

SURGICAL TREATMENT

Surgery is indicated for the patient with ulcerative colitis intractable to medical management or when complications such as persistent hemorrhage, perforation or strictures of the colon, or toxic megacolon are present (Long et al, 1987). Types of surgery that may be performed include proctocolectomy with permanent or continent ileostomy, total colectomy with ileorectal anastomosis, or total colectomy and mucosal proctectomy with ileoanal anastomosis. Surgery is considered curative, and recurrences are few (Long et al, 1987).

PSYCHOLOGICAL SUPPORT

Ulcerative colitis can be a lifetime illness with periods of exacerbation and remission that can disrupt the person's life situation. Because emotions and stress can play a role in exacerbation of the illness, psychological support may help to decrease the frequency of these attacks by helping the individual to recognize the stressors that precipitate exacerbations and identify more adaptive ways of coping. The person with ulcerative colitis often feels a lack of control over his or her life. Psychological support may help with feelings of insecurity, dependency, and depression. It is extremely important that the individual express feelings of repressed/suppressed anger and hostility.

Fears and anxieties associated with possible sexual dysfunction need to be explored. The individual who has undergone surgical intervention for ulcerative colitis may be experiencing a body image disturbance that could interfere with sexual functioning. The person must be given the opportunity to discuss these sexual concerns. He or she may require assistance in communicating these concerns to the sexual partner. Alternate ways of meeting sexual needs can be explored.

SUMMARY

Psychophysiological disorders are those in which psychological factors contribute to the initiation or exacerbation of the physical condition. There is evidence of either demonstrable organic pathology or a known pathophysiological process involved. The *DSM-III-R* identifies this category as "psychological factors affecting physical condition."

Virtually any organic disorder can be considered psychophysiological in nature. The following disorders were discussed in this chapter:

- Asthma
- Cancer
- Coronary heart disease
- Peptic ulcer disease
- Essential hypertension
- Migraine headache
- Obesity
- Rheumatoid arthritis
- Ulcerative colitis

It is thought that psychophysiological disorders occur when the body remains in a prolonged state of moderate-to-severe anxiety. This prolonged period of arousal may contribute to the initiation or exacerbation of the physical symptoms in otherwise predisposed individuals.

Predisposing factors to the development of psychophysiological disorders include heredity, allergies, environmental conditions, viruses, elevated serum lipoproteins, cigarette smoking, alcohol abuse, specific foods, and a dysfunctional immune system. The following personality characteristics have also been implicated in the predisposition to psychophysiological disorders:

- Asthma: unfulfilled dependency needs.
- Cancer: repressed anger and low self-esteem (type C).
- Coronary heart disease: competitive drive and continual sense of time urgency (type A personality).
- Peptic ulcer: unfulfilled dependency needs.
- Essential hypertension: repressed anger.
- Migraine headache: repressed anger, perfectionism.
- Obesity: unresolved dependency needs.
- Rheumatoid arthritis: repressed anger, self-sacrifice.
- Ulcerative colitis: repressed anger, dependency.

Nursing care of the patient with psychophysiological disorders is accomplished using the steps of the nursing process. Background assessment data were presented, along with nursing diagnoses common to each disorder as well as to the general psychophysiological condition. Interventions appropriate to selected general nursing diagnoses and relevant outcome criteria for each were included. An overview of current medical treatment modalities for each disorder was discussed.

Nurses in all areas of clinical practice should be aware of patient potential for psychophysiological responses and the possible psychosocial influences associated with these disorders. Nurses will most likely (at least initially) encounter these patients in areas other than psychiatry.

REVIEW QUESTIONS

Self-Examination/Learning Exercise

Match the following psychophysiological disorders to the psychosocial profile with which it has been associated:

_____ 1. Asthma

a. Competitive; aggressive; ambitious; no time for leisure; never satisfied with accomplishments; easily aroused hostility.

_____ 2. Cancer

b. Obsessive-compulsive by nature; anxious; rigid; excessively neat; repressed anger; depression is common.

_____ 3. Coronary heart disease

c. Unfulfilled dependency needs; views separation from significant other as abandonment or rejection.

_____ 4. Peptic ulcer disease

d. Fixed in oral stage of development; unresolved dependency needs; excessive optimism or pessimism.

_____ 5. Essential hypertension

e. Unfulfilled dependency needs; suppressed anxiety; resentment and frustration resulting in increased gastric secretion.

_____ 6. Migraine headache

f. Perfectionistic; somewhat rigid; compulsive; sets unrealistic expectations; suppresses or represses anger.

_____ 7. Obesity

g. "The nice guy"; suppresses anger; low self-esteem; depression is common; feelings of hopelessness.

_____ 8. Rheumatoid arthritis

h. Suppresses anger; longs for approval from others; stems from childhood fears of loss of love if showed anger toward parents.

_____ 9. Ulcerative colitis

i. Self-sacrificing; inhibited; perfectionistic; repressed anger; depression is common.

10. Which of the following is the primary nursing diagnosis for patients in the *general category* of psychophysiological disorders?
    a. Pain, evidenced by classic pain behaviors
    b. Ineffective individual coping, evidenced by exacerbation of physical symptoms
    c. Altered role performance, evidenced by inability to perform usual responsibilities
    d. Activity intolerance, evidenced by inability to participate in activities

REFERENCES

Ackerman, S. (1983). The management of obesity. *Hosp Pract, 18*(3), 117–135.

Alexander, F., French, T. M., & Pollack, G. H. (Eds.). (1968). *Psychosomatic specificity* (Vol. 1). Chicago: University of Chicago Press.

American Cancer Society (1981). *A cancer source book for nurses* (rev. ed.). New York: American Cancer Society.

American Cancer Society. (1989). *Cancer facts and figures.* New York: American Cancer Society.

American Psychiatric Association. (1987). *Diagnostic and statistical manual of mental disorders* (3rd ed., rev.). Washington, DC: American Psychiatric Association.

Ananth, J. (1989). Rheumatoid arthritis. In H. I. Kaplan & B. J. Sadock (Eds.), *Comprehensive textbook of psychiatry* (ed. 5). Baltimore: Williams & Wilkins.

Anderson, K. L. (1991). Obstructive respiratory disorders. In M. L. Patrick, S. L. Woods, R. F. Craven, J. S. Rokovsky, & P. M. Bruno (Eds.), *Medical-surgical nursing* (2nd ed.). Philadelphia: JB Lippincott.

Bakal, D. A. (1979). *Psychology and medicine: Psychobiological dimensions of health and illness.* New York: Springer Publishing.

Brucia, J, Phipps, W. J., & Daly, B. J. (1987). Interventions for persons with problems of the lower airway. In W. J. Phipps, B. C. Long, & N. F. Woods (Eds.), *Medical-surgical nursing: Concepts and clinical practice* (3rd ed.). St. Louis: CV Mosby.

Cicero, T. F. (1991). Musculoskeletal inflammation and connective tissue disorders. In M. L. Patrick, S. L. Woods, R. F. Craven, J. S. Rokovsky, & P. M. Bruno (Eds.), *Medical-surgical nursing* (2nd ed.). Philadelphia: JB Lippincott.

Cunningham, S. L. (1991). Hypertension. In M. L. Patrick, S. L. Woods, R. F. Craven, J. S. Rokovsky, & P. M. Bruno (Eds.), *Medical-surgical nursing* (2nd ed.). Philadelphia: JB Lippincott.

Dreher, H. (1988). *The complete guide to cancer prevention.* New York: Harper & Row.

Engel, G. L. (1955). Studies in ulcerative colitis: The nature of the psychologic process. *Am J Med, 19,* 231.

Friedman, M. & Rosenman, R. H. (1974). *Type A behavior and your heart.* New York: Alfred A. Knopf.

Gallagher, R. E. & Gallo, R. C. (1975). Type C RNA tumor virus isolated from cultured human acute myelogenous leukemia cells. *Science, 187,* 350–353.

Hackett, T. P., Rosenbaum, J. F., & Cassem, N. H. (1989). Cardiovascular disorders. In H. I. Kaplan & B. J. Sadock (Eds.), *Comprehensive textbook of psychiatry* (ed. 5). Baltimore: Williams & Wilkins.

Hagberg, J. M. et al. (1983). Effect of exercise training on the blood pressure and hemodynamic features of hypertensive adolescents. *Am J Cardiol, 52,* 763.

Harris, E. D., (1983). Evaluation of pathophysiology and drug effects on rheumatoid arthritis. *Am J Med, 31,* 56.

Heitkemper, M. & Brubacher, L. (1991). Nursing strategies for common gastrointestinal problems. In M. L. Patrick, S. L. Woods, R. F. Craven, J. S. Rokovsky, & P. M. Bruno (Eds.), *Medical-surgical nursing* (2nd ed.). Philadelphia: JB Lippincott.

Heitkemper, M. & Martin, D. L. (1991). Infectious and inflammatory gastrointestinal disorders. In M. L. Patrick, S. L. Woods, R. F. Craven, J. S. Rokovsky, & P. M. Bruno (Eds.), *Medical-surgical nursing* (2nd ed.). Philadelphia: JB Lippincott.

Hogan, R. & Xistris, D. M. (1987). Cancer. In W. J. Phipps, B. C. Long, & N. F. Woods (Eds.), *Medical-surgical nursing: Concepts and clinical practice* (3rd ed.). St. Louis: CV Mosby.

Kaplan, H. I. & Sadock, B. J. (1985). *Modern synopsis of comprehensive textbook of psychiatry* (4th ed.). Baltimore: Williams & Wilkins.

Kaplan, H. I. (1989). History of psychosomatic medicine. In H. I. Kaplan & B. J. Sadock (Eds.), *Comprehensive textbook of psychiatry* (5th ed.). Baltimore: Williams & Wilkins.

Kavanagh, J. M. (1987). Interventions for persons with problems of the cardiovascular system. In W. J. Phipps, B. C. Long, & N. F. Woods (Eds.), *Medical-surgical nursing: Concepts and clinical practice* (3rd ed.). St. Louis: CV Mosby.

Langford, G. H. et al. (1985). Dietary therapy slows the return of hypertension after stopping prolonged medication. *JAMA, 253,* 657.

LeShan, L. (1966). An emotional life-history pattern associated with neoplastic disease. *Ann NY Acad Sci, 3,* 780–793.

LeShan, L. (1977). *You can fight for your life.* New York: M. Evans and Company.

Lipsitt, D. R. (1989). Gastrointestinal disorders. In H. I. Kaplan & B. J. Sadock (Eds.), *Comprehensive textbook of psychiatry* (ed. 5). Baltimore: Williams & Wilkins.

Lomax, J. W. (1989). Obesity. In H. I. Kaplan & B. J. Sadock (Eds.), *Comprehensive textbook of psychiatry* (ed. 5). Baltimore: Williams & Wilkins.

Long, B. C. & Neville, J. (1987). Interventions for persons with problems of ingestion. In W. J. Phipps, B. C. Long, & N. F. Woods (Eds.), *Medical-surgical nursing: Concepts and clinical practice* (3rd ed.). St. Louis: CV Mosby.

Long, B. C., Roberts, R., & Broadwell, D. C. (1987). Interventions for persons with problems of intestinal elimination. In W. J. Phipps, B. C. Long, & N. F. Woods (Eds.), *Medical-surgical nursing: Concepts and clinical practice* (3rd ed.). St. Louis: CV Mosby.

Norman, K. (1984). Eating disorders. In H. H. Goldman (Ed.), *Review of general psychiatry.* Los Altos, CA: Lange Medical Publications.

Pelletier, K. R. (1977). *Mind as healer, mind as slayer.* New York: Dell Publishing.

Peplau, H. (1963). A working definition of anxiety. In S. Burd & M. Marshall (Eds.), *Some clinical approaches to psychiatric nursing.* New York: Macmillan.

Riley, V. (1975). Mouse mammary tumors: Alteration of incidence as apparent function of stress. *Science, 189,* 465–467.

Rosenman, R. H. et al (1975). Coronary heart disease in the Western Collaborative Group Study: Final follow-up experience of eight-and-one-half years. *JAMA, 8,* 233.

Saper, J. R. & Magee, K. R. (1981). *Freedom from headaches.* New York: Simon & Schuster.

Schenk, E. (1987). Interventions for persons with common neurologic manifestations. In W. J. Phipps, B. C. Long, & N. F. Woods (Eds.), *Medical-surgical nursing: Concepts and clinical practice* (3rd ed.). St. Louis: CV Mosby.

Selye, H. (1976). *The stress of life.* New York: McGraw-Hill.

Simmons, L. M. & Heitkemper, M. (1991). Ulcers of the gastrointestinal tract. In M. L. Patrick et al. (Eds.), *Medical-surgical nursing* (2nd ed.). Philadelphia: JB Lippincott.

Simonton, O. C. & Simonton, S. (1975). Belief systems and management of the emotional aspects of malignancy. *Journal of Transpersonal Psychology, 7,* 29–48.

Thompson, J. M., G. K. McFarland, J. E. Hirsch, S. M. Tucker, & A. C. Bowers (1986). *Clinical nursing.* St. Louis: CV Mosby.

Vachon, L. (1989). Respiratory disorders. In H. I. Kaplan & B. J. Sadock (Eds.), *Comprehensive textbook of psychiatry* (ed. 5). Baltimore: Williams & Wilkins.

Walsh, E. & Woloszyn, C. T. (1987). Interventions for persons with problems of the peripheral vascular system. In W. J. Phipps, B. C. Long, & N. F. Woods (Eds.), *Medical-surgical nursing: Concepts and clinical practice* (3rd ed.). St. Louis: CV Mosby.

Weiner, H. et al (1957). Etiology of duodenal ulcer: The relation of specific psychological characteristics to rate of gastric secretion. *Psychosom Med, 19,* 1.

Wheeler, V. (1991). Cancer therapy and principles of nursing management. In M. L. Patrick et al. (Eds.), *Medical-surgical nursing* (2nd ed.). Philadelphia: JB Lippincott.

Woods, S. L., Underhill, S. L., & Cowan, M. (1991). Coronary heart disease: Myocardial ischemia and infarction. In M. L. Patrick, S. L. Woods, R. F. Craven, J. S. Rokovsky, & P. M. Bruno (Eds.), *Medical-surgical nursing* (2nd ed.). Philadelphia: JB Lippincott.

BIBLIOGRAPHY

Droba, M. & Whybrow, P. C. (1989). Endocrine and metabolic disorders. In H. I. Kaplan & B. J. Sadock (Eds.), *Comprehensive textbook of psychiatry* (ed. 5). Baltimore: Williams & Wilkins.

26

PERSONALITY DISORDERS

KEY TERMS
histrionic
narcissism
object constancy
passive-aggressive
personality
schizoid
schizotypal
splitting

OBJECTIVES

After reading this chapter, the student will be able to:

1. Define *personality*.
2. Compare stages of personality development according to Sullivan, Erikson, and Mahler.
3. Identify various types of personality disorders.
4. Discuss historical and epidemiological statistics related to various personality disorders.
5. Describe symptomatology associated with borderline personality disorder and antisocial personality disorder, and use this data in patient assessment.
6. Identify predisposing factors to borderline personality disorder and antisocial personality disorder.
7. Formulate nursing diagnoses and goals of care for patients with borderline personality disorder and antisocial personality disorder.
8. Describe appropriate nursing interventions for behaviors associated with borderline personality disorder and antisocial personality disorder.
9. Evaluate nursing care of patients with borderline personality disorder and antisocial personality disorder.
10. Discuss various modalities relevant to treatment of personality disorders.

INTRODUCTION

The word "personality" is derived from the Greek term *persona*. It was used originally to describe the theatrical mask worn by some dramatic actors at the time. Over the years, it lost its connotation of pretense and illusion, and came to represent the person behind the mask—the "real" person. Millon (1981) defines personality as:

". . . a complex pattern of deeply embedded psychological characteristics that are largely unconscious, cannot be eradicated easily, and express themselves automatically in almost every facet of functioning. Intrinsic and pervasive, these traits emerge from a complicated matrix of biological dispositions and experiential learnings and now comprise the individual's distinctive pattern of perceiving, feeling, thinking, and coping."

The *Diagnostic and Statistical Manual of Mental Disorders, ed. 3, revised* (*DSM-III-R*) defines personality *traits* as "enduring patterns of perceiving, relating to, and thinking about the environment and oneself [that] are exhibited in a wide range of important social and personal contexts" (American Psychiatric Association [APA], 1987). Personality *disorders* occur when these traits become inflexible and maladaptive and cause either significant functional impairment or subjective distress. These disorders are coded on Axis II of the multiaxial diagnostic system used by the American Psychiatric Association (see Chapter 2 for an explanation of this system). Virtually all individuals exhibit some behaviors associated with the various personality disorders from time to time. Only when significant functional impairment occurs in response to these personality characteristics is the individual thought to have a personality disorder.

Personality development occurs in response to a number of biological and psychological influences. These variables include (but are not limited to) heredity, temperament, experiential learning, and social interaction. A number of theorists have attempted to provide information about personality development. Most suggest that it occurs in an orderly, stepwise fashion. These stages overlap, however, as maturation occurs at different rates in different individuals. The theories of Sullivan (1953), Erikson (1963), and Mahler and colleagues (1975) were presented at length in Chapter 3. A comparison of the stages of personality development according to these three theorists is presented in Table 26.1. The nurse should understand "normal" personality development before learning about what is considered dysfunctional.

Table 26.1 COMPARISON OF PERSONALITY DEVELOPMENT—SULLIVAN, ERIKSON, AND MAHLER

MAJOR DEVELOPMENTAL TASKS AND DESIGNATED AGES

Sullivan	Erikson	Mahler
Birth to 18 months: Relief from anxiety through oral gratification of needs	**Birth to 18 months:** To develop a basic trust in the mothering figure and be able to generalize it to others	**Birth to 1 month:** Fulfillment of basic needs for survival and comfort
18 months to 6 years: Learning to experience a delay in personal gratification without undo anxiety	**18 months to 3 years:** To gain some self-control and independence within the environment	**1 to 5 months:** Developing awareness of external source of need fulfillment
6 to 9 years: Learning to form satisfactory peer relationships	**3 to 6 years:** To develop a sense of purpose and the ability to initiate and direct own activities	**5 to 10 months:** Commencement of a primary recognition of separateness from the mothering figure
9 to 12 years: Learning to form satisfactory relationships with persons of the same sex; the initiation of feelings of affection for another person	**6 to 12 years:** To achieve a sense of self-confidence by learning, competing, performing successfully, and receiving recognition from significant others, peers, and acquaintances	**10 to 16 months:** Increased independence through locomotor functioning; increased sense of separateness of self
12 to 14 years: Learning to form satisfactory relationships with persons of the opposite sex; developing a sense of identity	**12 to 20 years:** To integrate the tasks mastered in the previous stages into a secure sense of self	**16 to 24 months:** Acute awareness of separateness of self; learning to seek "emotional refueling" from mothering figure to maintain feeling of security
14 to 21 years: Establishing self-identity; experiences satisfying relationships; working to develop a lasting, intimate opposite-sex relationship	**20 to 30 years:** To form an intense, lasting relationship or a commitment to another person, a cause, an institution, or a creative effort	**24 to 36 months:** Sense of separateness established; on the way to object constancy: able to internalize a sustained image of loved object/person when it is out of sight; resolution of separation anxiety
	30 to 65 years: To achieve the life goals established for oneself, while also considering the welfare of future generations	
	65 years to death: To review one's life and derive meaning from both positive and negative events, while achieving a positive sense of self-worth	

Historical and epidemiological aspects regarding personality disorders are discussed in this chapter. Predisposing factors that have been implicated in the etiology of personality disorders are presented. An explanation of the symptomatology is presented as background knowledge for assessing patients with personality disorders.

Individuals with personality disorders are not often treated in acute care settings for the personality disorder as their primary psychiatric diagnosis. However, many patients with other psychiatric and medical diagnoses manifest symptoms of personality disorders. Nurses are likely to encounter patients with these personality characteristics frequently in all health-care settings.

Nurses working in psychiatric settings are likely to encounter patients with borderline and antisocial personality characteristics. The behavior of borderline patients is very unstable, and hospitalization is often required for attempts at self-injury. The patient with antisocial personality disorder may enter the psychiatric arena as a result of a judicially ordered evaluation. Psychiatric intervention may be an alternative to imprisonment for antisocial behavior if it is deemed potentially helpful.

Nursing care of patients with borderline personality disorder or antisocial personality disorder is presented in this chapter in the context of the nursing process. Various medical treatment modalities for personality disorders are explored.

HISTORICAL ASPECTS

The concept of a personality disorder has been present throughout the history of medicine (Frances & Widiger, 1986; Millon, 1981). In the fourth century B.C., Hippocrates concluded that all disease stemmed from an excess of or imbalance among four bodily humors: yellow bile, black bile, blood, and phlegm. Hippocrates identified four fundamental personality styles that he concluded stemmed from excesses in the four humors: the irritable and hostile choleric (yellow bile); the pessimistic melancholic (black bile); the overly optimistic and extraverted sanguine (blood); and the apathetic phlegmatic (phlegm).

Within the profession of medicine, the first recognition that personality disorders, apart from psychosis, were cause for their own special concern was in 1801, with the recognition that an individual can behave irrationally even when the powers of intellect are intact (Perry & Vaillant, 1989). Nineteenth-century psychiatrists embraced the term *moral insanity*, which was introduced by an English physician who defined the concept of what we know today as personality disorders in the following manner:

> "Moral insanity is madness consisting in a morbid perversion of the natural feelings, affections, inclinations, temper, habits, moral disposition, and natural impulses, without any remarkable disorder or defect of the intellect or knowing and reasoning faculties, and particularly without any insane illusion or hallucination."

A major difficulty for psychiatrists has been the establishment of a classification of personality disorders. The *DSM-III-R* (APA, 1987) has been finetuned to provide specific criteria for diagnosing these disorders. The *DSM-III-R* groups the personality disorders into three clusters. These clusters, and the disorders classified under each, are described as follows:

1. Cluster A—behaviors are described as odd or eccentric
   a. Paranoid personality disorder
   b. Schizoid personality disorder
   c. Schizotypal personality disorder
2. Cluster B—behaviors are described as dramatic, emotional, or erratic
   a. Antisocial personality disorder
   b. Borderline personality disorder
   c. Histrionic personality disorder
   d. Narcissistic personality disorder
3. Cluster C—behaviors are described as anxious or fearful
   a. Avoidant personality disorder
   b. Dependent personality disorder
   c. Obsessive-compulsive personality disorder
   d. Passive-aggressive personality disorder

Historically, individuals with personality disorders have been labeled as "immoral or bad," as deviating from social norms, and as extremes on the continuum of normal personality dimensions (Perry & Vaillant, 1989). The events and sequences that result in pathology of the personality are complicated and difficult to unravel. Continued study is needed to facilitate understanding of this complex behavioral phenomenon.

APPLICATION OF THE NURSING PROCESS

Types of Personality Disorders

PARANOID PERSONALITY DISORDER

Definition and Epidemiological Statistics The *DSM-III-R* defines paranoid personality disorder as "a pervasive and unwarranted tendency, beginning by early adulthood and present in a variety of contexts, to interpret the actions of people as deliberately demeaning or threatening" (APA, 1987). Perry and Vaillant (1989) identify the characteristic feature as a long-standing suspiciousness and mistrust of people in general. Prevalence is difficult to establish, since individuals with the disorder seldom seek assistance for their problem or require hospitalization. When they present for treatment at the insistence of others, they may be able to pull themselves together sufficiently so that their behavior does not appear maladaptive. The disorder is more common in men than women by about 7 to 5 (Perry & Vaillant, 1989).

Clinical Picture Individuals with paranoid personality disorder are constantly on guard, hypervigilant, and ready for any real or imagined threat. They appear tense and irritable. They have developed a hard exterior and become immune or insensitive to the feelings of others. They avoid interactions with other people, lest they be forced to relinquish some of their own power. There is always the feeling that others are there to take advantage of them.

They are extremely oversensitive and tend to misinterpret even minute cues within the environment, magnifying and distorting them into thoughts of trickery and deception. Since they trust no one, they are constantly "testing" the honesty of others. Their intimidating manner provokes almost everyone with whom they come in contact into exasperation and anger.

Paranoid persons maintain their self-esteem by attributing their shortcomings to others. Millon (1981) states:

"Paranoids transform events to suit their self-image and aspirations. They do this by denial of any personal weakness and malevolence, the projection of these traits upon others, and the aggrandizement of self through grandiose and persecutory fantasies."

They are envious and hostile toward others who are highly successful and believe the only reason they are not as successful is because they have been treated unfairly. Paranoid persons are extremely vulnerable and constantly on the defensive. Any real or imagined threat can release hostility and anger that is fueled by animosities from the past. The desire for reprisal and vindication is so intense that a possible loss of control can result in aggression and violence. These outbursts are usually brief, and the paranoid person soon regains external control, rationalizes the behavior, and reconstructs the defenses central to his or her personality pattern.

The *DSM-III-R* diagnostic criteria for paranoid personality disorder are presented in Table 26.2.

Predisposing Factors Research has indicated a possible genetic link in paranoid personality disorder. One study revealed that paranoid personality was significantly more common in first-degree relatives of chronic schizophrenics than in the study control group (Perry & Vaillant, 1989).

Psychosocially, paranoid persons may have been subjected to parental antagonism and harassment. They likely served as scapegoats for displaced parental aggression and gradually relinquished all hope of affection and approval. They learned to perceive the world as harsh and unkind, a place calling for protective vigilance and mistrust. They entered the world with a chip-on-the-shoulder attitude and were met with many rebuffs and rejections from others. Anticipating of humiliation and betrayal by others, the paranoid person learned to attack first.

SCHIZOID PERSONALITY DISORDER

Definition and Epidemiological Statistics Schizoid personality disorder is characterized primarily

Table 26.2 DIAGNOSTIC CRITERIA FOR PARANOID PERSONALITY DISORDER

A. A pervasive and unwarranted tendency, beginning by early adulthood and present in a variety of contexts, to interpret the actions of people as deliberately demeaning or threatening, as indicated by at least four of the following:
1. Expects, without sufficient basis, to be exploited or harmed by others
2. Questions, without justification, the loyalty or trustworthiness of friends or associates
3. Reads hidden demeaning or threatening meanings into benign remarks or events (e.g., suspects that a neighbor put out trash early to annoy him)
4. Bears grudges or is unforgiving of insults or slights
5. Is reluctant to confide in others because of unwarranted fear that the information will be used against him or her
6. Is easily slighted and quick to react with anger or to counterattack
7. Questions, without justification, fidelity of spouse or sexual partner

B. Occurrence not exclusively during the course of schizophrenia or a delusional disorder.

Source: American Psychiatric Association (1987) with permission.

by a profound defect in the ability to form personal relationships or to respond to others in any meaningful, emotional way (Widiger & Frances, 1988). These individuals display a lifelong pattern of social withdrawal, their discomfort with human interaction being very apparent. Prevalence of schizoid personality disorder within the general population has been estimated at between 3.0 percent and 7.5 percent. Significant numbers of people with the disorder are never observed in a clinical setting. Sex ratio of the disorder is unknown, although it is more frequently diagnosed in men.

Clinical Picture Persons with schizoid personality disorder are indifferent to others, aloof, detached, and unresponsive to praise, criticism, or any other feelings expressed by others (Widiger & Frances, 1988). They have no close friends and prefer to be alone. In fact, they often do well in jobs that require seclusion, that others find difficult to tolerate. They are able to invest enormous affective energy in intellectual pursuits.

In the presence of others, they appear shy, anxious, or ill at ease. They are inappropriately serious about everything and have difficulty acting in a lighthearted manner. Their behavior and conversation exhibit little or no spontaneity. They are typically anhedonic, in that they experience little pleasure or pain and often appear affectively bland, constricted, and apathetic (Widiger & Frances, 1988).

The *DSM-III-R* diagnostic criteria for schizoid personality disorder are presented in Table 26.3.

Predisposing Factors Although the role of heredity in the etiology of schizoid personality disorder is unclear, the feature of introversion appears to be a highly inheritable characteristic (Perry & Vaillant, 1989). Further studies are required before definitive statements can be made.

Psychosocially, the development of schizoid personality is likely influenced by early patterns of object relations, familial interactive style, and culture (Perry & Vaillant, 1989). The childhoods of these individuals have often been characterized as bleak, cold, unempathic, and notably lacking in nurturing. This type of parenting may produce a schizoid adult when it interacts with a child who possesses a shy, anxious, and introverted temperament. Millon (1981) states:

> "It is clear that children learn to imitate the pattern of interpersonal relationships to which they are repeatedly exposed. Thus, learning to be reticent and undemonstrative is often but an incidental product of observing everyday relationships within a family setting. Families that are characterized by interpersonal reserve and formality, or that possess a bleak and cold atmosphere in which members relate to each other in a remote or disaffiliated way, are likely breeding grounds for schizoid-prone children who will acquire deeply ingrained habits of social ineptness or insensitivity."

SCHIZOTYPAL PERSONALITY DISORDER

Definition and Epidemiological Statistics Schizotypal personality disorder once described "latent schizophrenics." Their behavior is odd and eccentric but does not decompensate to the level of schizophrenia. Schizotypal personality is a graver form of the pathologically less severe schizoid personality pattern (Millon, 1981). Recent studies in-

---

Table 26.3 DIAGNOSTIC CRITERIA FOR SCHIZOID PERSONALITY DISORDER

A. A pervasive pattern of indifference to social relationships and a restricted range of emotional experience and expression, beginning by early adulthood and present in a variety of contexts, as indicated by at least four of the following:

1. Neither desires nor enjoys close relationships, including being part of a family
2. Almost always chooses solitary activities
3. Rarely, if ever, claims or appears to experience strong emotions, such as anger and joy
4. Indicates little if any desire to have sexual experiences with another person (age being taken into account)
5. Is indifferent to the praise and criticism of others
6. Has no close friends or confidants (or only one) other than first-degree relatives
7. Displays constricted affect, e.g., is aloof, cold, rarely reciprocates gestures or facial expressions, such as smiles or nods

B. Occurrence not exclusively during the course of schizophrenia or a pervasive developmental disorder.

Source: American Psychiatric Association (1987) with permission.

dicate that approximately 3 percent of the population have this disorder (APA, 1987).

Clinical Picture   Schizotypals are aloof and isolated and behave in a bland and apathetic manner, since they experience few pleasures and have need to avoid few discomforts (Millon, 1981). Magical thinking, ideas of reference, illusions, and depersonalization are part of his or her everyday world. Examples include superstitiousness, belief in clairvoyance, telepathy, or a "sixth sense," or beliefs that "others can feel my feelings" (APA, 1987).

The speech pattern is odd, sometimes bizarre. Schizotypals are frequently unable to orient their thoughts logically and become lost in personal irrelevancies and in tangential asides that seem vague, digressive, and with no pertinence to the topic at hand. This feature of their personality only further alienates them from others.

Under pressure of adversity, they may react with an intense discharge of primitive impulses, delusional thoughts, hallucinations, and bizarre behaviors, which may reflect a lifetime of repressed anxieties and hostilities. At other times, the pressure may cause them to drift off into another world. They may disconnect socially for prolonged periods, during which they may be confused and aimless, display inappropriate affect and paranoid thinking, and communicate in odd, circumstantial, and metaphorical ways (Millon, 1981).

The *DSM-III-R* diagnostic criteria for schizotypal personality disorder are presented in Table 26.4.

Predisposing Factors   Some evidence suggests that schizotypal personality disorder is more common among the first-degree biological relatives of people with schizophrenia than among the general population, indicating a possible hereditary factor (APA, 1987). Other biogenic factors that, although speculative, may contribute to the development of this disorder include anatomic deficits or neurochemical dysfunctions in either reticular, limbic, sympathetic, or synaptic control systems, resulting in diminished activation, minimal pleasure-pain sensibilities, and cognitive dysfunctions (Millon, 1981).

The early family dynamics of the individual with schizotypal personality disorder may have been characterized by indifference, impassivity, or formality, leading to a pattern of discomfort with personal affection and closeness. Early on, affective deficits made them unattractive and unrewarding social companions. They were likely shunned, overlooked, rejected, and humiliated by others, resulting in feelings of low self-esteem and a marked distrust of interpersonal relations. Having failed repeatedly to cope with these adversities, they began to withdraw, to "tune out" reality, and reduce contact with persons and events that evoked nothing but shame and agony (Millon, 1981). This new

---

Table 26.4   DIAGNOSTIC CRITERIA FOR SCHIZOTYPAL PERSONALITY DISORDER

A. A pervasive pattern of deficits in interpersonal relatedness and peculiarities of ideation, appearance, and behavior, beginning by early adulthood and present in a variety of contexts, as indicated by at least five of the following:

 1. Ideas of reference (excluding delusions of reference)

 2. Excessive social anxiety (e.g., extreme discomfort in social situations involving unfamiliar people)

 3. Odd beliefs or magical thinking, influencing behavior and inconsistent with subcultural norms (e.g., superstitiousness, belief in clairvoyance, telepathy, or "sixth sense," "others can feel my feelings" [in children and adolescents, bizarre fantasies or preoccupations])

 4. Unusual perceptual experiences (e.g., illusions, sensing the presence of a force or person not actually present [e.g., "I felt as if my dead mother were in the room with me"])

 5. Odd or eccentric behavior or appearance (e.g., unkempt, unusual mannerisms, talks to self)

 6. No close friends or confidants (or only one) other than first-degree relatives

 7. Odd speech (without loosening of associations or incoherence) (e.g., speech that is impoverished, digressive, vague, or inappropriately abstract)

 8. Inappropriate or constricted affect (e.g., silly, aloof, rarely reciprocates gestures or facial expressions, such as smiles or nods)

 9. Suspiciousness or paranoid ideation

B. Occurrence not exclusively during the course of schizophrenia or a pervasive developmental disorder.

Source: American Psychiatric Association (1987).

inner world would provide them with an existence that was more significant and potentially rewarding than the one experienced in reality.

ANTISOCIAL PERSONALITY DISORDER

Definition and Epidemiological Statistics Antisocial personality disorder is a pattern of socially irresponsible, exploitative, and guiltless behavior, evident in the tendency to fail to conform to the law, to sustain consistent employment, to exploit and manipulate others for personal gain, to deceive, and to fail to develop stable relationships (Widiger & Frances, 1988). It is one of the oldest and best researched of the personality disorders, and has been included in all editions of the *Diagnostic and Statistical Manual of Mental Disorders* of the American Psychiatric Association. In the United States, prevalence estimates range from 3 percent in men to less than 1 percent in women (APA, 1987). The disorder is more common among the lower socioeconomic classes, and particularly so among highly mobile residents of impoverished urban areas (Perry & Vaillant, 1989).

> NOTE: The clinical picture, predisposing factors, nursing diagnoses, and interventions for care of patients with antisocial personality disorder will be presented later in this chapter.

BORDERLINE PERSONALITY DISORDER

Definition and Epidemiological Statistics Borderline personality disorder is characterized by a pattern of intense and chaotic relationships, with affective instability, fluctuating and extreme attitudes regarding other people, impulsivity, directly and indirectly self-destructive behavior, and lack of a clear or certain sense of identity, life plan, or values (Widiger & Frances, 1988). Prevalence estimates of borderline personality range from 2 percent to 4 percent of the population. It is the most common form of personality disorder. Approximately two thirds of patients with borderline personality disorder are women.

> NOTE: The clinical picture, predisposing factors, nursing diagnoses, and interventions for care of patients with borderline personality disorder will be presented later in this chapter.

HISTRIONIC PERSONALITY DISORDER

Definition and Epidemiological Statistics This disorder is characterized by colorful, dramatic, and extroverted behavior in excitable, emotional persons (Perry & Vaillant, 1989). They have difficulty maintaining long-lasting relationships, although they require constant affirmation of approval and acceptance from others. Prevalence of the disorder is thought to be about 2.2 percent, and it is twice as common in women as in men.

Clinical Picture Histrionic persons have a tendency to be self-dramatizing, attention seeking, overly gregarious, seductive, manipulative, exhibitionistic, shallow, frivolous, labile, vain, and demanding (Widiger & Frances, 1988). They often demonstrate in mild pathological form what our society tends to foster and admire in its members: to be well liked, successful, popular, extroverted, attractive, and sociable (Millon, 1981). Beneath these surface characteristics, however, is a driven quality, a consuming need for approval, a desperate striving to be conspicuous and to evoke affection or attract attention at all costs. Failure to evoke the attention and approval they seek often results in dejection and anxiety.

They are highly distractible and flighty by nature. They have difficulty with attention to detail. They usually show little interest in intellectual achievement, but they are often creative and imaginative (APA, 1987). They have the ability to portray themselves as carefree and sophisticated on the one hand, and inhibited and naive on the other. They tend to be highly suggestible, impressionable, and rather easily influenced by others. They have a strongly dependent quality about their personality.

Interpersonal relationships are fleeting and superficial. The histrionic person lacks the ability to provide another with genuinely sustained affection. Having failed throughout life to develop the richness of inner feelings and lacking resources from which they can draw, histrionics have difficulty in maintaining a full, meaningful, and stable relationship with another (Millon, 1981).

Somatic complaints are not uncommon, and fleeting episodes of psychosis may occur during periods of extreme stress. The *DSM-III-R* diagnostic criteria for histrionic personality disorder are presented in Table 26.5.

Table 26.5 DIAGNOSTIC CRITERIA FOR HISTRIONIC PERSONALITY DISORDER

A pervasive pattern of excessive emotionality and attention-seeking, beginning by early adulthood and present in a variety of contexts, as indicated by at least four of the following:

1. Constantly seeks or demands reassurance, approval, or praise
2. Is inappropriately sexually seductive in appearance or behavior
3. Is overly concerned with physical attractiveness
4. Expresses emotion with inappropriate exaggeration (e.g., embraces casual acquaintances with excessive ardor, uncontrollable sobbing on minor sentimental occasions, has temper tantrums)
5. Is uncomfortable in situations in which he or she is not the center of attention
6. Displays rapidly shifting and shallow expression of emotions
7. Is self-centered, actions being directed toward obtaining immediate satisfaction; has no tolerance for the frustration of delayed gratification
8. Has a style of speech that is excessively impressionistic and lacking in detail (e.g., when asked to describe mother, can be no more specific than, "She was a beautiful person.")

Source: American Psychiatric Association (1987) with permission.

Predisposing Factors Biological hypotheses have been proposed regarding the predisposition to histrionic personality disorder. These include ease of sympathetic arousal, adrenal hyperreactivity, and neurochemical imbalances (Millon, 1981). Heredity may be a factor, as the disorder is apparently more common among first-degree biological relatives of people with the disorder than among the general population (APA, 1987).

Various learning experiences may also be implicated. As an infant, the future histrionic may have been exposed to a number of different sources that provided brief, highly charged, and irregular stimulus reinforcements. For example, many different caretakers might have given the infant intense, short-lived stimulus gratifications at irregular or haphazard intervals (Millon, 1981).

As the child matured, he or she may have come to learn that positive reinforcement was contingent upon the ability to perform parentally approved and admired behaviors. Rarely did the child receive criticism or punishment, but often he or she did not receive the positive reinforcement even when behaving acceptably. In other words, parental acceptance and approval came inconsistently and only when the behaviors met parental expectations. Millon (1981) states:

"These types of experiences have several consequences in terms of personality. They appear to create behaviors that are designed primarily to evoke rewards, create a feeling of competence and acceptance only if others acknowledge and

commend one's performances, and build a habit of seeking approval for its own sake. All three of these traits are characteristic of the histrionic personality."

NARCISSISTIC PERSONALITY DISORDER

Definition and Epidemiological Statistics Persons with narcissistic personality disorder have an exaggerated sense of self-worth. They lack empathy and are hypersensitive to the evaluation of others. They believe that they have the inalienable right to receive special consideration and that their desire is justification for possessing whatever they seek. It is a relatively new psychiatric diagnosis, having only appeared for the first time in the *DSM-III* (APA, 1980). However, the concept of narcissism has its roots in the 19th century. It was viewed by early psychoanalysts as a normal phase of psychosexual development. Epidemiological patterns have not been fully investigated, but anecdotal reports suggest the disorder is more common in men than in women (Perry & Vaillant, 1989).

Clinical Picture Narcissists appear to lack humility. They are overly self-centered and exploit others in an effort to fulfill their own desires. They often do not even conceive of their behavior being inappropriate or objectionable. Because they view themselves as "superior" beings, they believe they are entitled to special rights and privileges.

Their mood, though often grounded in grandiose distortions of reality, is generally optimistic, relaxed, cheerful, and carefree. This mood can easily change, however, due to their very fragile self-esteem. If they do not meet self-expectations, do not receive the positive feedback they expect from others, or draw criticism from others, they may respond with rage, shame, humiliation, or dejection. They may turn inward and fantasize rationalizations that convince them of their continued stature and perfection.

The exploitation of others for self-gratification results in impaired interpersonal relationships. In selecting a mate, narcissists frequently choose a person who will be obedient, solicitous, and subservient, without expecting anything in return except strength and assurances of fidelity (Millon, 1981).

The *DSM-III-R* diagnostic criteria for narcissistic personality disorder are presented in Table 26.6.

Predisposing Factors The family dynamics of a person with narcissistic personality disorder fosters feelings of omnipotence and grandiosity in the child. The family world revolves around the child, and the parents acquiesce to and indulge his or her every whim. There is no give-and-take on the part of the child—only taking. Millon (1981) states, "Every minor achievement of future narcissists is responded to with such favor as to give them a deluded sense of their own extraordinary self-worth." Adding to this predisposing influence is a minimal amount of parental guidance, discipline, and control. These conditions arise with high frequency among only children, who often experience few of the restrictions and learn few of the responsibilities of sharing acquired by youngsters with siblings (Millon, 1981).

Narcissism may also arise out of an environment in which parents attempt to live their lives vicariously through their child. They expect the child to achieve the things they did not achieve, possess that which they did not possess, and have life better and easier than they did. The child is not subjected to the requirements and restrictions that may have dominated the parents' lives and thereby grows up believing he or she is above that which is required for everyone else. Horney (1939) wrote:

"Parents who transfer their own ambitions to the child and regard the boy as an embryonic genius or the girl as a princess, thereby develop in the child the feeling that he is loved for imaginary qualities rather than for his true self."

AVOIDANT PERSONALITY DISORDER

Definition and Epidemiological Statistics The individual with avoidant personality disorder is extremely sensitive to rejection and because of this may lead a very socially withdrawn life. It is not that he or she is asocial. In fact, there may be a strong desire for companionship. But extreme shyness and fear of rejection create needs for unusually strong guarantees of uncritical acceptance (Perry &

Table 26.6 DIAGNOSTIC CRITERIA FOR NARCISSISTIC PERSONALITY DISORDER

A pervasive pattern of grandiosity (in fantasy or behavior), lack of empathy, and hypersensitivity to the evaluation of others, beginning by early adulthood and present in a variety of contexts, as indicated by at least five of the following:

1. Reacts to criticism with feelings of rage, shame, or humiliation (even if not expressed)
2. Is interpersonally exploitative: takes advantage of others to achieve his or her own ends
3. Has a grandiose sense of self-importance (e.g., exaggerates achievements and talents, expects to be noticed as "special" without appropriate achievement)
4. Believes that his or her problems are unique and can be understood only by other special people
5. Is preoccupied with fantasies of unlimited success, power, brilliance, beauty, or ideal love
6. Has a sense of entitlement: unreasonable expectation of especially favorable treatment (e.g., assumes that he or she does not have to wait in line when others must do so)
7. Requires constant attention and admiration (e.g., keeps fishing for compliments)
8. Lack of empathy: inability to recognize and experience how others feel (e.g., annoyance and surprise when a friend who is seriously ill cancels a date)
9. Is preoccupied with feelings of envy

Source: American Psychiatric Association (1987) with permission.

Vaillant, 1989). Although no statistics are available as to prevalence of the disorder, it is apparently fairly common, and more so in women than in men.

Clinical Picture   Individuals with this disorder are awkward and uncomfortable in social situations. They may be perceived by others from a distance as timid, withdrawn, or perhaps cold and strange. Those who have closer relationships with them, however, soon learn of their sensitivities, touchiness, evasiveness, and mistrustful qualities.

Their speech is generally slow and constrained, with frequent hesitations, fragmentary thought sequences, and occasional confused and irrelevant digressions. They are often lonely, and express feelings of being unwanted. They view others as critical, betraying, and humiliating. They desire to be close, show affection, and be warm with others, but they cannot shake themselves of the belief that such actions will result in pain and disillusion (Millon, 1981). Depression, anxiety, and anger at oneself for failing to develop social relations are commonly experienced. Specific phobias may also be present (APA, 1987). The *DSM-III-R* diagnostic criteria for avoidant personality disorder are presented in Table 26.7.

Predisposing Factors   Millon (1981) suggests that there may be a hereditary influence with avoidant personality disorder, as there appears to be a higher than chance correspondence rate among family members. Some infants who exhibit traits of hyperirritability, crankiness, tension, and withdrawal behaviors may possess a temperamental disposition toward an avoidant pattern.

The primary psychosocial predisposing influence to avoidant personality disorder is parental rejection and deprecation (Millon, 1981). These children are often reared in a family in which they are belittled, abandoned, and censured, such that any natural optimism is extinguished and replaced with feelings of low self-worth and social alienation. They learn to be suspicious and to view the world as hostile and dangerous.

The *DSM-III-R* suggests that having a disfiguring physical illness may predispose an individual to this disorder. Avoidant disorder of childhood or adolescence may also be a contributing factor (APA, 1987).

DEPENDENT PERSONALITY DISORDER

Definition and Epidemiological Statistics   Widiger and Frances (1988) identify dependent personality disorder as "a pattern of relying excessively on others for emotional support, advice, and reassurance." These characteristics are evident in the tendency to allow others to make decisions, to feel helpless when alone, to act submissively, to subordinate needs to others, to tolerate mistreatment by others, to demean oneself to gain acceptance, and to fail to function adequately in situations that require assertive or dominant behavior.

The disorder is relatively common. Perry and Vaillant (1989) discuss the results of one study in which 2.5 percent of the sample were diagnosed with dependent personality disorder. It is more common in women than men by about 3 to 1, and in

---

Table 26.7   DIAGNOSTIC CRITERIA FOR AVOIDANT PERSONALITY DISORDER

A pervasive pattern of social discomfort, fear of negative evaluation, and timidity, beginning by early adulthood and present in a variety of contexts, as indicated by at least four of the following:

1. Is easily hurt by criticism or disapproval
2. Has no close friends or confidants (or only one) other than first-degree relatives
3. Is unwilling to get involved with people unless certain of being liked
4. Avoids social or occupational activities that involve significant interpersonal contact (e.g., refuses a promotion that will increase social demands)
5. Is reticent in social situations because of a fear of saying something inappropriate or foolish, or of being unable to answer a question
6. Fears being embarrassed by blushing, crying, or showing signs of anxiety in front of other people
7. Exaggerates the potential difficulties, physical dangers, or risks involved in doing something ordinary but outside his or her usual routine (e.g., may cancel social plans because she anticipates being exhausted by the effort of getting there)

Source: American Psychiatric Association (1987) with permission.

the youngest children of a family than the older ones.

Clinical Picture Individuals with dependent personality disorder have a notable lack of self-confidence that is often apparent in their posture, voice, and mannerisms (Millon, 1981). They are typically passive and acquiescent to the desires of others. They are generous and thoughtful to a fault, all the while underplaying their own attractiveness and achievements. They are inclined to see the world "through rose-colored glasses," at least so far as allowing others to know how they feel. Once alone, they may feel pessimistic, discouraged, and dejected. However, others are not made aware of these feelings. Their "suffering" is done in silence.

Individuals with dependent personality disorder assume the passive and submissive role in relationships. They are willing to allow others to make their important decisions. They avoid positions of responsibility and become anxious when forced into them. They have feelings of low self-worth and are easily hurt by criticism and disapproval. They will do almost anything, even if it is unpleasant or demeaning, to earn the acceptance of others.

The *DSM-III-R* criteria for dependent personality disorder are presented in Table 26.8.

Predisposing Factors An infant may be genetically predisposed toward characteristics of a dependent temperament. Twin studies measuring submissiveness have shown a higher correlation between identical twins than fraternal twins (Perry & Vaillant, 1989).

Psychosocially, dependency is fostered in infancy when stimulation and nurturance are experienced exclusively from one source. The infant forms an attachment to one source to the exclusion of all others. If this exclusive attachment continues as the child grows, the dependency is nurtured. A problem may arise when parents become overprotective and discourage independent behaviors on the part of the child. Parents who make new experiences unnecessarily easy for the child and refuse to allow him or her to learn by experience encourage their children to give up their efforts at autonomy. Dependent behaviors may be subtly rewarded in this environment, and the child may come to fear a loss of love or attachment from the parental figure if independent behaviors are attempted.

OBSESSIVE-COMPULSIVE PERSONALITY DISORDER

Definition and Epidemiological Statistics Individuals with obsessive-compulsive personality disorder are very serious, formal and have difficulty expressing emotions. They are overly disciplined, perfectionistic, and preoccupied with rules. They are inflexible about the way in which things must be done and have a devotion to productivity at the exclusion of personal pleasure. An intense fear of making mistakes leads to difficulty with decision making. The disorder is relatively common and occurs more often in men than in women. In the family constellation, it appears to be most common in oldest children.

Clinical Picture Individuals with obsessive-compulsive personality disorder are inflexible and lack spontaneity. They are very meticulous and work diligently and patiently at tasks that require accuracy and discipline. They are especially con-

---

Table 26.8 DIAGNOSTIC CRITERIA FOR DEPENDENT PERSONALITY DISORDER

A pervasive pattern of dependent and submissive behavior, beginning by early adulthood and present in a variety of contexts, as indicated by at least five of the following:

1. Is unable to make everyday decisions without an excessive amount of advice or reassurance from others
2. Allows others to make most of his or her important decisions (e.g., where to live, what job to take)
3. Agrees with people even when he or she believes they are wrong, because of fear of being rejected
4. Has difficulty initiating projects or doing things on his or her own
5. Volunteers to do things that are unpleasant or demeaning in order to get other people to like him or her
6. Feels uncomfortable or helpless when alone, or goes to great lengths to avoid being alone
7. Feels devastated or helpless when close relationships end
8. Is frequently preoccupied with fears of being abandoned
9. Is easily hurt by criticism or disapproval

Source: American Psychiatric Association (1987) with permission.

cerned with matters of organization and efficiency, and tend to be rigid and unbending about rules and procedures (Millon, 1981).

Social behavior tends to be polite and formal. They are very "rank conscious," a characteristic that is reflected in their contrasting behaviors with "superiors" as opposed to "inferiors." They can be very solicitous and ingratiating with authority figures. However, with subordinates the compulsive person is quite autocratic and condemnatory, often appearing pompous and self-righteous.

Compulsives typify the "bureaucratic personality"—the company man. They see themselves as conscientious, loyal, dependable, and responsible. They are contemptuous of people whose behavior they consider frivolous and impulsive. Emotional behavior is considered immature and irresponsible.

Although these individuals appear very controlled on the surface, underneath this calm exterior lies a great deal of ambivalence, conflict, and hostile feelings. Compulsives commonly use the defense mechanism of reaction formation. Not daring to expose their true feelings of defiance and anger, they bind these feelings so tightly that their opposite comes forth (Millon, 1981). The defenses of isolation, intellectualization, displacement, and undoing are also commonly evident (Perry & Vaillant, 1989).

The *DSM-III-R* diagnostic criteria for obsessive-compulsive personality disorder are presented in Table 26.9.

Predisposing Factors The parenting style under which the individual with obsessive-compulsive personality disorder was reared is one of "overcontrol" (Millon, 1981). Parents of future compulsives expect their children to live up to their expectations and condemn them if they fail to achieve the imposed standards of conduct. Praise for positive behaviors is bestowed upon the child with much less frequency than punishment for undesirable behaviors. Future compulsives become experts in learning what they must *not* do, so as to avoid punishment and condemnation, rather than what they *can* do to achieve attention and praise. They learn to heed rigid restrictions and rules. Positive achievements are expected, taken for granted, and only occasionally acknowledged by their parents; comments and judgments are almost exclusively limited to pointing out infractions of rules and boundaries the child must never transgress (Millon, 1981).

PASSIVE-AGGRESSIVE PERSONALITY DISORDER

Definition and Epidemiological Statistics The *DSM-III-R* defines this disorder as a pervasive pattern of passive resistance, expressed indirectly rather than directly, to demands for adequate so-

---

Table 26.9 DIAGNOSTIC CRITERIA FOR OBSESSIVE-COMPULSIVE PERSONALITY DISORDER

A pervasive pattern of perfectionism and inflexibility, beginning by early adulthood and present in a variety of contexts, as indicated by at least five of the following:

1. Perfectionism that interferes with task completion (e.g., inability to complete a project because own overly strict standards are not met)
2. Preoccupation with details, rules, lists, order, organization, or schedules to the extent that the major point of the activity is lost
3. Unreasonable insistence that others submit to exactly his or her way of doing things, or unreasonable reluctance to allow others to do things because of the conviction that they will not do them correctly
4. Excessive devotion to work and productivity to the exclusion of leisure activities and friendships (not accounted for by obvious economic necessity)
5. Indecisiveness: decision making is either avoided, postponed, or protracted (e.g., the person cannot get assignments done on time because of ruminating about priorities [do not include if indecisiveness is due to excessive need for advice or reassurance from others])
6. Overconscientiousness, scrupulousness, and inflexibility about matters of morality, ethics, or values (not accounted for by cultural or religious identification)
7. Restricted expression of affection
8. Lack of generosity in giving time, money, or gifts when no personal gain is likely to result
9. Inability to discard worn-out or worthless objects even when they have no sentimental value

Source: American Psychiatric Association (1987) with permission.

cial and occupational performance. The name of the disorder is based on the assumption that such people are passively expressing covert aggression (APA, 1987). The passive-aggressive syndrome has been included in all editions of the APA's *Diagnostic and Statistical Manual of Mental Disorders*, and although there are no statistics on the prevalence of the disorder, it appears to be relatively common. It is thought to be somewhat more prevalent among women than men (Millon, 1981).

Clinical Picture Widiger and Frances (1988) profile the passive-aggressive personality in the following manner:

> "Passive-aggressive personality disorder is the tendency to be passively and indirectly resistant to authority, demands, obligations, and responsibilities by such behaviors as dawdling, procrastination, and "forgetting." These persons tend to be complaining, irritable, whining, argumentative, scornful, critical, discontented, disillusioned, and disgruntled. They may not acknowledge or express their anger directly, preferring instead to express it through resistant and negativistic behavior. Their generally hostile-submissive interpersonal stance can be observed not only at work, but also with friends and family (for example, spoiling the evening for others when their preferences are not fulfilled)."

Passive-aggressives feel cheated and unappreciated. They believe that life has been unkind to them, and they express envy and resentment over the "easy life" that they perceive others having. When they feel they have been "wronged" by an-

other, they may go to great lengths to seek retribution, or "get even," but always in a subtle and passive manner rather than by discussing their feelings with the "offending" individual. Passive-aggressives commonly switch among the roles of the martyr, the affronted, the aggrieved, the misunderstood, the contrite, the guilt-ridden, the sickly, and the overworked as a tactic of interpersonal behavior that gains them the attention, reassurance, and dependency they crave, while at the same time allowing them to subtly vent their angers and resentments (Millon, 1981).

The *DSM-III-R* diagnostic criteria for passive-aggressive personality disorder are presented in Table 26.10.

Predisposing Factors The family dynamics of the future passive-aggressive personality involve contradictory parental attitudes and inconsistent training methods (Millon, 1981). At any moment, and without provocation, they may receive the kindness and support they crave, or they may be the recipients of hostility and rejection. Parental responses to the child's behaviors are inconsistent and unpredictable. They internalize these conflicting attitudes toward themselves and others. For example, they do not know whether to think of themselves as competent or incompetent, and are unsure as to whether they love or hate those upon whom they depend. Double-bind communication may also be exhibited in these families. Expressions of concern and affection may be verbalized and then negated and undone through subtle and devious behavioral manifestations. This *approach-avoidance* pattern is modeled by the child, who

---

Table 26.10   DIAGNOSTIC CRITERIA FOR PASSIVE-AGGRESSIVE PERSONALITY DISORDER

A pervasive pattern of passive resistance to demands for adequate social and occupational performance, beginning by early adulthood and present in a variety of contexts as indicated by at least five of the following:

1. Procrastinates, that is, puts off things that need to be done so that deadlines are not met
2. Becomes sulky, irritable, or argumentative when asked to do something he or she does not want to do
3. Seems to work deliberately slowly or to do a bad job on tasks that he or she really does not want to do
4. Protests, without justification, that others make unreasonable demands on him or her
5. Avoids obligations by claiming to have "forgotten"
6. Believes that he or she is doing a much better job than others think he or she is doing
7. Resents useful suggestions from others concerning how he or she could be more productive
8. Obstructs the efforts of others by failing to do his or her share of the work
9. Unreasonably criticizes or scorns people in positions of authority

Source: American Psychiatric Association (1987) with permission.

then becomes equally equivocal and ambivalent in his or her own thinking and actions.

In this inconsistent environment, the child learns to control his or her anger for fear of provoking parental withdrawal and not receiving love and support even on an inconsistent basis. Overtly, the child appears polite and undemanding. Hostility and inefficiency are manifested only covertly and indirectly.

BORDERLINE PERSONALITY DISORDER

Historically, there have been a group of patients who did not classically conform to the standard categories of neuroses or psychoses. Stern (1938) first used the designation "borderline" to identify patients who seemed to fall on the border between the two categories. Other theorists who have attempted to identify this disorder have used terminology such as *ambulatory schizophrenia, pseudoneurotic schizophrenia*, and *emotionally unstable personality*. When the term *borderline* was first proposed for inclusion in the *DSM-III* (APA, 1980), some psychiatrists feared it might be used as a "wastebasket" diagnosis for difficult-to-treat patients. However, a specific set of criteria has been established for diagnosing what Schmideberg

(1959) emphasized as a consistent and "stable course of unstable behavior" (Table 26.11).

Background Assessment Data

CLINICAL PICTURE

The most striking characteristic of borderlines is the intensity of their affect and the changeability of their actions (Millon, 1981). These changes can occur within a matter of days, hours, or even minutes (Kernberg & Haran, 1984). Often they exhibit a single, dominant affective tone, such as depression, which may give way periodically to anxious agitation or inappropriate outbursts of anger.

Chronic Depression Depression is so common in borderline patients that prior to the inclusion of borderline personality disorder in the APA's *Diagnostic and Statistical Manual of Mental Disorders*, many of these patients were diagnosed as depressed. Depression occurs in response to feelings of abandonment by the mother in early childhood (see section on "Predisposing Factors"). Underlying the depression is a sense of rage that is sporadically turned inward on the self and externally on to the environment. Seldom is the individual aware of the true source of these feelings until well into long-term therapy.

Unable to Be Alone Out of this chronic fear of abandonment, borderline patients have little toler-

---

Table 26.11 DIAGNOSTIC CRITERIA FOR BORDERLINE PERSONALITY DISORDER

A pervasive pattern of instability of mood, interpersonal relationships, and self-image, beginning by early adulthood and present in a variety of contexts, as indicated by at least five of the following:

1. A pattern of unstable and intense interpersonal relationships characterized by alternating between extremes of overidealization and devaluation
2. Impulsiveness in at least two areas that are potentially self-damaging (e.g., spending, sex, substance use, shoplifting, reckless driving, binge eating [Do not include suicidal or self-mutilating behavior covered in (5).])
3. Affective instability: marked shifts from baseline mood to depression, irritability, or anxiety, usually lasting a few hours and only rarely more than a few days
4. Inappropriate, intense anger or lack of control of anger (e.g., frequent displays of temper, constant anger, recurrent physical fights)
5. Recurrent suicidal threats, gestures, or behavior, or self-mutilating behavior
6. Marked and persistent identity disturbance manifested by uncertainty about at least two of the following: self-image, sexual orientation, long-term goals or career choice, type of friends desired, preferred values
7. Chronic feelings of emptiness or boredom
8. Frantic efforts to avoid real or imagined abandonment (Do not include suicidal or self-mutilating behavior covered in [5].)

Source: American Psychiatric Association (1987) with permission.

ance for being alone. They prefer a frantic search for companionship, no matter how unsatisfactory, to sitting with feelings of loneliness, emptiness, and boredom (Kaplan & Sadock, 1985).

PATTERNS OF INTERACTION

Clinging and Distancing The borderline patient commonly exhibits a pattern of interaction with others that is characterized by clinging and distancing behaviors. When patients are clinging to another, they behave in a helpless, dependent, and regressive manner (Kerr, 1992). They overidealize a single individual with whom they want to spend all their time, express a frequent need to talk, or from whom they seek constant reassurance. Acting-out behaviors, even self-mutilation, may result when they cannot be with this chosen individual. Distancing behaviors are characterized by hostility, anger, and devaluation of others that arise out of a feeling of discomfort with closeness. Devaluation often occurs in response to separations, limits, or confrontations, and refers to the tendency to discredit or undermine the strengths and personal significance of important others (Gunderson, 1989).

Splitting Splitting is a primitive ego defense mechanism that is common in persons with borderline personality disorder. It arises out of their lack of achievement of object constancy and is manifested by an inability to integrate and accept both positive and negative feelings. In their view, people — including themselves — and life situations are either all good or all bad.

Manipulation In their efforts to prevent the separation they so desperately fear, borderlines become masters of manipulation. Virtually any behavior becomes an acceptable means to achieve the desired results: relief from separation anxiety. Playing one individual against another is a common ploy to allay these fears of abandonment.

Self-Destructive Behaviors Repetitive, self-mutilative behaviors are classic manifestations of borderline personality disorder. Even though these acts can be potentially fatal, most commonly they are manipulative gestures designed to elicit a rescue response from significant others (Gunderson, 1989). Suicide attempts are not uncommon and may be in response to feelings of abandonment following separation from a significant other. The endeavor is often attempted, however, in a place with a degree of "safety" to it (e.g., swallowing pills in an

area where the person will surely be discovered by others; or swallowing pills and making a phone call to report the deed to someone).

Other types of destructive behaviors include cutting, scratching, and burning. Various theories abound regarding the ability of these individuals to inflict pain upon themselves. One hypothesis suggests they may have higher levels of endorphins in their bodies than most people, thereby increasing their threshold for pain. Another theory relates to the individual's personal identity disturbance. It proposes that since much of the self-mutilating behaviors take place when the individual is in a state of depersonalization and derealization, he or she does not initially feel the pain. They continue to mutilate until the pain is felt in an effort to counteract the feelings of unreality. Some patients with borderline personality disorder have reported that, ". . . to feel pain is better than to feel nothing." Pain validates their existence.

Impulsivity Borderlines have poor impulse control based on primary process functioning. Impulsive behaviors associated with borderline personality disorder include running away, episodic substance abuse, gambling, promiscuity, fighting, and binging and purging (Gunderson, 1989). Many times, these acting-out behaviors occur in response to real or perceived feelings of abandonment.

Predisposing Factors

According to Mahler's Theory of Object Relations (Mahler et al, 1975), the infant passes through six phases from birth to 36 months, when a sense of separateness from the parenting figure is finally established. These phases are discussed below.

Phase 1 (birth to 1 month), Autistic Phase During this time, the baby spends most of his or her time in a half-waking, half-sleeping state. The main goal is fulfillment of needs for survival and comfort.

Phase 2 (1 to 5 months), Symbiotic Phase At this time, there is a type of psychic fusion of mother and child. The child views the self as an extension of the parenting figure, although there is a developing awareness of external sources of need fulfillment.

Phase 3 (5 to 10 months), Differentiation Phase The child is beginning to recognize that there is a separateness between the self and the parenting figure.

Phase 4 (10 to 16 months), Practicing Phase This

phase is characterized by increased locomotor functioning and the ability to explore the environment independently. Sense of separateness of the self is increased.

Phase 5 (16 to 24 months), Rapprochement Phase Awareness of separateness of self becomes acute. This is frightening to the child, who wants to regain some lost closeness but not return to symbiosis. The child wants the mother there as needed for "emotional refueling" and to maintain feelings of security.

Phase 6 (24 to 36 months), On the Way to Object Constancy Phase In this phase, the child completes the individuation process and learns to relate to objects in an effective, constant manner. A sense of separateness is established, and the child is able to internalize a sustained image of the loved object/person when out of sight. Separation anxiety is resolved.

The individual with borderline personality disorder becomes fixed in the rapprochement phase of development. This occurs when the child shows increasing separation and autonomy. The mother, who feels secure in the relationship as long as the child is dependent, begins to feel threatened by the child's increasing independence. The mother may indeed be experiencing her own fears of abandonment. In response to separation behaviors, the mother withdraws the emotional support that is so vital to the child at this time. The "emotional refueling" needed during this phase for the child to feel secure is not provided by the mother. Instead, she rewards clinging, dependent behaviors, while punishing (withholding emotional support) independent behaviors. With his or her sense of emotional survival at stake, the child learns to behave in a manner that satisfies the parental wishes. An internal conflict develops within the child based on fear of abandonment. He or she wants to achieve the independence common to this stage of development, but fears that the mother will withdraw emotional support as a result. This unresolved fear of abandonment remains with the child into adulthood. Unresolved grief for the nurturing they failed to receive results in internalized rage that manifests itself in the depression so common in borderline personality disorder.

Gunderson (1989) states:

"This pattern of a hostile and conflictual relationship with the mother is not counterbalanced by a positive relationship with the father: both parents usually have significant psychopathology. Mothers tend to be erratic and depressed, whereas fathers are often absent or characterologically disturbed. These families are frequently flawed by a variety of disruptive acts including incest, violence, and alcoholism."

Nursing Diagnosis, Planning/Implementation

Nursing diagnoses are formulated from the data gathered during the assessment phase and with background knowledge regarding predisposing factors to the disorder. Some common nursing diagnoses for the patient with borderline personality disorder include:

High risk for self-mutilation related to parental emotional deprivation (unresolved fears of abandonment)*

Dysfunctional grieving related to maternal deprivation during rapprochement phase of development (internalized as a loss, with fixation in anger stage of grieving process), evidenced by depressed mood, acting-out behaviors

Impaired social interaction related to extreme fears of abandonment and engulfment, evidenced by alternating clinging and distancing behaviors

Personal identity disturbance related to underdeveloped ego, evidenced by feelings of depersonalization and derealization

Anxiety (Severe to Panic) related to unconscious conflicts based on fear of abandonment, evidenced by transient psychotic symptoms (disorganized thinking; misinterpretation of the environment)

Self-esteem disturbance related to lack of positive feedback, evidenced by manipulation of others and inability to tolerate being alone

In Table 26.12, selected nursing diagnoses common to the patient with borderline personality disorder are presented in a plan of care. Goals of care and appropriate nursing interventions are included for each. Rationales are presented in italics.

---

*This nursing diagnosis was proposed for acceptance by the North American Nursing Diagnosis Association at its biennial conference in April 1992.

Table 26.12   CARE PLAN FOR THE PATIENT WITH BORDERLINE PERSONALITY DISORDER

Nursing Diagnoses	Objectives	Nursing Interventions
High risk for self-mutilation related to parental emotional deprivation (unresolved fears of abandonment)	Patient will not harm self.	Observe patient's behavior frequently. Do this through routine activities and interactions; avoid appearing watchful and suspicious. *Close observation is required so that intervention can occur if required to ensure patient's (and others') safety.* Secure a verbal contract from patient that he or she will seek out staff member when urge for self-mutilation is felt. *Discussing feelings of self-harm with a trusted individual provides a degree of relief to the patient. A contract gets the subject out in the open and places some of the responsibility for his or her safety with the patient. An attitude of acceptance of the patient as a worthwhile individual is conveyed.* If self-mutilation occurs, care for patient's wounds in matter-of-fact manner. Do not give positive reinforcement to this behavior by offering sympathy or additional attention. *Lack of attention to the maladaptive behavior may decrease repetition of its use.* Encourage patient to talk about feelings he or she was having just prior to this behavior. *To problem solve the situation with the patient, knowledge of the precipitating factors is important.* Act as a role model for appropriate expression of angry feelings and give positive reinforcement to patient when attempts to conform are made. *It is vital that the patient express angry feelings, as suicide and other self-destructive behaviors are often viewed as a result of anger turned inward on the self.* Remove all dangerous objects from patient's environment. *Patient safety is a nursing priority.* May need to assign staff on a one-to-one basis if warranted by the situation. *Because of their extreme fear of abandonment, leaving patients with borderline personality disorder alone at a stressful time may cause an acute rise in level of anxiety and agitation.*
Dysfunctional grieving related to maternal deprivation during rapprochement phase of development (internalized as a loss, with fixation in anger stage of grieving process), evidenced by depressed mood, acting-out behaviors.	Patient will be able to identify true source of anger, accept ownership of the feelings, and express them in a socially acceptable manner, in an effort to progress through the grief process.	Convey an accepting attitude—one that creates a nonthreatening environment for the patient to express feelings. Be honest and keep all promises. *An accepting attitude conveys to the patient that you believe he or she is a worthwhile person. Trust is enhanced.* Identify the function that anger, frustration, and rage serve for the patient. Allow him or her to express these feelings within reason. *Verbalization of feelings in a nonthreatening environment may help patient come to terms with unresolved issues.* Encourage patient to discharge pent-up anger through participation in large motor activities (e.g., brisk walks, jogging, volleyball, punching bag, exercise bike). *Physical exercise provides a safe and effective method for discharging pent-up tension.* Explore with patient the true source of the anger. This is a painful therapy that often leads to regression as the patient deals with the feelings of early abandonment. *Reconciliation of the feelings associated with this stage is necessary before progression through the grieving process can*

(continued)

Table 26.12 CONTINUED

Nursing Diagnoses	Objectives	Nursing Interventions
		continue. As anger is displaced onto the nurse or therapist, caution must be taken to guard against the negative effects of countertransference. These are very difficult patients who have the capacity for eliciting a whole array of negative feelings from the therapist. These feelings must be acknowledged *but not allowed to interfere with the therapeutic process.* Explain the behaviors associated with the normal grieving process. Help the patient recognize his or her position in this process. *Knowledge of the acceptability of the feelings associated with normal grieving may help to relieve some of the guilt that these responses generate.* Help patient to understand appropriate ways to express anger. Give positive reinforcement for behaviors used to express anger appropriately. Act as a role model. *Positive reinforcement enhances self-esteem and encourages repetition of desirable behaviors.* Set limits on acting-out behaviors and explain consequences of violation of those limits. Be supportive, yet consistent and firm in caring for this patient. *Patient lacks sufficient self-control to limit maladaptive behaviors, so assistance is required from staff. Without consistency on the part of all staff members working with this patient, however, a positive outcome will not be achieved.*
Impaired social interaction related to extreme fears of abandonment and engulfment, evidenced by alternating clinging and distancing behaviors and staff splitting.	Patient will exhibit no evidence of splitting or clinging/distancing behaviors in relationships with staff or peers.	Encourage patient to examine these behaviors (to recognize that they are occurring). *Patient may be unaware of splitting or of clinging/distancing pattern of interaction with others.* Help patient realize that you will be available, without reinforcing dependent behaviors. *Knowledge of your availability may provide needed security for the patient.* Give positive reinforcement for independent behaviors. *Positive reinforcement enhances self-esteem and encourages repetition of desirable behaviors.* Rotate staff who work with the patient to avoid patient's developing dependence on particular staff members. *Patient must learn to relate to more than one staff member in an effort to decrease use of splitting and diminish fears of abandonment.* Explore feelings that relate to fears of abandonment and engulfment with patient. Help patient understand that clinging and distancing behaviors are engendered by these fears. *Exploration of feelings with a trusted individual may help patient come to terms with unresolved issues.* Help patient understand how these behaviors interfere with satisfactory relationships. *Patient may be unaware of others' perception of him or her and why these behaviors are not acceptable to others.* Assist patient to work toward achievement of object constancy. Be available, without promoting dependency, *so that patient may resolve fears of abandonment and develop the ability to establish satisfactory intimate relationships.*

Outcome Criteria The following criteria may be used for measurement of outcomes in the care of patients with borderline personality disorder.

The patient:

1. Has not harmed self.
2. Is able to seek out staff when desire for self-mutilation is strong.
3. Is able to identify true source of anger.
4. Is able to express anger appropriately.
5. Is able to relate to more than one staff member.
6. Completes activities of daily living independently.
7. Does not manipulate one staff member against the other to fulfill own desires.

Evaluation

Reassessment is conducted to determine if the nursing actions have been successful in achieving the objectives of care. Evaluation of the nursing actions for the patient with borderline personality disorder may be facilitated by gathering information using the following types of questions.

Has the patient been able to seek out staff when feeling the desire for self-harm? Has the patient avoided self-harm? Can the patient correlate times of desire for self-harm to times of elevation in level of anxiety? Is the patient able to discuss feelings with staff (particularly feelings of depression and anger)? Is the patient able to identify true source toward whom the anger is directed? Can the patient verbalize understanding of the basis for anger? Is the patient able to express anger in an appropriate manner? Is the patient able to function in an independent manner? Can he or she relate to more than one staff member? Is he or she able to verbalize knowledge that staff will return and is not abandoning patient when leaving for the day? Can the patient separate from staff in an appropriate manner? Is the patient able to delay gratification and refrain from manipulating others to fulfill own desires? Can the patient name resources within the community from whom he or she may seek assistance in times of extreme stress?

Antisocial Personality Disorder

Millon (1981) suggests that the criteria for antisocial personality disorder described in the APA's *Diagnostic and Statistical Manual of Mental Disorders* is excessively focused on the criminal orientation of an individual. He states, "The write-up fails to deal with personality characteristics at all, but rather lists a series of antisocial behaviors that stem from such characteristics."

In the *DSM-I*, antisocial behavior was categorized as a "sociopathic or psychopathic" reaction that was symptomatic of any of several underlying personality disorders. The *DSM-II* represented it as a distinct personality type, and it has retained that distinction in subsequent editions. The *DSM-III-R* diagnostic criteria for antisocial personality disorder are presented in Table 26.13.

Individuals with antisocial personality disorder are not often seen in most clinical settings, and when they are it is commonly a way to avoid legal consequences. Sometimes they are admitted to the health-care system by court order for psychological evaluation. Most frequently, however, these individuals may be encountered in prisons, jails, and rehabilitation services.

Background Assessment Data

Clinical Picture Widiger and Frances (1988) describe antisocial personality disorder as a pattern of socially irresponsible, exploitative, and guiltless behavior, evident in the tendency to fail to conform to the law, to sustain consistent employment, to exploit and manipulate others for personal gain, to deceive, and to fail to develop stable relationships. These individuals appear cold and callous, often intimidating others with their brusque and belligerent manner. They tend to be argumentative, and at times cruel and malicious. They lack warmth and compassion, and are often suspicious of these qualities in others.

Individuals with antisocial personality disorder have a very low tolerance for frustration, they act impetuously, and they are unable to delay gratification. They are restless and easily bored, often taking chances and seeking thrills, acting as if they were immune from danger (Millon, 1981).

When things go their way, they act cheerful, even gracious and charming. Because of their low tolerance for frustration, this pleasant exterior can change very quickly. Faced with a challenge to pursue what they desire at the moment, they are likely to become furious and vindictive. Easily provoked

Table 26.13 DIAGNOSTIC CRITERIA FOR ANTISOCIAL PERSONALITY DISORDER

A. Current age at least 18.

B. Evidence of conduct disorder with onset before age 15, as indicated by a history of three or more of the following:

   1. Was often truant
   2. Ran away from home overnight at least twice while living in parental or parental surrogate home (or once without returning)
   3. Often initiated physical fights
   4. Used a weapon in more than one fight
   5. Forced someone into sexual activity with him or her
   6. Was physically cruel to animals
   7. Was physically cruel to other people
   8. Deliberately destroyed others' property (other than by fire setting)
   9. Deliberately engaged in fire setting
   10. Often lied (other than to avoid physical or sexual abuse)
   11. Has stolen without confrontation of a victim on more than one occasion (including forgery)
   12. Has stolen with confrontation of a victim (e.g., mugging, purse snatching, extortion, armed robbery)

C. A pattern of irresponsible and antisocial behavior since the age of 15, as indicated by at least four of the following:

   1. Is unable to sustain consistent work behavior, as indicated by any of the following (including similar behavior in academic settings if the person is a student):
      a. Significant unemployment for 6 months or more within 5 years when expected to work and work was available
      b. Repeated absences from work unexplained by illness in self or family
      c. Abandonment of several jobs without realistic plans for others
   2. Fails to conform to social norms with respect to lawful behavior, as indicated by repeatedly performing antisocial acts that are grounds for arrest (whether arrested or not) (e.g., destroying property, harassing others, stealing, pursuing an illegal occupation)
   3. Is irritable and aggressive, as indicated by repeated physical fights or assaults (not required by one's job or to defend someone or oneself), including spouse or child beating
   4. Repeatedly fails to honor financial obligations, as indicated by defaulting on debts or failure to provide child support or support for other dependents on a regular basis
   5. Fails to plan ahead, or is impulsive, as indicated by one or both of the following:
      a. Traveling from place to place without a prearranged job or clear goal for the period of travel or clear idea about when the travel will terminate
      b. Lack of a fixed address for a month or more
   6. Has no regard for the truth, as indicated by repeated lying, use of aliases, or "conning" others for personal profit or pleasure
   7. Is reckless regarding his or her own or others' personal safety, as indicated by driving while intoxicated or recurrent speeding
   8. If a parent or guardian, lacks ability to function as a responsible parent, as indicated by one or more of the following:
      a. Malnutrition of child
      b. Child's illness resulting from lack of minimal hygiene
      c. Failure to obtain medical care for a seriously ill child
      d. Child's dependence on neighbors or nonresident relatives for food or shelter
      e. Failure to arrange for a caretaker for young child when parent is away from home
      f. Repeated squandering, on personal items, of money required for household necessities
   9. Has never sustained a totally monogamous relationship for more than 1 year
   10. Lacks remorse (feels justified in having hurt, mistreated, or stolen from another)

D. Occurrence of antisocial behavior not exclusively during the course of schizophrenia or manic episodes.

Source: American Psychiatric Association (1987) with permission.

to attack, their first inclination is to demean and to dominate. They believe that "good guys come in last," and show contempt for the weak and underprivileged. They exploit others to fulfill their own desires, showing no tract of shame or guilt for their behavior.

Antisocial personalities see themselves as victims. Projection is the primary ego defense mechanism employed. They do not accept responsibility for the consequences of their behavior. Millon (1981) states, "Accustomed throughout life to anticipate hostility from others and exquisitely attuned to the subtlest signs of contempt and derision, they are everready to interpret the incidental behaviors and remarks of others as fresh attacks upon them." In their own minds, this perception justifies their malicious behavior, lest they be the recipient of unjust persecution and hostility from others.

Satisfying interpersonal relationships are not possible, for individuals with antisocial personalities have learned to place their trust only in themselves. Their basic philosophy of life allows that "only by acquiring power can one be assured of gaining the rewards of life. Only by usurping the powers that others command can one thwart them from misusing it" (Millon, 1981).

One of the most distinctive characteristics of antisocial personalities is their tendency to ignore conventional authority and rules. They act as though established social norms and guidelines for self-discipline and cooperative behavior do not apply to them. They are flagrant in their disrespect for the law and for the rights of others.

Predisposing Factors

Biological Influences Family and twin studies have demonstrated some degree of biogenetic predisposition to antisocial behavior (Brantley & Sutker, 1984). Although the principal biogenetic variables are unclear, low cortical arousal and reduced level of inhibitory anxiety may play a role (Fowles, 1984).

Genetics were also implicated in a study by Robins (1966) in which it was found that having a sociopathic or alcoholic father was a powerful predictor of antisocial personality disorder in adult life. The result was unrelated to whether the child had actually been reared in the presence of the father. Only adequate and strict discipline diminished the risk of antisocial behavior in these children with delinquent parents.

Characteristics associated with temperament in the newborn may be of some significance in the predisposition to antisocial personality. Parents who bring their behavior-disordered children to clinics often report that the child displayed temper tantrums from infancy and would get furious when frustrated, either when awaiting the bottle or feeling uncomfortable in a wet diaper (Millon, 1981). As these children mature, they commonly develop a bullying attitude toward other children. Parents report that they are undaunted by punishment and generally quite unmanageable. They are daring and foolhardy in their willingness to chance physical harm and seem unaffected by pain.

The *DSM-III-R* identifies attention-deficit hyperactivity disorder and conduct disorder during prepuberty as predisposing factors to antisocial personality disorder.

Family Dynamics Antisocial personality disorder frequently arises out of a chaotic home environment (Perry & Vaillant, 1989). Parental deprivation during the first 5 years of life appears to be a critical predisposing factor in the development of antisocial personality disorder. Separation due to parental delinquency appears to be more highly correlated with the disorder than is parental loss from other causes. The presence or intermittent appearance of inconsistent, impulsive parents, not the loss of a consistent parent, is environmentally *most* damaging.

A consistent finding in the histories of individuals with antisocial personality disorder is having been severely physically abused (Lewis, 1989). The abuse contributes to the development of antisocial behavior in several ways. First, it provides a model for behavior. Second, it may result in injury to the child's central nervous system, thereby impairing the child's ability to function appropriately. Finally, it engenders rage in the victimized child, which is then displaced onto others in the environment.

Townsend (1991) cites several sources that have implicated family functioning as an important factor in determining whether or not an individual develops antisocial personality disorder. The following circumstances may be influential in the predisposition to antisocial personality disorder:

1. Absence of parental discipline
2. Extreme poverty
3. Removal from the home
4. Growing up without parental figures of both sexes

5. Erratic and inconsistent methods of discipline
6. Being "rescued" each time they are in trouble (never having to suffer the consequences of their own behavior)
7. Maternal deprivation

Nursing Diagnosis, Planning/Implementation

Nursing diagnoses are formulated from the data gathered during the assessment phase and with background knowledge regarding predisposing factors to the disorder. Some common nursing diagnoses for the patient with antisocial personality disorder include:

High risk for violence: Directed at others related to rage reactions, negative role-modeling, or inability to tolerate frustration

Defensive coping related to dysfunctional family system, evidenced by disregard for societal norms and laws, absense of guilty feelings, or inability to delay gratification

Self-esteem disturbance related to repeated negative feedback resulting in diminished self-worth, evidenced by manipulation of others to fulfill own desires or inability to form close, personal relationships.

Impaired social interaction related to negative role modeling and low self-esteem, evidenced by inability to develop satisfactory, enduring, intimate relationship with another

Knowledge deficit (self-care activities to achieve and maintain optimal wellness) related to lack of interest in learning and denial of need for information, evidenced by demonstration of inability to take responsibility for meeting basic health practices

In Table 26.14, selected nursing diagnoses common to the patient with antisocial personality disorder are presented in a plan of care. Goals of care and appropriate nursing interventions are included for each. Rationales are presented in italics.

Outcome Criteria The following criteria may be used for measurement of outcomes in the care of the patient with antisocial personality disorder.

The patient:
1. Discusses angry feelings with staff and in group sessions.
2. Has not harmed self or others.
3. Is able to rechannel hostility into socially acceptable behaviors

4. Follows rules and regulations of the milieu environment
5. Is able to verbalize which of his or her behaviors are not acceptable.
6. Shows regard for the rights of others by delaying gratification of own desires when appropriate.
7. Does not manipulate others in an attempt to increase feelings of self-worth.
8. Verbalizes understanding of knowledge required to maintain basic health needs.

Evaluation

Reassessment is conducted to determine if the nursing actions have been successful in achieving the objectives of care. Evaluation of the nursing actions for the patient with antisocial personality disorder may be facilitated by gathering information using the following types of questions.

Does the patient recognize when anger is getting out of control? Is he or she able to seek out staff instead of expressing anger in an inappropriate manner? Does the patient demonstrate the ability to use other sources for rechanneling anger (e.g., physical activities)? Has harm to others been avoided? Is the patient able to follow rules and regulations of the milieu with little or no reminding? Can he or she verbalize which behaviors are appropriate and which are not? Does the patient express a *desire* to change? Is the patient able to delay gratifying own desires in deference to those of others when appropriate? Does the patient manipulate others in an attempt to have own desires fulfilled? Does he or she fulfill activities of daily living willingly and independently? Can the patient verbalize methods of achieving and maintaining optimal wellness? Can the patient name community resources from whom he or she can seek assistance with daily living and health-care needs when required?

TREATMENT MODALITIES

Few would argue that treatment of individuals with personality disorders can be described as difficult, and in some instances, may even seem impossible. Personality characteristics are learned very early in life and perhaps may even be genetic. It is not surprising, then, that these enduring patterns of behavior may take years to change, if change occurs. Widiger and Frances (1988) state,

Table 26.14 CARE PLAN FOR THE PATIENT WITH ANTISOCIAL PERSONALITY DISORDER

Nursing Diagnoses	Objectives	Nursing Interventions
High risk for violence: Directed at others related to rage reactions, negative role modeling, or inability to tolerate frustration.	Patient will not harm self or others.	Convey an accepting attitude toward this patient. Feelings of rejection are undoubtedly familiar to him or her. Work on development of trust. Be honest, keep all promises, and convey the message that it is not him or her but the behavior that is unacceptable. *An attitude of acceptance promotes feelings of self-worth. Trust is the basis upon which a therapeutic relationship is established.* Maintain low level of stimuli in patient's environment (low lighting, few people, simple decor, low noise level). *A stimulating environment may increase agitation and promote aggressive behavior.* Observe patient's behavior frequently during routine activities and interactions; avoid appearing watchful and suspicious. *Close observation is required so that intervention can occur if required to ensure patient's (and others') safety.* Remove all dangerous objects from patient's environment. *Patient safety is a nursing priority.* Help patient identify the true object of his or her hostility. *Because of weak ego development, patient may be misusing the defense mechanism of displacement. Helping him or her recognize this in a nonthreatening manner may help reveal unresolved issues so that they may be confronted.* Encourage patient to gradually verbalize hostile feelings. *Verbalization of feelings in a nonthreatening environment may help patient come to terms with unresolved issues.* Explore with patient alternative ways of handling frustration (e.g., large motor skills that channel hostile energy into socially acceptable behavior). *Physically demanding activities help to relieve pent-up tension.* Staff should maintain and convey a calm attitude. *Anxiey is contagious and can be transferred from staff to patient. A calm attitude provides patient with a feeling of safety and security.* Have sufficient staff available to present a show of strength to patient if necessary. *This conveys to the patient evidence of control over the situation and provides some physical security for staff.* Administer tranquilizing medications as ordered by physician or obtain an order if necessary. Monitor for effectiveness and for adverse side effects. *Antianxiety agents (e.g., diazepam, chlordiazepoxide, oxazepam) produce a calming effect and may help to allay hostile behaviors (NOTE: Medications are not often prescribed for patients with antisocial personality disorder because of these individuals' strong susceptibility to addictions.)* If patient is not calmed by "talking down" or by medication, use of mechanical restraints may be necessary. Be sure to have sufficient staff available to assist. Follow protocol established by the institution in executing this intervention. Most states require that the physician re-evaluate and issue a new order for

(continued)

Table 26.14 CONTINUED

Nursing Diagnoses	Objectives	Nursing Interventions
		restraints every 3 hours, except between the hours of midnight and 8:00 AM. If patient has refused medication, administer after restraints have been applied. Most states consider this intervention appropriate in emergency situations or in the event that a patient would likely harm self or others. Never use restraints as a punitive measure but rather as a protective measure for a patient who is out of control. Observe the patient in restraints every 15 minutes (or according to institutional policy). Ensure that circulation to extremities is not compromised (check temperature, color, pulse). Assist patient with needs related to nutrition, hydration, and elimination. Position patient so that comfort is facilitated and aspiration can be prevented. *Patient safety is a nursing priority.*
Defensive coping related to dysfunctional family system, evidenced by disregard for societal norms and laws, absence of guilty feelings, or inability to delay gratification.	Patient will be able to follow rules and delay personal gratification.	From the onset, patient should be made aware of which behaviors are acceptable and which are not. Explain consequences of violation of the limits. A consequence must involve something of value to the patient. All staff must be consistent in enforcing these limits. Consequences should be administered in a matter-of-fact manner immediately following the infraction. *Since patient cannot (or will not) impose own limits on maladaptive behaviors, they must be delineated and enforced by staff. Undesirable consequences may help to decrease repetition of these behaviors.* Do not attempt to coax or convince patient to do the "right thing." Do not use the words "You should (or shouldn't) . . ."; instead, use "You will be expected to . . ." The ideal would be for patient to eventually internalize societal norms, beginning with this step-by-step, "either/or" approach (EITHER you do [don't do] this, OR this will occur). *Explanations must be concise, concrete, and clear, with little or no capacity for misinterpretation.* Provide positive feedback or reward for acceptable behaviors. *Positive reinforcement enhances self-esteem and encourages repetition of desirable behaviors. To assist patient in the delay of gratification,* begin to increase the length of time requirement for acceptable behavior to achieve the reward. For example, 2 hours of acceptable behavior may be exchanged for a phone call; 4 hours of acceptable behavior for 2 hours of television; 1 day of acceptable behavior for a recreational therapy bowling activity; 5 days of acceptable behavior for a weekend pass. A milieu unit provides the appropriate environment for the patient with antisocial personality. *The democratic approach, with specific rules and regulations, community meetings, and group therapy sessions emulates the type of societal situation in which the patient must learn to live. Feedback from peers is often more effective than confrontation from an*

(*continued*)

Table 26.14 CONTINUED		
Nursing Diagnoses	**Objectives**	**Nursing Interventions**
		authority figure. The patient learns to follow the rules of the group as a positive step in the progression toward internalizing the rules of society. Help patient to gain insight into his or her own behaviors. Often these individuals rationalize to such an extent that they deny that what they have done is wrong (e.g., "The owner of this store has so much money, he'll never miss the little bit I take. He has everything, and I have nothing. It's not fair! I deserve to have some of what he has.") *Patient must come to understand that certain behaviors will not be tolerated within the society and that severe consequences will be imposed upon those individuals who refuse to comply. Patient must WANT to become a productive member of society before he or she can be helped.* Talk about past behaviors with patient. Discuss behaviors that are acceptable by society and those that are not. Help patient identify ways in which he or she has exploited others. Encourage patient to explore how he or she would feel if the circumstances were reversed. *An attempt may be made to enlighten the patient to the sensitivity of others by promoting self-awareness in an effort to assist the patient gain insight into his or her own behavior.* Throughout relationship with patient, maintain attitude of "It is not you, but your behavior, that is unacceptable." *An attitude of acceptance promotes feelings of dignity and self-worth.*

"In most cases it is unrealistic to set a goal of fundamental alteration of the personality style. A more practical goal would be to lessen the inflexibility of the maladaptive traits and to reduce their interference with everyday functioning and meaningful relationships."

Little research exists to guide the decision of which therapy is most appropriate in the treatment of personality disorders. Selection of intervention is generally based on the area of greatest dysfunction, such as cognition, affect, behavioral or interpersonal relations (Frances et al, 1984). Following is a brief description of various types of therapy and the disorders to which they are customarily suited.

Interpersonal Psychotherapy

Depending on the therapeutic goals, this treatment may be brief and time-limited or long-term exploratory psychotherapy. This type of therapy is particularly appropriate, since to a large extent personality disorders reflect problems in interpersonal style (Kiesler, 1986). Widiger and Frances (1988) suggest the following approach:

"the strategy is to adopt an interpersonal style that encourages more flexible and adaptive functioning in the patient to break the collusive pattern of mutually debilitating relationships. Oppositional and controlling patients may be directed toward more adaptive functioning by being explicitly encouraged to escalate their maladaptive personality traits."

Interpersonal psychotherapy is suggested for patients with paranoid, schizoid, schizotypal, borderline, dependent, narcissistic, and obsessive-compulsive personality disorders.

Psychoanalytical Psychotherapy

This therapy has been considered the treatment of choice for individuals with histrionic personality disorder (Perry & Vaillant, 1989; Widiger &

Frances, 1988). Treatment focuses on the unconscious motivation for seeking total satisfaction from others and for being unable to commit oneself to a stable, meaningful relationship.

Milieu or Group Therapy

This treatment is especially appropriate for individuals with antisocial personality disorder. Support and feedback from peers has been shown to be more effective with antisocial personality disorder patients than one-to-one interaction with a therapist. Group therapy is helpful in overcoming social anxiety and developing interpersonal trust and rapport in patients with avoidant personality disorder (Widiger & Frances, 1988). Feminist consciousness-raising groups can be useful in helping dependent patients struggling with social-role stereotypes.

Behavior Therapy

This therapy offers reinforcement for positive change. Social skills training and assertiveness training teach alternative ways to deal with frustration. This type of therapy may be useful for patients with obsessive-compulsive, passive-aggressive, antisocial, and avoidant personality disorders.

Psychopharmacology

Psychopharmacology may be helpful in some instances. Although medications have no effect in the direct treatment of the disorder itself, some symptomatic relief can be achieved. Thiothixine (Navane) has been shown to be useful with schizotypal patients in decreasing levels of illusions, ideas of reference, obsessive-compulsive symptoms, and phobic anxiety (Perry & Vaillant, 1989).

A variety of pharmacological interventions have been employed with borderline personality disorder. Both carbamazepine (Tegretol) and tranylcypromine (Parnate) have been associated with a decrease in impulsive, self-destructive acts in these patients (Perry & Vaillant, 1989). Haloperidol (Haldol) and thiothixine (Navane) have demonstrated significant improvement in illusions, ideas of reference, paranoid thinking, anxiety, and hostility in some patients. A number of antidepressants have been tried with varying degrees of success in alleviating the symptoms of depression common in borderline personality.

Lithium carbonate and propranolol (Inderal) have been found to be useful for the violent episodes found in antisocial patients when administered within a structured setting (Widiger & Frances, 1988). Medications are seldom prescribed outside the structured setting because of the high risk for abuse by patients with antisocial personality disorder.

For the patient with avoidant personality disorder, anxiolytics are sometimes helpful during times when previously avoided behavior is being attempted. Mere possession of the medication may be reassurance enough to help the patient through the stressful period. Antidepressants may be useful with these patients if panic disorder develops (Liebowitz, et al, 1986).

SUMMARY

Patients with personality disorders are undoubtedly some of the most difficult ones health-care workers are likely to encounter. Personality characteristics are formed very early in life and are difficult if not impossible to change. In fact, some clinicians believe the therapeutic approach is not to try to change the characteristics, but rather to decrease the inflexibility of the maladaptive traits and to reduce their interference with everyday functioning and meaningful relationships.

This chapter presents a review of the development of personality according to Sullivan, Erikson, and Mahler. The stages identified by these theorists represent the "normal" progression and establish a foundation for studying dysfunctional patterns.

The concept of a personality disorder has been present throughout the history of medicine. Problems have arisen in the attempt to establish a classification system for these disorders. The *DSM-III-R* groups them into three clusters. Cluster A (behaviors described as odd or eccentric) includes paranoid, schizoid, and schizotypal personality disorders. Cluster B (behaviors described as dramatic, emotional, or erratic) includes antisocial, borderline, histrionic, and narcissistic personality disorders. Cluster C (behaviors described as anxious or fearful) includes avoidant, dependent, obsessive-compulsive, and passive-aggressive personality disorders.

Nursing care of the patient with a personality disorder is accomplished using the steps of the nursing process. Background assessment data were presented along with information regarding possible etiological implications for each disorder. An overview of current medical treatment modalities for each disorder was presented.

Care of patients with borderline personality disorder and antisocial personality disorder was described at length. Individuals with borderline personality disorder may enter the health-care system because of their instability and frequent attempts at self-destructive behavior. Individuals with antisocial personality disorder find their way into the health-care system as a way to avoid legal consequences or because of a court order for psychological evaluation. Nursing diagnoses common to each disorder were presented, along with appropriate interventions and relevant outcome criteria for each.

Nurses who work in all types of clinical settings should be familiar with the characteristics associated with personality-disordered individuals. Nurses working in psychiatry must be knowledgeable regarding appropriate intervention with these patients, for it is unlikely that many of their other patients can or will match the challenge presented by patients with personality disorders.

REVIEW QUESTIONS
Self-Examination/Learning Exercise

*Select the answer that is **most** appropriate for each of the following questions:*

1. Kim has a diagnosis of borderline personality disorder. She often exhibits alternating clinging and distancing behaviors. The most appropriate nursing intervention with this type of behavior would be:
   a. encourage Kim to establish trust in one staff person, with whom all therapeutic interaction should take place.
   b. secure a verbal contract from Kim that she will discontinue these behaviors.
   c. withdraw attention if behaviors continue.
   d. rotate staff members who work with the patient so that she will learn to relate to more than one person.

2. Kim manipulates the staff in an effort to fulfill her own desires. All of the following may be examples of manipulative behaviors in the borderline patient *except*:
   a. refusal to stay in room alone, stating, "It's so lonely."
   b. asking Nurse Jones for cigarettes after 30 minutes, knowing the assigned nurse has explained she must wait 1 hour.
   c. stating to Nurse Jones, "I really like having you for my nurse. You're the best one around here."
   d. cutting arms with razor blade after discussing dismissal plans with physician.

3. "Splitting" by the patient with borderline personality disorder denotes:
   a. evidence of precocious development.
   b. a primitive defense mechanism in which the patient sees objects as all good or all bad.
   c. a brief psychotic episode in which the patient loses contact with reality.
   d. two distinct personalities within the borderline patient.

4. According to Margaret Mahler, predisposition to borderline personality disorder occurs when developmental tasks go unfulfilled in which of the following phases?

a. Autistic phase, during which the child's needs for security and comfort go unfulfilled

b. Symbiotic phase, during which the child fails to bond with the mother

c. Differentiation phase, during which the child fails to recognize a separateness between self and mother

d. Rapprochement phase, during which the mother withdraws emotional support in response to the child's increasing independence

Jack was arrested for breaking into a jewelry store and stealing thousands of dollars worth of diamonds. At his arraignment, the judge ordered a psychological evaluation. He has just been admitted by court order to the locked unit. Based on a long history of maladaptive behavior, he has been given the diagnosis of antisocial personality disorder.

5. Which of the following characteristics would you expect to assess in Jack?
   a. Lack of guilt for wrongdoing
   b. Insight into his own behavior
   c. Ability to learn from past experiences
   d. Compliance with authority

6. Milieu therapy is a good choice for patients with antisocial personality disorder because it:
   a. provides a system of punishment and rewards for behavior modification.
   b. emulates a social community in which the patient may learn to live harmoniously with others.
   c. provides mostly one-to-one interaction between the patient and therapist.
   d. provides a very structured setting in which the patients have very little input into the planning of their care.

7. In evaluating Jack's progress, which of the following behaviors would be considered the *most* significant indication of positive change?
   a. Jack only got angry once in group this week.
   b. Jack was able to wait a whole hour for a cigarette without verbally abusing the staff.
   c. On his own initiative, Jack sent a note of apology to a man he had injured in a recent fight.
   d. Jack stated that he wasn't going to start any more fights.

8. Donna and Katie work in the secretarial pool of a large organization. It is 30 minutes until quitting time when a supervisor hands Katie a job that will take an hour and says he wants it before she leaves. She then says to Donna, "I can't stay over! I'm meeting Bill at 5:00 P.M.! Be a doll, Donna. Do this job for me!" Donna agrees, although silently she is furious at Katie since this is the third time this has happened in 2 weeks. Katie leaves and Donna says to herself, "This is crazy. I'm not finishing this job for her. Let's see how she likes getting in trouble for a change." Donna leaves without finishing the job. This is an example of which type of personality characteristic?
   a. Antisocial
   b. Paranoid
   c. Passive-aggressive
   d. Obsessive-compulsive

9. Carol is a new nursing graduate being oriented on a medical/surgical unit by the head nurse, Mrs. Carey. When Carol describes a new

technique she has learned for positioning immobile patients, Mrs. Carey states, "What are you trying to do . . . tell me how to do my job? We have always done it this way on this unit, and we will continue to do it this way until I say differently!" This is an example of which type of personality characteristic?

a. Antisocial
b. Paranoid
c. Passive-aggressive
d. Obsessive-compulsive

10. Which of the following behavioral patterns is characteristic of individuals with histrionic personality disorder?

a. They belittle themselves and their abilities.
b. They inappropriately overreact to minor stimuli.
c. They are suspicious and mistrustful of others.
d. They have a lifelong pattern of social withdrawal.

REFERENCES

American Psychiatric Association. (1980). *Diagnostic and statistical manual of mental disorders* (3rd ed.). Washington, DC: American Psychiatric Association.

American Psychiatric Association. (1987). *Diagnostic and statistical manual of mental disorders* (3rd ed., rev.), Washington, DC: American Psychiatric Association.

Brantley, P. & Sutker, P. (1984). Antisocial behavior disorders. In H. Adams & P. Sutker (Eds.), *Comprehensive handbook of psychopathology*. New York: Pergamon Press.

Erikson, E. (1963). *Childhood and society* (2nd ed.). New York: WW Norton & Co.

Fowles, D. (1984). Biological variables in psychopathology. In H. Adams & P. Sutker (Eds.), *Comprehensive handbook of psychopathology*. New York: Pergamon Press.

Frances, A., Clarkin, J., & Perry, S. (1984). *Differential therapeutics in psychiatry*. New York: Brunner/Mazel.

Frances, A. & Widiger, T. (1986). A critical review of four *DSM-III* personality disorders: An overview of problems and solutions. In A. Frances & R. Hales (Eds.), *Psychiatry update: The American Psychiatric Association annual review* (Vol. 5.). Washington, DC: American Psychiatric Press.

Gunderson, J. G. (1989). Borderline personality disorder. In H. I. Kaplan & B. J. Sadock (Eds.), *Comprehensive textbook of psychiatry* (Vol. 2), (5th ed.). Baltimore: Williams & Wilkins.

Horney, K. (1939). *New ways in psychoanalysis*. New York: WW Norton & Co.

Kaplan, H. I. & Sadock, B. J. (1985). *Modern synopsis of comprehensive textbook of psychiatry* (4th ed.). Baltimore: Williams & Wilkins.

Kernberg, O. F. & Haran, C. (1984). Milieu treatment with borderline patients: The nurse's role. *J Psychosoc Nurs, 22*(4), 20–36.

Kerr, N. J. (1992). Management of borderline and antisocial personality disorders. In J. Haber, A. L. McMahon, P. Price-Hoskins, & B. F. Sidelau (Eds.), *Comprehensive psychiatric nursing* (4th ed.). St. Louis: Mosby-Year Book.

Kiesler, D. (1986). The 1982 interpersonal circle: An analysis of *DSM-III* personality disorders. In T. Millon & G. Klerman (Eds.), *Contemporary directions in psychopathology*. New York: Guilford Press.

Lewis, D. O. (1989). Adult antisocial behavior and criminality. In H. I. Kaplan & B. J. Sadock (Eds.), *Comprehensive textbook of psychiatry* (Vol. 2) (5th ed.). Baltimore: Williams & Wilkins.

Liebowitz, M., Stone, M., & Turkat, I. (1986). Treatment of personality disorders. In A. Frances & R. Hales (Eds.), *Psychiatry update: The American Psychiatric Association annual review* (Vol. 5). Washington, DC: American Psychiatric Press.

Mahler, M. et al (1975). *The psychological birth of the human infant*. New York: Basic Books.

Millon, T. (1981). *Disorders of personality*. New York: John Wiley & Sons.

Perry, J. C. & Vaillant, G. E. (1989). Personality disorders. In H. I. Kaplan & B. J. Sadock (Eds.), *Comprehensive textbook of psychiatry* (Vol. 2) (5th ed.). Baltimore: Williams & Wilkins.

Robins, L. N. (1966). *Deviant children grown up: A sociological and psychiatric study of sociopathic personality*. Baltimore: Williams & Wilkins.

Schmideberg, M. (1959). The borderline patient. In S. Arieti (Ed.), *American handbook of psychiatry* (Vol. 1). New York: Basic Books.

Stern, A. (1938). Psychoanalytic investigation of and therapy in the borderline group of neuroses. *Psychoanal Q, 7,* 467–489.

Sullivan, H. S. (1953). *The interpersonal theory of psychiatry.* New York: WW Norton & Co.

Townsend, M. C. (1991). *Nursing diagnoses in psychiatric nursing: A pocket guide for care plan construction* (2nd ed.). Philadelphia: FA Davis.

Widiger, T. A. & Frances, A. J. (1988). Personality disorders. In J. A. Talbott et al. (Eds.), *The American Psychiatric Press textbook of psychiatry.* Washington, DC: American Psychiatric Press.

BIBLIOGRAPHY

Gallop, R. (1985). The patient is splitting: Everyone knows and nothing changes. *J Psychosocial Nurs, 23*(4), 6–10.

Hickey, B. A. (1985). The borderline experience: Subjective impressions. *J Psychosoc Nurs, 23*(4), 24–29.

Kernberg, O. F. et al. (1989). *Psychodynamic psychotherapy of borderline patients.* New York: Basic Books.

Lacy, L. L. & Pitts, W. M. (1983). A comment on hospitalization. *American J Nurs, 83*(12), 1670–1671.

Mark, B. (1980). Hospital treatment of borderline patients: Toward a better understanding of problematic issues, *J Psychosoc Nurs, 18*(8), 25–31.

McEnany, G. W. & Tescher, B. E. (1985). Contracting for care: One nursing approach to the hospitalized borderline patient. *J Psychosoc Nurs, 23*(4)4, 11–18.

O'Brien, P., Caldwell, C., & Transeau, G. (1985). Destroyers: Written treatment contracts can help cure self-destructive behaviors of the borderline patient. *J Psychosoc Nurs, 23*(4), 19–23.

Platt-Koch, L. M. (1983). Borderline personality disorder: A therapeutic approach. *Am J Nurs, 83*(12), 1666–1671.

Wester, J. M. (1991). Rethinking inpatient treatment of borderline clients. *Perspect Psychiatr Care, 27*(2), 17–20.

Witherspoon, V. (1985). Using Lakovic's system: Countertransference classifications. *J Psychosoc Nurs, 23*(4), 30–34.

SPECIAL TOPICS IN PSYCHIATRIC/MENTAL HEALTH NURSING

THE AGING INDIVIDUAL

SPECIAL CONCERNS OF THE
    ELDERLY
Retirement
Long-Term Care
Elder Abuse
Suicide
APPLICATION OF THE NURSING
    PROCESS
Assessment
Nursing Diagnosis,
    Planning/Implementation
        Outcome Criteria
Evaluation
SUMMARY

OBJECTIVES

After reading this chapter, the student will be able to:

1. Discuss societal perspectives on aging.
2. Describe an epidemiological profile of aging in the United States.
3. Discuss various theories of aging.
4. Describe aspects of the normal aging process:
    a. Biological
    b. Psychological
    c. Sociocultural
    d. Sexual
5. Discuss retirement as a special concern to the aging individual.
6. Explain personal and sociological perspectives of long-term care of the aging individual.
7. Describe the problem of elder abuse as it exists in today's society.
8. Discuss the implications of the increasing number of suicides among the elderly population.
9. Apply the steps of the nursing process to the care of aging individuals.

INTRODUCTION

What is it like to grow old? Many people in America likely would state that it is something they do not want to do. Most would agree, however, that it is "better than the alternative."

Bowen (1944) tells the following often-told tale of Supreme Court Justice Oliver Wendell Holmes, Jr. In the year before he retired at 91 as the oldest justice ever to sit on the Supreme Court of the United States, Holmes and his close friend Justice Louis Brandeis, then a mere 74, were out for one of their frequent constitutionals on Washington's Capitol Hill. On this particular day, the justices spotted a very attractive young woman approaching them. As she passed, Holmes paused, sighed, and said to Brandeis, "Oh, to be 70 again!" Obviously, being old is relative to the individual experiencing it.

Growing old has not been a popular phenomenon in the youth-oriented American culture. However, with 66 million "baby-boomers" reaching their 65th birthdays by the year 2030, greater emphasis is being placed on the needs of an aging population. Growing old in a society that has been obsessed with youth may have a critical impact on the mental health of many people. This situation has serious implications for psychiatric nursing.

What is it like to grow old? More and more people will be able to answer this question as the turn of the century approaches. Perhaps they will be asking the question that Roberts (1991) asks: "How did I get here so fast?"

This chapter focuses on the physical and psychological changes associated with the aging process, as well as special concerns of the elderly, such as retirement, long-term care, elder abuse, and rising suicide rates. The nursing process is presented as the vehicle for delivery of nursing care to elderly individuals.

HOW OLD IS *OLD*?

The concept of "old" has changed drastically over the years. Our prehistoric ancestors probably had a life span of 40 years, with the average life span around 18 years (Hendricks & Hendricks, 1977). As civilization developed, mortality rates remained high as a result of periodic famine and frequent malnutrition. An improvement in standard of living was not truly evident until around the mid-17th century. Since that time, assured food supply, changes in food production, better housing conditions, and more progressive medical and sanitation facilities have contributed to population growth, declining mortality rates, and substantial increases in longevity.

In 1900, the average life expectancy in the United States was 47 years, and only 4 percent of the population was age 65 or older. By 1985, the average life expectancy at birth was 71.2 years for men and 78.2 years for women (Butler, 1989).

The United States Census Bureau has created a system for classification of older Americans. Their categories are as follows:

Older	55 through 64
Elderly	65 through 74
Aged	75 through 84
Very old	85 and older

Some gerontologists have elected to use a simpler classification system:

Young old	60 through 74
Middle old	75 through 84
Old old	85 and older

So how old is *old?* Obviously, the term cannot be defined by a number. Myths and stereotypes of aging have long obscured our understanding of the aged and the process of aging. Kermis (1986) identifies the following potentially damaging myths of old age:

1. Old people are all alike.
2. Old people are all poor.
3. Old people are all sick.
4. Old people are incapable of change.
5. Old people are all depressed.
6. Old people always think about death.
7. If we live long enough, we will all become senile.

Myths and stereotypes of this type affect the way in which elderly people are treated. They even shape the pattern of aging of the people who believe them. They can become self-fulfilling prophecies, in which persons believe they should behave in certain ways, and therefore act according to their beliefs. Generalized assumptions can in fact be demeaning and interfere with the quality of life for older individuals.

Just as there are many differences in individual adaptation at earlier stages of development, so is it true in the elderly individual. Erikson (1963) has suggested that the mentally healthy older person possesses a sense of ego integrity and self-acceptance that will help in adapting to the ambiguities of the future with a sense of security and optimism. Goldfarb (1974) states:

"The well-adjusted aged appear to have carried into their late life the capacity to gain gratifications, to relieve their tensions, so as to maintain their self-esteem, self-confidence, purposivity and a satisfying sense of personal identity and social role despite losses that may occur with aging. This differs from the maladjusted who, either because of earlier influences upon their personality adjustment or differences in life experience at whatever age, do not have the resources to deal constructively and efficiently with life problems."

Everyone, particularly health-care workers, should see aging persons as individuals, each with specific needs and abilities, rather than as a stereotyped group. Some individuals may seem "old" at 40, while others may not seem "old" at 70. Variables such as attitude, mental health, physical health, and degree of independence strongly influence how an individual perceives himself or herself. Surely, in the final analysis, whether or not one is considered "old" must be self-determined.

EPIDEMIOLOGICAL STATISTICS

The Population

In 1980, Americans 65 years of age or older numbered 25.5 million. By 1990, these numbers had increased to approximately 31.2 million, represent-

ing 12.6 percent of the population (Fowles, 1991). This trend is expected to continue, with a projection for 2030 at approximately 66 million, or 21.8 percent of the population.

Marital Status

In 1990, of individuals age 65 and older, 77 percent of men and 42 percent of women were married (Fowles, 1991). Forty-nine percent of all women in this age group were widowed. There were five times as many widows as widowers. This is due to the fact that women live longer than men and tend to marry men who are older than they (Butler, 1989).

Living Arrangements

The majority of individuals age 65 or older live alone, with a spouse, or with relatives (Fowles, 1991). At any one time, only about 5 percent of people in this age group live in institutions (Butler, 1989). See Figure 27.1 for a distribution of living arrangements.

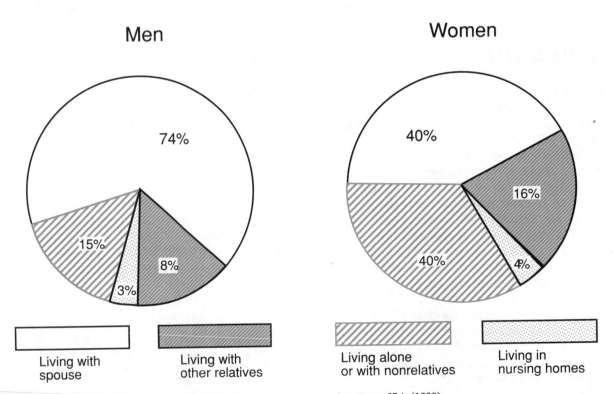

Figure 27.1 Living arrangements of persons 65+ (1990).

Economic Status

Approximately 3.7 million persons age 65 or older were below the poverty level in 1990 (Fowles, 1991). Older women, and particularly black women, had a higher poverty rate than older men. Poor people who have worked all their lives can expect to become poorer in old age, and others will become poor only after becoming old (Butler, 1989). However, a substantial number of affluent and middle-income older persons do enjoy a high quality of life.

Seventy-five percent of individuals in this age group own their own homes (Butler, 1989). However, the housing of older Americans is generally older and less adequate than that of the younger population, and a higher percentage of income is spent on maintenance and repairs.

Employment

With the passage of the Age Discrimination in Employment Act in 1967, forced retirement has been virtually eliminated in the workplace. Evidence suggests that involvement in purposive activity is vital to successful adaptation and even to survival (Butler, 1989). Individuals age 65 or older constituted 2.8 percent of the United States labor force in 1990 (Fowles, 1991).

Health Status

The number of days in which usual activities are restricted because of illness or injury increases with age. Persons 65 years of age or older averaged 31 such days in 1989 and accounted for 33 percent of all hospital stays. Most older individuals have at least one chronic condition and many have more than one. The most commonly occurring conditions for the elderly in 1989 (in descending order of frequency) were: arthritis, hypertension, hearing impairments, heart disease, cataracts, orthopedic impairments, sinusitis, diabetes, visual impairments, and varicose veins (Fowles, 1991).

Emotional and mental illnesses increase over the life cycle. Depression is particularly prevalent, and suicide is increasing among elderly Americans. Organic mental disease increases dramatically in old age (Butler, 1989).

THEORIES OF AGING

Biological Theories

Busse (1989) has identified the following eight biological theories regarding the aging process. Despite these propositions, a single, satisfactory biological theory has yet to be empirically demonstrated.

1. *The exhaustion theory.* This theory suggests that the body contains a finite amount of energy that is gradually used up over time. When the energy is gone, the body dies.
2. *The accumulation theory.* According to this theory, harmful material, such as lipofuscin, develops late in life and destroys cells.
3. *The biological programming theory.* This theory says that cells are genetically programmed to live for a specific period, leading to inevitable death.
4. *The error theory.* This theory states that, in senescence, alterations occur in the structure of the deoxyribonucleic acid (DNA) molecule. When the errors are transmitted to messenger ribonucleic acid, there is a buildup of defective enzymes, leading ultimately to cell and organismic death.
5. *The cross-linkage or eversion theory.* This theory suggests that the linkages holding together the polypeptide strands of collagen change, thus rendering collagen less permeable and elastic and therefore less capable of sustaining normal life.
6. *The immunologic theory.* This theory postulates that with time the protective mechanisms of the immune system are reduced. Consequently, the system may become autoaggressive, leading to destruction of the body tissue.
7. *The "aging clock" theory.* This "clock" is said to reside in the hypothalamus. The hypothalamus is central to a variety of brain and endocrine functions, and cell loss at this site has a particularly important role in decline of homeostatic mechanisms with age.
8. *The free radical theory.* Free radicals are molecules with unpaired electrons that exist normally in the body, as well as being produced by ionizing radiation, ozone, and chemical toxins. According to this theory, these free radicals cause DNA damage, cross-linkage of

collagen, and the accumulation of age pigments.

Psychosocial Theories

1. *The activity theory of aging.* Roscow (1967) has suggested that social integration is the prime factor in determining psychosocial adaptation in later life. Social integration refers to how the aging individual is included and takes part in the life and activities of his or her society. This theory holds that the maintenance of activities is important to most people as a basis for deriving and sustaining satisfaction, self-esteem, and health.
2. *Continuity theory.* Atchley (1989) proposed that while the basic structure of the individual remains intact over time, a variety of adaptive changes occur that require the aging person to make choices. Choices are made based on the preservation of inner psychological continuity and external continuity of social behaviors. Maintenance of internal continuity is motivated by the need for preservation of self-esteem, ego integrity, cognitive function, and social support. As they age, individuals maintain their self-concept by reinterpreting their current experiences so that old values can take on new meanings in keeping with present circumstances (Kaufman, 1986). Internal self-concepts and beliefs are not readily vulnerable to environmental change; and external continuity in skills, activities, roles, and relationships remains remarkably stable into the 70s (Lieberman & Tobin, 1983; Lawton, 1983).

Personality Theories

Personality theories of aging are influenced by the fact that, as they traverse life experiences, people become increasingly different (Sadavoy et al, 1991). In extreme old age, however, people show greater similarity in certain characteristics, probably because of similar declines in biological functioning and societal opportunities.

Neugarten and associates (1964) found that when comparing 60 year olds with 40 year olds, the older individuals seem to see the environment as more complex and more dangerous. Their world becomes more internally oriented. In addition, older men seem to be more receptive than younger men to their nurturing and sensual capacities, while older women become more accepting of their own "aggressive and egocentric impulses."

In a study by Reichard and colleagues (1962), the personalities of older men were classified into five major categories according to their patterns of adjustment to aging:

1. *Mature men* are those well-balanced types who maintain close personal relationships. They accept both the strengths and weaknesses of their age, finding little to regret about retirement and approaching most problems in a relaxed or convivial manner without having to continually assess blame.
2. *Rocking chair* personalities are passive-dependent agers who are content to lean on others for support, disengage, and let most of life's activities pass by their doors.
3. *Armored men* have well-integrated defense mechanisms, which serve as adequate protection. Rigid and stable, they present a strong, silent front and often rely on activity as an expression of their continuing independence.
4. *Angry men* are bitter about life, themselves, and other people. Aggressiveness is a common response, as is suspicion of others, especially of minorities or women. With little tolerance for ambiguity or frustration, they have always shown some instability in work and their personal lives, and now feel extremely threatened by age.
5. *Self-haters* are similar to angry men, except most of their animosity is turned inward on themselves. Seeing themselves as dismal failures, being old only depresses them all the more.

The investigators identified the mature, rocking chair, or armored categories as healthy, adjusted individuals, while the angry men and self-haters were characterized as less successful agers. In all cases, the evidence suggested that the personalities of the subjects, though distinguished by age-specific criteria, had not changed appreciably throughout most of adulthood.

THE NORMAL AGING PROCESS

Biological Aspects of Aging

Individuals are unique in their physical and psychological aging processes, as influenced by their predisposition or resistance to illness; the effects of their external environment and behaviors; their exposure to trauma, infections, and past diseases; and the health and illness practices they have adopted during their life span (Leventhal, 1991). As the individual ages, there is a quantitative loss of cells as well as changes in many of the enzymatic activities within cells, resulting in a diminished responsiveness to biological demands made on the body. Age-related changes occur at different rates for different individuals, although in actuality, when growth stops, aging begins. Virtually all growth ceases with puberty (Leventhal, 1991). This section presents a brief overview of the normal biological changes that occur with the aging process.

SKIN

One of the most dramatic changes that occurs in aging is the loss of elastin in the skin. The effects of elastin, as well as changes occurring to collagen, result in the wrinkling and sagging of aged skin. Solar exposure accelerates this process. People with prolonged tanning exposure have more wrinkles at earlier ages as well as a greater incidence of skin malignancies (Kligman et al, 1985).

Fat redistribution results in a loss of the subcutaneous cushion of adipose tissue. Thus older people lose "insulation" and are more sensitive to extremes of ambient temperature than younger people (Kenney, 1989). Fewer blood vessels to the skin result in a slower rate of healing.

CARDIOVASCULAR SYSTEM

The age-related decline in the cardiovascular system has been thought to be the major determinant of decreased tolerance for exercise and loss of conditioning, and thus the major factor contributing to feelings of agedness and overall decline in energy reserve (Leventhal, 1991). The aging heart is characterized by modest hypertrophy, with reduced ventricular compliance and diminished cardiac output (Shader & Kennedy, 1989). This results in a decrease in response to work demands, and some diminishment of blood flow to the brain, kidneys, liver, and muscles. Heart rate also slows with time. If arteriosclerosis is present, cardiac function is further compromised.

RESPIRATORY SYSTEM

Thoracic expansion is diminished by an increase in fibrous tissue and loss of elastin. Pulmonary vital capacity decreases and the amount of residual air increases. Scattered areas of fibrosis in the alveolar septae interfere with exchange of oxygen and carbon dioxide. These changes are accelerated by use of cigarettes or other inhaled substances. Cough and laryngeal reflexes are reduced, resulting in decreased ability to defend the airway. Decreased pulmonary blood flow and diffusion ability result in reduced efficiency in responding to sudden respiratory demands.

MUSCULOSKELETAL SYSTEM

Skeletal aging involving the bones, muscles, ligaments, and tendons probably generates the most frequent limitations on activities of daily living experienced by aging individuals (Leventhal, 1991). Loss of muscle mass is significant, although this occurs more slowly in men than in women. Demineralization of the bones occurs at a rate of about 1 percent per year throughout the life span in both men and women. However, this increases to approximately 10 percent in women around menopause, making them particularly vulnerable to osteoporosis.

Individual muscle fibers become thinner and less elastic with age. Muscles become less flexible following disuse. There is diminished storage of muscle glycogen, resulting in loss of energy reserve for increased activity. These changes are accelerated by nutritional deficiencies and inactivity.

GASTROINTESTINAL SYSTEM

In the oral cavity, the teeth show a reduction in dentine production, shrinkage and fibrosis of root pulp, gingival retraction, and loss of bone density in the alveolar ridges (Leventhal, 1991). There is some loss of peristalsis in the stomach and intestines, and gastric acid production decreases.

Levels of intrinsic factor may also decrease, resulting in vitamin B_{12} malabsorption in some aging individuals. A significant decrease in absorptive surface area of the small intestine may be associated with some decline in nutrient absorption. Motility slowdown of the large intestine, combined with poor dietary habits, dehydration, lack of exercise, and some medications, may give rise to problems with constipation.

There is a modest decrease in size and weight of the liver. This decrease in liver mass results in losses in enzyme activity that function in the deactivation of certain medications by the liver. These age-related changes can influence the metabolism and excretion of these medications. These changes, along with the pharmacokinetics of the drug, must be considered when giving medications to aging individuals.

ENDOCRINE SYSTEM

A decreased level of thyroid hormones results in a lowered basal metabolic rate. Decreased amounts of adrenocorticotropic hormone may result in a less efficient stress response.

Impairments in glucose tolerance are evident in aging individuals (Leventhal, 1991). Studies of glucose challenges show that insulin levels are equivalent or slightly higher than those from younger challenged individuals, although peripheral insulin resistance appears to play a significant role in carbohydrate intolerance. The observed glucose clearance abnormalities and insulin resistance in older people may be related to many factors other than biological aging (e.g., obesity, family history of diabetes) and may be influenced substantially by diet or exercise (Marchesini et al, 1987; Pacini et al, 1988).

GENITOURINARY SYSTEM

Age-related declines in renal function occur because of a steady attrition due to sclerosis of nephrons over time (Leventhal, 1991). Clinical evidence from morphology and urinalysis suggests a decline of more than 45 percent of glomerular filtration between maturity and the ninth decade (Hendricks & Hendricks, 1977). The elderly are prone to develop the syndrome of inappropriate antidiuretic hormone secretion, and levels of blood urea nitrogen and creatinine may be elevated slightly. The overall decline in renal functioning has serious implications for physicians in prescribing medications for elderly individuals.

In men, enlargement of the prostate gland is common. Prostatic hypertrophy is associated with an increased risk for urinary retention and may also be a cause of urinary incontinence (Shader & Kennedy, 1989). Loss of muscle and sphincter control, as well as various medications, may result in urinary incontinence in women. Not only is this problem a cause of social stigma, but left untreated it increases the risk of urinary tract infection and local skin irritation.

Normal changes in the genitalia will be discussed in the section on "Sexual Aspects of Aging, p. 608."

IMMUNE SYSTEM

With the aging process, the actual numbers of some immune cells decline. The result is a decline in cellular functions and a slowing of metabolic reactions (Hausman & Weksler, 1985). Atrophy of the thymus gland and reticuloendothelial system results in a weak antibody response to new antigens. The inflammatory response is diminished and healing is delayed. These responses may be aggravated by nutritional deficiencies.

The incidence of autoimmune responses increases with age (Sigel & Good, 1972). The prevalence of rheumatoid arthritis is testimony to the effects of impairment in autoimmune regulation.

Because of the overall decrease in efficiency of the immune system, the proliferation of abnormal cells is facilitated in the elderly individual. Cancer is the best example of aberrant cells allowed to proliferate because of the ineffectiveness of the immune system.

NERVOUS SYSTEM

With aging, there is an absolute loss of neurons, which correlates with decreases in brain weight of about 10 percent for men and about 5 percent for women at age 70 (Shader & Kennedy, 1989). Gross morphological examination reveals gyral atrophy in the frontal, temporal, and parietal lobes; widening of the sulci; and ventricular enlargement. However, it must be remembered that these changes have been identified in careful study of adults with normal intellectual function (Shader & Kennedy, 1989).

The brain has enormous reserve, and little cerebral function is lost over time, although greater functional decline is noted in the periphery (Leventhal, 1991). There appears to be a disproportionately greater loss of cells in the cerebellum, the locus ceruleus, the substantia nigra, and olfactory bulbs, accounting for some of the more characteristic aging behaviors, such as mild gait disturbances, sleep disruptions, and decreased smell and taste perception (Brody, 1976).

Some of the age-related changes within the nervous system may be due to alterations in neurotransmitter release, uptake, turnover, catabolism, or receptor functions (Shader & Kennedy, 1989). A great deal of attention is being given to brain biochemistry, and in particular the neurotransmitters acetylcholine, dopamine, norepinephrine, and epinephrine. These biochemical changes may be responsible for the altered responses of many older persons to stressful events and some biological treatments.

SENSORY SYSTEMS

Vision Visual acuity begins to decrease in midlife. Presbyopia is the standard marker of aging of the eye. It occurs as the muscles and ligaments supporting the lens become less taut and stretchable, compromising accommodation (Fisher, 1973).

Cataract development is inevitable if the individual lives long enough for the changes to occur. Cataracts are formed when pigment is laid down in specific patterns in the lens over time and is coupled with increased rigidity of the lenticular proteins (Leventhal, 1991).

The color in the iris may fade, and the pupil may become irregular in shape. A decrease in production of secretions by the lacrimal glands may cause dryness and result in increased irritation and infection. The pupil may become constricted, requiring an increase in the amount of light needed for reading.

Hearing There is significant change in hearing with the aging process. Gradually over time, the ear loses its sensitivity in discriminating sounds as a result of damage to the hair cells of the cochlea. The most dramatic decline appears to be in perception of high-frequency sounds.

Although hearing loss is significant in all aging individuals, the decline is more dramatic in men than in women. This may be related to deterioration resulting from occupational exposure to noise (Leventhal, 1991).

Taste and Smell Taste sensitivity decreases over the life span. There is a loss of discrimination, with bitter taste sensations predominating. Sensitivity to sweet and salty tastes is diminished.

With a deterioration of the olfactory bulbs, there is an accompanying loss of smell acuity. The "aromatic" component of taste perception diminishes.

Touch and Pain There is a continuous decrease in organized sensory nerve receptors on the skin throughout the life span. Thus the touch threshold increases as a function of age (Leventhal, 1991). The ability to feel pain also decreases in response to these changes, as well as alterations in the ability to perceive and interpret painful stimuli. These changes have critical implications for the elderly in their potential lack of ability to use sensory warnings for escaping serious injury.

Psychological Aspects of Aging

MEMORY FUNCTIONING

Age-related memory deficiencies have been widely reported in the psychological literature (Hendricks & Hendricks, 1977). While short-term memory seems to deteriorate with age, perhaps as a consequence of poorer sorting strategies, long-term memories of remote events do not show similar changes. However, in nearly every instance, well-educated, mentally active people do not exhibit the same decline in memory functioning as their age peers who do not have similar opportunities to flex their minds. Nevertheless, with few exceptions, the time required for memory scanning is longer for both recent and remote recall among older people, perhaps more because of social and health factors than any irreversible effects of age (Eriksen et al, 1973; Taub, 1973).

INTELLECTUAL FUNCTIONING

There appears to be a high degree of regularity in intellectual functioning across the adult age span.

Crystallized abilities, or knowledge acquired in the course of the socialization process, tend to remain stable over the adult life span. Fluid abilities, or abilities involved in the solution of novel problems, tend to decline gradually from young to old adulthood (Schaie, 1990). In other words, intellectual abilities of older people do not decline, although they do become obsolete. The age of their formal educational experiences is reflected in their intelligence scoring.

LEARNING ABILITY

The ability to learn is not diminished by age. Studies, however, have shown that some aspects of learning do change with age. The ordinary slowing of reaction time with age for nearly all tasks or the overarousal of the central nervous system may account for lower performance levels on tests requiring rapid responses. Under conditions that allow self-pacing by the respondent, the magnitude of the age decrements is lessened considerably (Hendricks & Hendricks, 1977). Thus, ability to learn remains intact. Adjustments need to be made in teaching methodology and time allowed for learning.

ADAPTATION TO THE TASKS OF AGING

Loss and Grief Individuals experience losses from the very beginning of life. By the time individuals reach the 60s and 70s, they have experienced numerous losses, and mourning has become a lifelong process. Those who are most successful at adapting earlier in life will similarly cope better with the losses and grief inherent in aging (Cath & Sadavoy, 1991). Unfortunately, with the aging process comes a convergence of losses, the timing of which makes it impossible for the aging individual to complete the grief process in response to one loss before another occurs. Because grief is cumulative, this can result in *bereavement overload*, which has been implicated in the predisposition to depression in the elderly.

Attachment and Disengagement Many studies have confirmed the importance of interpersonal relationships at all stages in the life cycle. So important is the need for attachments, that having a confidant has been shown to be the greatest single factor discriminating between those elderly who remained in the community and those who were institutionalized (Lowenthal & Haven, 1968). These findings are consistent with the activity theory of aging that correlates the degree of social integration with successful adaptation in later life (Roscow, 1967).

A contrasting theory, the disengagement theory, suggests that 1) the process of mutual withdrawal of aging persons and society from each other is typical of most aging persons, 2) this process is biologically and psychologically intrinsic and inevitable, and 3) the disengagement process is not only correlated with successful aging, but also is usually necessary for aging (Cummings & Henry, 1961). There have been many critics of this theory, and greater acceptance of the attachment theory over the disengagement theory currently exists.

Maintenance of Self-Identity Several authors have asserted that self-concept and self-image remain stable and do not become impoverished or negative in old age (Cath & Sadavoy, 1991). A study by Vaillant and Vaillant (1990) found that the factors that favored good psychosocial adjustment in later life were sustained family relationships, maturity of ego defenses, absence of alcoholism, and absence of depressive disorder. Studies show that the elderly have a strong need for and remarkable capability of retaining a persistent self-concept in the face of the many changes that create the instability so evident in later life.

Dealing with Death Death anxiety among the aging is apparently more of a myth than a reality. Studies have not supported the negative view of death as an overriding psychological factor in the aging process (Cath & Sadavoy, 1991). Various investigators who have worked with dying patients report that it is not death itself, but rather abandonment, pain, and confusion that is feared. What many desire most is someone to talk with, to tell them their life's meaning is not shattered merely because they are about to die (Sudnow, 1967; Kübler-Ross, 1969).

Psychiatric Disorders in Later Life The later years constitute a time of especially high risk for emotional distress. Developmental stresses appear to be of a cumulative nature, often taking years to become clinically observable (Hendricks & Hendricks, 1977).

Dementing disorders are the most common causes of psychopathology in the elderly (Small,

1989a). About half of these disorders are of the Alzheimer's type, which is characterized by an insidious onset and a gradually progressive course of cognitive impairment. No curative treatment is currently available. Symptomatic treatments, including pharmacological interventions, attention to the environment, and family support, can help to maximize the patient's level of functioning and minimize the suffering of patients and family members (Small, 1989b).

Delirium has been described as one of the most common and important forms of psychopathology in later life. Lipowski (1989) described a number of factors that predispose the elderly to delirium, including structural brain disease, reduced capacity for homeostatic regulation, impaired vision and hearing, a high prevalence of chronic disease, reduced resistance to acute stress, and age-related changes in the pharmacokinetic and pharmacodynamics of drugs. Delirium needs to be recognized and the underlying condition treated as soon as possible. A high mortality is related to this condition (Rabins & Folstein, 1982).

Depressive disorders are the most common affective illness found after the middle years. The incidence of increased depression among the elderly is influenced by the variables of physical illness, functional disability, and cognitive impairment (Berkman et al, 1986). Hypochondriacal symptoms are frequent in the depressed elderly, and symptomatology often mimics that of dementia. Suicide is more prevalent in the elderly, with economic status being considered an important influencing factor. Treatment is with psychotropic medications or electroconvulsive therapy (Gerner, 1989).

Schizophrenia and delusional disorders may continue into old age or may manifest themselves for the first time only during senescence (Post, 1989). In most instances, individuals who manifest psychotic disorders early in life show a decline in psychopathology as they age. Late-onset schizophrenia (after age 60) is not common and is often characterized by delusions or hallucinations of a persecutory nature (Jeste et al, 1991). The course is chronic, and treatment is with neuroleptics and supportive psychotherapy.

Most anxiety disorders begin early in life, and problems appearing in the elderly are usually of long standing (Guterman & Eisdorfer, 1989). Seventy-five percent to eighty percent of the aged do not appear to react to trauma with typical neurotic symptoms, suggesting that expression of anxiety neurosis may be correlated to a younger age group.

Personality disorders are also uncommon in the elderly. The incidence peaks between ages 25 and 44 years, and declines thereafter, with an incidence of less than 5 percent after age 65 (Guterman & Eisdorfer, 1989). These investigators suggest the following three explanations for this decline: 1) personality disorders improve with increasing age past middle age, 2) behavior patterns undergo deterioration to more severe states (e.g., psychoses), and 3) persons with such psychopathology do not survive to old age. Most elderly people with personality disorder have likely manifested the symptomatology for many years.

Sleep disorders are common in the aging individual. Epidemiological surveys have reported as many as 30 percent of persons aged 60 and older suffer from and complain of poor sleep quality on a chronic basis (Reynolds, 1991). Some common causes of sleep disturbances among the elderly include age-dependent decreases in the ability to sleep ("sleep decay"); increased prevalence of sleep apnea; depression; dementia; anxiety; pain; impaired mobility; medications; and psychosocial factors such as loneliness, inactivity, and boredom. Benzodiazepines are often used as sleep aids with the elderly, along with nonpharmacological approaches. Changes in aging associated with metabolism and elimination must be considered when maintenance benzodiazepine therapy is administered for chronic insomnia in the aging patient.

Sociocultural Aspects of Aging

Old age brings many important socially induced changes, some of which have the potential for negative effect on both the physical and mental well-being of older persons (Warheit et al, 1991). In American society, old age is arbitrarily defined as being 65 or older, because that is the age at which the majority of persons can retire with full Social Security and other pension benefits.

The elderly in virtually all cultures share some basic needs and interests. Palmore and Maddox (1977) have summarized these into the following five categories:

1. To live as long as possible or at least until life's

satisfactions no longer compensate for its privations.

2. To get some release from the necessity of wearisome exertion at humdrum tasks and to have protection from too great exposure to physical hazards.

3. To safeguard or even strengthen any prerogatives acquired in midlife, such as skills, possessions, rights, authority, and prestige.

4. To remain active participants in the affairs of life in either operational or supervisory roles, any sharing in group interests being preferred to idleness and indifference.

5. To withdraw from life when necessity requires it, as timely, honorably, and comfortably as possible.

From the beginning of human culture, the aged have had a special status in society. Even today, in some cultures the aged are the most powerful, the most engaged, and the most respected members of the society. This has not been the case in modern industrial societies, although trends in the status of the aged differ widely between one industrialized country and another. For example, the status and integration of the aged in Japan have remained relatively high when compared with the other industrialized nations (Palmore & Maddox, 1977).

Many negative stereotypes color the perspective on aging in the United States. Ideas that elderly individuals are always tired or sick, slow and forgetful, isolated and lonely, unproductive and angry determine the way younger individuals relate to the elderly in this society. Increasing disregard for the elderly has resulted in a type of segregation, as aging individuals voluntarily seek out or are involuntarily placed in special residences for the aged. The growing segregation of the aged has been described by Breen (1960) as follows:

"Homes for the aged, public housing projects, medical institutions, recreation centers, and communities which are devoted to the exclusive use of the retired have been increasing in number and size in recent years. Retirement "villages" have been sponsored by philanthropic organizations, unions, church groups, and others. Even established communities which are now known as "retirement centers" have become inundated by older migrants seeking identification and spatial contiguity with "the clan."

Since this description was written, the concept has blossomed. The 1990 census showed that about half (52 percent) of persons 65 and older lived in nine states, with the majority in California, Florida, and New York (Fowles, 1991). It is important for elderly individuals to feel part of an integrated group, and they are migrating to these areas in an effort to achieve this integration. This phenomenon provides additional corroboration for Roscow's (1967) activity theory and the need for attachment to others.

Employment is another area in which the elderly experience discrimination. Even though compulsory retirement has been virtually eliminated, discrimination still exists in hiring and promotion practices. Not only in our nation, but also apparently throughout the world, most employers are generally not eager to retain or hire older workers (Palmore & Maddox, 1977). It is difficult to determine how much of the failure to hire and promote is a result of discrimination based on age alone and how much of it is related to a realistic and fair appraisal of the aged employee's ability and efficiency. Undoubtedly, many elderly individuals are no longer capable of doing as good a job as a younger worker. However, surveys have shown that many employers accept the negative stereotypes of the elderly and believe that older workers are hard to please, set in their ways, less productive, frequently absent, and involved in more accidents (Palmore & Maddox, 1977).

The status of the elderly may improve with time and as their numbers increase with the aging of the "baby boomers." As older individuals gain political power, the benefits and privileges designed for the elderly will increase. There is power in numbers, and the 21st century promises power for individuals 65 and older.

Sexual Aspects of Aging

Sexuality and the sexual needs of elderly people are frequently misunderstood, condemned, stereotyped, ridiculed, repressed, and ignored (Kermis, 1986). Americans have grown up in a society that has liberated sexual expression for all other age groups but still retains certain Victorian standards regarding sexual expression by the elderly. Kermis (1986) describes some stereotyped notions that younger individuals possess concerning sexual interest and activity of the elderly:

1. Old people do not have sexual desires or engage in sexual activity.
2. Older people could not engage in intercourse, even if they wanted to, because they are too fragile physically and might hurt themselves.
3. Elderly people are unattractive, which makes them sexually undesirable.
4. Sexuality among the aged is shameful and perverse.

These cultural stereotypes undoubtedly play a large part in the misperception many people hold regarding sexuality of the aged, and they may be reinforced by the common tendency of the young to deny the inevitability of aging. Masters and Johnson (1966) have stated that reasonable good health and an interesting and interested partner should ensure an active sexual life even into the 80s.

PHYSICAL CHANGES ASSOCIATED WITH SEXUALITY

Many of the changes in sexuality that occur in later years are related to the physical changes that are taking place during that period of the life cycle.

Changes in the Female   Although there is a great deal of individual variability, most studies indicate that menopause occurs at approximately 48 to 51 years of age (Kolodny et al, 1979). At this time, there is a gradual decline in the functioning of the ovaries and the subsequent production of estrogen, which results in a number of changes. The walls of the vagina become thin and inelastic, the vagina itself shrinks in both width and length, and the amount of vaginal lubrication decreases noticeably. Orgastic uterine contractions may become spastic. All of these changes can result in painful penetration, vaginal burning, pelvic aching, or irritation on urination. In some women, the discomfort may be severe enough to result in an avoidance of intercourse. Paradoxically, these symptoms are more likely to occur with infrequent intercourse of only one time a month or less. Regular and more frequent sexual activity results in a greater capacity for sexual performance (Masters & Johnson, 1966). Other symptoms that are associated with menopause in some women include hot flashes, night sweats, sleeplessness, irritability, mood swings, short-term memory loss, migraine headaches, urinary incontinence, and weight gain (Beck et al, 1992).

About 15 percent of menopausal American women take hormone replacement therapy for relief of these changes and symptoms (Seligmann et al, 1992). With estrogen therapy, the symptoms of menopause are minimized or do not occur at all. However, some women choose not to take the hormone because of an increased risk of breast cancer, and when given alone, an increased risk of endometrial cancer. To combat this latter effect, most women also take a second hormone, progesterone. Taken for 7 to 10 days during the month, progesterone decreases the risk of estrogen-induced endometrial cancer.

Changes in the Male   Testosterone production declines gradually over the years, beginning between ages 40 and 60. A major change resulting from this hormone reduction is that erections occur more slowly and require more direct genital stimulation to achieve. There may also be a modest decrease in the firmness of the erection in men older than age 60. The refractory period lengthens with age, increasing the amount of time following orgasm before the man can achieve another erection. The volume of ejaculate generally decreases, and the force of ejaculation lessens. The testes become somewhat smaller, but viable sperm are produced by some men well into their 90s (Hyde, 1986). Prolonged control over ejaculation in middle-aged and elderly men may bring increased sexual satisfaction for both partners.

SEXUAL BEHAVIOR IN THE ELDERLY

Masters and Johnson (1966) found that coital frequency in early marriage and the overall quantity of sexual activity between age 20 and 40 correlate significantly with frequency patterns of sexual activity during aging. While sexual interest and behavior do appear to decline somewhat with age, studies show that significant numbers of elderly men and women have active and satisfying sex lives well into their 80s. A survey by Brecher et al (1984) presented a revealing depiction of sexual behavior among the elderly population. Some statistics from the survey are summarized in Table 27.1.

Table 27.1 SEXUAL BEHAVIOR IN THE ELDERLY

Sex	Ages	Percentage of Respondents (n = ~4200)
Women		
Women who have sex with their husbands (frequency):	50–59	88 (1.3 times/wk)
	60–69	76 (1.0 times/wk)
	70+	65 (0.7 times/wk)
Women who masturbate (frequency):	50–59	47 (0.7 times/wk)
	60–69	37 (0.6 times/wk)
	70+	33 (0.7 times/wk)
Engaged in extramarital sex after age 50:		8
Engaged in homosexual experience after age 50:		2
Men		
Men who have sex with their wives (frequency):	50–59	87 (1.3 times/wk)
	60–69	78 (1.0 times/wk)
	70+	59 (0.6 times/wk)
Men who masturbate (frequency):	50–59	66 (1.2 times/wk)
	60–69	50 (0.8 times/wk)
	70+	43 (0.7 times/wk)
Engaged in extramarital sex after age 50:		24
Engaged in homosexual experience after age 50:		4

Source: Adapted from Brecher et al. (1984).

The information from this survey clearly indicates that sexual activity in all forms can and does continue well past the 70s for those individuals who are healthy and active and have regular opportunities for sexual expression. As Hogan (1980) states:

"Aging individuals can have satisfying sexual activity if they can compensate for physical changes that occur, if sex has been a positive force in their lives in the past, and if they have reasonably good health and an interested and interesting partner."

SPECIAL CONCERNS OF THE ELDERLY

Retirement

Statistics reflect that a larger percentage of Americans of both sexes are living longer and that many of them are retiring earlier. The reasons given most often for the increasing pattern of early retirement include health problems, Social Security and other pension benefits, social expectations, and long-held plans (Fields & Mitchell, 1983). Even eliminating the mandatory retirement age and the possibility of delaying the age of eligibility for Social Security benefits from 65 to 67 by 2027 is not expected to have a significant effect on the trend toward earlier retirement.

In 1986, nearly 90 percent of men in their early 50s participated in the labor force while only about 45 percent of men between the ages of 62 and 64 were still working (Schulz, 1988). This rate declines remarkably with age; after age 70, only about 10 percent of men and 4 percent of women are in the labor force.

Retirement has both social and economic implications for elderly individuals. The role is fraught with a great deal of ambiguity and requires many adaptations on the part of those involved.

SOCIAL IMPLICATIONS

Retirement is regarded as an achievement in principle, but is dreaded as a crisis when it actually occurs (Back, 1977). Our society places a great deal of importance on productivity, making money (as much as possible!), and doing it at as young an age as possible. These types of values contribute to the ambiguity associated with retirement. Although leisure has been acknowledged as a legitimate reward for workers, leisure during retirement has never been accorded the same value (Hendricks & Hendricks, 1977). Adjustment to this life cycle event becomes more difficult in the face of societal values that are in direct conflict with the new life-style.

Historically, many women have derived a good deal of their self-esteem from their families — birthing them, rearing them, and being a "good mother." Likewise, many men have achieved self-esteem through work-related activities — creativity, productivity, and earning money. With the termination of these activities comes a loss of self-worth. Depression may be the result for some individuals who are unable to adapt satisfactorily. Hendricks and Hendricks (1977) describe an adaptive pattern that focuses on continuity of environmental factors that serve to *reinforce* appropriate responses. They state:

> "If the positive reinforcements present during early life and working adulthood are removed by retirement, the likelihood of adjustment is jeopardized. If a worker perceived money to be the most important reward for working, the significant decline in income after retirement will complicate the process of adjustment. If friends or feelings of autonomy were the reinforcing component of work, then retirement may pose markedly fewer problems."

American society often identifies an individual by his or her occupation. This is reflected in the conversation of people who are meeting each other for the first time. Undoubtedly, most everyone has either asked or been asked at some point in time, "What do you do?" or "Where do you work?" Occupation determines status, and retirement represents a significant change in status. The basic ambiguity of retirement occurs in an individual's or society's definition of this change. Is it undertaken voluntarily or involuntarily? Is it desirable or undesirable? Is one's status made better or worse by the change?

In looking at the trend of the past 2 decades, we may presume that retirement is becoming, and will continue to become, more accepted by societal standards. With more and more individuals retiring earlier and living longer, the growing number of aging persons will spend a significantly longer time in retirement. At present, retirement has become more of an institutionalized expectation, and there appears to be increasing acceptance of it as a social status (Atchley, 1984).

ECONOMIC IMPLICATIONS

Because retirement is generally associated with a one third to one half reduction in personal income, the standard of living after retirement may be adversely affected (Soldo & Agree, 1988). Most older adults derive postretirement income from a combination of Social Security benefits, public and private pensions, and income from savings or investments.

In 1985, the median income of families with a head of household aged 25 to 64 was $30,504. For those with a head of household 65 or older it was $19,117, or about one third less (Warheit et al, 1991). In 1990, about 3.7 million elderly persons were below the poverty level (Fowles, 1991). The rate of those living in poverty was higher among blacks and Hispanics than whites, and among women than men.

The Social Security Act of 1935 promised assistance with financial security for the elderly. Since then the original legislation has been modified, yet the basic philosophy remains intact. Its effectiveness however, is now being questioned. Faced with staggering deficits, the program is forced to pay benefits to those presently retired from both the reserve funds and monies currently being collected. How, then, can this benefit the elderly of the future, when undoubtedly there will be no reserve funds? Because many of the programs that benefit older adults depend on contributions from the younger population, the growing ratio of older Americans to younger persons may affect society's ability to supply the goods and services necessary to meet this expanding demand (Gottlieb, 1991).

The Medicare and Medicaid systems were established by the government to provide medical-care benefits for elderly and indigent Americans. Medicaid funds are matched by the states, and coverage varies significantly from state to state. Medicare covers only about 75 percent of elderly hospital care, 2 percent to 3 percent of nursing home care, and about 58 percent of physician services, totaling slightly less than half of geriatric health-care costs (Physician Payment Review Commission, 1989). To reduce risk related to out-of-pocket expenditures, 71 percent of older adults purchase private medigap policies designed to cover charges in excess of those approved by Medicare (Gottlieb, 1991).

The magnitude of retirement earnings depends almost entirely on preretirement income. The poor will remain poor and the wealthy are unlikely to lower their status during retirement. But for many in the middle classes, the relatively fixed income sources may be inadequate, forcing them to suffer the consequences of poverty for the first time in their lives (Furino & Fogel, 1990).

Long-Term Care

Long-term care refers to a variety of formal and informal services needed for an extended period by people with limitations in function, as a result of one or more chronic illnesses or conditions, that interfere with daily living (Schecter & Butler, 1989). Long-term care facilities are defined by the level of care they provide. They may be skilled nursing facilities (SNF) or intermediate care facilities (ICF), or an institution may provide both types of care. Some nursing homes provide convalescent care for individuals recovering from acute illness or injury, and some provide long-term care for individuals with chronic illness or disabilities. Others may provide a combination of both types of assistance.

Most elderly individuals prefer to remain in their own homes or in the homes of family members for as long as this can meet their needs without deterioration of family or social patterns. Many elderly are placed in institutions as a last resort only after heroic efforts have been made to keep them in their own or a relative's home. The increasing emphasis on home health care has served to extend the period of independence for aging individuals.

In 1987, approximately 5 percent of the population aged 65 and older lived in nursing homes (Fowles, 1991). The percentage increased dramatically with age, ranging from 1 percent for persons aged 65 to 74 to 5 percent for persons aged 75 to 84, and 25 percent for persons aged 85 and older. A profile of the "typical" elderly nursing home resident is about 78 years of age, white, female, widowed, with multiple chronic health conditions (Eustis et al, 1984).

Who in our society will need long-term care? Eustis and associates (1984) have identified the following factors that appear to place people at risk of requiring institutionalization. These risk factors are used to increase understanding of types of services required, to predict potential need for services, to estimate future costs, and to allocate resources.

- *Age.* Because people grow older in very different ways, and the range of differences becomes greater with the passage of time, age is becoming a less relevant characteristic than it was historically (Neugarten, 1979). However, because of the high prevalence of chronic health conditions and disabilities, as well as the greater chance of diminishing social supports associated with advancing age, the 65 and older population is often viewed as an important long-term care target group.
- *Health.* Level of functioning, as determined by ability to perform various behaviors or activities such as bathing, eating, mobility, meal preparation, handling finances, judgment, and memory, is a measurable risk factor. The need for ongoing assistance from another person is critical in determining the need for long-term care.
- *Mental health status.* Mental health problems are risk factors in assessing need for long-term care. Many of the symptoms associated with certain mental disorders (especially the dementias), such as memory loss, impaired judgment, impaired intellect, and disorientation, would render the individual incapable of meeting the demands of daily living independently.
- *Socioeconomic and demographic factors.* Low income is generally associated with greater physical and mental health problems among the elderly. Because of limited finances, these individuals are less able to purchase noninstitutional long-term care and thus are at greater risk of being institutionalized (Butler & Newacheck, 1981). Women are at greater risk of being institutionalized than men, not because they are less healthy, but because they live longer and thus are older and more likely to be unmarried. Whites have a higher rate of institutionalization than nonwhites. This may be related to cultural and financial influences.

- *Marital status, living arrangement, and the informal support network.* Those who are married and live with a spouse are the least likely of all disabled people to be institutionalized (Eustis et al., 1984). Living alone without resources for home care and few or no relatives living nearby to provide informal care are high-risk factors for institutionalization.

ATTITUDINAL FACTORS

Elderly people in general are opposed to the use of institutions (Goldfarb, 1977). Goldfarb (1977) states, "Those who seem to need protective care the most want it the least and may oppose it the most vigorously, whereas those who may need it the least are less resistant to accepting the change in residence." Many elderly individuals and their families perceive nursing homes as a place to go to die, and the fact that many of these institutions are poorly equipped, staffed, and organized keeps this societal perception alive. There are, however, many excellent nursing homes that strive to go beyond the minimum federal regulations for Medicaid and Medicare reimbursement. In addition to medical, nursing, rehabilitation, and dental services, social and recreational services are provided to increase the quality of life for the elderly living in nursing homes. These activities include cards, bingo, and other games; parties; church activities; books; television; movies; arts and crafts and other classes. Some nursing homes provide occupational and professional counseling. These facilities strive to enhance opportunities for improving quality of life and for becoming "places to live" rather than "places to die."

Elder Abuse

Abuse of the elderly, sometimes referred to by the media as "granny bashing," is a prevalent and serious form of family violence. Approximately 700,000 to 1 million elderly persons experience physical, verbal, sexual, or other kinds of abuse every year (Adelman & Butler, 1989). The abuser is most often a relative who lives with the elderly person and is likely to be the assigned caregiver. Typical caregivers who were likely to be abusers of the elderly were described by O'Malley and colleagues (1983) as being isolated, under severe stress, sub-

stance abusers, themselves the victims of previous family violence, and as having refused outside services despite frustration in dealing with the elderly person. The same investigators identified risk factors for abuse as being age 75 and older, mentally or physically impaired, unable to meet daily self-care needs, and having care needs that exceeded the caretaker's ability to respond.

Adelman and Butler (1989) define three general categories of abuse of elderly persons — psychological, physical, and financial — and two categories of neglect — intentional and unintentional. Psychological abuse includes yelling, insulting, harsh commands, threats, silence, and social isolation. Physical abuse is described as striking, shoving, beating, or restraint. Financial abuse refers to misuse or theft of finances, property, or material possessions. Neglect implies failure to do the obviously necessary things that the elderly person cannot do independently. Unintentional neglect is inadvertent, while intentional neglect is deliberate. Additionally, elderly individuals may be the victims of sexual abuse, which refers to sexual intimacy between two persons that occurs without the consent of one of the persons involved. Another type of abuse, called "granny dumping" by the media, involves abandoning elderly individuals at emergency departments, nursing homes, or other facilities — literally leaving them in the hands of others when the strain of caregiving becomes intolerable.

Elder victims often deny that abuse has occurred, even when confronted with its evidence (King, 1984). The elderly person may be unwilling to disclose information because of fear of retaliation, embarrassment about the existence of abuse in the family, protectiveness toward a family member, or an unwillingness to institute legal action. Adding to this unwillingness to report is the fact that infirm elders are often isolated, and therefore their mistreatment is less likely to be noticed by those who might be alert to symptoms of abuse. For these reasons, detection of abuse of the elderly is difficult at best.

FACTORS THAT CONTRIBUTE TO ABUSE

King (1984) describes a number of factors that contribute to abuse of elderly individuals.

Longer Life The 65 and older age group has become the fastest-growing segment of the population, and within this segment, the number of elderly older than age 75 has increased most rapidly. This trend is expected to continue into the 21st century. The 75 and older age group is the one most likely to be physically or mentally impaired, requiring assistance and care from family members. This group also is the most vulnerable to abuse from caregivers.

Dependency Dependency is the most common precondition in domestic abuse (King, 1984). Changes associated with normal aging or changes induced by chronic illness often result in loss of self-sufficiency in the elderly, requiring that they become dependent on another for assistance with daily functioning. Long life may also consume finances to the point that the elderly individual becomes financially dependent on another as well. This dependence increases the elderly person's vulnerability to abuse.

Stress The stress inherent in the caregiver role is a factor in most abuse cases. Some clinicians believe that elder abuse occurs as a result of individual or family psychopathology. Others suggest that even psychologically healthy family members can become abusive as the result of the exhaustion and acute stress caused by overwhelming caregiving responsibilities (King, 1984). This is compounded in an age group that has been dubbed the "sandwich generation"—those individuals who elected to delay childbearing so that they are now at a point in their lives when they are "sandwiched" between providing care for their children and providing care for their aging parents.

Learned Violence Children who have been abused or witnessed abusive and violent parents are more likely to evolve into abusive adults. Renvoise (1978) found that children who abuse their parents were most likely to have been abused by them as children. She also found that drinking was associated with violence in almost half the cases she studied.

IDENTIFYING ELDER ABUSE

Because so many elderly individuals are reluctant to report personal abuse, health-care workers need to be able to detect signs of mistreatment when they are in a position to do so. Adelman and Butler (1989) have identified the following signs and symptoms of the various categories of abuse:

- Indicators of psychological abuse include a broad range of behaviors, such as the symptoms associated with pathological depression, excessive anxiety, increased confusion or agitation.
- Indicators of physical abuse may include bruises, welts, lacerations, burns, punctures, evidence of hair pulling, and skeletal dislocations and fractures.
- Neglect may be manifested as inadequate warm clothing or heat in the home; lack of necessary supervision; substandard living conditions in relation to financial assets; failure to obtain eyeglasses, hearing aids, dentures, or prostheses; and failure to provide food and water, leading to malnutrition and dehydration.
- Possible sexual abuse may be suspected when the elderly person presents with unexplained venereal disease or unusual genital infections.
- Financial abuse may be occurring when there is an obvious disparity between assets and satisfactory living conditions or when the elderly person complains of a sudden lack of sufficient funds for daily living expenses.

Health-care workers often feel intimidated when confronted with cases of elder abuse. In these instances, referral to an individual experienced in management of victims of such abuse may be the most effective approach to evaluation and intervention. Intervention generally takes into consideration each individual case and ranges from counseling and court advocacy to supplying homemaker support or nursing home placement (Adelman & Butler, 1989). A family-oriented approach to intervention is favorable.

Increased efforts need to be made to provide health-care workers with comprehensive training in the detection of and intervention in elder abuse. More research is needed to increase knowledge and understanding of the phenomenon of elder abuse and ultimately to effect more sophisticated strategies for prevention, intervention, and treatment.

Suicide

Although persons older than age 65 comprise only 12 percent of the population, they represent a disproportionately high percentage of individuals who commit suicide. Of all suicides, 17 percent are committed by this age group, and suicide is the 10th most common cause of death in the elderly (Blazer et al, 1986).

The group especially at risk appears to be white men who are recently bereaved, living alone, in frail health, and fearful of becoming a financial burden on their relatives (Kermis, 1986). The major indirect indicator of suicide risk is depression, as evidenced by insomnia, agitation, hypochondriasis, self-neglect, or evidence of impaired memory (Gurland & Cross, 1983).

The number of suicides among this age group dropped steadily from 1930 to 1980. Investigators who study these trends surmised that this decline was due to increases in services for older people and an understanding of their problems in society. However, from 1980 to 1986 the number of suicides among those 65 and older increased by 25 percent. This suggests that other factors are contributing to the problem. Dr. Richard Sattin, a researcher at the Centers for Disease Control in Atlanta, suggests that increased social isolation may be a contributing factor to suicide among the elderly (Kaufman, 1991). The number of elderly individuals who are divorced, widowed, or otherwise living alone has increased. Divorce is a clear risk factor for elderly suicide, with the suicide rate for divorced men older than 65 three times as great as for married men older than 65 (Kaufman, 1991).

The American Association of Suicidology, however, suggests that isolation itself is not the key determinant, but the presence of a psychiatric disorder is the most important factor (Kaufman, 1991). A study conducted by the association revealed the presence of depression, alcoholism, or drug dependence (usually to prescription drugs) to be a factor in a great majority of cases. Approximately one third suffered from a terminal illness or a severe and chronic medical condition.

Sadly, many elderly individuals express symptoms associated with depression that are never recognized as such. Any sign of helplessness or hopelessness should elicit a supportive intervening response. In assessing suicide intention, direct questions should be asked, but with concern and compassion:

- Have you ever had thoughts of suicide in the past?
- Have you ever attempted suicide?
- Are you currently experiencing thoughts of suicide?
- Do you have a plan for committing suicide?
- Do you have the means to carry out your plan?

(Stevenson, 1988)

Components of intervention with a suicidal elderly person should include demonstrations of genuine concern, interest, and caring; indications of empathy for their fears and concerns; identification and clarification of the focal problem; and help in formulating a plan of action to resolve the precipitating situation (Altrocchi, 1980). If it appears that the elderly person's behavior is particularly lethal, additional family or staff coverage and contact should be arranged to prevent isolation.

APPLICATION OF THE NURSING PROCESS

Assessment

Assessment of the elderly individual may follow the same framework used for all adults, but with consideration of the possible biological, psychological, sociocultural, and sexual changes that occur in the normal aging process described previously in this chapter. In no other area of nursing is it more important for nurses to practice holistic nursing than with the elderly. Older adults are likely to have multiple physical problems that contribute to problems in other areas of their lives. Obviously, these components cannot be addressed as separate entities. Nursing the elderly is a multifaceted, challenging process as a result of the multiple changes occurring at this time in the life cycle and the way in which each change affects every aspect of the individual.

Several considerations are unique to assessment of the elderly. A primary responsibility exists to assess the older person's thought processes. Knowledge about the presence and extent of disorientation or confusion will influence the way in which the nurse approaches elder care.

Information about sensory capabilities is also extremely important. Because hearing loss is common, the nurse should lower the pitch and loudness of his or her voice when addressing the older person. Looking directly into the face of the older person when talking facilitates communication. By asking questions that require a declarative sentence in response, the nurse is able to assess if there is a problem with speech discrimination (Stone, 1977). Visual acuity can be determined by assessing adaptation to the dark, color matching, and the perception of color contrast. Knowledge about these aspects of sensory functioning is essential in the development of an effective care plan.

The nurse should be familiar with the normal physical changes associated with the aging process. Examples of some of these changes include:

- Less effective response to changes in environmental temperature, resulting in hypothermia.
- Decreases in oxygen use and the amount of blood pumped by the heart, resulting in cerebral anoxia or hypoxia.
- Skeletal muscle wasting and weakness, resulting in difficulty in physical mobility.
- Limited cough and laryngeal reflexes, resulting in high risk for aspiration.
- Demineralization of bones, resulting in spontaneous fracturing.
- Decrease in gastrointestinal motility, resulting in constipation.
- Decrease in the ability to interpret painful stimuli, resulting in high risk for injury.

Common psychosocial changes associated with aging include:

- Prolonged and exaggerated grief, resulting in depression.
- Physical changes, resulting in altered body image.
- Changes in status, resulting in loss of self-worth.

This list is by no means exhaustive. The nurse will have to consider many other alterations in his or her assessment of the patient. Knowledge of the patient's functional capabilities is essential for determining the physiological, psychological, and sociological needs of the elderly individual. Age alone does not preclude that all of these changes have occurred. The aging process progresses at a wide range of variance, and each patient must be assessed as a unique individual.

Nursing Diagnosis, Planning/Implementation

Virtually any nursing diagnosis may be applicable to the aging patient, depending on individual needs for assistance. Based on normal changes that occur in the elderly, the following nursing diagnoses may be considered:

Physiologically Related Diagnoses

High risk for trauma related to confusion, disorientation, muscular weakness, spontaneous fractures, falls.

Hypothermia related to loss of adipose tissue under the skin, evidenced by increased sensitivity to cold and body temperature below 98.6°F.

Decreased cardiac output related to decreased myocardial efficiency secondary to age-related changes, evidenced by decreased tolerance for activity and decline in energy reserve.

Ineffective breathing pattern related to increase in fibrous tissue and loss of elasticity in lung tissue, evidenced by dyspnea and activity intolerance.

High risk for aspiration related to diminished cough and laryngeal reflexes.

Impaired physical mobility related to muscular wasting and weakness, evidenced by need for assistance in ambulation.

Altered nutrition, less than body requirements, related to inefficient absorption from gastrointestinal tract, difficulty chewing and swallowing, anorexia, difficulty in feeding self, evidenced by wasting syndrome, anemia, or weight loss.

Constipation related to decreased motility; inadequate diet; insufficient activity or exercise, evidenced by decreased bowel sounds; hard, formed stools; or straining at stool.

Stress incontinence related to degenerative changes in pelvic muscles and structural supports associated with increased age, evidenced by reported or observed dribbling with increased abdominal pressure or urinary frequency.

Urinary retention related to prostatic enlargement, evidenced by bladder distention, frequent voiding of small amounts, dribbling, or overflow incontinence.

Sensory-perceptual alteration related to age-related alterations in sensory transmission, evidenced by decreased visual acuity, hearing loss, diminished sensitivity to taste and smell, or increased touch threshold.

Sleep pattern disturbance related to age-related decrease in ability to sleep ("sleep decay"), dementia, or medications, evidenced by interrupted sleep, early awakening, or falling asleep during the day.

Pain related to degenerative changes in joints, evidenced by verbalization of pain or hesitation to use weight-bearing joints.

Self-care deficit (specify) related to weakness, confusion, or disorientation, evidenced by inability to feed self, maintain hygiene, dress/groom self, or toilet self without assistance.

High risk for impaired skin integrity related to alterations in nutritional state, circulation, sensation, or mobility.

Psychosocially Related Diagnoses

Altered thought processes related to age-related changes that result in cerebral anoxia, evidenced by short-term memory loss, confusion, or disorientation.

Dysfunctional grieving related to bereavement overload, evidenced by symptoms of depression.

High risk for self-directed violence related to depressed mood and feelings of low self-worth.

Powerlessness related to life-style of helplessness and dependency on others, evidenced by depressed mood, apathy, or verbal expressions of having no control or influence over life situation.

Self-esteem disturbance related to loss of preretirement status, evidenced by verbalization of negative feelings about self and life.

Fear related to nursing home placement, evidenced by symptoms of severe anxiety and statement, "Nursing homes are places to go to die."

Body image disturbance related to age-related changes in skin, hair, and fat distribution, evidenced by verbalization of negative feelings about body.

Altered sexuality patterns related to dyspareunia, evidenced by reported dissatisfaction with decrease in frequency of sexual intercourse.

Sexual dysfunction related to medications (e.g., antihypertensives), evidenced by inability to achieve an erection.

Social isolation related to total dependence on others, evidenced by expression of inadequacy in or absence of significant purpose in life.

High risk for trauma (elder abuse) related to caregiver role strain.

Caregiver role strain related to severity and duration of the care receiver's illness; lack of respite and recreation for the caregiver, evidenced by feelings of stress in relationship with care receiver; feelings of depression and anger; or family conflict around issues of providing care.

In Table 27.2, selected nursing diagnoses are presented for the elderly patient. Goals of care and appropriate nursing interventions are included for each. Rationales are presented in italics.

OUTCOME CRITERIA

The following criteria may be used for measurement of outcomes in the care of the elderly patient.

The patient:
1. Has not experienced injury.
2. Maintains reality orientation consistent with cognitive level of functioning.
3. Manages own self-care with assistance.
4. Expresses positive feelings about self, past accomplishments, and hope for the future.
5. Compensates adaptively for diminished sensory perception.

Caregivers:
1. Are able to problem solve effectively regarding care of elderly patient.
2. Demonstrate adaptive coping strategies for dealing with stress of caregiver role.
3. Openly express feelings.
4. Express desire to join support group of other caregivers.

Evaluation

Reassessment is conducted to determine if the nursing actions have been successful in achieving the objectives of care. Evaluation of the nursing actions for the elderly patient may be facilitated by gathering information using the following types of questions.

Has the patient escaped injury from falls, burns, or other means to which he or she is vulnerable because of age? Are caregivers able to verbalize means of providing a safe environment for the patient? Does the patient maintain reality orientation at an optimum for his or her cognitive functioning? Can the patient distinguish between reality-based and nonreality-based thinking? Can caregivers ver-

Table 27.2 CARE PLAN FOR THE ELDERLY PATIENT

Nursing Diagnoses	Objectives	Nursing Interventions
Potential for trauma related to confusion, disorientation, muscular weakness, spontaneous fractures, falls.	Patient will not experience injury.	The following measures may be instituted *to ensure patient safety:* a. Arrange furniture and other items in the room to accommodate patient's disabilities. b. Store frequently used items within easy access. c. Keep bed in unelevated position. Pad siderails and headboard if patient has history of seizures. Keep bedrails up when patient is in bed. d. Assign room near nurses' station; observe frequently. e. Assist patient with ambulation. f. Keep a dim light on at night. g. If patient is a smoker, cigarettes and lighter or matches should be kept at the nurses' station and dispensed only when someone is available to stay with patient while he or she is smoking. h. Frequently orient patient to place, time, and situation. i. Soft restraints may be required if patient is very disoriented and hyperactive.
Altered thought processes related to age-related changes that result in cerebral anoxia, evidenced by short-term memory loss, confusion, or disorientation.	Patient will interpret the environment accurately and maintain reality orientation to the best of his or her cognitive ability.	Frequently orient patient to reality. Use clocks and calendars with large numbers that are easy to read. Notes and large, bold signs may be useful as reminders. Allow patient to have personal belongings. *All of these items serve to help maintain orientation and aid in memory and recognition.* Keep explanations simple. Use face-to-face interaction. Speak slowly and do not shout. *These interventions facilitate comprehension. Shouting may create discomfort, and in some instances, may provoke anger.* Discourage rumination of delusional thinking. Talk about real events and real people. *Rumination promotes disorientation. Reality orientation increases sense of self-worth and personal dignity.* Monitor for medication side effects. *Physiological changes in the elderly can alter the body's response to certain medications. Toxic effects may intensify altered thought processes.*
Self-care deficit (specify) related to weakness, disorientation, confusion, or memory deficits, evidenced by inability to fulfill activities of daily living.	Patient will accomplish activities of daily living to the best of his or her ability. Unfulfilled needs will be met by caregivers.	Provide a simple, structured environment *to minimize confusion:* a. Identify self-care deficits and provide assistance as required. Promote independent actions as able. b. Allow plenty of time for patient to perform tasks. c. Provide guidance and support for independent actions by talking the patient through the task one step at a time. d. Provide a structured schedule of activities that do not change from day to day. e. Activities of daily living should follow home routine as closely as possible. f. Allow consistency in assignment of daily caregivers.

(continued)

Table 27.2 CONTINUED

Nursing Diagnoses	Objectives	Nursing Interventions
Caregiver role strain related to severity and duration of the care receiver's illness; lack of respite and recreation for the caregiver, evidenced by feelings of stress in relationship with care receiver; feelings of depression and anger; family conflict around issues of providing care.[1]	Caregivers will achieve effective problem-solving skills and develop adaptive coping mechanisms to regain equilibrium.	Assess prospective caregivers' ability to anticipate and fulfill patient's unmet needs. Provide information to assist caregivers with this responsibility. Ensure that caregivers are aware of available community support systems from whom they can seek assistance when required. Examples include: adult day-care centers, housekeeping and homemaker services, respite care services, or perhaps a local chapter of the Alzheimer's Disease and Related Disorders Association (ADRDA). This organization sponsors a nationwide 24-hour hot line to provide information and link families who need assistance with nearby chapters and affiliates. The hot-line number is 1-800-621-0379. *Caregivers require relief from the pressures and strain of providing 24-hour care for their loved one. Studies have shown that elder abuse arises out of caregiving situations that place overwhelming stress on the caregivers.* Encourage caregivers to express feelings, particularly anger. *Release of these emotions can serve to prevent psychopathology, such as depression or psychophysiological disorders from occurring.* Encourage participation in support groups comprised of members with similar life situations. *Hearing others who are experiencing the same problems discuss ways in which they have coped may help caregiver adopt more adaptive strategies. Individuals who are experiencing similar life situations provide empathy and support for each other.*
Self-esteem disturbance related to loss of preretirement status, evidenced by verbalization of negative feelings about self and life.	Patient will demonstrate increased feelings of self-worth by expressing positive aspects of self and past accomplishments.	Encourage patient to express honest feelings in relation to loss of prior status. Acknowledge pain of loss. Support patient through process of grieving. *Patient may be fixed in anger stage of grieving process, which is turned inward on the self, resulting in diminished self-esteem.* If lapses in memory are occurring, devise methods for assisting patient with memory deficit. Examples: a. Name sign on door identifying patient's room. b. Identifying sign on outside of dining room door. c. Identifying sign on outside of restroom door. d. Large clock, with oversized numbers and hands, appropriately placed. e. Large calendar, indicating one day at a time, with month, day, and year in bold print. f. Printed, structured daily schedule, with one copy for patient and one posted on unit wall. g. "News board" on unit wall where current news of national and local interest may be posted. *These aids may assist patient to function more independently, thereby increasing self-esteem.* Encourage patient's attempts to communicate. If verbalizations are not understandable, express to patient what you think he or she intended to say. It may be necessary to reorient patient frequently. *The ability to communicate effectively with others*

(continued)

Table 27.2 CONTINUED

Nursing Diagnoses	Objectives	Nursing Interventions
		may enhance self-esteem. Encourage reminiscence and discussion of life review. Also discuss present-day events. Sharing picture albums, if possible, is especially good. *Reminiscence and life review help the patient resume progression through the grief process associated with disappointing life events and increase self-esteem as successes are reviewed.* Encourage participation in group activities. May need to accompany patient at first, until he or she feels secure that the group members will be accepting, regardless of limitations in verbal communication. *Positive feedback from group members will increase self-esteem.* Encourage patient to be as independent as possible in self-care activities. Provide written schedule of tasks to be performed. Intervene in areas where patient requires assistance. *The ability to perform independently preserves self-esteem.*
Sensory-perceptual alteration related to age-related alterations in sensory transmission, evidenced by decreased visual acuity, hearing loss, diminished sensitivity to taste and smell, and increased touch threshold.[2]	Patient will attain optimal level of sensory stimulation. Patient will not experience injury due to diminished sensory-perception.	*In an effort to assist patient with diminished sensory perception and because patient safety is a nursing priority, the following nursing strategies are indicated:* • Provide meaningful sensory stimulation to all special senses through conversation, touch, music, or pleasant smells. • Encourage wearing of glasses, hearing aids, prostheses, and other adaptive devices. • Use bright, contrasting colors in the environment. • Provide large-print reading materials, such as books, clocks, calendars, and educational materials. • Maintain room lighting that distinguishes day from night and that is free of shadows and glare. • Teach patient to scan the environment to locate objects. • Help patient to locate food on plate using "clock" system, and describe food if patient is unable to visualize; assist with feeding as needed. • Arrange physical environment to maximize functional vision. • Place personal items, call light, and so forth within patient's field of vision. • Teach patient to watch the person who is speaking. • Reinforce wearing of hearing aid; if patient does not have an aid, use a communication device. • Communicate clearly, distinctly, and slowly, using a low-pitched voice and facing patient; avoid overarticulation. • Remove as much unnecessary background noise as possible. • Do not use slang or extraneous words. • As speaker, position self at eye level and no farther than 6 feet away. • Get the patient's attention before speaking. • Avoid speaking directly into the patient's ear. • If the patient does not understand what is being said, rephrase the statement rather than simply repeating it.

(continued)

Table 27.2 CONTINUED		
Nursing Diagnoses	**Objectives**	**Nursing Interventions**
		• Help patient select foods from the menu that will ensure a discrimination between various tastes and smells. • Ensure that food has been properly cooled so that patient with diminished pain threshold is not burned. • Ensure that bath or shower water is appropriate temperature. • Use backrubs and massage as therapeutic touch to stimulate sensory receptors.

[1]This nursing diagnosis was proposed at the 10th conference of the North American Nursing Diagnosis Association in April 1992.
[2]The interventions for this nursing diagnosis were adapted from Rogers-Seidl (1991), with permission.

balize ways in which to orient patient to reality, as needed? Is the patient able to accomplish self-care activities independently to his or her optimum level of functioning? Does the patient seek assistance for aspects of self-care that he or she is unable to perform independently? Does the patient express positive feelings about himself or herself? Does the patient reminisce about accomplishments that have occurred in his or her life? Does the patient express some hope for the future? Does the patient wear eyeglasses or a hearing aid, if needed, to compensate for sensory deficits? Does the patient consistently look others in the face to facilitate hearing when they are talking to him or her? Does the patient use helpful aids, such as signs identifying various rooms, to help maintain orientation? Are the caregivers able to work through problems and make decisions regarding care of the elderly patient? Do they include the elderly patient in the decision-making process, if appropriate? Are the caregivers able to demonstrate adaptive coping strategies for dealing with the strain of long-term caregiving? Are they open and honest in expression of feelings? Are they able to name community resources to whom they can go for assistance with their caregiving responsibilities? Have they joined a support group?

SUMMARY

Care of the aging individual presents one of the greatest challenges for nursing. The growing population of individuals 65 and older suggests that the challenge will progress well into the 21st century.

America is a youth-oriented society. It is not desirable to be old. In fact, to some it is repugnant. Most, however, if faced with a choice, choose growing old to the alternative, death. In some cultures, the elderly are revered and hold a special place of honor within the society. But in highly industrialized countries such as the United States, status declines with the decrease in productivity and participation in the mainstream of society.

Individuals experience many changes as they age. Physical changes occur in virtually every body system. Psychologically, there may be age-related memory deficiencies, particularly for recent events. Intellectual functioning does not decline with age, but the length of time required for learning increases.

Aging individuals experience many losses, potentially leading to bereavement overload. They are vulnerable to depression and to feelings of low self-worth. The number of suicides increased 25 percent in the 65 and older age group from 1980 to 1986. Dementing disorders are the most frequent causes of psychopathology in the elderly. Sleep disorders are very common.

The need for sexual expression by the elderly is often misunderstood within our society. Although many physical changes occur at this time of life that alter an individual's sexuality, if he or she has reasonably good health and a willing partner, sexual activity can continue well past the 70s for most people.

Retirement has both social and economic implications for elderly individuals. Society often equates an individual's status with his or her occupation, and loss of employment results in the need for adjustment in the standard of living, sometimes by as much as one third to one half of preretirement earnings.

In 1987, approximately 5 percent of the population aged 65 and older lived in nursing homes. A profile of the "typical" elderly nursing home resident is about 78 years of age, white, female, widowed, and with multiple chronic health conditions. A great deal of stigma is attached to what some still call "rest" homes or "old age" homes. Many elderly people still equate them with a place "to go to die."

The strain of the caregiver role has become a major dilemma in our society. Elder abuse is sometimes the result of caregivers for whom the role has become overwhelming and intolerable. There is an intense need to find assistance for these people, who must provide care for their loved ones on a 24-hour basis. Home health care, respite care, support groups, and financial assistance are needed to ease the burden of this role strain.

Nursing of the elderly individual is accomplished through the five steps of the nursing process. Assessment requires that changes occurring in the normal aging process — biological, psychological, sociocultural, and sexual — be taken into consideration before an accurate plan of care can be formulated.

Nursing of elderly individuals requires a special kind of inner strength and compassion. The following poem, which has undoubtedly become very familiar over the years, is excellent in eliciting empathy for what the elderly must feel. I thank the anonymous author for sharing. It has a powerful message.

WHAT DO YOU SEE, NURSE?

What do you see, nurse, what do you see?
What are you thinking when you look at me?
A crabbed old woman, not very wise.
Uncertain of habit, with faraway eyes.
Who dribbles her food and makes no reply
When you say in a loud voice, "I do wish you'd try."
Who seems not to notice the things that you do
And forever is losing a stocking or shoe.
Who unresisting or not, lets you do as you will
With bathing and feeding, the long day to fill.
Is that what you're thinking, is that what you see?
Then open your eyes, you're not looking at me.
I'll tell you who I am as I sit here so still.
As I move at your bidding, as I eat at your will.
I'm a small child of ten with a father and mother,
Brothers and sisters who love one another.
A young girl at sixteen with wings on her feet
Dreaming that soon now a lover she'll meet.
A bride soon at twenty — my heart gives a leap
Remembering the vows that I promised to keep.
At twenty-five, now, I have young of my own
Who need me to build a secure happy home.
A woman of thirty, my young now grow fast
Bound to each other with ties that should last.
At forty my young now will soon be gone,
But my man stays beside me to see I don't mourn.
At fifty once more babies play round my knee.
Again we know children, my loved one and me.
Dark days are upon me, my husband is dead.
I look at the future, I shudder with dread.
For my young are all busy rearing young of their own.
And I think of the years and the love I have known.
I'm an old woman now and nature is cruel.
Tis her jest to make old age look like a fool.
The body it crumbles, grace and vigor depart.
There is now just a stone where I once had a heart.
But inside this old carcass a young girl still dwells.
And now and again my battered heart swells.
I remember the joys, I remember the pain.
And I'm loving and living life all over again.
I think of the years all too few — gone so fast.
And accept the stark fact that nothing can last.
So open your eyes, nurse, open and see.
Not a crabbed old woman — look closer — SEE ME.

— Author unknown

REVIEW QUESTIONS
Self-Examination/Learning Exercise

*Select the answer that is **most** appropriate for each of the following questions.*

Situation: Stanley, a 72-year-old widower, was brought to the hospital by his son, who reports that Stanley has become increasingly withdrawn. He has periods of confusion and forgetfulness, but most of the time his thought processes are intact. He eats very little and has lost some weight. His wife died 5 years ago and the son reports, "He did very well. Didn't even cry." Stanley attended the funeral of his best friend 1 month ago, after which these symptoms began. Stanley has been admitted for testing and evaluation.

1. In her admission assessment, the nurse notices an open sore on Stanley's arm. When she questions him about it he says, "I scraped it on the fence 2 weeks ago. It's smaller than it was." How might the nurse analyze this data?
   a. Stanley was trying to commit suicide.
   b. The delay in healing may indicate that Stanley has developed cancer of the skin.
   c. A diminished inflammatory response in the elderly increases healing time.
   d. Age-related skin changes and distribution of adipose tissue delay healing in the elderly.

2. Stanley is deaf on his right side. Which is the most appropriate nursing intervention for communicating with Stanley?
   a. Speak loudly into his left ear.
   b. Speak to him from a position on his left side.
   c. Speak face-to-face in a high-pitched voice.
   d. Speak face-to-face in a low-pitched voice.

3. Why is it important to have the nurse check the temperature of the water before Stanley takes a shower?
   a. Stanley may catch cold if the water is too cold.
   b. Stanley may burn himself due to higher pain threshold.
   c. Stanley has difficulty discriminating between hot and cold.
   d. The water must be exactly 98.6°F.

4. From the information provided in the situation, which would be the priority nursing diagnosis for Stanley?
   a. Dysfunctional grieving
   b. Altered nutrition: less than body requirements
   c. Social isolation
   d. High risk for injury

5. The physician diagnoses Stanley with major depression. A suicide assessment is conducted. Why is Stanley at high risk for suicide?
   a. All depressed people are at high risk for suicide.
   b. Stanley is in the age group in which the highest percentage of suicides occur.
   c. Stanley is a white man, recently bereaved, living alone.
   d. His son reports that Stanley owns a gun.

6. Which of the following would be a priority nursing intervention with Stanley?
   a. Take blood pressure once each shift.
   b. Ensure that Stanley attends group activities.
   c. Encourage Stanley to eat all of the food on his food tray.
   d. Encourage Stanley to talk about his wife's death.

7. In group exercise, Stanley becomes tired and short of breath very quickly. This is most likely due to:
   a. age-related changes in the cardiovascular system.
   b. Stanley's sedentary life-style.
   c. the effects of pathological depression.
   d. medication the physician has prescribed for depression.

8. Stanley says to the nurse, "I'm all alone now. My wife is gone. My best friend is gone. My son is busy with his work and family. I might as well just go, too." Which is the best response by the nurse?
   a. "Are you thinking that you want to die, Stanley?"
   b. "You have lots to live for, Stanley."
   c. "Cheer up, Stanley. It's almost time for activity therapy."
   d. "Tell me about your family, Stanley."

9. Stanley says to the nurse, "I don't want to go to that crafts class. I'm too old to learn anything." Based on knowledge of the aging process, which of the following is a true statement?
   a. Memory functioning in the elderly most likely reflects loss of long-term memories of remote events.
   b. Intellectual functioning declines with advancing age.
   c. Learning ability remains intact, but time required for learning increases with age.
   d. Cognitive functioning is rarely affected in aging individuals.

10. According to the literature, which of the following is most important for Stanley to maintain a healthy, adaptive old age?
    a. To remain socially interactive.
    b. To disengage slowly in preparation of the last stage of life.
    c. To move in with his son and family.
    d. To maintain total independence and accept no help from anyone.

REFERENCES

Adelman, R. D. & Butler, R. N. (1989). Elder abuse and neglect. In H. I. Kaplan & B. J. Sadock (Eds.), *Comprehensive textbook of psychiatry* (Vol. 2) (5th ed.). Baltimore: Williams & Wilkins.

Altrocchi, J. (1980). *Abnormal Behavior.* New York: Harcourt Brace Jovanovich.

Atchley, R. C. (1984). The process of retirement: Comparing women and men. In M. Szinovacz (Ed.), *Women's retirement.* Beverly Hills, CA: Sage.

Atchley, R. C. (1989). A continuity theory of normal aging. *Gerontologist, 29,* 183–190.

Back, K. W. (1977). The ambiguity of retirement. In E. W. Busse & E. Pfeiffer (Eds.), *Behavior and adaptation in late life* (2nd ed.). Boston: Little, Brown and Co.

Beck, M. et al. (1992, May 25). Menopause. *Newsweek,* Vol. CXIX, No. 21, 38–42.

Berkman, W. F., Berkman, C. S., & Kaol, S. (1986). Depression symptoms in relation to physical health and functioning in the elderly. *Am J Epidemiology, 124,* 372–388.

Blazer, D. et al. (1986). Suicide in late life: Review and commentary. *J Am Geriatr Soc, 34,* 519–525.

Bowen, C. D. (1944). *Yankee from Olympus.* Boston: Little, Brown and Co.

Brecher, E. M. et al (1984). *Love, sex, and aging.* Mount Vernon, NY: Consumers Union.

Breen, L. A. (1960). The aging individual. In C. Tibbits (Ed.), *Handbook of social gerontology.* Chicago: University of Chicago Press.

Brody, H. (1976). *Development and aging in the nervous system.* New York: Academic.

Busse, E. W. (1989). The myth, history, and science of aging. In E. W. Busse & D. G. Blazer (Eds.), *Geriatric psychiatry.* Washington, DC: American Psychiatric Press.

Butler, L. H. & Newacheck, P. W. (1981). Health and social factors relevant to long-term care policy. In J. Meltzer et al. (Eds.), *Policy options in long-term care.* Chicago: University of Chicago Press.

Butler, R. N. (1989). Psychosocial aspects of aging. In H. I. Kaplan & B. J. Sadock (Eds.), *Comprehensive textbook of psychiatry* (Vol. 2) (5th ed.). Baltimore: Williams & Wilkins.

Cath, S. H. & Sadavoy, J. (1991). Psychosocial aspects. In J. Sadavoy et al. (Eds.), *Comprehensive review of geriatric psychiatry.* Washington, DC: American Psychiatric Press.

Cummings, E. & Henry, W. E. (1961). *The process of disengagement.* New York: Basic Books.

Eriksen, C. W., Hamlin, R. M., & Daye, C. (1973). Aging adults and rate of memory scan. *Bulletin of the Psychonomic Society, 1*(4), 259–260.

Erikson, E. H. (1963). *Childhood and society* (2nd ed.). New York: WW Norton & Co.

Eustis, N., Greenberg, J., & Patten, S. (1984). *Long-term care for older persons: A policy perspective.* Monterey, CA: Brooks/Cole Publishing Co.

Fields, G. & Mitchell, O. (1983). *Restructuring social security: How will retirement ages respond?* Washington, DC: National Commission on Employment Policy.

Fisher, R. F. (1973). Presbyopia and changes with age in the crystalline lens. *J Physiol (Lond), 228,* 765–779.

Fowles, D. G. (1991). *A profile of older Americans.* Washington, DC: American Association of Retired Persons (AARP) and the Administration of Aging (AOA), US Department of Health and Human Services.

Furino, A. F. & Fogel, B. S. (1990). The economic perspective. In B. S. Fogel et al. (Eds.), *Mental health policy for older Americans: Protecting minds at risk.* Washington, DC: American Psychiatric Press.

Gerner, R. H. (1989). Mood disorders (of late life). In H. I. Kaplan & B. J. Sadock (Eds.), *Comprehensive textbook of psychiatry* (Vol. II) (5th ed.). Baltimore: Williams & Wilkins.

Goldfarb, A. I. (1974). Minor adjustments in the aged. In S. Arieti & E. B. Brody (Eds.), *American handbook of psychiatry* (Vol. 3). New York: Basic Books.

Goldfarb, A. I. (1977). Institutional care of the aged. In E. W. Busse & E. Pfeiffer (Eds.), *Behavior and adaptation in late life.* Boston: Little, Brown and Co.

Gottlieb, G. L. (1991). Financial issues. In J. Sadavoy et al. (Eds.), *Comprehensive review of geriatric psychiatry.* Washington, DC: American Psychiatric Press.

Gurland, B. J. & Cross, P. S. (1983). Suicide among the elderly. In M. K. Aronson et al. (Eds.), *The acting-out elderly.* New York: Haworth Press.

Guterman, A. & Eisdorfer, C. (1989). Other psychiatric conditions of the elderly. In H. I. Kaplan & B. J. Sadock (Eds.), *Comprehensive textbook of psychiatry* (Vol. 2) (5th ed.). Baltimore: Williams & Wilkins.

Hausman, P. B. & Weksler, M. E. (1985). Changes in the immune response with age. In C. E. Finch & E. L. Schneider (Eds.), *Handbook of the biology of aging* (2nd ed.). New York: Van Nostrand Reinhold.

Hendricks, J. & Hendricks, C. D. (1977). *Aging in mass society.* Cambridge, MA: Winthrop Publishers, Inc.

Hogan, R. (1980). Sexual problems of aging. In R. Hogan (Ed.), *Human sexuality: A nursing perspective.* New York: Appleton-Century-Crofts.

Hyde, J. S. (1986). *Understanding human sexuality* (3rd ed.). New York: McGraw-Hill.

Jeste, D. V. et al. (1991). Psychoses. In J. Sadavoy et al. (Eds.), *Comprehensive review of geriatric psychiatry.* Washington, DC: American Psychiatric Press.

Kaufman, M. (1991, October 2). Elderly suicide increase baffling. *The Wichita Eagle,* 1a.

Kaufman, S. R. (1986). *The ageless self: Sources of meaning in late life.* Madison, WI: University of Wisconsin Press.

Kenney, A. R. (1989). *Physiology of aging: A synopsis* (2nd ed.). Chicago: Year Book Medical Publishers.

Kermis, M. D. (1986). *Mental health in late life: The adaptive process.* Boston: Jones and Bartlett Publishers.

King, N. R. (1984). Exploitation and abuse of older family members: An overview of the problem. In J. J. Costa (Ed.), *Abuse of the elderly.* Lexington, MA: D.C. Heath and Company.

Kligman, A. M., Grove, G. L., & Balin, A. K. (1985). Aging of human skin. In C. E. Finch & E. L. Schneider (Eds.), *Handbook of biology of aging* (Vol. 2). New York: Van Nostrand Reinhold.

Kolodny, R. C., Masters, W. H., & Johnson, V. E. (1979). Geriatric sexuality. In *Textbook of sexual medicine.* Boston: Little, Brown and Co.

Kübler-Ross, E. (1969). *On death and dying.* New York: The Macmillan Co.

Lawton, M. P. (1983). Environmental and other determinants of well-being in older people. *Gerontologist, 23,* 348–357.

Leventhal, E. A. (1991). Biological aspects. In J. Sadavoy et al. (Eds.), *Comprehensive review of geriatric psychiatry.* Washington, DC: American Psychiatric Press.

Lieberman, M. A. & Tobin, S. S. (1983). *The experience of old age.* New York: Basic Books.

Lipowski, Z. J. (1989). Delirium in the elderly patient. *N Engl J Med, 320,* 578–582.

Lowenthal, M. F. & Haven, C. (1968). Interaction and adaptation: Intimacy as a critical variable. In B. L. Neugarten (Ed.), *Middle-age and aging.* Chicago, IL: University of Chicago Press.

Marchesini, G. et al. (1987). Insulin resistance in aged man: Relationship between impaired glucose tolerance and decreased insulin activity on branched-chain amino acids. *Metabolism, 36,* 1096–1100.

Masters, W. H. & Johnson, V. E. (1966). *Human sexual response.* Boston: Little, Brown and Co.

Neugarten, B. L. (1979). Policy for the 1980s: Age or need entitlement. In *Aging agenda for the eighties.* Washington, DC: National Journal.

Neugarten, B. L. et al. (1964). *Personality in middle and late life.* New York: Atherton.

O'Malley, TA et al. (1983). Identifying and preventing family-mediated abuse and neglect of elderly persons. *Ann Intern Med, 98*, 998–1005.

Pacini, G. M. et al. (1988). Insulin sensitivity and beta-cell responsivity are not decreased in elderly subjects with normal OGTT. *J Am Geriatr Soc, 36*, 317–323.

Palmore, E. & Maddox, G. L. (1977). Sociological aspects of aging. In E. W. Busse & E. Pfeiffer (Eds.), *Behavior and adaptation in late life.* Boston: Little, Brown and Co.

Physician Payment Review Commission. (1989). *Annual report to Congress.* Washington, DC: US Government Printing Office.

Post, F. (1989). Schizophrenia and delusional disorders (of late life). In H. I. Kaplan & B. J. Sadock (Eds.), *Comprehensive textbook of psychiatry* (Vol. 2) (5th ed.). Baltimore: Williams & Wilkins.

Rabins, P. & Folstein, M. F. (1982). Delirium and dementia: Diagnostic criteria and fatality rates. *Br J Psychiatry, 140*, 149–153.

Reichard, S., Livson, F., & Peterson, P. G. (1962). *Aging and personality.* New York: John Wiley & Sons.

Renvoise, J. (1978). *Web of violence: A study of family violence.* London: Routledge and Kegan Paul.

Reynolds, C. F. (1991). Sleep disorders. In J. Sadavoy et al. (Eds.), *Comprehensive review of geriatric psychiatry.* Washington, DC: American Psychiatric Press.

Roberts, C. M. (1991). *How did I get here so fast?* New York: Warner Books.

Rogers-Seidl, F. F. (1991). *Geriatric nursing care plans.* St. Louis: Mosby Year Book.

Roscow, I. (1967). *Social integration of the aged.* New York: Free Press.

Sadavoy, J., Lazarus, L. W., & Jarvik, L. F. (1991). *Comprehensive review of geriatric psychiatry.* Washington, DC: American Psychiatric Press.

Schaie, K. W. (1990). Intellectual development in adulthood. In J. E. Birren & K. W. Schaie (Eds.), *Handbook of the psychology of aging* (3rd ed.). New York: Academic.

Schechter, M. & Butler, R. N. (1989). Long-term care. In H. I. Kaplan & B. J. Sadock (Eds.), *Comprehensive textbook of psychiatry* (Vol. 2) (5th ed.). Baltimore: Williams & Wilkins.

Schulz, J. (1988). *Economics of aging* (4th ed.). Dover, MA: Auburn House Publications.

Seligmann, J. et al. (1992, May 25). Every woman for herself. *Newsweek.*

Shader, R. I. & Kennedy, J. S. (1989). Biological treatments. In H. I. Kaplan & B. J. Sadock (Eds.), *Comprehensive textbook of psychiatry* (Vol. 2) (5th ed.). Baltimore: Williams & Wilkins.

Sigel, M. M. & Good, R. A. (1972). *Tolerance, autoimmunity and aging.* Springfield, IL: Charles C. Thomas.

Small, G. W. (1989a) Alzheimer's disease and other dementing disorders. In H. I. Kaplan & B. J. Sadock (Eds.), *Comprehensive textbook of psychiatry (Vol. 2)* (5th ed.). Baltimore: Williams & Wilkins.

Small, G. W. (1989b) Psychiatric problems of the medically ill geriatric patient. In H. I. Kaplan & B. J. Sadock (Eds.), *Comprehensive textbook of psychiatry (Vol. 2)* (5th ed.). Baltimore: Williams & Wilkins.

Soldo, B. J. & Agree, E. M. (1988). America's elderly population. *Population Bulletin, 43*(3), 1–53.

Stevenson, J. M. (1988). Suicide. In J. A. Talbott et al. (Eds.), *Textbook of psychiatry.* Washington, DC: American Psychiatric Press.

Stone, V. (1977). Nursing of old people. In E. W. Busse & E. Pfeiffer (Eds.), *Behavior and adaptation in late life* (2nd ed.). Boston: Little, Brown and Co.

Sudnow, D. (1967). *Passing on.* Englewood Cliffs, NJ: Prentice-Hall.

Taub, H. A. (1973). Memory span, practice and aging. *J Gerontology, 28*(3), 335–338.

Vaillant, G. & Vaillant, C. O. (1990). Natural history of male psychosocial health: A 45-year study of predictors of successful aging at age 65. *Am J Psychiatry, 147*, 31–37.

Warheit, G. J., Longino, C. F., & Bradsher, J. E. (1991). Sociocultural aspects. In J. Sadavoy et al. (Eds.), *Comprehensive review of geriatric psychiatry.* Washington, DC: American Psychiatric Press.

BIBLIOGRAPHY

Beck, C. et al. (1991). Dressing for success: Promoting independence among cognitively impaired elderly. *J Psychosoc Nurs, 29*(7), 30–35.

Busse, E. W. & Pfeiffer, E. (1977). *Behavior and adaptation in late life* (2nd ed.). Boston: Little, Brown and Co.

Caroselli-Karinja, M. (1985). Drug abuse and the elderly. *J Psychosoc Nurs, 23*(6), 25–30.

Chaisson, M. et al. (1984). Treating the depressed elderly. *J Psychosoc Nurs, 22*(5), 25–30.

Costa, J. J. (1984). *Abuse of the elderly: A guide to resources and services.* Lexington, MA: Lexington Books, D.C. Heath and Co.

Dellasega, C. (1991). Meeting the mental health needs of elderly clients. *J Psychosoc Nurs, 29*(2), 10–14.

Eth, S. & Mills, M. J. (1989). Ethical and legal considerations. In H. I. Kaplan & B. J. Sadock (Eds.), *Comprehensive textbook of psychiatry* (Vol. 2) (5th ed.). Baltimore: Williams & Wilkins.

Gunter, L. M. & Estes, C. A. (1979). *Education for gerontic nursing.* New York: Springer Publishing Co.

Gurland, B. J. & Meyers, B. S. (1988). Geriatric psychiatry. In J. A. Talbott, R. E. Hales, & S. C. Yudofsky (Eds.), *Textbook of psychiatry.* Washington, DC: American Psychiatric Press.

Jarvik, L. F. & Small, G. W. (1989). Geriatric psychiatry. In H. I. Kaplan & B. J. Sadock (Eds.), *Comprehensive textbook of psychiatry* (Vol. 2) (5th ed.). Baltimore: Williams & Wilkins.

Keith, J. (1982). *Old people as people: Social and cultural influences on aging and old age.* Boston: Little, Brown and Co.

Lazarus, L. W. (1989). Psychotherapy with the elderly. In H. I. Kaplan & B. J. Sadock (Eds.), *Comprehensive textbook of psychiatry* (Vol. 2) (5th ed.). Baltimore: Williams & Wilkins.

Markley, V. J. (1982). Sexuality and aging. *Human sexuality in nursing process.* New York: John Wiley & Sons.

McCullough, P. K. (1992). Evaluation and management of anxiety in the older adult. *Geriatrics, 47*(4), 35–38.

Plotkin, D. A. (1989). Psychiatric examination of the older patient. In H. I. Kaplan & B. J. Sadock (Eds.), *Comprehensive textbook of psychiatry* (Vol. 2) (5th ed.). Baltimore: Williams & Wilkins.

Seligman, J., Friday, C., & Wingert, P. (1992, May 25). Every woman for herself. Newsweek, Vol. CXIX, No. 21, 43–44.

Unruh, P. (1991). Hints for successful aging. *The Prairie View, 30*(1), 1–3.

Vander Zyl, S. (1983). Psychotherapy with the Elderly. *J Psychosoc Nurs, 21*(10), 25–29.

Van Gorp, W. G. & Satz, P. (1989). Neuropsychological examination of the older patient, In H. I. Kaplan & B. J. Sadock (Eds.), *Comprehensive textbook of psychiatry* (Vol. 2) (5th ed.). Baltimore: Williams & Wilkins.

Zerhusen, J. D., Boyle, K., & Wilson, W. (1991). Out of the darkness: Group cognitive therapy for depressed elderly. *J Psychosoc Nurs, 29*(9), 16–21.

THE INDIVIDUAL WITH HIV/AIDS

KEY TERMS
acquired immunodeficiency syndrome
AIDS dementia complex
AIDS-related complex
azidothymidine
HIV wasting syndrome
hospice
human immunodeficiency virus
Kaposi's sarcoma
opportunistic infection
persistent generalized
  lymphadenopathy
pneumocystis pneumonia
seroconversion
T4 lymphocytes
universal precautions

TREATMENT MODALITIES
Pharmacology
Universal Infection Precautions
Hospice Care
SUMMARY

OBJECTIVES

After reading this chapter, the student will be able to:

1. Differentiate between human immunodeficiency virus (HIV), acquired immunodeficiency syndrome (AIDS), and AIDS-related complex (ARC).
2. Describe the pathophysiology incurred by HIV.
3. Discuss historical perspectives associated with AIDS.
4. Relate epidemiological statistics associated with AIDS.
5. Identify predisposing factors to AIDS.
6. Describe symptomatology associated with HIV, AIDS, and ARC, and use this data in patient assessment.
7. Formulate nursing diagnoses and goals of care for patients with AIDS.
8. Describe appropriate nursing interventions for patients with AIDS.
9. Evaluate nursing care of patients with AIDS.
10. Discuss various modalities relevant to treatment of patients with AIDS.

INTRODUCTION

Acquired immunodeficiency syndrome (AIDS) was recognized as a lethal clinical syndrome in 1981 (Wolcott et al, 1989). Since that time, it has grown in epidemic proportions and has been declared the number one health priority in the United States today. Much research is now focused on the treatment and prevention of human immunodeficiency virus (HIV) infection as a possible means of altering the course of the epidemic.

The human immunodeficiency virus is the etiological agent that produces the immunosuppression resulting in AIDS and AIDS-related complex (ARC). Individuals are diagnosed as having HIV infection when the virus is directly identified in host tissues by virus isolation, or indirectly identified by the presence of HIV antibodies in body fluid using laboratory immunoassay testing (Osmond, 1990a). Individuals who have HIV infection may or may not exhibit clinical manifestations. The current median incubation period from HIV infection until the emergence of AIDS is 9.8 years (Osmond, 1990b).

AIDS-related complex includes those HIV-infected individuals with persistent generalized lymphadenopathy (involving two or more extrainguinal sites for 3 or more months), oral candidiasis, single or multidermatomal herpes zoster, biopsy-proven hairy leukoplakia, persistent unexplained fever for more than 2 weeks, or persistent unexplained diarrhea for more than 30 days (Wolcott et al, 1989). AIDS-related complex is no longer recognized as a useful diagnosis. It was used in the past to identify cases that did not fit the criteria for AIDS according to the Centers for Disease Control (CDC). A definition is presented here since the term is still used in the literature.

In 1986, AIDS was defined by the CDC as:

". . . a disease, at least moderately predictive of a defect in cell-mediated immunity, occurring in a person with no known cause for diminished resistance to that disease. Such diseases include Kaposi's sarcoma (KS), *Pneumocystis carinii* pneumonia (PCP), and other serious opportunistic infections."

A 1987 revision of the definition now includes other diseases indicative of the presence of AIDS. The CDC classification system is presented in Table 28.1.

This chapter presents physical and psychological manifestations of AIDS. Delivery of nursing care is described in terms of the nursing process. Various medical treatment modalities are discussed.

PATHOPHYSIOLOGY INCURRED BY THE HIV VIRUS

Normal Immune Response

Cells responsible for nonspecific immune reactions include neutrophils, monocytes, and macrophages. They work to destroy the invasive organism and initiate and facilitate damaged tissue. If these cells are not effective in accomplishing a satisfactory healing response, specific immune mechanisms take over.

Specific immune mechanisms are divided into two major types: the cellular response and the humoral response. The controlling elements of the cellular response are the T lymphocytes (T cells); those of the humoral response are called B lymphocytes (B cells). When the body is invaded by a specific antigen, the T cells, and particularly the T4 lymphocytes (also called *T helper cells*), become sensitized to and specific for the foreign antigen. These antigen-specific T4 cells divide many times, producing antigen-specific T4 cells with other functions. One of these, the T killer cell, destroys viruses that reproduce inside other cells by puncturing the cell membrane of the host cell and allowing the contents of the cell, including viruses, to spill out into the bloodstream, where they can be engulfed by macrophages (Perdew, 1990). Another cell produced through division of the T4 cells is the suppressor T cell, which serves to stop the immune response once the foreign antigen has been destroyed (Scanlon & Sanders, 1991).

The humoral response is activated when antigen-specific T4 cells communicate with B cells in the spleen and lymph nodes. These B cells in turn produce the antibodies specific to the foreign antigen. Antibodies attach themselves to foreign antigens so that they are unable to invade body cells. These invader cells are then destroyed without being able to multiply.

The Immune Response to HIV

The most conspicuous immunologic abnormality associated with HIV infection is a striking depletion of T4 cells (Rosenberg & Fauci, 1989). The HIV infects the T4 lymphocyte, thereby destroying the very cell the body needs to direct an attack on the virus.

An individual with a healthy immune system may present with a T4 count between 600 and 1200 mm³. The individual with HIV infection may experience a drop at the time of acute infection with a subsequent increase when the acute stage subsides. Typically, the T-cell count is around 500 to 600 when the individual begins to develop chronic persistent generalized lymphadenopathy (PGL). With symptoms characteristic of ARC, the T-cell count is commonly about 400. Opportunistic infections are common when the T-cell count reaches 200 (Sweet, 1992). For someone with advanced HIV disease, it is not uncommon to find fewer than 10 T4 cells mm³ (Grady, 1992).

When an individual is infected with HIV, T4 lymphocytes become the main target of attack by the virus. Rapid viral production within the cell causes destruction of the lymphocyte that has either direct or indirect control over virtually every other response of the human immune system (Roitt et al. 1989). The remaining T4 cells seem to lose the ability to function at full capacity and are therefore unable to initiate responses by various other components of the immune system. Because of this, the B cells demonstrate a decreased ability to mount an antibody response to a *new* antigen (Lane & Fauci, 1985).

Table 28.1   CDC CLASSIFICATION SYSTEM FOR HIV INFECTION

Group I. Acute Infection

These individuals have transient signs and symptoms, often somewhat like mononucleosis, that appear at the time of, or shortly after, initial infection with HIV, which is diagnosed by laboratory tests. Symptoms may include fever, malaise myalgias, enlarged lymph nodes, fatigue, and skin rash. The symptoms usually occur about 2 to 3 weeks after exposure and resolve in about a week. Patients usually then test HIV positive at that time. When the symptoms subside, these individuals are reclassified to another diagnostic group.

Group II. Asymptomatic Infection

This group is comprised of individuals with HIV infection, but who have no signs or symptoms. They may be reclassified based upon results of hematologic or immunologic laboratory studies. Probably the largest number of HIV-infected individuals fall within this group (Abrams, 1988).

Group III. Persistent Generalized Lymphadenopathy

These individuals have HIV infection, and their only symptom is persistent generalized lymphadenopathy, a palpable disease of the lymph nodes lasting longer than 3 months with no other etiological explanation. Nodal enlargement is greater than 1 cm at more than one extrainguinal site.

Group IV. Other Disease

Individuals in this group are HIV-infected, and have other clinical symptoms or opportunistic diseases, other than or in addition to lymphadenopathy. Group IV is divided into five subgroups. Individuals may be assigned to one or more subgroups at any given time based on clinical findings. The subgroups are:

Subgroup A: Constitutional Disease

This subgroup includes individuals who have one or more of the following with absence of concurrent illness other than HIV infection to explain the symptom(s):

· Fever persisting for more than 1 month
· Involuntary weight loss of greater than 10 percent of baseline
· Diarrhea persisting more than 1 month

Subgroup B: Neurologic Disease

This subgroup includes individuals who have one or more of the following with absence of concurrent illness other than HIV infection to explain the symptom(s):

· Dementia
· Myelopathy
· Peripheral neuropathy

Subgroup C: Secondary Infectious Diseases

This subgroup includes individuals diagnosed with an infectious disease associated with HIV infection or at least moderately indicative of a defect in cell-mediated immunity. It is further divided into two categories:

Category C-1: Includes individuals with one of the opportunistic infections listed in the new CDC surveillance definition of AIDS: PCP, cryptosporidiosis, toxoplasmosis, strongyloidosis, isosporiasis, candidiasis, cryptococcosis, histoplasmosis, mycobacteriosis, cytomegalovirus, herpes simplex, or progressive multifocal leukoencephalopathy.

Category C-2: Includes individuals with one of the six other specified secondary infectious diseases: oral hairy leukoplakia, multidermatomal herpes zoster, recurrent salmonella bacteremia, nocardiosis, tuberculosis, or oral candidiasis (thrush).

Subgroup D. Secondary Cancers

This subgroup includes individuals with one or more kinds of cancer known to be associated with HIV infection as listed in the new CDC surveillance definition of AIDS: KS, non-Hodgkin's lymphoma, or primary lymphoma of the brain.

Subgroup E. Other Conditions in HIV Infection

Individuals in this subgroup have other clinical findings or diseases that are not classifiable above, and that may be attributed to HIV infection or may be indicative of a defect in cell-mediated immunity. An example is chronic lymphoid interstitial pneumonitis.

Source: Centers for Disease Control (1986a).

The HIV continues to infiltrate new T4 cells, reproducing until they burst out of the cell membrane and begin to float freely in the blood, infecting other T4 cells, of which the body has a limited supply. B cells are stimulated by free-floating HIVs to start producing antibodies. Unfortunately, by the time enough antibodies to HIV are produced to mount an effective attack, the viruses have invaded other cells where they are safe from the attacking antibodies (Perdew, 1990). Protection by monocytes and macrophages is also compromised as a result of lack of stimulation by T4 cells and additionally because some monocytes and macrophages are directly infected by HIV.

Investigators and clinicians require a great deal more knowledge about the effects of HIV on the immune system. Currently, researchers are actively trying to develop a vaccine against HIV that could prevent infection or clinical progression. Until there is a greater understanding of what type of immunity will provide a protective response to HIV, development of a vaccine remains in the future.

HISTORICAL ASPECTS

The first description of what was later to be called AIDS appeared in the CDC's *Morbidity and Mortality Weekly Report* of June 5, 1981. The report described unusual outbreaks of PCP and KS among specific groups of young homosexual men in California and New York. Appearance of these syndromes was considered unusual because of the frequency with which they were occurring and the population being affected. Historically, these conditions were seen infrequently and generally only in severely immunosuppressed individuals (Essex, 1988).

Because these first cases were identified only in homosexual and bisexual men, investigators assumed that the immune deficiency was etiologically related to the gay life-style. The disease was even referred to as gay-related immune deficiency (Flaskerud, 1992a).

Numbers of reported cases were mounting rapidly. Within a brief period, AIDS cases began appearing in other special populations: heterosexual intravenous (IV) drug users and hemophiliacs. Soon after, the first AIDS cases associated with blood transfusions were suspected. These individuals were found to have a history of receiving blood transfusions within the preceding 3 to 5 years (Essex, 1988).

Meanwhile, a number of researchers began to postulate that a mutant variant of the human T-lymphotropic retrovirus (HTLV) might be the etiologic agent of AIDS (Essex et al, 1984; Gallo et al, 1983). Soon after, Gallo and associates (1984) confirmed the link to a T-lymphotropic retrovirus, which they called human T-lymphotropic virus type III (HTLV-III). Today, the term has been standardized worldwide and is called human immunodeficiency virus type 1 (HIV-1). Once the virus had been isolated, a test for identifying HIV antibodies in the blood was developed, making it possible to determine if individuals had been infected by HIV. Screening of blood and blood products also became possible, curbing transmission of the virus through blood transfusion (Najera et al, 1987).

The HTLV may have originated in Africa with a virus called simian T-cell leukemia virus (STLV) found in more than 30 species of monkeys and apes. Spread of the virus progressed from subprimate to African humans. Early reports of its presence were cited in Africans living in southwestern Japan (Gallo et al, 1986). The virus then reportedly moved at elevated rates to the Caribbean, northern South America, and at lower rates to North America and Europe. Recent cultural changes, such as gay liberation, relaxed heterosexual sexual mores, and post-1960 increases in IV drug use, may have amplified the spread of HIV in the United States (Osmond, 1990c).

In the early 80s, Haitians were considered to be a distinct high-risk group for the development of AIDS. They did indeed comprise approximately 5 percent of all cases (Steis & Broder, 1985). However, they have since been reclassified by the CDC into the "heterosexual contact" group and are no longer considered a separate group at risk for AIDS. According to Landesman et al (1985), it does not appear that "being of Haitian extraction by itself, in isolation from other risk factors, increases the relative risk of being exposed to HTLV-III [HIV-1]."

The AIDS epidemic has assumed major proportions, with the numbers of cases continuing to grow internationally. Virtually every major country in the world is confronting what has become the major health crisis of modern times. If progression is not curtailed, it will undoubtedly come to be ranked among history's greatest killers.

EPIDEMIOLOGICAL STATISTICS

Worldwide, HIV infects approximately 8 to 10 million adults and a million children (CDC, June 1991). Projections are that by 2000, 50 to 100 million people could be infected unless effective measures are taken to slow the transmission (Wolcott et al, 1989). The World Health Organization's (WHO) projection for 1991 predicted that between 500,000 and 3 million cases of AIDS would have developed since the beginning of the epidemic (WHO, April 1990).

In the United States, about 1 million people are infected with HIV, and more than 160,000 cases of AIDS have been reported (CDC, April 1991). This number is expected to increase to 365,000 by the end of 1992 (AIDS Update, 1989).

Worldwide, the largest number of AIDS cases are reported to be in Africa and the United States (WHO, November 1990). In the United States, the disease has now been reported in all 50 states and in the District of Columbia (CDC, November 1990). Geographic distribution shows the highest number of cases in New York and California, and the lowest number of cases in North Dakota and South Dakota.

Behavioral changes have resulted in a decline in the number of cases among homosexual men (Osmond & Moss, 1989). However, the number of cases transmitted through heterosexual contact and by perinatal transmission, primarily through contact with IV drug users, has increased (Meyer, 1991).

Nursing care of AIDS patients is moving away from the acute care hospitals. Length of acute care hospital stays is decreasing, and a greater focus is being placed on home care, extended care institutions, and hospice care (Scitovsky, 1989).

The epidemiology of HIV/AIDS changes rapidly, and current information becomes outdated almost before it is published. Nurses must maintain awareness of the latest available information about the disease and the issues that affect provision and outcome of nursing care of patients with HIV/AIDS.

PREDISPOSING FACTORS

The etiological agent associated with AIDS is HIV. It is currently known to have two subtypes known as type 1 and type 2 (HIV-1 and HIV-2). Most of the cases of AIDS worldwide are linked to HIV-1 with the exception of West Africa, where HIV-2 is prevalent (Cohen, 1991a).

The major routes for transmission of HIV are sexual, bloodborne, and perinatal transmission. There has been a shift in the identification of at-risk populations from that of merely belonging to a specific group to having characteristic behaviors that place individuals at risk. According to Barnes (1991), "the risk for AIDS is having sex with someone who is infected or being exposed to blood that is infected. The risk is not being a homosexual man or being a member of any group."

Sexual Transmission

It is now clear that both homosexual and heterosexual activity play major roles in the transmission of HIV infection worldwide (Osmond, 1990d). In the United States and Europe, most AIDS cases are homosexual men. In Africa, most cases result from heterosexual transmission of HIV.

HETEROSEXUAL TRANSMISSION

The virus is found in greater concentration in semen than in vaginal secretions, which more readily facilitates transmission from men to women than from women to men (Osmond, 1990d). Male-to-female transmission has been reported in cases of HIV positive female partners of hemophiliacs, bisexual men, and male IV drug users, and in women artificially inseminated by specimens from infected men.

The HIV may be transmitted from an infected man to his female sexual partner by vaginal or anal intercourse (Osmond, 1990d). It appears that the possibility of oral transmission through sexual practices such as fellatio is relatively low. Although data on female-to-male transmission in the United States has been limited, it is biologically plausible, since HIV has been isolated from vaginal secretions (Wofsy et al, 1986). Cases of female-to-male transmission have been documented (Flaskerud, 1992b).

HOMOSEXUAL TRANSMISSION

The most significant risk factors for homosexual transmission of HIV is receptive anal intercourse and the number of male sexual partners (Osmond, 1990d). Other behaviors that may injure rectal mucosa (e.g., fisting, rectal douching, rectal enemas) increase the risk of viral invasion. Concomitant infections with other diseases, such as hepatitis, herpes, and other sexually transmitted diseases, increases the risk of infection with HIV due to antigenic overload in the host resulting in acceleration of pathogenesis of immunodeficiency (Flaskerud, 1992b).

Bloodborne Transmission

TRANSFUSION WITH BLOOD PRODUCTS

Transmission of HIV-1 has been documented after transfusion of the following single-donor blood and blood components: whole blood, packed red cells, fresh-frozen plasma, cryoprecipitate, and platelets (Donegan, 1990). An estimated 12,000 living transfusion recipients are HIV-infected (Peterman et al, 1987). Almost all of these received transfusions between 1978 and March 1985, when antibody testing for HIV-1 became available. Although laboratory tests are more than 99 percent sensitive, screening problems occur when donations are received from recently HIV-1–infected individuals who have not yet developed antibody or from persistently antibody-negative HIV-1–infected donors (Donegan, 1990). Donors of blood products are asked to self-exclude if they are at risk for HIV-1 infection; however, self-exclusion is still voluntary.

Individuals at highest risk for HIV infection from blood transfusion are hemophiliacs simply because of their massive requirements for blood products. Other individuals who require blood because of temporary illness or surgery are also at risk.

TRANSMISSION BY NEEDLES INFECTED WITH HIV-1

The highest number of cases occurring via this route are among IV drug users who share needles and other equipment contaminated with HIV-1–infected blood. In some areas of the country, this is the most prevalent mode of transmission. Intravenous drug abusers are also at higher risk because of the immunosuppressive factors associated with many of the drugs of abuse (Des Jarlais et al, 1988) and the common underlying existence of malnutrition (Karan, 1989). Some regions (e.g., New York City) have established programs to provide drug users with clean needles in an effort to diminish the spread of HIV.

A second bloodborne mode of transmission of HIV with contaminated needles is through accidental needle sticks by health-care workers, as well as by other means and with other contaminated equipment used for therapeutic purposes. Some examples include:

- Needle sticks caused by recapping needles and by improper disposal of syringes
- Coming in contact with blood or other body fluids during treatments without wearing gloves and while having chapped hands or cuts on the hands
- Having blood or other body fluids splashed on the face during treatments, causing entry through ocular, nasal, or oral mucous membranes
- Being cut with a sharp object that has been contaminated with the blood of an HIV positive patient
- Dressing open wounds without wearing gloves

Perinatal Transmission

Thirty to fifty percent of infants born to HIV-infected women are infected with the virus (Valente & Main, 1990). Modes of transmission include transplacental, exposure to maternal blood and vaginal secretions during delivery, and through breast milk. Intrauterine exposure is possible through transplacental transmission of HIV or of HIV-infected maternal lymphocytes (Maury et al, 1989). The method of delivery (vaginal or cesarean) appears to play no significant role in HIV transmission; however, advanced stage of HIV infection with evidence of clinical illness may be influential (Nokes, 1992). Because breast milk has been implicated as a mode of transmission, women should be counseled to use other forms of infant feeding when possible.

Other Possible Modes of Transmission

To date, HIV has been isolated from blood, semen, vaginal secretions, saliva, tears, breast milk, cerebrospinal fluid, amniotic fluid, and urine. However, only blood, semen, vaginal secretions, and breast milk have been epidemiologically linked to transmission of the virus (CDC, 1987). Anecdotal accounts have described isolated cases of casual transmission. Some examples of these include:

- A mother who was infected by her infant son who had received contaminated blood at birth. Apparently the mother failed to follow recommended precautions when exposing herself to the child's secretions (CDC, 1986b).
- A child who was infected by a sibling through a bite that did not break the skin (Allen & Curran, 1988).
- A woman who was infected by her HIV positive husband through passionate kissing and with small lesions in her oral mucous membranes. The man had been infected through blood transfusion and was known to be impotent (Haverkos & Edelman, 1988).

Cohen (1991a) states, "The exchange of saliva during intimate kissing has not been completely exonerated as a route of HIV transmission, although if it exists, its actual occurrence is very rare."

The risk of being infected with HIV through casual, nonsexual contact is so low as to be virtually nonexistent. Even in those isolated cases that have been reported, most consistently exhibit additional risk factors that may account for the infection (Gershon et al, 1990).

APPLICATION OF THE NURSING PROCESS

Background Assessment Data

The CDC (1986a) now identifies HIV infection as a continuous and progressive process (see Table 28.1). Symptoms characteristic of each stage in the disease progression are presented here.

ACUTE HIV INFECTION

The acute HIV infection is identified by a characteristic syndrome of symptoms that occur from 6 days to 6 weeks after exposure to the virus. The symptoms have an abrupt onset, are somewhat vague, and are similar to those sometimes seen in mononucleosis. Symptoms of acute HIV infection include fever, myalgia, malaise, lymphadenopathy, sore throat, anorexia, nausea and vomiting, headaches, photophobia, skin rash, and diarrhea (Crowe & McGrath, 1990). Most symptoms resolve themselves in 1 to 3 weeks, with the exception of fever, myalgia, lymphadenopathy, and malaise,

which may continue for several months. Seroconversion, the detectability of antibodies to the HIV, usually occurs from a few weeks to as long as 2 to 3 months after the onset of acute illness (Steckelberg & Cockerill, 1988).

ASYMPTOMATIC INFECTION

The acute infection progresses to an asymptomatic stage. Probably the largest number of HIV-infected individuals fall within this group (Abrams, 1988). Individuals may remain in this asymptomatic stage for 10 or more years. The median incubation period from HIV infection until the emergence of full-blown AIDS is currently 9.8 years (Osmond, 1990b). The time is often shorter in children and longer in individuals with hemophilia.

These asymptomatic HIV-infected persons may develop immunological and hematological abnormalities of varying severity, including leukopenia, anemia, thrombocytopenia, hypergammaglobulinemia, decreased T4 lymphocytes, or any combination of these conditions (Wolcott et al, 1989).

PERSISTENT GENERALIZED LYMPHADENOPATHY

A high percentage of patients with HIV infection have PGL, that is, lymph nodes greater than 1 cm in diameter at two extrainguinal sites persisting for 3 months or longer, not attributable to other causes, and not associated with other substantial constitutional symptoms (CDC, 1986a). This syndrome often occurs within a few months of seroconversion for HIV antibody. In addition to swollen, sometimes painful lymph nodes, symptoms may include fever, night sweats, weight loss, and an enlarged spleen (Flaskerud, 1992a). Persistent generalized lymphadenopathy may persist for several years, even in the absence of symptoms other than nodal enlargement (Cohen, 1991b).

AIDS-RELATED COMPLEX

AIDS-related complex is gradually being abandoned as a clinical description. However, since it was an important concept in early descriptions of HIV disease, and because it is still referred to in the literature, it will be discussed here.

AIDS-related complex was considered a disease of HIV-infected individuals that did not fit the CDC's classification of full-blown AIDS. Flaskerud (1992a) states,

> "The term 'ARC' was used when a person infected by HIV had at least two well-developed symptoms of immunodeficiency with at least two laboratory abnormalities. Symptoms such as fever, drenching night sweats, weight loss, fatigue, and lymphadenopathy in the absence of an opportunistic infection or Kaposi's sarcoma were known formerly as ARC."

Today, HIV infection itself is considered a disease with various clinical manifestations as a gradient of host responses. AIDS-related complex is no longer considered a separate and nonoverlapping syndrome (Abrams, 1990).

HIV WASTING SYNDROME

The CDC (1986a) identifies this syndrome as having one or more of the following with absence of concurrent illness other than HIV infection:

- Fever and weakness for more than 30 days
- Involuntary weight loss of more than 10 percent of baseline body weight
- Chronic diarrhea (at least two loose stools per day) for more than 1 month

Patients in this group may be classified with AIDS if they meet the definition for HIV wasting syndrome and have laboratory evidence of HIV infection (Cohen, 1991b).

OPPORTUNISTIC INFECTIONS

Opportunistic infections have long been a defining characteristic of AIDS. Descriptions of the common ones follow.

Protozoans

Pneumocystis carinii *pneumonia* The most common, life-threatening opportunistic infection seen in patients with AIDS is PCP (Cook, 1987). Symptoms include fever, exertional dyspnea, and nonproductive cough (Wolcott et al, 1989).

Cryptosporidiosis This parasitic infection may cause chronic profuse watery diarrhea in AIDS patients. Some patients may have up to 20 or more bowel movements a day.

Isosporiasis Caused by the protozoan *Isospora belli*, this infection causes chronic intermittent en-teritis in AIDS patients. Symptoms are similar to those caused by cryptosporidiosis.

Toxoplasmosis This protozoan infection frequently causes central nervous system (CNS) disease in AIDS patients (Wolcott et al, 1989). Common presenting symptoms include impaired level of consciousness, fever, headache, seizures, and focal neurological signs, such as hemiparesis, cognitive deficits, ataxia, aphasia, movement disorders, and visual field loss (Israelski & Remington, 1988).

Fungal Infections

Candidiasis Most commonly caused by the fungus *Candida albicans*, this infection generally occurs in the oral cavity and esophagus of the HIV-infected individual. Vaginal and anal infections are seen less frequently. Oral candidiasis, commonly called *thrush*, is characterized by white plaques on the oral mucosa. Esophageal candidiasis presents with painful lesions in the esophagus, making swallowing difficult.

Cryptococcosis This yeast infection, caused by *Cryptococcus neoformans*, most commonly causes meningitis in AIDS patients (Wolcott et al, 1989). Symptoms include fever, headache, and altered mental status.

Histoplasmosis The causative organism, *Histoplasma capsulatum*, is endemic to the central and southern United States. Presenting symptoms include fever, chills, sweats, weight loss, nausea, vomiting, diarrhea, pneumonitis, and occasionally skin lesions and lymphadenopathy (Kovacs & Masur, 1988).

Coccidioidomycosis Endemic to the southwestern United States, especially southern California and Arizona, *Coccidioides immitis* is derived from contaminated soil. Symptoms include fever, malaise, and weight loss. Cough, possibly associated with pulmonary nodules, may be prominent (Kovacs & Masur, 1988).

Viral Infections

Cytomegalovirus Cytomegalovirus (CMV) is common in most human populations. In most instances, it is latent and asymptomatic. Immunosuppression by HIV reactivates the virus. In about 30 percent of AIDS patients, CMV is recognized as a major contributor to death (Kovacs & Masur, 1988). Cytomegalovirus causes retinitis (and possible blindness), enteritis (manifested by profuse watery diarrhea), pneumonitis, cerebral disease, myelitis, pericarditis, endometritis, glomerulitis, epididymitis, hepatitis, and adrenal necrosis.

Herpes Simplex The most common manifestations of herpes simplex disease in homosexual men with HIV infection are colitis and perirectal lesions that are prone to ulcerate (Siegel et al, 1981). Chronic genital lesions may also be observed. Herpes simplex colitis is usually confined to the rectum and may result in itching, burning, pain, bloody stool, and fever (Kovacs & Masur, 1988).

Herpes Zoster Herpes zoster has been found to cause both dermatomal (shingles) and disseminated disease in patients with HIV infection. It has been estimated that within 4 years of diagnosis of dermatomal zoster, nearly 50 percent of HIV-infected patients will have developed AIDS (Kovacs & Masur, 1988). After initial infection (usually in childhood), herpes zoster lies latent in the dorsal root ganglia of the peripheral nerves. Reactivation results in painful lesions on the skin area supplied by the affected nerve (Cohen, 1991b). Dissemination to the lung or CNS can result in pneumonia or encephalitis. Ophthalmic nerve involvement can result in blindness (Andiman & Leicht, 1988).

Epstein-Barr Virus Virtually all AIDS patients have serologic evidence of infection with Epstein-Barr virus (EBV) (Rogers et al, 1983). The role that EBV plays in HIV disease is not clearly understood. The virus has been found in oral hairy leukoplakia lesions, in conjunction with papillomavirus (Greenspan et al, 1985). Symptoms of EBV include fever, lymphadenopathy, and fatigue.

J-C Virus J-C virus has been implicated as the etiological agent for progressive multifocal leukoencephalopathy (PML) in HIV-infected patients. Common manifestations of PML include weakness in the extremities, cognitive impairments, headache, visual disturbances, ataxia, altered mental status, and hemiparesis (Berger et al, 1987). Progressive multifocal leukoencephalopathy is relatively rare, but diagnosis of the disease in HIV-infected individuals presents a poor prognosis. Survival after onset of PML may only be a matter of weeks or months (Cohen, 1991b).

Bacterial Infections

Mycobacteria *Mycobacterium avium-intracellulare* complex (MAC) and *M. tuberculosis* occur with great frequency among HIV-infected patients (Kovacs & Masur, 1988). MAC may contribute to the AIDS "wasting" syndrome with symptoms of diarrhea and malabsorption. Other symptoms include high, swinging fever; weight loss; malaise; anorexia; weakness; myalgia; night sweats; cough; and headache (Cohen, 1991b). *M. tuberculosis* is associated with the development of tuberculosis in HIV-infected patients. The primary manifestation is pulmonary lesions. Extrapulmonary lesions involving bone, kidney, brain, lymph nodes, and virtually every other site have been reported (Kovacs & Masur, 1988).

Salmonella AIDS patients with salmonellosis usually present with nonspecific symptoms: fever, malaise, fatigue, anorexia, cachexia, myalgias, weight loss, and watery diarrhea (Jacobs et al, 1985). There is a high incidence of bacteremia in AIDS patients with salmonellosis (Glaser et al, 1985).

Nocardiosis Primary infections by the bacterium *Nocardia* occur in the lung. However, disseminated disease is not uncommon. Lung involvement presents with pneumonitis, and possibly lesions or abscesses. Other clinical manifestations include fever, chills, cough with sputum production, malaise, weakness, weight loss, and compromised respiratory function (Cohen, 1991b).

AIDS-RELATED MALIGNANCIES

Kaposi's Sarcoma The etiology of KS is unknown, but may be caused by a yet unidentified virus that is transmitted through intimate sexual contact or exposure to blood or blood products (Krigel & Friedman-Kien, 1988). Lesions associated with KS may appear on any body surface or in the viscera. They are usually painless, nonpruritic, pigmented (red to blue), and nonblanching (Heyer et al, 1990). Flat "patchy" lesions become elevated and develop into papules or plaques. Eventually the plaques enlarge, coalesce, and form tumor nodules. Skin lesions may form anywhere on the body, although characteristic sites include the tip of the nose, the eyelid, the hard palate and posterior pharynx, the glans penis, and the sole of the foot (Heyer et al, 1990). Virtually any organ system, including the heart and lungs, may be affected. Gastrointestinal involvement is common and may result in impaired swallowing, obstruction, or perforation. Pulmonary KS may present with symptoms similar to pneumonia, thereby creating some difficulty with differential diagnosis. Kaposi's sarcoma rarely involves the CNS. Lymphedema from lymphatic obstruction is common in the face, lower extremities, scrotum, and abdomen. In the lower extremities, the collecting fluid is usually very firm and nonpitting (Heyer et al, 1990). Karposi's sarcoma is not viewed as a metastatic disease, but rather one with multifocal origin. A poor prognosis is associated with visceral involvement (Heyer et al, 1990).

Other Malignancies HIV-positive individuals are at increased risk for developing non-Hodgkin's lymphoma (Wolcott et al, 1989). Extranodal sites, including the CNS and bone marrow, are frequently involved. Major primary extranodal sites have been identified as the brain, anus, rectum, head, neck, lung, and liver (Biggar, 1990). Clinical features are consistent with regional involvement. Hodgkin's disease, squamous-cell carcinomas, malignant melanoma, testicular cancers, and primary hepatocellular carcinoma have been reported in association with AIDS; however, a direct correlation with HIV-induced immune deficiency has not been established (Volberding, 1990a).

ALTERED MENTAL STATES

Delirium Delirium is one of the most common organic mental syndromes seen in AIDS patients (Dilley et al, 1990). Clinical manifestations may include a fluctuating level of consciousness, reversal of sleep-wake cycle, abnormal vital signs, and psychotic phenomena (e.g., hallucinations). Contributing factors to the development of delirium include CNS infections, CNS neoplastic disease, side effects of various chemotherapeutic agents, hypoxemia from respiratory compromise, electrolyte imbalance, and sensory deprivation. In AIDS patients, delirium is frequently superimposed on, or evolves into, dementia (Dilley et al, 1990).

Depressive Syndromes Anticipatory or actual grief, which may be acute or chronic, normal or pathological, is an important cause of depressive symptoms in AIDS patients (Wolcott et al, 1989). Transient suicidal ideation on learning of HIV positivity is quite common, although serious suicidal behavior is relatively rare. Depression in AIDS patients may be related to receiving a new diagnosis of HIV positivity or AIDS, perceiving rejection by

loved ones, multiple losses of friends to the disease, an inadequate social and financial support system, and presence of an early organic mental disorder.

AIDS Dementia Complex AIDS dementia complex (ADC) is identified as a neuropathological syndrome, possibly caused by chronic HIV encephalitis and myelitis (Wolcott et al, 1989). Early clinical manifestations include subtle cognitive, behavioral, and motor symptoms that become more severe with progression of the disease (Table 28.2). The incidence of ADC in AIDS patients is probably between 70 and 95 percent, although the clinical severity of the dementia varies considerably (Wolcott et al, 1989). AIDS dementia complex is thought to be the most common CNS complication of HIV infection (Navia et al, 1985).

Table 28.2 SIGNS AND SYMPTOMS OF AIDS DEMENTIA COMPLEX

Early	Late
Cognitive	**Cognitive**
Forgetfulness	Severe cognitive deficits
Loss of concentration	Mutism
Confusion	
Slowness of thought	
Motor	**Motor**
Loss of balance	Psychomotor retardation
Leg weakness	Ataxia
Deterioration in handwriting	Hypertonia
	Paraparesis
	Quadriparesis
	Hemiparesis
	Tremors
	Vegetative state
Behavioral	**Behavioral**
Apathy	Organic psychosis—persistent
Social withdrawal	Vacant staring
Dysphoric mood	Lethargy
Organic psychosis	Hypersomnolence
Regressed behavior	
Other	**Other**
Headache	Bowel and bladder incontinence
Seizures	Myoclonus
	Seizures

Source: Adapted from Navia et al. (1985); Navia & Price (1986); and Price & Brew (1988).

PSYCHOSOCIAL IMPLICATION OF HIV/AIDS

The psychosocial problems that confront a person with AIDS can be overwhelming. Health-care workers still face a number of unknowns related to the disease, thereby setting AIDS patients apart from individuals with other life-threatening illnesses. Persons with AIDS (PWAs) are often the victims of discrimination, due to fear of contagion, prejudices, and stigmatization founded in societal attitudes toward groups most commonly afflicted. Dilley (1990) lists the following facts that contribute to the psychosocial problems experienced by PWAs:

1. AIDS is a new and complicated disease that is not well understood by the general population. Well-intentioned but uninformed individuals can have unfounded fears of contagion and be restrained toward people with AIDS.
2. AIDS is most frequently a venereal disease. In addition, it is commonly found among IV drug users, who spread it through sharing "dirty needles." Both of these issues, sexuality and illicit drug use, can raise moral issues, thereby making it easy for patients and nonpatients alike to develop an attitude of "blaming the victim" for the illness.
3. Gay people have historically been stigmatized solely on the basis of their homosexuality. Similarly, individuals who use IV drugs share, at best, a public image of being troubled, difficult, or frightening.
4. At this time, AIDS is an incurable disease that in the United States predominantly strikes men in their early adult years.

The individual with newly diagnosed HIV seropositivity commonly responds with shock and disbelief, followed by guilt, anger, and depression. In some instances, a symptom complex similar to post-traumatic stress disorder is common in the first few weeks after notification of HIV positivity (Wolcott et al, 1989). The person may become extremely anxious and hypervigilant about physical symptoms, exhibiting marked dependence on health-care workers. Feelings of guilt prevail over previous life activities and there is self-blame for becoming infected. Depressive thoughts are common, and acute suicidal crises may occur. Other responses to initial diagnosis of HIV seropositivity have included transient or chronic sexual dysfunction and social withdrawal due to fear of infecting others or of social rejection (Wolcott et al, 1989). Crisis intervention with newly diagnosed HIV-positive persons is aimed at promoting accurate cognitive understanding of the meaning of the test results, restoration of a positive psychological equilibrium, and making the necessary sexual behavior changes to protect self and others (Wolcott et al, 1989).

Denial is a common defense mechanism among individuals with high-risk behaviors. Denial prevents individuals from undergoing HIV testing; it delays some HIV-positive individuals from seeking early medical care; and it prevents some HIV-positive individuals from changing their behavior to prevent HIV transmission.

Significant others of patients with HIV disease face a great many stresses associated with the patient's illness. Initially they may experience emotions typical of the grief response. Reality comes with accepting the immense responsibility for the physical and emotional care of their loved one. They may experience financial concerns and lack of social support.

When the significant other is a gay lover, there may be guilt over having infected the partner or fear of having been infected by the partner (Wolcott et al, 1989). The gay lover may be rejected by the patient's family members, who themselves may be experiencing unique stresses associated with learning for the first time of their child's life-style. Parents may blame themselves and their childrearing practices. The family may experience a lack of social support because of the stigma attached to their child's illness. Grief responses by family members are common.

Nursing Diagnosis, Planning/Implementation

Nursing diagnoses are formulated from the data gathered during the assessment phase and with background knowledge regarding predisposing factors to the disorder. The following nursing diagnoses may be used for the patient with AIDS:

Altered protection related to compromised immune status secondary to diagnosis of AIDS evidenced by laboratory values indicating decreased numbers of T4 cells and presence of opportunistic infections manifested by fever, night sweats, copious watery diarrhea, weight loss, fatigue, malaise, swollen lymph glands, cough, dyspnea, rash, skin lesions, white patches in mouth, headache, ataxia, anorexia, bleeding, bruising, and various neurological effects.

Altered family processes related to crisis associated with having a family member diagnosed with AIDS evidenced by difficulty making decisions that affect all family members; inability to meet physical, emotional, spiritual, and security needs of its members.

Knowledge deficit (prevention of transmission and protection of the patient) related to lack of exposure to accurate information evidenced by inaccurate statements by patient and family.

Altered thought processes related to primary HIV infection (ADC), opportunistic infections that invade the CNS, and/or adverse effects of therapy evidenced by confusion, disorientation, memory deficits, and inappropriate nonreality-based thinking. (Refer to Table 16.3, Care Plan for Patient with Dementia.)

High risk for self-directed violence related to new diagnosis of AIDS evidenced by statements of taking own life and would rather die than face future with AIDS. (Refer to Table 19.6, Care Plan for Depressed Patient.)

In Table 28.3, selected nursing diagnoses are presented in a plan of care for the patient with HIV/AIDS. Goals of care and appropriate nursing interventions are included for each. Rationales are presented in italics.

OUTCOME CRITERIA

The following criteria may be used for measurement of outcomes in the care of the patient with HIV/AIDS.

The patient:
1. Shows no new signs or symptoms of infection.
2. Does not experience respiratory distress.
3. Maintains optimal nutrition and hydration.
4. Has experienced no further weight loss.
5. Maintains integrity of skin and mucous membranes.

6. Manifests evidence of wound healing.
7. Attains and maintains normal fluid and electrolyte balance.
8. Has fewer bowel movements, with increased stool consistency.
9. Explores feelings about self and illness.
10. Verbalizes understanding about disease process, modes of transmission, and prevention of infection.

The family/significant others:
1. Discuss feelings regarding patient's diagnosis and prognosis.
2. Are able to make rational decisions regarding care of their loved one and the effect on family function.
3. Are able to verbalize precautions for preventing transmission of HIV to themselves and others and infection of the patient.
4. Verbalize knowledge of resources within the community from whom they may seek support and assistance.

Evaluation

Reassessment is conducted to determine if the nursing actions have been successful in achieving the objectives of care. Evaluation of the nursing actions for the patients with HIV/AIDS may be facilitated by gathering information using the following types of questions.

Have precautions been successful in preventing new infection of the patient? Have fever and night sweats been controlled? Has there been a decrease in frequency and increase in consistency of stools? Have weight and nutritional status stabilized? Are fluid and electrolyte values within normal limits? Does the patient experience respiratory distress? Have bleeding and bruising been avoided? Are skin and mucous membranes intact? Do family members/significant others verbalize feelings (including anger) regarding patient's diagnosis and prognosis? Are members able to identify areas of dysfunction within the family? If patient has a homosexual lover, has any conflict been resolved? Have caregiving responsibilities been defined and distributed in a manner acceptable to all? Have parents worked through feelings of guilt and shame? Are patient and family/significant other(s) able to verbalize educational information presented re-

Table 28.3 CARE PLAN FOR THE PATIENT WITH HIV/AIDS

Nursing Diagnoses	Objectives	Nursing Interventions*

Altered protection related to compromised immune status secondary to diagnosis of AIDS evidenced by laboratory values indicating decreased numbers of T4 cells and presence of opportunistic infections manifested by fever, night sweats, diarrhea, weight loss, fatigue, malaise, swollen lymph glands, cough, dyspnea, rash, skin lesions, white patches in mouth, headache, ataxia, anorexia, bleeding, bruising, and various neurological effects	Patient safety and comfort will be maximized.	*In an effort to prevent infection in an immunocompromised individual:*
		1. Implement universal blood and body fluid precautions
		2. Wash hands with antibacterial soap before entering and on leaving patient's room
		3. Monitor vital signs at regular intervals.
		4. Monitor CBCs for leukopenia/neutropenia.
		5. Monitor for signs and symptoms of specific opportunistic infections.
		6. Protect patient from individuals with infections.
		7. Maintain meticulous sterile technique for dressing changes and any invasive procedure.
		8. Administer antibiotics as ordered.
		
		In an effort to restore nutritional status and decrease nausea/vomiting and diarrhea:
		1. Provide low-residue, high-protein, high-calorie, soft, bland diet. Maintain hydration with adequate fluid intake.
		2. Obtain daily weight and record intake/output.
		3. Monitor serum electrolytes and CBCs.
		4. If patient is unable to eat, provide isotonic tube feedings as tolerated. Check for gastric residual frequently.
		5. If patient is unable to tolerate oral intake/tube feedings, consult physician regarding possibility of parenteral hyperalimentation. Observe hyperalimentation administration site for signs of infection.
		6. Administer antidiarrheals and antiemetics as ordered.
		7. Perform frequent oral care. Promote prevention and healing of lesions in the mouth.
		8. Have the patient eat small, frequent meals with high-calorie snacks rather than three large meals/day.
		
		In an effort to prevent impairment of skin and mucous membrane integrity:
		1. Monitor skin condition for signs of redness and breakdown.
		2. Reposition patient every 1 to 2 hr.
		3. Encourage ambulation and chair activity as tolerated.
		4. Use egg crate or air mattress on bed.
		5. Wash skin daily with soap and rinse well with water.
		6. Apply lotion to skin to maintain skin softness.
		7. Provide wound care as ordered for existing pressure sores or lesions.
		8. Cleanse skin exposed to diarrhea thoroughly and protect rectal area with ointment.
		9. Apply artificial tears to eyes as appropriate.
		10. Perform frequent oral care; apply ointment to lips.
		
		In an effort to maximize oxygen consumption and minimize respiratory distress:
		1. Assess respiratory status frequently:
		  a. Monitor depth, rate, and rhythm of respirations.
		  b. Auscultate lung fields every 2 hr and prn.

(continued)

Table 28.3 CONTINUED

Nursing Diagnoses	Objectives	Nursing Interventions*

    c. Monitor arterial blood gases.
    d. Check color of skin, nail beds, and sclerae.
    e. Assess sputum for color, odor, and viscosity.
2. Encourage coughing and deep-breathing exercises.
3. Provide humidified oxygen as ordered.
4. Suction as needed using sterile technique.
5. Space nursing care to allow patient adequate rest periods between procedures.
6. Administer analgesics or sedatives judiciously to prevent respiratory depression.
7. Administer bronchodilators and antibiotics as ordered.

In an effort to minimize the potential for easy bleeding due to HIV-induced thrombocytopenia:

1. Follow protocol for maintenance of skin integrity.
2. Provide safe environment to minimize falling or bumping into objects.
3. Provide soft toothbrush or "toothette" swabs for cleaning teeth and gums.
4. Ensure that patient does not take aspirin or other medications that increase the potential for bleeding.
5. Clean up areas contaminated by patient's blood with household bleach (5.25% sodium hypochlorite) diluted 1:10 with water (Carpenito, 1991; Ungvarski, 1992).

In an effort to maintain near-normal body temperature:

1. Provide frequent tepid water sponge baths.
2. Provide antipyretic as ordered by physician (avoid aspirin).
3. Place patient in cool room, with minimal clothing and bed covers.
4. Encourage intake of cool liquids (if not contraindicated.)

Nursing Diagnoses	Objectives	Nursing Interventions*
Altered family processes related to crisis associated with having a family member diagnosed with AIDS evidenced by difficulty making decisions that affect all family members; inability to meet physical, emotional, spiritual, and security needs of its members.	Family will verbalize areas of dysfunction and demonstrate ability to cope more effectively. Family members will express feelings regarding loved one's diagnosis and prognosis.	Create an environment that is comfortable, supportive, private, and promotes trust. *Basic needs of the family must be met before crisis resolution can be attempted.* Encourage each individual member to express feelings regarding loved one's diagnosis and prognosis. *Each individual is unique and must feel that his or her private needs can be met within the family constellation.* If the patient is homosexual, and this is family's first awareness, help them deal with guilt and shame they may experience. Help parents to understand they are not responsible, and their child is still the same individual they have always loved. *Resolving guilt and shame enables family members to respond adaptively to the crisis. Their response can affect the patient's remaining future and the family's future as well* (Christ et al, 1988). Serve as facilitator between patient's family and homosexual lover. The family may have difficulty accepting the lover as a person who is as significant as a spouse. Clarify roles and responsibilities of family and lover. Do this by bringing both parties together to define and distribute the tasks involved in the patient's care. *By minimizing the lack of legally defined roles, and by focusing on the need for making realistic decisions about the patient's care, communication*

(*continued*)

Table 28.3 CONTINUED

Nursing Diagnoses	Objectives	Nursing Interventions*
		and resolution of conflict is enhanced (Christ et al, 1988). **Encourage use of stress management techniques (e.g., relaxation exercises, guided imagery, attendance at support group meetings for significant others of AIDS patients).** *Reduction of stress and support from others who share similar experiences enables individuals to begin to think more clearly and develop new behaviors to cope with this situational crisis.* **Provide educational information about AIDS and opportunity to ask questions and express concerns.** *Many misconceptions about the disease abound within the public domain. Clarification may calm some of the family's fears and facilitate interaction with the patient.* **Make family referrals to community organizations that provide supportive help or financial assistance to AIDS patients.** *Extended care can place a financial burden on patient and family members. Respite care may provide family members with occasional much-needed relief away from the stress of physical and emotional caregiving responsibilities.*

Knowledge deficit (prevention of transmission and protection of the patient) related to lack of exposure to accurate information evidenced by inaccurate statements by patient and family.	Patient and family will be able to verbalize accurate information regarding transmission of HIV, as well as protection of the immunodeficient patient.	*In an effort to clarify misconceptions, calm fears, and support an environment of appropriate interventions for care of the AIDS patient, provide patient and significant others with the following information:*
		
		1. Teach that AIDS cannot be contracted from:
		  a. Casual or household contact with an AIDS patient.
		  b. Shaking hands, hugging, social (dry) kissing, holding hands, or other nonsexual physical contact.
		  c. Touching unsoiled linens or clothing, money, furniture, or other inanimate objects.
		  d. Being near someone who has AIDS at work, school, stores, restaurants, elevators.
		  e. Toilet seats, bathtubs, towels, showers, or swimming pools.
		  f. Dishes, silverware, or food handled by a person with AIDS.
		  g. Animals (pets may transmit opportunistic organisms).
		  h. (Very unlikely spread by) coughing, sneezing, spitting, kissing, tears, saliva.
		2. AIDS virus dies quickly outside the body because it requires living tissue to survive. It is readily killed by soap, cleansers, hot water, and disinfectants.
		3. Teach patient to protect self from infections by taking the following precautions:
		  a. Avoid unpasteurized milk or milk products.
		  b. Cook all raw vegetables and fruits before eating. *Raw or improperly washed foods may transmit microbes.*
		  c. Cook all meals well before eating.
		  d. Avoid direct contact with persons with known contagious illnesses.
		  e. Consult physician before getting a pet. *Pets require extra infection control precautions due to the opportunistic organisms carried by animals.*

(continued)

Table 28.3 CONTINUED

Nursing Diagnoses	Objectives	Nursing Interventions*

f. Avoid touching animal feces, urine, emesis, litter boxes, aquariums, or bird cages. Always wear mask and gloves when cleaning up after a pet.

g. Avoid traveling in countries with poor sanitation.

h. Avoid vaccines or vaccinations. *These may be fatal to immunosuppressed persons.*

i. Exercise regularly.

j. Control stress factors. A counselor or support group may be helpful.

k. Stop smoking. *Smoking predisposes to respiratory infections.*

l. Maintain good personal hygiene.

4. Teach patient/significant others about prevention of transmission:

   a. Do not donate blood, plasma, body organs, tissues, or semen.

   b. Inform physician, dentists, and anyone providing care that you have AIDS.

   c. Do not share needles or syringes.

   d. Do not share personal items, such as tooth brushes, razors, or other implements that may be contaminated with blood or body fluids.

   e. Do not eat or drink from the same dinnerware and utensils without washing them between use.

   f. Avoid becoming pregnant if at risk for AIDS or HIV infection.

   g. Engage in only "safe" sexual practices (those *not* involving exchange of body fluids).

   h. Avoid sexual practices medically classified as "unsafe," such as anal or vaginal intercourse and oral sex.

   i. Avoid the use of recreational drugs because of their immunosuppressive effects.

5. Teach the home caregiver(s) to protect self from HIV infection by taking the following precautions:

   a. Wash hands thoroughly with liquid antibiotic soap before and after each patient contact. Use moisturizing lotion afterward to prevent dry, cracking skin.

   b. Wear gloves when hands have cuts or when in contact with blood or body fluids (e.g., open wounds, suctioning, feces). Gown or aprons may be worn if soiling is likely.

   c. Wear a mask:

      (1) When patient has a productive cough and tuberculosis has not been ruled out.

      (2) To protect patient if caregiver has a cold.

      (3) During suctioning.

   d. Bag disposable gloves and masks with patient's trash.

(continued)

Table 28.3 CONTINUED		
Nursing Diagnoses	**Objectives**	**Nursing Interventions***
		e. Dispose of the following in the toilet: (1) Organic material on clothes or linen before laundering. (2) Blood or body fluids. (3) Soiled tissue or toilet paper. (4) Cleaners or disinfectants used to clean contaminated articles. (5) Solutions contaminated with blood or body fluids. f. Double-bag patient's trash and soiled dressings in an impenetrable, plastic bag. *Tie* the bag shut and discard with household trash. g. Do not recap needles, syringes, and other sharp items. Use puncture-proof covered containers for disposal (e.g., coffee cans, jars). h. Place soiled linen and clothing in a plastic bag and tie shut until washed. Launder these separately from other laundry. Use bleach or other disinfectant in hot water. i. When house cleaning, all equipment used in care of the patient, as well as bathroom and kitchen surfaces, should be cleaned with 1:10 dilute bleach solutions. j. Mops, sponges, and other items used for cleaning should be reserved specifically for that purpose.

*The interventions for this care plan have been adapted from "Nursing Care Plan for the AIDS Patient," written by the nursing staff of Hospice, Inc., Wichita, KS, 1989, with permission.

garding ways in which HIV can and cannot be transmitted, ways to protect patient from infections, and ways to prevent transmission to caregivers and others? Can patient and family/significant other(s) identify resources within the community from whom they may seek support and assistance (e.g., AIDS support groups, home care, respite care, hospice, financial support)?

TREATMENT MODALITIES

Pharmacology

ANTIVIRAL THERAPY

Yarchoan and Broder (1988) base the rationale for use of antiretroviral therapy in patients with AIDS on the following premises that they consider to be true in *most* cases:

1. That active replication of HIV is important in the pathogenesis and maintenance of the disease state.

2. That at any one point in time, most helper T cells (or other relevant cells) are not infected with HIV.
3. That infected cells die in a relatively short period.
4. That it is possible to stop the replication of HIV and thus to block the spread of the virus.
5. That the damaged organs have at least some regenerative potential.

Azidothymidine The most widely used antiviral agent in the treatment of HIV infection is azidothymidine (AZT). Marketed under the generic name zidovudine and the brand name Retrovir, it was initially prescribed for patients with severe symptomatic HIV disease (less than 200 T4 cells). More recent data provide justification for treating all patients who have T4 counts less than 500 (Volberding, 1990b). Studies have shown that AZT inhibits progression to AIDS in HIV-infected persons with T4 counts between 200/mm^3 and 500/mm^3. Adverse effects of AZT include mild nausea and occasional mild-to-moderate agitational or confused states (Volberding, 1990b). Objective side effects are more problematic and include anemia and neutropenia. Recommendations are to decrease dosage or interrupt therapy when neutrophil counts fall below 500 (Volberding, 1990b). Individuals with HIV-related neurological disorders, including ADC, appear to show a sometimes rapid and striking improvement with AZT (Yarchoan & Broder, 1988).

At the time of publication, a number of other antiretroviral agents were in various stages of clinical trials. The role for most of these drugs in the treatment of HIV infection and AIDS has yet to be defined. There is hope and optimism that these research efforts will contribute to the successful control of this epidemic.

OTHER CHEMOTHERAPEUTIC AGENTS

Various other drugs are used in HIV-infected individuals to treat the opportunistic infections and malignancies associated with the disease. Some examples include antibiotics, antifungal agents, antiviral agents, and antineoplastic agents. Table 28.4 presents a list of selected medications within these classifications and the disease process they are used to counteract.

Universal Infection Precautions

In 1987, the CDC in Atlanta published guidelines for prevention of HIV transmission in health-care settings. The following section includes the recommendations that the CDC set forth in the care of HIV-infected individuals to prevent HIV transmission:

"Since medical history and examination cannot reliably identify all patients infected with HIV or other bloodborne pathogens, blood and body-fluid precautions should be consistently used for *all* patients. This approach, previously recommended by the CDC, and referred to as "universal blood and body-fluid precautions" or "universal precautions," should be used in the care of *all* patients, especially including those in emergency-care settings in which the risk of blood exposure is increased and the infection status of the patient is usually unknown.

1. All health-care workers should routinely use appropriate barrier precautions to prevent skin and mucous-membrane exposure when contact with blood or other body fluids of any patient is anticipated. Gloves should be worn for touching blood and body fluids, mucous membranes, or nonintact skin of all patients, for handling items or surfaces soiled with blood or body fluids, and for performing venipuncture and other vascular access procedures. Gloves should be changed after contact with each patient. Masks and protective eyewear or face shields should be worn during procedures that are likely to generate droplets of blood or other body fluids to prevent exposure of mucous membranes of the mouth, nose, and eyes. Gowns or aprons should be worn during procedures that are likely to generate splashes of blood or other body fluids.

2. Hands and other skin surfaces should be washed immediately and thoroughly if contaminated with blood or other body fluids. Hands should be washed immediately after gloves are removed.

3. All health-care workers should take precautions to prevent injuries caused by needles, scalpels, and other sharp instruments or devices during procedures; when cleaning used instruments; during disposal of used needles; and when handling sharp instruments after procedures. To prevent needlestick injuries, needles should not be recapped, purposely bent or broken by hand, removed from disposable syringes, or otherwise manipulated by hand. After they are used, disposable syringes and needles, scalpel blades, and other sharp items should be placed in puncture-resistant containers for disposal; the puncture-resistant containers should be located as close as practical to the use area. Large-bore reusable needles should be placed in a puncture-resistant container for transport to the reprocessing area.

4. Although saliva has not been implicated in HIV transmission, to minimize the need for emergency mouth-to-mouth resuscitation, mouthpieces, resuscitation bags, or other ventilation devices should be available for use in areas in which the need for resuscitation is predictable.

5. Health-care workers who have exudative lesions or weeping dermatitis should refrain from all direct patient care and from handling patient-care equipment until the condition resolves.

6. Pregnant health-care workers are not known to be at greater risk of contracting HIV infection than health-care workers who are not pregnant; however, if a health-care worker develops HIV infection during pregnancy, the infant is at risk of infection resulting from perinatal transmission.

Table 28.4 DRUGS USED TO TREAT OPPORTUNISTIC INFECTIONS IN HIV-INFECTED PATIENTS

Etiologic Agent/Clinical Manifestation	Drugs Commonly Used Generic (Trade) Name	Classification of Drug	Common Side Effects
Protozoans			
Pneumocystis carinii pneumonia	Pentamidine (Pentam)	Antiprotozoal	Hypotension; hypoglycemia/ hyperglycemia; nausea/vomiting; nephrotoxicity
	Dapsone (Avlosulfon)	Anti-infective; antileprosy agent	Nausea/vomiting; anorexia; fever; hemolytic anemia
	Trimethoprim/ sulfamethoxazole (Septra, Bactrim)	Anti-infective	Nausea/vomiting; anorexia; rash; agranulocytosis; Stevens-Johnson syndrome
Toxoplasma encephalitis	Pyrimethamine (Daraprim)	Anti-infective	Anorexia; vomiting; glossitis, skin rash; folic acid deficiency
Isospora enteritis	Trimethoprim/ sulfamethoxazole (Septra, Bactrim)	Anti-infective	(Same as pneumocystis)
Fungi			
Candida stomatitis, esophagitis	Nystatin (Nilstat, Mycostatin)	Antifungal agent, anti-infective	Nausea/vomiting; diarrhea; gastric distress
	Clotrimazole (Mycelex troches)	Antifungal agent, anti-infective	Nausea/vomiting; diarrhea; gastric distress
	Ketoconazole (Nizoral)	Antifungal agent, anti-infective	Nausea/vomiting; diarrhea; headache; dizziness
Cryptococcosis histoplasmosis coccidioidomycosis	Amphotericin B (Fungizone)	Antifungal agent, anti-infective, antibiotic	Nausea/vomiting; fever; diarrhea; tinnitis; chills; blurred vision; hypokalemia; seizures
Bacteria			
Mycobacterium tuberculosis	Isoniazid (INH)	Antituberculosis; anti-infective	Nausea/vomiting; anorexia; fever; malaise; peripheral neuropathy; blurred vision
Salmonellosis	Ampicillin (Omnipen, Polycillin)	Anti-infective, antibiotic	Anaphylaxis; serum sickness; bone marrow depression; nausea/ vomiting; epigastric distress; diarrhea
	Trimethoprim/ sulfamethoxazole (Septra, Bactrim)	Anti-infective	(Same as pneumocystis)
	Chloramphenicol (Chloromycetin)	Anti-infective, antibiotic	Bone marrow depression; nausea/ vomiting; diarrhea; headache; confusion; abdominal distention
Viruses			
Cytomegalovirus	Ganciclovir (Cytovene)	Antiviral	Neutropenia; thrombocytopenia; malaise; nausea/vomiting; fever; tremor
Herpes simplex Herpes zoster	Acyclovir (Zovirax)	Antiviral	Dizziness; headache; diarrhea; Nausea/vomiting; anorexia; abdominal pain
Malignancies			
Kaposi's sarcoma Non-Hodgkin's lymphoma	Bleomycin (Blenoxane)	Antineoplastic; antibiotic	Headache; confusion; nausea/vomiting; diarrhea; weight loss; pneumonitis
	Doxorubicin (Adriamycin)	Antineoplastic, antibiotic	Myocardial toxicity; leukopenia; fever; chills; nausea/vomiting; thrombocytopenia; stomatitis

(continued)

Table 28.4 CONTINUED			
Etiologic Agent/Clinical Manifestation	**Drugs Commonly Used Generic (Trade) Name**	**Classification of Drug**	**Common Side Effects**
	Etoposide (VePesid)	Antineoplastic	Nausea/vomiting; anorexia; diarrhea; leukopenia; thrombocytopenia; alopecia; bronchospasm
	Vincristine (Oncovin)	Antineoplastic	Nausea/vomiting; alopecia; peripheral neuropathy; constipation; polyuria; ptosis; fever; headache; ataxia
Kaposi's sarcoma	Alpha-interferons (Intron-A; Roferon-A)	Antineoplastic, antiviral	Flulike syndrome; fatigue; weakness; Nausea/vomiting; diarrhea; anorexia; leukopenia; neutropenia; alopecia
	Vinblastine (Velban)	Antineoplastic	Nausea/vomiting; diarrhea; anorexia; leukopenia; agranulocytosis; alopecia
Non-Hodgkins lymphoma	Cyclophosphamide (Cytoxan)	Antineoplastic	Nausea/vomiting; anorexia; diarrhea; leukopenia; neutropenia; alopecia amenorrhea
	Cytarabine (Ara-C)	Antineoplastic	Headache; neurotoxicity; nausea/vomiting; diarrhea; conjuctivitis; leukopenia; thrombocytopenia; rash; fever
	Methotrexate (Folex, Mexate)	Antineoplastic	Headache; blurred vision; nausea/vomiting; diarrhea; leukopenia; thrombocytopenia; alopecia; hepatotoxicity; gastrointestinal ulceration and hemorrhage; stomatitis

Source: Adapted from Kovacs & Masur (1988); Deglin et al. (1991); Durham & Cohen (1991); Flaskerud & Ungvarski (1992); Wong, 1990.

Because of this risk, pregnant health-care workers should be especially familiar with and strictly adhere to precautions to minimize the risk of HIV transmission.

Implementation of universal blood and body-fluid precautions for *all* patients eliminates the need for use of the isolation category of 'Blood and Body Fluid Precautions' previously recommended by the CDC for patients known or suspected to be infected with bloodborne pathogens. Isolation precautions (e.g., enteric or tuberculosis) should be used as necessary if associated conditions, such as infectious diarrhea or tuberculosis, are diagnosed or suspected."

Hospice Care

Hospice is a program that provides palliative and supportive care to meet the special needs arising out of the physical, psychosocial, spiritual, social, and economic stresses that are experienced during the final stages of illness and during bereavement (Lemus, 1990). Various models of hospice exist, including freestanding institutions that provide both inpatient and home care; those affiliated with hospitals in which hospice services are provided within the hospital setting; and hospice organizations that provide home care only. Historically, the hospice movement in the United States has evolved mainly as a system of home-based care.

Candace and Walter (1988) state:

"The goal of hospice care is to enable persons who are dying to function optimally, in spite of the devastating effects of their physical condition, by preventing pain and other symptoms, anticipating and minimizing the side effects of drugs and fatigue, and allowing control and independent decision making by the patient and [significant others] of caregivers."

The National Hospice Organization (1979) has published guidelines for standards of care that are directed at the hospice program concept. These standards of care are presented in Table 28.5.

Table 28.5 NATIONAL HOSPICE ORGANIZATION STANDARDS OF A PROGRAM OF CARE

1. Appropriate therapy is the goal of hospice care.
2. Palliative care is the most appropriate form of care when cure is no longer possible.
3. The goal of palliative care is the prevention of distress from chronic signs and symptoms.
4. Admission to a hospice program of care is dependent on patient and family needs.
5. Hospice care consists of a blending of professional and nonprofessional services.
6. Hospice care considers all aspects of the lives of patients and their families as valid areas of therapeutic concern.
7. Hospice care is respectful of all patient and family belief systems and will employ resources to meet the personal philosophical, moral, and religious needs of patients and their families.
8. Hospice care provides continuity of care.
9. A hospice-care program considers the patient and the family together as the unit of care.
10. The patient's family is considered to be a central part of the hospice-care team.
11. Hospice-care programs seek to identify, coordinate, and supervise persons who can give care to patients who do not have a family member available to take on the responsibility of giving care.
12. Hospice care for the family continues into the bereavement period.
13. Care is available 24 hours a day, 7 days a week.
14. Hospice care is provided by an interdisciplinary team.
15. Hospice programs will have structured and informal means of providing support to staff.
16. Hospice programs will be in compliance with the Standards of the National Hospice Organization and the applicable laws and regulations governing the organization and delivery of care to patients and families.
17. The services of the hospice program are coordinated under a central administration.
18. The optimal control of distressful symptoms is an essential part of a hospice-care program requiring medical, nursing, and other services of the interdisciplinary team.
19. The hospice-care team will have:
   a. A medical director on staff
   b. Physicians on staff
   c. A working relationship with the physicians
20. Based on patients' needs and preferences as determining factors in the setting and location for care, a hospice program provides inpatient care and care in the home setting.
21. Education, training, and evaluation of hospice services is an ongoing activity of a hospice-care program.
22. Accurate and current records are kept on all patients.

Source: NHO (1979).

Hospice follows a multidisciplinary team approach to provide care for the individual with AIDS in the familiar surroundings of the home environment. The multidisciplinary team consists of nurses, attendants (homemakers, home health aides), physicians, social workers, volunteers, and other health-care workers from other disciplines as required for individual patients (Martin, 1986).

Candace and Walter (1988) identify seven components on which the hospice approach is based. They include the multidisciplinary team, pain and symptom management, emotional support to patient and family, pastoral and spiritual care, bereavement counseling, 24-hour on-call nurse/counselor, and staff support. These are the ideal, and not all hospice programs may include all of these services.

MULTIDISCIPLINARY TEAM

Nurses A registered nurse usually acts as case manager for care of hospice patients. The nurse assesses the patient's and family's needs, establishes the goals of care, supervises and assists caregivers, evaluates care, serves as patient advocate, and provides educational information as needed to patient, family, and caregivers. He or she also provides physical care when needed, including IV therapy.

Attendants These individuals are usually the members of the team who spend the most time with the patient. They assist with personal care as well as all activities of daily living. Without these daily attendants, many AIDS patients would be unable to spend their remaining days in their home. Attendants may be noncertified and provide basic housekeeping services; they may be certified nursing assistants who assist with personal care or licensed vocational or practical nurses who provide more specialized care, such as dressing changes or tube feedings (Lewis, 1988).

Physicians The patient's primary physician, as well as the hospice medical consultant, have input into the care of the AIDS hospice patient. Orders may continue to come from the primary physician, while pain and symptom management may come from the hospice consultant. Ideally, these physicians attend weekly patient care conferences and provide inservice education for hospice staff as well as others in the medical community.

Social Workers The social worker assists the patient and family members with psychosocial issues, including those associated with the diagnosis of AIDS and its prognosis, financial issues, legal needs, and bereavement concerns. The social worker provides information on community resources from which patient and family may receive support and assistance. Some of the functions of the nurse and social worker may overlap at times.

Trained Volunteers Volunteers are vital to the hospice concept. They provide services that may otherwise be financially impossible. They are specially selected and extensively trained, and provide such services as transportation, companionship, respite care, recreational activities, light housekeeping, and in general are sensitive to the needs of families in stressful situations (Martin, 1990a).

Rehabilitation Therapists Physical therapists may assist hospice patients in an effort to minimize physical disability. They may assist with strengthening exercises, and provide assistance with special equipment needs. Occupational therapists may help the debilitated patient learn to accomplish activities of daily living as independently as possible. Other consultants, such as speech therapists, may be called upon for the patient with special needs.

Dietitian A nutritional consultant may be helpful to the AIDS patient who is experiencing nausea and vomiting, diarrhea, anorexia, and weight loss. A nutritionist can ensure that the patient is receiving the proper balance of calories and nutrients.

Counseling Services The hospice patient may require the services of a psychiatrist or psychologist if there is a history of mental illness, or if AIDS-related dementia or depressive syndrome has become evident. The AIDS patient with a history of substance abuse may benefit from the services of a substance abuse counselor to provide assistance in dealing with these special needs.

PAIN AND SYMPTOM MANAGEMENT

Improved quality of life at all times is a primary goal of hospice care. Thus, a major intervention for all caregivers is to ensure that the patient is as comfortable as possible, whether experiencing pain or nausea, vomiting, and diarrhea, which are commonly associated with the AIDS patient.

EMOTIONAL SUPPORT

Members of the hospice team encourage patients and families to discuss the eventual outcome of the disease process. Some individuals find discussing issues associated with death and dying uncomfortable, and if so, their decision is respected. However, honest discussion of these issues provides a sense of relief for some people, and they are more realistically prepared for the future. It may even draw some patients and families closer together during this stressful time.

PASTORAL AND SPIRITUAL CARE

Hospice philosophy supports the individual's right to seek guidance or comfort in the spiritual practices most suited to that person (Martin, 1990). Treatment team members must be aware and accepting of the fact that many AIDS patients seek spiritual support from various alternatives to traditional Western religions or spiritual practices. In the gay population, this may be partly due to the rejection they have experienced from some traditional religious organizations. The hospice team members provide assistance to the patient in obtaining the spiritual support and guidance for which he or she expresses a preference.

BEREAVEMENT COUNSELING

Hospice provides a service to surviving family members or significant others following the death of their loved one. This is usually provided by a bereavement counselor, but when one is not available, volunteers with special training in bereavement care may be of service. A grief support group may be helpful for the bereaved and provide a safe place for them to discuss their own fears and concerns about the death of a loved one (Martin, 1990).

TWENTY-FOUR-HOUR ON-CALL

The standards of care set forth by the National Hospice Organization state that care shall be available 24 hours a day, 7 days a week. A nurse or counselor is usually available either by phone or for home visits around the clock. The knowledge that emotional or physical support is available at any time, should it be required, provides considerable support and comfort to significant others or family caregivers.

STAFF SUPPORT

Team members (all who work closely and frequently with the patient) often experience emotions similar to those of the person with AIDS or their family/significant others. They may experience anger, frustration, or fears of contagion or of death and dying, all of which must be addressed through staff support groups, team conferences, time off, and adequate and effective supervision (Martin, 1990). Burnout is a common problem among hospice staff. Stress can be reduced, trust enhanced, and team functioning more effective if lines of communication are kept open between all members (medical director through volunteer), if information is readily accessible through staff conferences and inservice education, and if staff know they are appreciated and feel good about what they are doing (Candace & Walter, 1988).

SUMMARY

Acquired immunodeficiency syndrome is likely to be one of this century's major killers. The disease is the terminal end of a continuum of syndromes identified by HIV infection. The continuum begins with the acute response that occurs when the individual is initially infected with the virus, and progresses to a period of asymptomatic infection that may last for as long as 10 years. Advanced stages of the disease present with lymphadenopathy, neurological involvement, opportunistic infections, HIV wasting syndrome, malignancies, and finally death.

The HIV invades the T4 cells (normal range 600/mm^3 to 1200/mm^3) until in the very advanced stage of the disease the individual may have fewer than 10/mm^3. Examples of opportunistic infections that attack the body of an individual with AIDS include PCP, candidiasis, histoplasmosis, CMV, EBV, *M. tuberculosis*, and salmonellosis. Many of these were rarely observed before the AIDS epidemic. Common malignancies associated with AIDS include KS and non-Hodgkin's lymphoma. Any infectious or other disease process can prove fatal to an individual with AIDS whose immune system is so severely depressed.

Approximately 70 percent to 95 percent of AIDS patients develop a syndrome called ADC, which is thought to be the most common CNS complication of HIV infection. Cognitive, motor, and behavioral processes are affected to a point at which the individual may become totally vegetative.

Transmission of HIV infection is via three major routes: sexual, bloodborne, and perinatal. Sexual transmission can occur through any activity in which there is an exchange of body fluids with an infected individual. Although most sexual transmission in the past has occurred within the homosexual population, increasing numbers of cases are occurring from heterosexual contact. Bloodborne transmission can occur when an individual is transfused with blood or blood products that have been contaminated with HIV. Other modes of bloodborne transmission include sharing of contaminated needles by IV drug users and accidental sticks with contaminated needles by health-care workers. Perinatal transmission occurs in infants born to HIV-infected women through exposure to maternal blood and vaginal secretions during delivery. It can also occur transplacentally and through infant feeding with breast milk.

This chapter discussed delivery of care to the HIV/AIDS patient via the steps of the nursing process. Background assessment data included a description of the predisposing factors as well as symptomatology associated with various aspects of the disease. Nursing diagnoses and a plan of care for the patient with HIV/AIDS were presented, along with outcome criteria and guidelines for evaluation of nursing care. Other treatment modalities including pharmacology, universal precautions, and hospice care were discussed.

REVIEW QUESTIONS
Self-Examination/Learning Exercise

*Select the answer that is **most** appropriate for each of the following questions.*

Situation: Joe is a 34-year-old homosexual man. He and his partner were both tested and found to be HIV positive 8 years ago. His partner died 2 years ago. Joe had taken care of him until his death. Joe has seen his primary physician, who is admitting him to the hospital with a loss of 15 lb in the past 2 weeks, fever, night sweats, persistent diarrhea, and enlarged cervical, axillary, and inguinal lymph nodes. His laboratory T4 count is 400/mm³. Oral candidiasis (thrush) is evident upon examination. This is his third hospitalization in 15 months. He previously had a diagnosis of PGL.

1. Opportunistic infections are common in AIDS patients with T4 counts at 400/mm³ or below. Laboratory results show that Joe has enteritis from the protozoan *Isospora*. The physician is likely to order which medication for Joe?
   a. Pentamidine (Pentam)
   b. Amphotericin B (Fungizone)
   c. Isoniazid (INH)
   d. Trimethoprim-sulfamethoxazole (Septra)

2. Oral candidiasis presents with which of the following symptoms?
   a. Bleeding gums
   b. Dry, cracking lips
   c. White patches on the oral mucosa
   d. Blisters on the tongue

3. What type of organism is *Candida*?
   a. Fungus
   b. Protozoan
   c. Bacterium
   d. Virus

4. Joe's physician prescribed the antiviral agent AZT for him 5 years ago. What is the rationale behind administration of this medication?
   a. It cures HIV infection.
   b. It prevents the HIV-infected person from getting other viruses.
   c. It slows down the progression from HIV infection to full-blown AIDS.
   d. It prevents entry of HIV into the CNS.

5. In providing nursing care for Joe, which of the following interventions would be most appropriate for preventing tranmission to the caregiver?
   a. Wear a gown to carry in Joe's food tray
   b. Do not recap Joe's medication injection needles
   c. Wear a mask when changing the linen on Joe's bed
   d. Wear gloves to change the bag on Joe's continuous IV fluids

6. Which of the following interventions would be most appropriate for prevention of infection to Joe?
   a. Allow only one staff person to provide care for Joe.
   b. Place Joe in protective isolation.
   c. Put a "no visitors" sign on Joe's door.
   d. Wash hands before entering Joe's room.

7. Joe is discharged from the hospital after 2 weeks. Which of the following would be appropriate to teach Joe and his caregivers?
   a. Joe should cook all vegetables and fruits before eating them.
   b. Joe should abstain from all sexual activities.
   c. Joe should refrain from exercising due to weakness and fatigue.
   d. Joe should not kiss anyone on the mouth.

8. Fourteen months later Joe is readmitted. He has lost a great deal more weight. He is unable to take nourishment by mouth and has apparent

difficulty breathing. He has numerous raised, purplish lesions over his body. The physician diagnoses advanced visceral KS with obstruction of the upper gastrointestinal tract and tumors in his lungs. What might be the most probable medical intervention for Joe?
a. Chemotherapy with vinblastine
b. Surgery to remove the obstructive tumors
c. Radiation therapy for the dermal lesions
d. Bone marrow transplant to restore the immune system

9. Joe's condition continues to deteriorate and he is transferred to hospice care. The primary goal of hospice care is:
a. to assist with legal and financial problems of long-term care and dying.
b. to provide quality of life for the terminally ill person until death occurs.
c. to assist family and significant others through their loved one's dying process.
d. to fulfill the emotional and spiritual needs of the patient and family/significant others.

10. Which of the following is *NOT* necessarily true about hospice care?
a. Joe's family will be able to call someone from hospice on a 24-hour basis.
b. Hospice services to Joe and his family will be discontinued upon Joe's death.
c. Joe will be allowed to remain in his home during his terminal illness.
d. Psychiatric services may be provided through the hospice program if deemed necessary.

REFERENCES

Abrams, D. (1988). The pre-AIDS syndromes. *Infectious Disease Clinics of North America, 2*(2), 343–351.

Abrams, D. (1990). Definition of ARC. In P. T. Cohen, M. A. Sande, & P. A. Volberding (Eds.), *The AIDS knowledge base.* Waltham, MA: The Medical Publishing Group.

AIDS Update. (November, 1989). *Caring, 8*(11), 50.

Allen, J. R. & Curran, J. W. (1988). Prevention of AIDS and HIV-Infection: Needs and priorities for epidemiologic research. *Am J Public Health, 78,* 381–386.

Andiman, R. M. & Leicht, S. S. (1988). Herpes zoster on the increase. *Patient Care, 22*(8), 71–92.

Berger, J. R. et al. (1987). Progressive, multifocal leukoencephalopathy associated with human immunodeficiency virus infection: A review of the literature with a report of sixteen cases. *Ann Intern Med, 107*(1), 78–87.

Biggar, R. J. (1990). Cancer in acquired immunodeficiency syndrome: An epidemiological assessment. *Seminars in Oncology, 17,* 251–260.

Candace, R. & Walter, M. (1988). The hospice approach to care. In A. Lewis (Ed.), *Nursing care of the person with AIDS/ARC.* Rockville, MD: Aspen Publishers, Inc.

Carpenito, L. J. (1991). Acquired immunodeficiency syndrome. In *Nursing care plans and documentation.* Philadelphia: JB Lippincott.

Centers for Disease Control. (1991, April). *AIDS Weekly Surveillance Report.* Atlanta: United States AIDS Program.

Centers for Disease Control. (1991, June 7). The HIV/AIDS epidemic: The first ten years. *Morbidity and Mortality Weekly Report, 40,* 357.

Centers for Disease Control. (1990, November). HIV/AIDS surveillance report, pp. 1–18.

Centers for Disease Control. (1987, August 21). Recommendations for prevention of HIV transmission in health care settings. *Mobidity and Mortality Weekly Report, 36*(2S), 1–18.

Centers for Disease Control. (1986a, May 23). Classification system for human T-lymphotropic virus type III/lymphadenopathy-asociated virus infections. *Morbidity and Mortality Weekly Report, 35*(20), 1–5.

Centers for Disease Control. (1986b). Apparent transmission of human T-lymphotrophic virus type

III/lymphadenopathy-associated virus from a child to a mother providing health care. *Morbidity and Mortality Weekly Report, 35,* 76–79.

Christ, G. H., Siegel, K. & Moynihan, R. T. (1988). Psychosocial issues: Prevention and treatment. In V. T. DeVita, S. Hellman, & S. A. Rosenberg. (Eds.), *AIDS: Etiology, diagnosis, treatment, and prevention* (2nd ed.). Philadelphia: JB Lippincott.

Centers for Disease Control. (1981, June 5). Pneumocystic Pneumonia. Morbidity and Mortality Weekly Report, (30), 205.

Cohen, F. L. (1991a). The etiology and epidemiology of HIV infection and AIDS. In J. D. Durham & F. L. Cohen, *The person with AIDS: Nursing perspectives.* New York: Springer.

Cohen, F. L. (1991b). The clinical spectrum of HIV infection and its treatment. In J. D. Durham & F. L. Cohen (Eds.), *The person with AIDS: Nursing perspectives.* New York: Springer.

Cook, G. C. (1987). Opportunistic parasitic infections associated with the acquired immune deficiency syndrome (AIDS): Parasitology, clinical presentation, diagnosis and management. *Q J Med, 65,* 967–983.

Crowe, S. M. & McGrath, M. S. (1990). Acute HIV infection. In P. T. Cohen, M. A. Sande, & P. A. Volberding. (Eds.), *The AIDS knowledge base.* Waltham, MA: The Medical Publishing Group.

Des Jarlais, D. C. et al. (1988). HIV infection and intravenous drug use: Critical issues in transmission dynamics, infection outcomes, and prevention. *Rev Infect Dis, 10*(1), 151–158.

Dilley, J. (1990). Psychosocial impact of AIDS: Overview. In P. T. Cohen, M. A. Sande, & P. A. Volderbing (Eds.), *The AIDS knowledge base.* Waltham, MA: The Medical Publishing Group.

Dilley, J. et al., (1990). Altered mental states: Clinical syndromes and diagnosis. In Cohen et al. (Eds.), *The AIDS knowledge base.* Waltham, MA: The Medical Publishing Group.

Donegan, E. (1990). Transmission of HIV in blood products. In P. T. Cohen, M. A. Sande, & P. A. Volderbing. (Eds.), *The AIDS knowledge base.* Waltham, MA: The Medical Publishing Group.

Durham, J. D. & Cohen, F. L. (Eds.). (1991). *The person with AIDS: Nursing perspectives* (2nd ed.). New York: Springer.

Essex, M. (1988). Origins of AIDS. In V. T. DeVita, S. Hellman, & S. A. Rosenberg. (Eds.), *AIDS: Etiology, diagnosis, treatment, and prevention.* Philadelphia: JB Lippincott.

Essex, M. et al. (1984). Seroepidemiology of HTLV in relation to immunosuppression and the acquired immunodeficiency syndrome. In R. C. Gallo et al. (Eds.), *Human T-cell leukemia viruses.* Cold Spring Harbor, NY: Cold Spring Harbor Press.

Flaskerud, J. H. (1992a). Overview: HIV disease and nursing. In J. H. Flaskerud & P. J. Ungvarski (Eds.), *HIV/AIDS: A guide to nursing care* (2nd ed.). Philadelphia: WB Saunders.

Flaskerud, J. H. (1992b). Cofactors of HIV and public health education. In J. H. Flaskerud & P. J. Ungvarski (Eds.), *HIV/AIDS: A guide to nursing care* (2nd ed.). Philadelphia: WB Saunders.

Gallo, R. C. et al. (1983). Isolation of human T-cell leukemia virus in acquired immune deficiency syndrome (AIDS). *Science, 220,* 865.

Gallo, R. C. et al. (1984). Frequent detection and isolation of cytopathic retroviruses (HTLV-III) from patients with AIDS and at risk for AIDS. *Science, 224,* 500–502.

Gallo, R. C. et al. (1986). Origins of human T-lymphotropic viruses. *Nature, 320,* 219.

Gershon, R. R. M., Vlahov, D., & Nelson, K. E. (1990). The risk of transmission of HIV-1 through non-percutaneous, non-sexual modes. A review. *AIDS, 4,* 645–650.

Glaser, J. B. et al. (1985). Recurrent *Salmonella typhimurium* bacteremia associated with the acquired immunodeficiency syndrome. *Ann Intern Med, 102,* 189.

Grady, C. (1992). HIV disease: Pathogenesis and treatment. In J. H. Flaskerud & P. J. Ungvarski (Eds.), *HIV/AIDS: A guide to nursing care* (2nd ed.). Philadelphia: WB Saunders.

Greenspan, J. S. et al. (1985). Replication of Epstein-Barr virus within the epithelial cells of oral "hairy" leukoplakia, an AIDS-associated lesion. *N Engl J Med, 313,* 1564.

Haverkos, H. W. & Edelman, R. (1988). The epidemiology of acquired immunodeficiency syndrome among heterosexuals. *J Am Med Assoc, 260,* 1922–1929.

Heyer, D. M. et al. (1990). HIV-related Kaposi's sarcoma. In P. T. Cohen, M. A. Sande, & P. A. Volderbing. (Eds.), *The AIDS knowledge base.* Waltham, MA: The Medical Publishing Group.

Israelski, D. M. & Remington, J. S. (1988). Toxoplasmic encephalitis in patients with AIDS. *Infectious Disease Clinics of North America, 2*(2), 429–445.

Jacobs, J. L. et al. (1985). Salmonella infections in patients with the acquired immunodeficiency syndrome. *Ann Intern Med, 102,* 86.

Karan, L. D. (1989). AIDS prevention and chemical dependence treatment needs of women and their children. *J Psychoactive Drugs, 21*(4), 395–399.

Kovacs, J. A. & Masur, H. (1988). Opportunistic infections. In V. T. DeVita, S. Hellman, & S. A. Rosenberg. (Eds.), *AIDS: Etiology, diagnosis, treatment and prevention* (2nd ed.). Philadelphia: JB Lippincott.

Krigel, R. L. & Friedman-Kien, A. E. (1988). Kaposi's sarcoma in AIDS: Diagnosis and treatment. In V. T. DeVita, S. Hellman, & S. A. Rosenberg. (Eds.), *AIDS: Etiology, diagnosis, treatment, and prevention* (2nd ed.). Philadelphia: JB Lippincott.

Landesman, S. H., Ginzburg, H. M., & Weiss, S. H. (1985). The AIDS epidemic. *N Engl J Med, 312,* 521–525.

Lane, H. & Fauci, A. (1985). Immunologic abnormalities in the acquired immunodeficiency syndrome. *Ann Rev Immunol, 3,* 477–500.

Lemus, E. (1990). Definition and standards of hospice care. In P. T. Cohen, M. A. Sande, & P. A. Volderbing. (Eds.), *The AIDS knowledge base.* Waltham, MA: The Medical Publishing Group.

Lewis, A. (Ed.). (1988). *Nursing care of the person with AIDS/ARC.* Rockville, MD: Aspen Publishers.

Martin, J. (1986). The AIDS home care and hospice program: A multidisciplinary approach to caring for persons with AIDS. *Am J Hospice Care, 3,* 35–37.

Martin, J. (1990). Psychosocial and spiritual concerns. In P. T. Cohen, M. A. Sande & P. A. Volderbing. (Eds.), *The AIDS knowledge base.* Waltham, MA: The Medical Publishing Group.

Maury, W., Potts, B. J., & Rabson, A. B. (1989). HIV-1 infection of first-trimester and term human placental tissue: A possible mode of maternal-fetal transmission. *J Infect Dis, 160,* 583–588.

Meyer, C. (1991). Nursing and AIDS: A decade of caring. *AJN. 191*(12), 26–31.

Najera, R. et al. (1984). Human immunodeficiency virus and related retroviruses. *West J Med, 147,* 694–701.

National Hospice Organization. (1979). *Standards of a program of care.* McLean, VA: National Hospice Organization.

Navia, B. A., Jordon, B. D., & Price, R. W. (1985). The AIDS dementia complex: I: Clinical features. *Ann Neurol, 19*(6), 517.

Navia, B. A. & Price, R. W. (1986). Central and peripheral nervous system complications of AIDS. *Clinics in Immunology and Allergy, 6*(3), 543–558.

Nokes, K. M. (1992). HIV infection in women. In J. H. Flaskerud & P. J. Ungvarski (Eds.), *HIV/AIDS: A guide to nursing care* (2nd ed.). Philadelphia: WB Saunders.

Osmond, D. (1990a). Definitions and codes for HIV infection and AIDS. In P. T. Cohen, M. A. Sande, & P. A. Volderbing. (Eds.), *The AIDS knowledge base.* Waltham, MA: The Medical Publishing Group.

Osmond, D. (1990b). Progression to AIDS in persons testing seropositive for antibody to HIV. In P. T. Cohen, M. A. Sande, & P. A. Volderbing. (Eds.), *The AIDS knowledge base.* Waltham, MA: The Medical Publishing Group.

Osmond, D. (1990c). AIDS in Africa. In P. T. Cohen, M. A. Sande, & P. A. Volderbing. (Eds.), *The AIDS knowledge base.* Waltham, MA: The Medical Publishing Group.

Osmond, D. (1990d). Sexual transmission of HIV infection: Overview, homosexual, and heterosexual. In P. T. Cohen, M. A. Sande, & P. A. Volderbing. (Eds.), *The AIDS knowledge base.* Waltham, MA: The Medical Publishing Group.

Osmond, D. & Moss, A. R. (1989). The prevalence of HIV infection in the United States: A reappraisal of the Public Health Service estimate. In P. Volberding & M. A. Jacobson (Eds.), *AIDS clinical review 1989.* New York: Marcel Dekker.

Perdew, S. (1990). *Facts about AIDS: A guide for health care providers.* Philadelphia: JB Lippincott.

Peterman, T. A. et al. (1987). Estimating the risk of transfusion-associated acquired immune deficiency syndrome and human immunodeficiency virus infection. *Transfusion, 27,* 371–374.

Price, R. W. & Brew, B. (1988). The AIDS dementia complex. *J Infect Dis, 158,* 1079–1083.

Rogers, M. F. et al. (1983). National case-control study of Kaposi's sarcoma and *Pneumocystis carinnii* pneumonia in homosexual men: Part 2, laboratory results. *Ann Intern Med, 99,* 151.

Roitt, I, Brostoff, J., & Male, D. (1989). *Immunology* (2nd ed.). St. Louis: CV Mosby.

Rosenberg, Z. & Fauci, A. (1989). The immunopathogenesis of HIV infection. *Adv Immunol, 47,* 377–431.

Scanlon, V. C. & Sanders, T. (1991). *Essentials of anatomy and physiology.* Philadelphia: F. A. Davis.

Scitovsky, A. A. (1989). The cost of AIDS: An agenda for research. *Health Policy, 11,* 197–208.

Siegel, F. P. et al. (1981). Severe acquired immunodeficiency syndrome in male homosexuals manifested by chronic perianal ulcerative *Herpes simplex* lesions, *N Engl J Med, 305,* 1439.

Steckelberg, J. & Cockerill, F. (1988). Serological testing for human immunodeficiency virus antibodies. *Mayo Clin Proc, 63,* 373–380.

Steis, R. & Broder, S. (1985). AIDS: A general overview. In V. T. DeVita, S. Hellman, & S. A. Rosenberg. (Eds.), *AIDS: Etiology, diagnosis, treatment, and prevention* Philadelphia: JB Lippincott.

Sweet, D. (1992, April 4). AIDS information: Understanding the disease. Continuing education conference: On psychosocial aspects of HIV/AIDS, University of Kansas School of Medicine, Wichita.

Ungvarski, P. J. (1992). Nursing management of the adult client. In J. H. Flaskerud & P. J. Ungvarski (Eds.), *HIV/AIDS: A guide to nursing care.* Philadelphia: WB Saunders.

Valente, P. & Main, E. (1990). Role of the placenta in perinatal transmission of HIV. *Obstetrics and Gynecology Clinics of North America, 17*(3), 607–616.

Volberding, P. A. (1990a). Other cancers in HIV-infected patients. In P. T. Cohen, M. A. Sande, & P. A. Volderbing. (Eds.), *The AIDS knowledge base*. Waltham, MA: The Medical Publishing Group.

Volberding, P. A. (1990b). Clinical applications of antiviral therapy: Use of zidovudine. In Cohen et al. (Eds.), *The AIDS knowledge base*. Waltham, MA: The Medical Publishing Group.

Wofsy, C. B. et al. (1986). Isolation of AIDS associated retrovirus from genital secretions of women with antibodies to the virus. *Lancet, 1*, 527–529.

Wolcott, D. L., Dilley, J. W., & Mitsuyasu, R. T. (1989). Psychiatric aspects of acquired immune deficiency syndrome. In H. I. Kaplan & B. J. Sadock (Eds.), *Comprehensive textbook of psychiatry* (Vol. 2) (5th ed.). Baltimore: Williams & Wilkins.

Wong, R. J. (1990). HIV-related pharmacology. In P. T. Cohen, M. A. Sande, & P. A. Volderbing. (Eds.), *The Aids knowledge base*. Waltham, MA: The Medical Publishing Group.

World Health Organization. (1990, April 30). *AIDS/HIV Record, 4*(1), 10.

World Health Organization. (1990, November 2). Acquired immunodeficiency syndrome. *Weekly Epidemiological Record, 65*(44), 337–344.

Yarchoan, R. & Broder, S. (1988). Pharmacologic treatment of HIV infection. In V. T. DeVita et al. (Eds.), *AIDS: Etiology, diagnosis, treatment, and prevention* (2nd ed.). Philadelphia: JB Lippincott.

BIBLIOGRAPHY

Barnes, D. M. (1986). Grim projections for AIDS epidemic. *Science, 232*, 1589–1590.

Barrick, B. (1990). AIDS: Light at the end of a decade. *AJN, 90*(11), 36–40.

Brennan, L. (1988, April). The battle against AIDS. *Nursing 88*, 60–64.

Centers for Disease Control. (1991, July 12). Recommendations for preventing transmission of human immunodeficiency virus and hepatitis B virus to patients during exposure-prone invasive procedures. *Morbidity and Mortality Weekly Report, 40*(8), 1–9.

Chaisson, R. E. (1990). Transmission of HIV in intravenous drug users. In Cohen et al. (Eds.), *The AIDS knowledge base*. Waltham, MA: The Medical Publishing Group.

Cohen, P. T., Sande, M. A., & Volberding, P. A. (Eds.). (1990). *The AIDS knowledge base*. Waltham, MA: The Medical Publishing Group.

Craig, D. An AIDS update: The challenge. *The Kansas Nurse, 65*(1), 1–3.

Deglin, J. H., Vallerand, A. H., & Russin, M. M. (1991). *Davis's drug guide for nurses* (2nd ed.). Philadelphia: FA Davis.

DeVita, V. T., Hellman, S., & Rosenberg, S. A. (Eds.). (1988). *AIDS: Etiology, diagnosis, treatment, and prevention* (2nd ed.). Philadelphia: JB Lippincott.

Fitzhugh, Z. & Shubin, S. (1989, October). Caring for AIDS patients: The stress will be on you. *Nursing 89*, pp 43–46.

Graham, L. L. & Cates, J. A. (1992). How to reduce the risk of HIV infection for the seriously mentally ill. *J Psychosoc Nurse, 30*(6), 9–13.

Kopp, M. Preparing the person with AIDS for discharge: A nursing directive. *The Kansas Nurse, 65*(1), 6–7.

Lee, S. (1990). Women and children and HIV infection. *The Kansas Nurse, 65*(1), 8–9.

Marshall, P. & Green-Nigro, C. (1992). AIDS dilemma: Risk vs. responsibility in nursing care. *The Kansas Nurse, 67*(5), 3–5.

Martin, E. (1990). The pathophysiology of AIDS. *The Kansas Nurse, 65*(1), 4–5.

Martin, J. (1990a). A multidisciplinary team approach to case management. In P. T. Cohen, M. A. Sande, & P. A. Volderbing. (Eds.), *The AIDS knowledge base*. Waltham, MA: The Medical Publishing Group.

Nokes, K. M. (1989). Nursing care plan for the AIDS patient. Wichita, KS: Nursing Staff, Hospice, Inc.

Regan-Kubinski, M. J. & Sharts-Engel, N. (1992). The HIV-infected woman. *J Psychosoc Nurs, 30*(2), 11–15.

Saunders, J. M. & Buckingham, S. L. (1988, July). When the depression turns deadly: Suicidal AIDS patients. *Nursing 88*, pp. 59–64.

Scherer, P. (1990). How AIDS attacks the brain. *AJN, 90*(1), 44–53.

Swanson, B., Cronin-Stubbs, D., & Colletti, M. A. (1990). Dementia and depression in persons with AIDS: Causes and care. *J Psychosoc Nurs, 28*(10), 33–39.

Taber, J. (1989). Nutrition in HIV infection. *AJN, 89*(11), 1446–1453.

Trudeau, M. (1991). Dark nights and bright mornings: Caring for a person with AIDS. *J Psychosoc Nurs, 29*(1), 32–33.

Weaver, K. (1991). Reversible malnutrition in AIDS. *AJN, 91*(9), 24–31.

Wofsy, C. B. (1990). Transmission of HIV by prostitutes and prevention of spread. In P. T. Cohen, M. A. Sande, & P. A. Volderbing. (Eds.), *The AIDS knowledge base*. Waltham, MA: The Medical Publishing Group.

29

VICTIMS OF VIOLENCE

KEY TERMS
battering
child sexual abuse
compounded rape reaction
controlled response pattern
cycle of battering
date rape
emotional injury
emotional neglect
expressed response pattern
incest
marital rape
physical neglect
rape
safe house/shelter
sexual exploitation of a child
silent rape reaction
statutory rape

OBJECTIVES

After reading this chapter, the student will be able to:

1. Discuss historical perspectives associated with woman battering, child abuse, and sexual assault.
2. Describe epidemiological statistics associated with woman battering, child abuse, and sexual assault.
3. Discuss characteristics of victims and victimizers.
4. Identify predisposing factors to victimization.
5. Describe the physical and psychological effects on the victim of woman battering, child abuse, and sexual assault.
6. Identify nursing diagnoses, goals of care, and appropriate nursing interventions for care of victims of woman battering, child abuse, and sexual assault.
7. Evaluate nursing care of victims of woman battering, child abuse, and sexual assault.
8. Discuss various modalities relevant to the treatment of victims of violence.

INTRODUCTION

Violence—the victimization of one person by another—is on the rise in this society (Gest, 1989). Books, newspapers, movies, and television inundate their audiences with stories of "man's inhumanity to man" (no gender bias intended).

According to statistics, a woman is battered in this country every 15 seconds (Meierhoffer, 1992). Battering is the single most common cause of injury to women, more frequent than auto accidents, muggings, and rape combined ("The Battered Woman," 1989). Rape is vastly underreported in the United States; however, West (1983) reported that in 1980 the rate of reported rape and attempted rape in the United States was 18 times higher than the corresponding rate for England and Wales.

An increase in the incidence of child abuse and related fatalities has also been documented. In 1989, there were 1,237 child abuse and neglect-related fatalities reported to child protection service agencies in the United States (National Committee for the Prevention of Child Abuse, 1990).

Violence affects all populations equally. Abuse occurs among all races, religions, economic classes, ages, and educational backgrounds (Meierhoffer, 1992). The phenomenon is cyclical in that many victimizers were victims of abuse themselves as children.

This chapter discusses battering of partners, child abuse (including neglect), and sexual assault. Factors that predispose individuals to commit acts of violence against others, as well as the physical and psychological effects on the victims, are examined.

Nursing of individuals who have experienced violent behavior from others is presented within the context of the nursing process. Various treatment modalities are described.

HISTORICAL PERSPECTIVES

Family violence is not a new problem; in fact, it is probably as old as humankind and has been documented back to Biblical times (Dickstein & Nadelson, 1989). In the United States, spouse and child abuse arrived with the Puritans; however, it was not until 1973 that public outrage initiated an active movement against the practice. Child abuse became a mandatory reportable occurrence in the United States in 1968, and in 1985, elder abuse was added to federal statutes as H.R. 1674 (Dickstein & Nadelson, 1989). These events have made it possible for individuals who once felt powerless to stop the abuse against themselves to come forward and seek advice, support, and protection.

Historically, violence against women partners (whether in a married or unmarried intimate relationship) has not been considered a social problem but rather a fact of life. Most individuals have been socialized within their cultural context to the acceptance of violence against women in their relationships (Martin, 1988).

From Roman times until the beginning of the 20th century, the notion existed of women as the personal property of men. Very early on in Roman times, women were purchased as brides, and their status, as well as that of their children, was closely akin to that of slaves. Violent beatings and even death occurred if women acted contrary to their husbands' wishes or to the social code of the time (Martin, 1988).

Women have historically been socialized to view themselves as sexual objects. Even in early Biblical times, women were expected to subjugate themselves to the will of men, and those who refused were seen as witches (Hays, 1964). Rape is largely a crime against women, although men and children also fall victim to this heinous act. Rape is the extreme manifestation of the domination of one individual over another. Rape is a ritual of power (Moynihan, 1988).

During the Puritan era, "spare the rod and spoil the child" was a theme supported by the Bible. Children were considered to be property of their parents and could be treated accordingly. Harsh treatment by parents was justified by the belief that severe physical punishment was necessary to maintain discipline, transmit educational decisions, and expel evil spirits (Hamilton, 1988). Change began in the mid-19th and early 20th century with the child welfare movement and the passage of laws for the protection of children.

Historical examination reveals an inclination toward violence among human beings from very early in civilization. Little has changed, for violence permeates every aspect of today's society, the victims of which are inundating the health-care system. Campbell (1992) states:

> "[Violence] is costing all of us, in terms of health-care dollars, human potential squandered, and even in terms of our personal sense of security and well being."

PREDISPOSING FACTORS

What predisposes individuals to be violent? No one really knows for sure. A number of theories have been espoused. A brief discussion of ideas as-

sociated with biological, psychological, and sociocultural views is presented here.

Biological Theories

NEUROPHYSIOLOGICAL INFLUENCES

Various components of the neurological system in both humans and animals have been implicated in both the facilitation and inhibition of aggressive impulses. The limbic system in particular appears to be involved, as stimulation of this area in humans has produced evidence of hostile and aggressive responses (Goldstein, 1974). Higher brain centers also play an important role in humans by constantly interacting with the aggression centers.

BIOCHEMICAL INFLUENCES

Goldstein (1974) suggests that various neurotransmitters (e.g., epinephrine, norepinephrine, dopamine, acetylcholine, and serotonin) may play a role in the facilitation and inhibition of aggressive impulses. This theory is consistent with the "fight or flight" arousal described by Selye (1956) in his theory of the response to stress.

GENETIC INFLUENCES

Various genetic components related to aggressive behavior have been investigated. Some studies have linked increased aggressiveness with selective inbreeding in mice, suggesting the possibility of a direct genetic link. Another genetic characteristic that was thought at one time to have some implication for aggressive behavior was the genetic karyotype XYY. A large sampling of XYY individuals was found in men who had been institutionalized for criminal activity (Kaplan & Sadock, 1985). The evidence linking this chromosomal aberration to aggressive and deviant behavior has not been firmly established.

DISORDERS OF THE BRAIN

Organic brain syndromes associated with various cerebral disorders have been implicated in the predisposition to aggressive and violent behavior (Mark & Ervin, 1970). Tumors in the brain, particularly in the areas of the limbic system and the temporal lobes; trauma to the brain, resulting in cerebral changes; diseases, such as encephalitis (or medications that may effect this syndrome) and epilepsy, particularly temporal lobe epilepsy, have all been implicated.

Psychological Theories

PSYCHOANALYTIC THEORY

The psychoanalytic theorists imply that unmet needs for satisfaction and security result in an underdeveloped ego and a poor self-concept. May (1972) suggests that aggression and violence supply this individual with a dose of power and prestige that boosts the self-image and validates a significance to his or her life that is lacking. Other psychoanalytic theorists have also supported the hypothesis that aggression and violence are the overt expressions of powerlessness and low self-esteem (Horney, 1939; Kaplan, 1975; Bromberg, 1965).

LEARNING THEORY

Children learn to behave by imitating their role models, which in most instances are their parents. Models are more likely to be imitated when they are perceived as prestigious, influential, or when the behavior is followed by positive reinforcement (Bandura, 1969). Children may have an idealistic perception of their parents during the very early developmental stages, but as they mature, may begin to imitate the behavior patterns of their teachers, friends, and others. Individuals who were abused as children or whose parents disciplined with physical punishment are more likely to behave in a violent manner as adults (Owens & Straus, 1975).

Adults and children alike model many of their behaviors after individuals whom they observe on television and in movies. Unfortunately, modeling can result in maladaptive as well as adaptive behavior, particularly when children view heroes triumphing over villains by using violence. Some theorists believe that those individuals who have a biological influence toward aggressive behavior are more likely to be affected by external models than those without this predisposition (Laborit, 1978).

Sociocultural Theories

SOCIETAL INFLUENCES

Although they agree that perhaps some biological and psychological aspects are influencial, social scientists believe that aggressive behavior is primarily a product of one's culture and social structure (West, 1979).

American society was essentially founded upon a general acceptance of violence as a means of solving problems. Wrightsman (1977) states:

> "One explanation for the origin of revolutions and other collective violence uses the concept of relative deprivation. When a group suffers an abrupt shift away from past increases in socioeconomic and political satisfaction, its members are more likely to revolt or express collective violence."

Indeed, the United States was populated by the violent actions of one group of people over another. Since that time, much has been said and written, and laws have been passed, regarding the civil rights of all people. However, to this day it is unlikely that many people would disagree that the statement "All men are created equal" remains a hypocrisy in our society.

Societal influences may also contribute to violence when individuals come to realize that their needs and desires cannot be met through conventional means (Toch, 1979). When poor and oppressed people find that they have limited access through legitimate channels, they are more likely to resort to delinquent behaviors in an effort to obtain desired ends (Cloward & Ohlin, 1960). This lack of opportunity and subsequent delinquency may even contribute to a subculture of violence within a society (Hepburn, 1971).

APPLICATION OF THE NURSING PROCESS

Background Assessment Data

BATTERED WOMEN

Definition   A number of definitions have been set forth for the term *battering*. Martin (1988) offers the following:

> "The infliction of physical pain or injury with the intent to cause harm which may include slaps,

punches, biting, and hair pulling, but in frequency or occurrence generally involves more serious assaults including choking, kicking, breaking bones, stabbing, or shooting; or forcible restraint which may include locking in homes or closets, being tied or handcuffed."

Campbell and Humphreys (1984) define wife abuse as:

". . . severe, deliberate and repeated demonstrable physical violence inflicted on a woman by a man with whom she has or has had an intimate relationship."

Finally, a definition by Sadock (1989) states:

"Spouse abuse is the mistreatment or misuse of one spouse by the other. It can range from shoving and pushing to choking and severe battering, involving broken limbs, broken ribs, internal bleeding, and brain damage. The face and breasts are the most frequent sites of assault, and when the woman is pregnant, her husband often batters her abdomen."

Profile of the Victim   Battered women represent all age, racial, religious, cultural, educational, and socioeconomic groups (Dickstein & Nadelson, 1989). They are married and single, housewives and business executives. According to Walker (1979), many women who are battered have low self-esteem. They commonly adhere to feminine sex-role stereotypes and typically accept self-blame for the batterer's actions. Feelings of guilt, anger, fear, and shame are common. They may be isolated from family and support systems.

Approximately one-half of the women who are in such relationships grew up in violent homes and may have left those homes, even married, at a very young age in an effort to escape the violence (Sadock, 1989). The battered woman views her relationship as male dominant, and as the battering continues, her ability to see the options available to her and to make decisions concerning her life (and possibly that of her children) decreases. Walker (1979) relates the phenomenon of *learned helplessness* to the woman's progressing inability to act in her own behalf. Learned helplessness occurs when an individual comes to understand that regardless of his or her behavior, the outcome is unpredictable, and usually undesirable.

Profile of the Victimizer   Men who batter are generally characterized as persons with low self-esteem. Pathologically jealous, they present a "dual personality," exhibit limited coping ability, and have severe stress reactions (Hutchings, 1988). The typical abuser is very possessive, and perceives his spouse as a possession. He becomes very threatened when she shows any sign of independence or attempts to share herself and her time with others. Small children are often ignored by the abuser; however, they too become the target of abuse as they grow older, and particularly when they attempt to protect their mother from abuse (Sadock, 1989).

The abusing man wages a continuous campaign of degradation against his female partner. He insults and humiliates her and everything she does at every opportunity. He strives to keep her isolated from others and totally dependent upon him. He demands to know where she is at every moment, and when she tells him he questions her honesty. He achieves power and control through intimidation.

A Cycle of Battering   Walker (1979), in her work with battered women and analysis of their battering relationships, has identified a cycle of predictable behaviors that are repeated over time. The behaviors can be discriminated into three distinct phases that vary in time and intensity both within the same relationship and between different couples.

Phase I. The Tension-Building Phase   During this phase, the woman senses that the man's tolerance for frustration is declining. Anger occurs with little provocation, although after lashing out at her he may be quick to apologize. The woman may become very nurturing and compliant, anticipating his every whim in an effort to prevent his anger from escalating. She may just try to stay out of his way.

Minor battering incidents may occur during this phase, and in a desperate effort to avoid more serious confrontations, the woman accepts the abuse as legitimately directed toward her. She denies her anger and rationalizes his behavior: "I need to do better." "He's under so much stress at work." "It's the alcohol. If only he didn't drink." She assumes the guilt for the abuse, even reasoning that perhaps she did deserve the abuse as her aggressor suggests.

The minor battering incidents continue and the

tension mounts as the woman waits for the impending explosion to occur. The abuser becomes fearful that his partner will leave him. His jealousy and possessiveness increase, and he uses threats and brutality to keep her in his captivity. Battering incidents become more intense, after which the woman becomes less and less psychologically capable of restoring equilibrium. She withdraws from him, which he misinterprets as rejection, further escalating his anger toward her. Phase I may last for a few weeks to many months or even years.

Phase II. The Acute Battering Incident This phase is the most violent and the shortest—usually lasting up to 24 hours. It usually begins with the batterer justifying his behavior to himself. However, by the end of the incident, he cannot understand what has happened—only that in his rage he has lost control over his behavior.

The incident may begin with the batterer wanting to "just teach her a lesson." In some instances, the woman may intentionally provoke the behavior. Having come to a point in Phase I in which the tension is unbearable, long-term battered women know that once the acute phase is behind them, things will be better.

During Phase II, women feel their only option is to find a safe place to hide from the batterer. The beating is severe, and many women are able to describe the violence in great detail, almost as if a dissociation from their bodies had occurred. The batterer generally minimizes the severity of the violence. Help is usually sought only in the event of severe injury or if the woman fears for her life or that of her children.

Phase III. Calm, Loving, Respite (Honeymoon) Phase In this phase, the batterer becomes extremely loving, kind, and contrite. He promises that the violence will never recur and begs her forgiveness. He is afraid she will leave him, and uses every bit of charm he can muster to ensure this does not happen. He believes he can now control his behavior, and besides, since he has now "taught her a lesson, she won't act up again."

He plays upon her feelings of guilt, and she desperately wants to believe him. She wants to believe that he *can* change, and that she will no longer have to suffer abuse. During this phase, the woman is able to relive her original dream of ideal love and chooses to believe that *this* is what her man is *really* like.

This loving phase becomes the focus of her perception of the relationship. She bases her reason for remaining in the relationship on this magical, ideal phase, and hopes against hope that the previous phases will not be repeated. This hope is evident even in those women who have lived through a number of horrendous cycles.

Phase III usually lasts somewhere between the lengths of time associated with Phases I and II. However, it can be so short as to almost pass undetected. In most instances, the cycle all too soon begins again with renewed tensions and minor battering incidents. In an effort to "steal" a few precious moments of the Phase III kind of loving, the battered woman becomes a collaborator in her own abusive life-style.

Why Does She Stay? Probably the most frequent response that battered women give for staying is that they fear for their life and/or the lives of their children. As the battering progresses, the man gains power and control through intimidation and instilling fear with threats such as, "I'll kill you and the kids if you don't do as I say." (Smith, 1987b). Challenged by these threats and compounded by her low self-esteem and sense of powerlessness, the woman sees no way out. In fact, she may try to leave, only to return when confronted by her partner and the psychological power he holds over her. Moss (1991) lists the following other reasons for the woman's staying in the marriage:

1. Lack of a support network for leaving. Our society glorifies the position of marriage and family, and some women report that family members encourage them to stay in the relationship and "try to work things out."
2. Religious beliefs. Many religious organizations denounce divorce and encourage the cohesion of the family. Some women have reported that their clergy told them this was "their cross to bear."
3. Lack of financial independence to support herself and her children.

Martin (1988) states,

"While some women have limited access to 'legitimate' resources, such as cash, a supportive network of family or friends, or strong assertive and communication skills, to assist them in leaving an abusive partner, almost all battered women seek help from traditional institutions or systems. The medical, mental health, and criminal justice/legal systems are the traditional formal sources of assistance sought by battered women. Yet each of these systems has reflected the pervasive cultural myths and stereotypes about battering and have generally been unresponsive to the needs of battered women."

CHILD ABUSE

Erik Erikson (1963) has stated, "The worst sin is the mutilation of a child's spirit." Children are vulnerable and relatively powerless, and the effects of maltreatment are infinitely deep and long lasting. Child abuse is typically defined as any physical or emotional injury, physical or emotional neglect, or sexual act inflicted upon a child by a caregiver (Kansas Child Abuse Prevention Council [KCAPC], 1992).

Physical Injury Physical injury to a child includes any *nonaccidental* physical injury caused by the parent or caretaker. The most obvious way to detect it is by outward physical signs. However, behavioral indicators may also be evident.

Physical Signs Indicators of physical abuse may include any of the following (KCAPC, 1992; Tower, 1987);

1. Bruises, especially numerous bruises of different colors (indicating various stages of healing) over multiple parts of the body; bruises around the head and face
2. Bite marks; skin welts
3. Burns, such as:
   a. glove-like burns that indicate the hand has been immersed in hot liquid
   b. cigarette burns
   c. burns in the shape of an object such as a poker or iron
4. Fractures, scars, or serious internal injuries
5. Lacerations, abrasions, or unusual bleeding
6. Bald spots indicative of severe hair pulling

Behavioral Signs Following are common behavioral indicators of physical abuse (KCAPC, 1992; Tower, 1987). These behaviors alone do not necessarily indicate physical abuse.

1. Behavioral extremes, including very aggressive or demanding conduct

2. Fear of the parent or caretaker
3. Extreme rage or passivity and withdrawal
4. Apprehension when other children cry
5. Verbal reporting of abuse
6. Extreme hyperactivity, distractibility, or irritability
7. Disorganized thinking; self-injurious or suicidal behavior
8. Running away from home or engaging in illegal behavior such as drug abuse or stealing
9. Displaying severe depression, flashbacks (including hallucinatory experiences), and dissociative disorders
10. Cheating, lying, or low achievement in school
11. Inability to form satisfactory peer relationships
12. Wearing clothing that covers the body and that may be inappropriate for warm weather
13. Regressiveness; demonstrating age-inappropriate behavior

Emotional Injury Emotional injury involves a pattern of behavior on the part of the parent or caretaker that results in serious impairment of the child's social, emotional, or intellectual functioning. Examples of emotional injury include belittling or rejecting the child, ignoring the child, blaming the child for things over which he or she has no control, isolating the child from normal social experiences, and using harsh and inconsistent discipline. Behavioral indicators of emotional injury may include (KCAPC, 1992; Tower, 1987):

1. Age-inappropriate behaviors
2. Daytime anxiety and unrealistic fears
3. Sleep problems; nightmares
4. Behavioral extremes (e.g., overly happy or affectionate)
5. Social isolation
6. Self-destructive behavior
7. Inappropriate affect (e.g., laughing at something sad)
8. Vandalism, stealing, cheating, substance abuse
9. Rocking, thumb sucking, enuresis, or other habitual problems
10. Anorexia nervosa (especially in adolescents)

Neglect

Physical Neglect Physical neglect of a child refers to the failure on the part of the parent or caregiver to provide for that child's basic needs, such as food, clothing, shelter, medical/dental care, and supervision (KCAPC, 1992). Tower (1987) describes the following physical and behavioral characteristics associated with physical neglect of a child:

1. Clothing may be soiled and in need of repair; often fit is too small or too large; may be inappropriate for weather.
2. Always seems hungry; steals and hoards food from others
3. Often appears listless and tired
4. May demonstrate poor hygiene, with bad breath and body odor
5. Medical problems, such as infected sores, and dental problems, such as decayed or abscessed teeth, may be evident.
6. Delinquent behavior, such as stealing and vandalism
7. Poor school performance and attendance record
8. Poor peer relationships
9. May be emaciated or have distended abdomens indicative of malnutrition

Emotional Neglect Emotional neglect refers to a chronic failure by the parent or caretaker to provide the child with the hope, love, and support necessary for the development of a sound, healthy personality. The KCAPC (1992) identifies the following behavioral indicators of emotional neglect by the parent or caretaker of a child:

1. Ignoring the child's presence
2. Rebuffing attempts by the child to establish meaningful interaction
3. Ignoring the child's social, educational, recreational, and developmental needs
4. Denying the child opportunities to receive positive reinforcement.

Sexual Abuse of a Child

Various definitions of sexual abuse are available in the literature. Sanford (1980) defines child sexual abuse as "sexual involvement imposed upon a child by an adult who has greater power, knowledge, and resources."

The KCAPC (1992) provides the following definition for sexual abuse of a child:

"Sexual abuse is any sexual act, such as indecent exposure, improper touching to penetration (sexual intercourse) that is carried out with a child."

Included in the definition is *sexual exploitation of a child*, in which a child is induced or coerced into engaging in sexually explicit conduct for the purpose of promoting any performance, and *sexual abuse*, in which a child is being used for the sexual pleasure of an adult (parent or caretaker) or any other person.

Incest has been defined as sexual exploitation of a child under 18 years of age by a relative or a nonrelative who holds a position of trust in the family (Courtois, 1988).

Indicators of Sexual Abuse Towers (1987) and the KCAPC (1992) list the following indicators of child sexual abuse:

Physical Indicators:
1. Frequent urinary infections
2. Any venereal disease or gonorrhea infection of the throat
3. Difficulty or pain in walking or sitting
4. Foreign matter in the bladder, rectum, urethra, or vagina
5. Sleep problems (e.g., nightmares, insomnia)
6. Rashes or itching in the genital area; scratching the area a great deal or fidgeting when seated
7. Frequent vomiting

Behavioral Indicators:
1. Seductive behavior, advanced sexual knowledge for the child's age, promiscuity, prostitution
2. Expressing fear of a particular person or place
3. Compulsive masturbation, precocious sex play, excessive curiosity about sex
4. Sexually abusing another child
5. Appearance of an inordinate number of gifts or money from a questionable source
6. A drop in school performance or sudden nonparticipation in school activities
7. Sudden onset of enuresis
8. Excessive anxiety
9. Expression of low self-worth; verbalizations of being "damaged"
10. Excessive bathing
11. Runnning away from home
12. Suicide attempts

Characteristics of the Abuser A number of factors have been associated with adults who abuse or neglect their children. Many investigators agree that parents who abuse their children were likely abused as children themselves (Bradshaw, 1988; Berger, 1980; Sadock, 1989; Helfer, 1973). Other characteristics of abusive parents include retarded ego development (accounting for immaturity and poor impulse control), lack of knowledge of adequate childrearing practices, lack of empathy, and low self-esteem (Humphreys, 1984). Environmental factors that may be influential in the predisposition to child abuse include numerous stresses, poverty, social isolation, and an absence of adequate support systems. Although there appears to be some correlation between substance abuse and child abuse, the exact relationship is unclear (Humphreys, 1984).

The Incestuous Relationship A great deal of attention has been given to the study of father-daughter incest. Commonly, there is an impaired sexual relationship between the parents. Communication is ineffective, thereby preventing the father and mother from correcting their problems. The father is often domineering, impulsive, and physically abusing. The mother is commonly passive, submissive, and denigrates her role as wife and mother. She is often aware of, or at least strongly suspects, the incestuous behavior between the father and daughter but may believe in or be fearful of her husband's absolute authority over the family. She may deny that her daughter is being harmed and may actually be grateful that her husband's sexual demands are being met by someone other than herself.

Onset of the incestuous relationship typically occurs when the daughter is around 8 to 10 years of age and commonly begins with genital touching and fondling. In the beginning, the child may accept the sexual advances from her father as signs of affection and "specialness" (Mrazek, 1981). As the incestuous behavior continues and progresses, she becomes more bewildered, confused, and frightened, never knowing whether her father will be paternal or sexual in his interactions toward her (Sadock, 1989).

The relationship may become a love-hate situation on the part of the daughter. She continues to strive for the ideal father-daughter relationship but is fearful and hateful of the sexual demands he places on her. The mother may be alternately car-

ing and competitive as she witnesses the possessiveness and affections directed toward her daughter by her husband. Out of fear that his daughter may expose their relationship, the father may attempt to interfere with her normal peer relationships (Sadock, 1989).

Some fathers who participate in incestuous relationships may have unconscious homosexual tendencies and have difficulty in achieving a stable heterosexual orientation (Mrazek, 1981). On the other hand, some men have frequent sex with their wives and several of their own children, but they are unwilling to seek sexual partners outside the nuclear family because of a need to maintain the public facade of a stable and competent patriarch. Although the oldest daughter in a family is most vulnerable to becoming a participant in father-daughter incest (Mrazek, 1981), some fathers form sequential relationships with several daughters, each lasting for an extended period, often over many years (Sadock, 1989).

The Adult Survivor of Incest Several common characteristics have been identified in adult individuals who have experienced incest as children. Basic to these characteristics is a fundamental lack of trust that arises out of an unsatisfactory mother-child relationship. This inadequate relationship results in low self-esteem and a poor sense of identity (Steele & Alexander, 1981). Children of incest often feel trapped, for they have been admonished not to talk about the experience and may fear, even for their lives, if they are exposed. If they do muster the courage to report the incest, particularly to the mother, they are frequently not believed. This is confusing to the child, who is then left with a sense of self-doubt and the inability to trust his or her own feelings. Guilt is engendered as the child comes to realize that over the years he or she is being used by the parents in attempts to solve their own problems.

Childhood sexual abuse is likely to distort the development of a normal association of pleasure with sexual activity (Steele & Alexander, 1981). Peer relationships are often delayed, altered, inhibited, or perverted. In some instances, individuals who were sexually abused as children completely retreat from sexual activity and avoid all close interpersonal relationships throughout life. Other adult manifestations of childhood sexual abuse in women include diminished libido, vaginismus, nymphomania, and promiscuity. In men, impotence, premature ejaculation, exhibitionism, and compulsive sexual conquests are common (Steele & Alexander, 1981). Kreidler and Carlson (1991) report the results of various studies suggesting that adult survivors of incest are at risk for flashbacks, nightmares, drug and alcohol abuse, anxiety attacks, denial, avoidance, emotional numbing, prostitution, depression, suicide, feelings of powerlessness, guilt, victimization, eating and sleeping disorders, sexual dysfunction, problems with trust and nonsexual intimacy, and for being abusers themselves.

The conflicts experienced by sexually abused children associated with pain (either physical or emotional) and sexual pleasure are commonly manifested symbolically in adult relationships. Steel and Alexander (1981) state,

> "It is not uncommon to find women who were physically or sexually abused as children repeatedly involved as sexual or marital partners with men who abuse them physically or emotionally."

Adult survivors of incest who decide to come forward with their stories are commonly estranged from nuclear family members. They are blamed by family members for disclosing the family secret and often accused of overreacting to the incest. Frequently the estrangement becomes permanent when family members continue to deny the behavior, and the individual is accused of lying. Recently, a number of celebrities have come forward with stories of their childhood sexual abuse. Some have chosen to make the disclosure only after the death of their parents. Revelation of these past activities can be one way of contributing to the healing process for which incest survivors so desperately strive.

SEXUAL ASSAULT

Definitions   Over the years, a number of definitions have emerged regarding the crime of rape, but one theme is common: rape is an act of aggression, not passion. One author defines rape as the expression of power and dominance by means of sexual violence, most commonly by men over women, although men may also be rape victims (Hoff, 1985). Sexual assault is identified by the use of force and executed against the person's will. It occurs over a broad spectrum of experiences rang-

ing from the surprise attack by a stranger, to insistence on sexual intercourse by an acquaintance or spouse (Moynihan, 1988).

Date rape is a term applied to situations in which the rapist is known to the victim (Sadock, 1989). They may be out on a first date, may have been dating for a number of months, or merely be acquaintances or schoolmates. College campuses are the location for a staggering number of these types of rapes, which are for the most part not reported (Moynihan, 1988).

Marital rape has only recently become recognized as a legal category, in which a spouse may be held liable for sexual violence directed at a marital partner against that person's will. Historically, with societal acceptance of the concept of women as marital property, the legal definition of rape held an exemption within the marriage relationship. However, since the 1982 conviction of a Florida man for raping his wife, 25 states have eliminated this legal exemption of marital rape (Sadock, 1989).

Statutory rape is defined as unlawful intercourse between a man older than age 16 and a female younger than the age of consent (Sadock, 1989). The age of consent varies from state to state, and ranges from 14 to 21. A man who has intercourse with a woman under the age of consent can be arrested for statutory rape, even though the interaction is likely to have occurred between consenting individuals. The charges, when they occur, are usually brought by the young woman's parents.

Profile of the Victimizer   One of the older profiles of the individual who rapes has been described by Abrahamsen (1960), who identifies the rapist's mother as "seductive but rejecting." Macdonald (1971) also supports the mother-dominated childhood as influential. The behavior of the mother toward the son is described as overbearing, with seductive undertones. They share little secrets, and she rescues him when his delinquent acts create problems with others. She is quick to withdraw her "love" and attention when he goes against her wishes. Her rejection can be powerful and unyielding. She is domineering and possessive of the son, and this dominance often continues into his adult life. Macdonald (1971) states:

> "The seductive mother arouses overwhelming anxiety in her son with great anger which may be expressed directly toward her but more often is displaced onto other women. When this seductive

behavior is combined with parental encouragement of assaultive behavior, the setting is provided for personality development in the child which may result in sadistic, homicidal sexual attacks on women in adolescence or adult life."

Many rapists report growing up in abusive homes (Scully, 1990). Even when the parental brutality is discharged by the father, the anger may be directed toward the mother who did not protect her child from physical assault (Macdonald, 1971).

Statistics show that the greatest number of rapists are between the ages of 25 and 44. Fifty-one percent are white; 42 percent are black; and the remaining 7 percent come from all other races (Sadock, 1989). Many are either married or cohabiting at the time of their offenses (Scully, 1990). For those with previous criminal activity, the majority of their convictions are for crimes against property rather than against people. The majority of rapists do not have histories of mental illness.

The Victim Rape can occur at virtually any age. Sadock (1989) reports cases in which the victim was as young as 15 months old and as old as 82. The high-risk age group appears to be 16 to 24 years (Macdonald, 1971; Sadock, 1989). Seventy percent to seventy-five percent of rape victims are single women, and the attack frequently occurs in or close to the victim's own neighborhood.

Scully (1990), in a study of a prison sample of rapists, found that in "stranger rapes," victims were not chosen for any reason having to do with appearance or behavior, but simply because the victim happened to be in that place at that particular time. Scully states:

"The most striking and consistent factor in all the stranger rapes, whether committed by a lone assailant or a group, is the unfortunate fact that the victim was "just there" in a location unlikely to draw the attention of a passerby. Almost every one of these men said exactly the same thing, "It could have been any woman," and a few added that because it was dark, they could not even see what their victim looked like very well."

In her study, Scully found that 62 percent of the rapists used a weapon, most frequently a knife. The majority suggested that they used the weapon to terrorize and subdue the victim, but not to inflict serious injury. The presence of a weapon (real or perceived) appears to be the principal measure of the degree to which a woman resists her attacker.

Rape victims who present themselves for care shortly after the crime has occurred may likely be experiencing an overwhelming sense of violation and helplessness that is a continuation of the powerlessness and intimidation experienced during the rape (Hutchings, 1988). Burgess (1984) identifies two emotional patterns of response that may occur within hours after a rape and with which health-care workers may be confronted in the emergency department or rape crisis center. In the *expressed response* pattern, the victim expresses feelings of fear, anger, and anxiety through such behavior as crying, sobbing, smiling, restlessness, and tenseness. In the *controlled response* pattern, the feelings are masked or hidden, and a calm, composed, or subdued affect is seen.

The following manifestations may be evident in the subsequent days and weeks following the attack (Burgess, 1984):

1. Contusions and abrasions about various parts of the body
2. Headaches, fatigue, sleep-pattern disturbances
3. Stomach pains, nausea, and vomiting
4. Vaginal discharge and itching, burning upon urination, rectal bleeding and pain
5. Rage, humiliation, embarrassment, desire for revenge, self-blame
6. Fear of physical violence and death

The long-term effects of sexual assault depend to a great degree upon the individual's ego strength, social support system, and the way they are treated as victims (Burgess, 1984). Various long-term effects include increased restlessness, dreams and nightmares, and phobias (particularly those having to do with sexual interaction). A number of women report that it takes many years to get over the experience (Sadock, 1989). They describe a sense of vulnerability and a loss of control over their own lives. They feel defiled and unable to wash themselves clean, and some women are unable to remain living alone in their home or apartment.

Some victims develop a *compounded reaction*, in which additional symptoms such as depression and suicide, substance abuse, and even psychotic behaviors may be noted (Burgess, 1984). Still another variation has been called the *silent rape reaction*, in which the victim tells no one about the assault. Anxiety is suppressed, and the emotional burden may become overwhelming. The unresolved sexual trauma may not be revealed until the woman is forced to face another sexual crisis in her life that reactivates the previously unresolved feelings.

Nursing Diagnoses, Planning/Implementation

Nursing diagnoses are formulated from the data gathered during the assessment phase and with background knowledge regarding predisposing factors to the situation. Some common nursing diagnoses for victims of violence include:

> Rape-trauma syndrome related to sexual assault evidenced by verbalizations of the attack; bruises and lacerations over areas of body; severe anxiety.
>
> Powerlessness related to cycle of battering evidenced by verbalizations of abuse; bruises and lacerations over areas of body; fear for her safety and that of her children; verbalizations of no way to get out of relationship.
>
> Altered growth and development related to abusive family situation evidenced by sudden onset of enuresis, thumb sucking, nightmares, inability to perform self-care activities appropriate for age.

In Table 29.1, these nursing diagnoses are presented in a plan of care for the patient who has been a victim of violence. Goals of care and appropriate nursing interventions are included for each. Rationales are presented in italics.

OUTCOME CRITERIA

The following criteria may be used for measurement of outcomes in the care of victims of violence.

The Patient Who Has Been Sexually Assaulted:
1. Is no longer experiencing panic anxiety.
2. Demonstrates a degree of trust in the primary nurse.
3. Has received immediate attention to physical injuries.
4. Has initiated behaviors consistent with the grief response.

The Patient Who Has Been Physically Battered:
1. Has received immediate attention to physical injuries.
2. Verbalizes assurance of her immediate safety.
3. Discusses life situation with primary nurse.
4. Is able to verbalize choices available to her from which she may receive assistance.

The Child Who Has Been Abused:
1. Has received immediate attention to physical injuries.
2. Demonstrates trust in primary nurse by discussing abuse through the use of play therapy.
3. Is demonstrating a decrease in regressive behaviors.

Evaluation

Evaluation of nursing actions to assist victims of violence must be considered both on a short- and long-term basis.

Short-term evaluation may be facilitated by gathering information using the following types of questions. Has the individual been reassured of his or her safety? Is this evidenced by a decrease in panic anxiety? Have wounds been properly cared for and provision made for follow-up care? Have emotional needs been attended to? Has trust been established with at least one person to whom the patient feels comfortable relating the abusive incident? Have available support systems been identified and notified? Have options for immediate circumstances been presented?

Long-term evaluation may be conducted by health-care workers who have contact with the individual long after management of the immediate crisis. Is the individual able to conduct activities of daily living satisfactorily? Have physical wounds healed properly? Is the patient appropriately progressing through the behaviors of grieving? Is the patient free of sleep disturbances (nightmares, insomnia), psychosomatic symptoms (headaches, stomach pains, nausea/vomiting), regressive behaviors (enuresis, thumb sucking, phobias), and psychosexual disturbances? Is the individual free from problems with interpersonal relationships? Has the individual considered the alternatives for change in his or her personal life? Has a decision been made relative to the choices available? Is he or she satisfied with the decision that has been made?

Table 29.1 CARE PLAN FOR VICTIMS OF VIOLENCE

Nursing Diagnoses	Objectives	Nursing Interventions
Rape-trauma syndrome related to sexual assault evidenced by verbalizations of the attack; bruises and lacerations over areas of body; severe anxiety.	The patient will begin a healthy grief resolution, initiating the process of healing (both physically and psychologically).	Smith (1987a). relates the importance of communicating the following four phrases to the rape victim: 1) I am very sorry this happened to you. 2) You are safe here. 3) I am very glad you are alive. 4) You are not to blame. You are a victim. It was not your fault. Whatever decisions you made at the time of the victimization were the right ones because you are alive. *The woman who has been sexually assaulted fears for her life and must be reassured of her safety. She may also be overwhelmed with self-doubt and self-blame, and these statements instill trust and validate self-worth.* Explain every assessment procedure that will be conducted and why. Ensure that data collection is conducted in a caring, nonjudgmental manner *to decrease fear/anxiety and increase trust.* Ensure that the patient has adequate privacy for all immediate postcrisis interventions. Try to have as few people as possible providing the immediate care or collecting immediate evidence. *The post-trauma patient is extremely vulnerable. Additional people in the environment increase this feeling of vulnerability and serve to escalate anxiety.* Encourage the patient to give an account of the assault. Listen, but do not probe. *Nonjudgmental listening provides an avenue for catharsis that the patient needs to begin healing. A detailed account may be required for legal follow-up, and a caring nurse, as patient advocate, may help to lessen the trauma of evidence collection.* Discuss with the patient whom to call for support or assistance. Provide information about referrals for aftercare. *Because of severe anxiety and fear, the patient may need assistance from others during this immediate postcrisis period. Provide referral information in writing for later reference (e.g., psychotherapist, mental health clinic, community advocacy group).*
Powerlessness related to cycle of battering evidenced by verbalizations of abuse; bruises and lacerations over areas of body; fear for her safety and that of her children; verbalizations of no way to get out of relationship.	Patient will recognize and verbalize choices that are available to her and her children, thereby perceiving some control over her life situation.	In collaboration with physician, ensure that all physical wounds, fractures, and burns receive immediate attention. It is a good idea to take photographs if the victim will permit (Smith, 1987b, Burgess, 1990). *Patient safety is a nursing priority. Photographs may be called in as evidence if charges are filed.* Take the woman to a private area to do the interview. *If the patient is accompanied by the man who did the battering, she is not likely to be truthful about her injuries.* If she has come alone or with her children, assure her of her safety. Encourage her to discuss the battering incident. Ask questions about whether this has happened before, whether the abuser takes drugs, whether the woman has a safe place to go, and whether she is interested in pressing charges. *Some women*

(continued)

Table 29.1 CONTINUED		
Nursing Diagnoses	**Objectives**	**Nursing Interventions**
		will attempt to keep secret how their injuries occurred in an effort to protect the partner, or because they are fearful that the partner will kill them if they tell. Ensure that "rescue" efforts are not attempted by the nurse. Offer support, but remember that the final decision must be made by the patient. *Making her own decision will give the patient a sense of control over her life situation. Imposing judgments and giving advice are nontherapeutic.* Stress the importance of safety. Smith (1987b). suggests a statement such as, "Yes, it has happened. Now where do you want to go from here?" Burgess (1990). states, "The victim needs to be made aware of the variety of resources that are available to her. These may include crisis hot lines, community groups for women who have been abused, shelters, a variety of counseling opportunities (i.e., couples, individual, or group), and information regarding the victim's rights in the civil and criminal justice system." Following a discussion of these available resources, the woman may choose for herself. If her decision is to return to the marriage and home, this choice, too, must be respected. *Knowledge of available choices can serve to decrease the victim's sense of powerlessness, but true empowerment comes only when she chooses to use that knowledge for her own benefit.*
Altered growth and development related to abusive family situation evidenced by sudden onset of enuresis, thumb sucking, nightmares, inability to perform self-care activities appropriate for age.	Patient will develop trusting relationship with nurse and report how evident injuries were sustained. Negative regressive behaviors (enuresis, thumb sucking, nightmares). will diminish.	Perform complete physical assessment of the child. Take particular note of bruises (in various stages of healing), lacerations, and patient complaints of pain in specific areas. Do not overlook or discount the possibility of sexual abuse. Assess for nonverbal signs of abuse: aggressive conduct, excessive fears, extreme hyperactivity, apathy, withdrawal, age-inappropriate behaviors. *An accurate and thorough physical assessment is required to provide appropriate care for the patient.* Conduct an in-depth interview with the parent or adult who accompanies the child. Consider: If the injury is being reported as an accident, is the explanation reasonable? Is the injury consistent with the explanation? Is the injury consistent with the child's developmental capabilities? *Fear of imprisonment or loss of child custody may place the abusive parent on the defensive. Discrepancies may be evident in the description of the incident, and lying to cover up involvement is a common defense that may be detectable in an in-depth interview.* Use games or play therapy to gain child's trust. Use these techniques to assist in describing his or her side of the story. *Establishing a trusting relationship with an abused child is extremely difficult. They may not even want to be touched. These types of play activities can provide a nonthreatening environment that may enhance the child's attempt to discuss these*

(continued)

Table 29.1 CONTINUED		
Nursing Diagnoses	**Objectives**	**Nursing Interventions**
		painful issues (Celano, 1990). Determine whether nature of the injuries warrants reporting to authorities. Specific state statutes must enter into the decision of whether or not to report suspected child abuse. *A report is commonly made if there is reason to suspect that a child has been injured as a result of physical, mental, emotional, or sexual abuse (KCAPC, 1992). "Reason to suspect" exists when there is evidence of a discrepancy or inconsistency in explaining a child's injury. Most states require that the following individuals report cases of suspected child abuse: all health-care workers, all mental health therapists, teachers, child-care providers, firefighters, emergency medical personnel, and law enforcement personnel. Reports are made to the Department of Social and Rehabilitative Services or a law enforcement agency.*

TREATMENT MODALITIES

Crisis Intervention

The focus of the initial interview and follow-up with the patient who has been sexually assaulted is on the rape incident alone. Problems identified but unassociated with the rape are not dealt with at this time. The goal of crisis intervention is to aid victims to return to their previous life-style as quickly as possible (Burgess, 1990).

The patient should be involved in the intervention from the beginning. This promotes a sense of competency, control, and decision making. Because an overwhelming sense of powerlessness accompanies the rape experience, active involvement by the victim is both an affirmation of competency and the beginning of recovery (Moynihan, 1988). Crisis intervention is usually time limited, generally 6 to 8 weeks. If problems resurface beyond this time, the victim is referred for assistance from other agencies (e.g., long-term psychotherapy from a psychiatrist or mental health clinic).

During the crisis period, attention is given to coping strategies for dealing with the symptoms common to the posttrauma patient. Initially, the individual undergoes a period of disorganization during which there is difficulty making decisions, extreme or irrational fears, and general mistrust.

Observable manifestations may range from stark hysteria to expression of anger and rage to silence and withdrawal. Guilt and feelings of responsibility for the rape as well as numerous physical manifestations are common. The crisis counselor will attempt to help the victim draw upon previous successful coping strategies to regain control over his or her life.

If the patient is a victim of battering, the counselor ensures that various resources and options are made known to the victim so that she may make a personal decision regarding what she wishes to do with her life. Support groups provide a valuable forum for reducing isolation and learning new strategies for coping with the aftermath of physical or sexual abuse (Moynihan, 1988). Particularly for the rape victim, the peer support group provides a therapeutic forum for reducing the sense of isolation she may feel in the aftermath of predictable social and interpersonal responses to her experience. Moynihan (1988) states:

"Rape affects almost every aspect of the victim's life, emotional, physical and social, and influences her future level of functioning as well. The manner in which a victim is treated at the moment of disclosure has a profound effect on recovery. Thus, the victim whose request for help is responded to by skepticism and doubt may respond by withdrawing, and closing communications. Feelings of guilt and self-blame may be exaggerated, and significant long-term effects will almost predictably occur."

The Safe House or Shelter

Most major cities in the United States now have safe houses or shelters where a woman can go to be assured of protection for themselves and their children. These shelters provide a variety of services, and best of all the women receive emotional support from staff and from each other. Campbell (1984a) identifies the following services that most shelters provide: individual and group counseling; help with bureaucratic institutions such as the police, legal representation, and social services; child care and children's programming; and aid for the woman in making future plans, such as employment counseling and contact with housing authorities.

The shelters are usually run by a combination of professional and volunteer staff, including nurses, psychologists, lawyers, and others. Volunteers often include women who have been previously abused themselves.

Group work is an important part of the service of shelters. Women in residence will range from those in the immediate crisis phase to those who have progressed through a variety of phases of the grief process. Those newer members can learn a great deal from the women who have successfully resolved similar problems. Length of stay varies a great deal from individual to individual, depending upon a number of factors, such as outside support network, financial situation, and personal resources.

The shelter not only provides a haven of physical safety for the battered woman, but also promotes expression of the intense emotions she may be experiencing regarding her situation. A woman will commonly show symptoms of depression, extreme fears, or even violent expressions of anger and rage. In the shelter, she learns that these feelings are normal and that others have also experienced these same emotions in similar situations. She is allowed to grieve for that which has been lost and that which was expected but was not achieved. Help is provided in overcoming the tremendous guilt associated with self-blame. This is a difficult step for someone who has accepted responsibility for another's behavior over a long period.

New arrivals at the shelter are given time to experience the relief from the safety and security provided. Decisions are discouraged during the period of immediate crisis and disorganization. Once the woman's emotions have become more stable, planning for the future begins. Through information from staff and peers, she learns what resources are available to her within the community. Feedback is provided, but the woman makes her own decision about "where she wants to go from here." She is accepted and supported in whatever she chooses to do.

Family Therapy

Campbell (1984b) states, "Any family which uses physical punishment or any form of physical aggression can be considered at risk to become violent, because violence tends to escalate under stress." The focus of therapy with families who use violence is to help them develop democratic ways of solving problems. Steinmetz (1977) found that the more the family used democratic means of conflict resolution, the less likely they were to engage in physical violence. Families need to learn to deal with problems in ways that can produce mutual benefits for all concerned, rather than engaging in power struggles between family members.

Parents also need to learn more effective methods of disciplining children, aside from physical punishment. Methods that emphasize the importance of positive reinforcement for acceptable behavior can be very effective. Family members must be committed to consistent use of this behavior modification technique for it to be successful.

Teaching parents about expectations for various developmental levels may serve to alleviate some of the stress that accompanies these changes. Knowledge of what to expect from individuals at various stages of development may provide needed anticipatory guidance to deal with the crises commonly associated with these various stages.

Therapy sessions with all family members together may focus on problems with family communications. Members are encouraged to express honest feelings in a manner that is nonthreatening to other family members. Active listening, assertiveness techniques, and respect for the rights of others are taught and encouraged. Barriers to effective communication are identified and resolved.

Referrals to agencies that promote effective parenting skills may be made (e.g., Parent Effectiveness Training). Alternative agencies that may provide relief from the stress of parenting may also be considered. Examples include "Mom's Day Out" programs, sitter-sharing organizations, and day-care institutions. Support groups for abusive parents may also be helpful and assistance in locating or initiating such a group may be provided.

SUMMARY

This chapter provided a discussion of violence —the victimization of one person by another. The incidence of woman battering, child abuse, and sexual assault are all on the rise in this country, and all populations are equally affected.

Abuse of women and children began early in the development of this country, when these individuals were considered to be property of their hussbands and fathers, and physical violence toward them was considered acceptable. Women came to believe that they were deserving of any physical or sexual abuse they encountered.

Various factors have been theorized as influential in the predisposition to violent behavior. Physiological and biochemical influences within the brain have been suggested, as has the possibility of a direct genetic link. Organic brain syndromes associated with various cerebral disorders have been implicated in the predisposition to aggressive and violent behavior.

Psychoanalytical theorists relate the predisposition to violent behavior to underdeveloped ego and a poor self-concept. Learning theorists suggest that children imitate the violent behavior of their parents. This theory has been substantiated by studies that show that individuals who were abused as children or whose parents disciplined with physical punishment are more likely to behave in a violent manner as adults. Societal influences, such as general acceptance of violence as a means of solving problems, have also been implicated.

Battered women generally take blame for their situation. They were often reared in abusive families and come to expect this type of behavior. The battered woman often see no way out of their present situation and is encouraged by their social support network (family, friends, clergy) to remain in the abusive relationship.

Child abuse includes physical and emotional injury, physical and emotional neglect, and sexual abuse of a child. A child may experience many years of abuse without reporting it, out of fear of retaliation by the abuser. Some children report incest experiences to their mothers only to be rebuffed by them and told to remain secretive about the abuse. Adult survivors of incest often experience a number of physical and emotional manifestations relating back to the incestual relationship.

Sexual assault is identified as an act of aggression, not passion. Many rapists report growing up in abusive homes, and some theorists relate the predisposition to rape to a "seductive, but rejecting, mother." Rape is a crisis situation from which some women experience sequellae for many years. Flashbacks, nightmares, rage, physical symptoms, depression, and thoughts of suicide are common.

Nursing implementation with victims of violence was discussed in the context of the nursing process. Assessment data, nursing diagnoses, outcome criteria, appropriate nursing interventions with rationale, and standards for evaluation were presented. Additional treatment modalities were described, including crisis intervention with the sexual assault victim, safe shelter for battered women, and therapy for families who use violence.

Violence is emerging as a national crisis in this country. Nurses are in a unique position to intervene at the primary, secondary, and tertiary levels of prevention with victims of violence.

REVIEW QUESTIONS
Self-Examination/Learning Exercise

*Select the answer that is **most** appropriate for each of the following questions:*

Situation: Sharon is a 32-year-old woman who arrives at the emergency department with her three small children. She has multiple bruises around her face and neck. Her right eye is swollen shut.

1. Sharon says to the nurse, "I didn't want to come. I'm really okay. He only does this when he has too much to drink. I just shouldn't have yelled at him." The best response by the nurse would be:
   a. "How often does he drink too much?"
   b. "It is not your fault. You did the right thing by coming here."
   c. "How many times has he done this to you?"
   d. "He is not a good husband. You have to leave him before he kills you."

2. In the interview, Sharon tells the nurse, "He's been getting more and more violent lately. He's been under a lot of stress at work the last few weeks, and so he drinks a lot when he gets home. He always gets mean when he drinks. I was getting scared. So I just finally told him I was going to take the kids and leave. He got furious when I said that and began beating me with his fists." With knowledge about the cycle of battering, what does this situation represent?
   a. Phase I. Sharon was desperately trying to stay out of his way and keep everything calm.
   b. Phase I. A minor battering incident for which Sharon assumes all the blame.
   c. Phase II. The acute battering incident that Sharon provoked with her threat to leave.
   d. Phase III. The honeymoon phase where the husband believes that he has "taught her a lesson and she won't act up again."

3. The *priority* nursing intervention for Sharon in the emergency department is:
   a. tending to the immediate care of her wounds.
   b. providing her with information about a safe place to stay.
   c. administering the prn tranquilizer ordered by the physician.
   d. explaining how she may go about bringing charges against her husband.

4. Sharon goes with her children to stay at a women's shelter. She participates in group therapy and receives emotional support from staff and peers. She is made aware of the alternatives open to her. Nevertheless, she decides to return to her home and marriage. The best response by the nurse upon Sharon's departure is:
   a. "I just can't believe you have decided to go back to that horrible man."
   b. "I'm just afraid he will kill you or the children when you go back."
   c. "What makes you think things have changed with him?"
   d. "I hope you have made the right decision. Call this number if you need help."

Situation: Carol is a school nurse. Five-year-old Jana has been sent to her office complaining of nausea. She lies down on the office cot, but eventually vomits and soils her blouse. When Carol removes Jana's blouse to clean it, she notices that Jana has a number of bruises on her arms and torso. Some are bluish in color; others are various shades of green and yellow. She also notices some small scars. Jana's abdomen protrudes on her small, thin frame.

5. From the objective physical assessment, the nurse suspects that:
   a. Jana is experiencing physical and sexual abuse.
   b. Jana is experiencing physical abuse and neglect.
   c. Jana is experiencing emotional neglect.
   d. Jana is experiencing sexual and emotional abuse.

6. Carol tries to talk to Jana about her bruises and scars, but Jana refuses to say how she received them. Another way in which Carol may be able to obtain information from Jana is:
   a. have her evaluated by the school psychologist.
   b. tell her she may select a "treat" from the treat box (e.g., sucker, balloon, junk jewelry) if she answers the nurse's questions.
   c. explain to her that if she answers the questions, she may stay in the nurse's office and not have to go back to class.
   d. use a "family" of dolls to role play Jana's family with her.

7. Carol strongly suspects that Jana is being abused. What would be the best way for Carol to proceed with this information?
   a. As a health-care worker, report the suspicion to Social and Rehabilitative Services.
   b. Check Jana again in a week and see if there are any new bruises.
   c. Meet with Jana's parents and ask them how Jana got the bruises.
   d. Initiate paperwork to have Jana placed in foster care.

Situation: Lana is an 18-year-old freshman at the state university. She was extremely flattered when Don, a senior star football player, invited her to a party. On the way home, he parked the car in a secluded area by the lake. He became angry when she refused his sexual advances. He began to beat her and finally raped her. She tried to fight him, but his physical strength overpowered her. He dumped her in the dorm parking lot and left. The dorm supervisor rushed Lana to the emergency department.

8. Lana says to the nurse, "It's all my fault. I shouldn't have allowed him to stop at the lake." The nurse's best response is:
   a. "Yes, you're right. You put yourself in a very vulnerable position when you allowed him to stop at the lake."
   b. "You are not to blame for his behavior. You obviously made some right decisions, because you survived the attack."
   c. "There's no sense looking back now. Just look forward, and make sure you don't put yourself in the same situation again."
   d. "You'll just have to see that he is arrested so he won't do this to anyone else."

9. The priority nursing intervention with Lana would be:
   a. help her to bathe and clean herself up.
   b. provide physical and emotional support during evidence collection.
   c. provide her with a written list of community resources for rape victims.
   d. discuss the importance of a follow-up visit to evaluate for sexually transmitted diseases.

10. Lana is referred to a support group for rape victims. She has been attending regularly for 6 months. From this group, she has learned that the most likely reason Don raped her was:
    a. He had had too much to drink at the party and was not in control of his actions.
    b. He had not had sexual relations with a girl in many months.
    c. He was predisposed to become a rapist by virtue of the poverty conditions under which he was reared.
    d. He was expressing power and dominance by means of sexual aggression and violence.

REFERENCES

Abrahamsen D. (1960). *The psychology of crime.* New York: John Wiley & Sons.

Bandura, A. (1969). Social-learning theory of identificatory processes. In D. A. Goslin (Ed.), *Handbook of socialization theory and research.* Chicago: Rand McNally.

The battered woman: Breaking the cycle of abuse. (1989, June 15). *Emerg Med Clin North Am.* pp, 104–115.

Berger, A. (1980, Fall). The child abusing family: I. Methodological issues and parent-related characteristics of abusing families. *Am J Fam Therapy, 8*(3), 53–66.

Bradshaw, J. (1988). *Bradshaw on: The family.* Deerfield Beach, FL: Health Communications.

Bromberg, W. (1965). *Crime and the mind.* New York: Macmillan.

Burgess, A. (1984). Intra-familial sexual abuse. In J. Campbell & J. Humphreys (Eds.), *Nursing care of victims of family violence.* Reston, VA: Reston Publishing.

Burgess, A. (1990). Victims of family violence: Incest and battering. In A. W. Burgess (Ed.), *Psychiatric nursing in the hospital and the community* (5th ed.). Norwalk, CT: Appleton & Lange.

Campbell, J. (1984a). Nursing care of abused women. In J. Campbell & J. Humphreys (Eds.), *Nursing care of victims of family violence.* Reston, VA: Reston Publishing.

Campbell, J. (1984b). Nursing care of families using violence. In J. Campbell, & J. Humphreys (Eds.), *Nursing care of victims of family violence.* Reston, VA: Reston Publishing.

Campbell, J. (1992). Violence demands nursing solutions. *The American Nurse, 24*(4), 4.

Campbell, J. & Humphreys, J. (1984). *Nursing care of victims of family violence.* Reston, VA: Reston Publishing.

Celano, M. P. (1990). Activities and games for group psychotherapy with sexually abused children. *Int J Group Psychother 40*(4), 419–428.

Cloward, M. & Ohlin, L. (1960). *Delinquency and opportunity.* Glencoe, IL: Free Press.

Courtois, C. (1988). *Healing the incest wound.* New York: WW Norton.

Dickstein, L. J. & Nadelson, C. C. (Eds.). (1989). *Family violence: Emerging issues of a national crisis.* Washington, DC: American Psychiatric Press.

Erikson, E. H. (1963). *Childhood and society* (2nd ed.). New York: WW Norton & Co.

Gest, T. (1989, July 31). Victims of crime. *U.S. News and World Report, 107,* 16–19.

Goldstein, M. (1974). Brain research and violent behavior. *Arch Neurol, 30*(1), 1–35.

Hamilton, J. (1988). Child abuse and family violence. In N. Hutchings (Ed.), *The violent family: Victimizatin of women, children, and elders.* New York: Human Sciences Press.

Hays, H. R. (1964). *The dangerous sex: The myth of feminine evil.* New York: Putnam.

Helfer, R. E. (1973, April). The etiology of child abuse. *Pediatr, 51*(4), 777–779.

Hepburn, J. (1971, May). Subcultures, violence, and the subculture of violence: An old rut or a new road. *Criminology, 9,* 87–98.

Hoff, L. A. (1985). Rape and sexual assault: Evaluation and treatment. *Surgeon General's workshop on violence and public health* (DHHS Publication No. HRS-D-MC86-1). Washington DC: US Government Printing Office.

Horney, K. (1939). *New ways in psychoanalysis.* New York: WW Norton.

Humphreys, J. (1984). Child abuse. In J. Campbell & J. Humphreys (Eds.), *Nursing care of victims of family violence.* Reston, VA: Reston Publishing.

Hutchings, N. (Ed.). (1988). *The violent family: Victimization of women, children, and elders.* New York: Human Sciences Press.

Kansas Child Abuse Prevention Council (1992). *A guide about child abuse and neglect.* Wichita, KS: National Committe for Prevention of Child Abuse and Parents Anonymous, Inc.

Kaplan, H. B. (1975). *Self-attitudes of deviant behavior.* Pacific Palisades, CA: Goodyear Publishing.

Kaplan, H. I. & Sadock, B. J. (1985). *Modern synopsis of comprehensive textbook of psychiatry* (4th ed.). Baltimore: Williams and Wilkins.

Kreidler, M. C. & Carlson, R. E. (1991). Breaking the incest cycle: The group as a surrogate family. *J Psychosoc Nurs, 29*(4), 28–32.

Laborit, H. (1978). The biological and sociological mechanisms of aggression. *Int Soc Science J, 30,* 727–749.

Macdonald, J. M. (1971). *Rape: Offenders and their victims.* Springfield, IL: Charles C. Thomas.

Mark, V. H. & Ervin, F. A. (1970). *Violence and the brain.* New York: Harper and Row.

Martin, M. (1989). Battered women. In N. Hutchings (Ed.), *The violent family: Victimization of women, children, and elders.* New York: Human Sciences Press.

May, R. (1972). *Power and innocence.* New York: WW Norton.

Meierhoffer, L. L. (1992, April). Nurses battle family violence. *The American Nurse, 24*(4), 1, 7–8.

Mims, F. H. & Chang, A. S. (1984). Unwanted sexual experiences of young women. *J. Psychosoc Nurs, 22*(6), 6–14.

Moss, V. A. (1991). Battered women and the myth of masochism. *J Psychosoc Nurs, 29*(7), 18–23.

Moynihan, B. (1988). The rape victim. In N. Hutchings (Ed.), *The violent family: Victimization of women, children and elders*. New York: Human Sciences Press.

Mrazek, P. B. (1981). The nature of incest: A review of contributing factors. In P. B. Mrazek & C. H. Kempe (Eds.), *Sexually abused children and their families*. Oxford: Pergamon Press.

Mrazek, P. B. & Kempe, C. H. (Eds.). (1981). *Sexually abused children and their families*. Oxford: Pergamon Press.

National Committee for the Prevention of Child Abuse (1990, July). *NCPCA Newsletter*.

Nikstaitis, G. (1985). Therapy for men that batter. *J Psychosoc Nurs, 23*(7), 33–36.

Owens, D. J. & Straus, M. A. (1975). The social structure of violence in childhood and approval of violence as an adult. *Aggressive Behavior, 1*, 193–211.

Sadock, V. A. (1989). Rape, spouse abuse, and incest. In H. I. Kaplan & B. J. Sadock (Eds.), *Comprehensive textbook of psychiatry*, Vol. I (5th ed). Baltimore: Williams and Wilkins.

Sanford, L. T. (1980). *The silent children: A parent's guide to the prevention of child sexual abuse*. Garden City, NY: Anchor Press/Doubleday.

Scully, D. (1990). *Understanding sexual violence: A study of convicted rapists*. Boston: Unwin Hyman.

Selye, H. (1956). *The stress of life*. New York: McGraw-Hill.

Smith, L. S. (1987a). Sexual assault: The nurse's role. *AD Nurse, 2*(2), 24–28.

Smith, L. S. (1987b). Battered women: The nurse's role. *AD Nurse, 2*(5), 21–24.

Steele, B. F. & Alexander, H. (1981). Long-term effects of sexual abuse in childhood. In P. B. Mrazek & C. H. Kempe (Eds.), *Sexually abused children and their families*. Oxford: Pergamon Press.

Steinmetz, S. K. (1977). *The cycle of violence: Assertive, aggressive, and abusive family interaction*. New York: Praeger.

Toch, H. (1979). *Psychology of crime and criminal justice*. New York: Holt, Rinehart and Winston.

Tower, C. C. (1987). *Child abuse and neglect* (2nd ed.). Washington, DC: National Education Association.

Walker, L. E. (1979). *The battered woman*. New York: Harper and Row.

West, D. J. (1979). The response to violence. *J Med Ethics, 5*, 128–131.

West, D. J. (1983). Sex offenses and offending. In M. Tonry & N. Morris (Eds.), *Crime and justice: An annual review of research*. Chicago: University of Chicago Press.

Wrightsman, L. B. (1977). *Social psychology*, (2nd ed.). Monterey, CA: Brooks/Cole.

BIBLIOGRAPHY

Ackley, M. D. (1987). Innocent victims. *AD Nurse, 2*(2), 29–33.

Bouza, A. V. (1987). This epidemic of family violence. *AD Nurse, 2*(5), 25–27.

Bowers, J. J. (1992). Therapy through art: Facilitating treatment of sexual abuse. *J Psychosoc Nurs, 30*(6), 15–24.

Burgess, A. (1985). Advancing the science of victimology. *J Psychosoc Nurs, 23*(1), 35–38.

Burgess, A, Hartman, C. R., Grant, C. A., Clover, C. L., Snyder, W., & King, L. A. (1991). Drawing a connection from victim to victimizer. *J Psychosoc Nurs, 29*(12), 9–14.

deChesnay, M. (1984). Father-daughter incest: Issues in treatment and research. *J Psychosoc Nurs, 22*(9), 8–16.

DiVasto, P. (1985). Measuring the aftermath of rape. *J Psychosoc Nurs, 23*(2), 33–35.

Draucker, C. B. (1992). The healing process of female adult incest survivors: Constructing a personal residence. *Image, 24*(1), 4–8.

Freeman-Longo, R. E. & Wall, R. V. (1986). Changing a lifetime of sexual crime. *Psychology Today, 20*(3), 58–64.

Germain, C. P. (1984). Sheltering abused women: A nursing perspective. *J Psychosoc Nurs, 22*(9), 24–31.

Glaister, J. A. & McGuinness, T. (1992). The art of therapeutic drawing: Helping chronic trauma survivors. *J Psychosoc Nurs, 30*(5), 9–17.

Kelley, S. J. (1984). The use of art therapy for sexually abused children. *J Psychosoc Nurs, 22*(12), 12–18.

Polk-Walker, G. C. (1990). What really happened? Incidence and factor assessment of abused children and adolescents, *J Psychosoc Nurs, 28*(11), 17–22.

Roy, M. (Ed.). (1982). *The abusive partner: An analysis of domestic battering*. New York: Van Nostrand Reinhold.

Weingourt, R. (1985). Never to be alone: Existential therapy with battered women. *J Psychosoc Nurs, 23*(3), 24–29.

30

ETHICAL AND LEGAL ISSUES IN PSYCHIATRIC/MENTAL HEALTH NURSING

Legal Issues in Psychiatric/Mental
   Health Nursing
      Confidentiality and Right to
         Privacy
      Informed Consent
      Restraints and Seclusion
      Commitment Issues
Nursing Liability
      Malpractice and Negligence
      Types of Lawsuits That Occur in
         Psychiatric Nursing
      Avoiding Liability

OBJECTIVES

After reading this chapter, the student will be able to:

1. Differentiate between ethics, morals, values, and rights.
2. Discuss ethical theories, including utilitarianism, Kantianism, Christian ethics, natural-law theories, and ethical egoism.
3. Define *ethical dilemma.*
4. Discuss the ethical principles of autonomy, beneficence, nonmaleficence, and justice.
5. Use an ethical decision-making model to make an ethical decision.
6. Describe ethical issues relevant to psychiatric/mental health nursing.
7. Define *statutory law* and *common law.*
8. Differentiate between civil and criminal law.
9. Discuss legal issues relevant to psychiatric/mental health nursing.
10. Differentiate between *malpractice* and *negligence.*
11. Identify behaviors relevant to the psychiatric/mental health setting for which specific malpractice action could be taken.

INTRODUCTION

In the education of mental health-care professionals, the teaching of ethical issues is inadequate (McGovern, 1991). This chapter provides a reference for the student and practicing nurse of the basic ethical and legal concepts and their relationship to psychiatric/mental health nursing.

Nurses are constantly faced with the challenge of making difficult decisions regarding good and evil or life and death. A discussion of ethical theory is presented as a foundation upon which ethical decisions may be made. The American Nurses' Association [ANA, (1985)] has established a code of ethics for nurses to use as a framework within which to make ethical choices and decisions (Table 30.1).

Because legislation determines what is "right" or "good" within a society, legal issues pertaining to psychiatric/mental health nursing are also discussed. Definitions are presented, along with rights of psychiatric patients of which nurses must be aware. Nursing competency and patient care accountability are compromised when the nurse has inadequate knowledge about the laws that regulate the practice of nursing.

Knowledge of the legal and ethical concepts presented in this chapter will enhance the quality of care the nurse provides in his or her psychiatric/mental health nursing practice, while also providing protection to the nurse within the parameters of legal accountability. Indeed, the very "right" to practice nursing carries with it the responsibility

Table 30.1 AMERICAN NURSES' ASSOCIATION CODE OF ETHICS FOR NURSES

1. The nurse provides services with respect for human dignity and the uniqueness of the client unrestricted by considerations of social or economic status, personal attributes, or the nature of health problems.
2. The nurse safeguards the client's right to privacy by judiciously protecting information of a confidential nature.
3. The nurse acts to safeguard the client and the public when health care and safety are affected by the incompetent, unethical, or illegal practice of any person.
4. The nurse assumes responsibility and accountability for individual nursing judgments and actions.
5. The nurse maintains competence in nursing.
6. The nurse exercises informed judgment and uses individual competence and qualifications as criteria in seeking consultations, accepting responsibilities, and delegating nursing activities to others.
7. The nurse participates in activities that contribute to the ongoing development of the profession's body of knowledge.
8. The nurse participates in the profession's efforts to implement and improve standards of nursing.
9. The nurse participates in the profession's efforts to establish and maintain conditions of employment conducive to high-quality nursing care.
10. The nurse participates in the profession's effort to protect the public from misinformation and misrepresentation and to maintain the integrity of nursing.
11. The nurse collaborates with members of the health profession and other citizens in promoting community and national efforts to meet the health needs of the public.

Source: ANA (1985).

to maintain a specific level of competency and to practice in accordance with certain ethical and legal standards of care.

DEFINITIONS

King (1984) defines *ethics* as "a branch of philosophy dealing with values related to human conduct, to the rightness and wrongness of certain actions, and to the goodness and badness of the motives and ends of such actions." *Bioethics* is the term applied to these principles when they refer to concepts within the scope of medicine, nursing, and allied health.

Moral behavior is defined as conduct that results from serious critical thinking about how individuals ought to treat others. Moral behavior reflects the way a person interprets basic respect for other persons, such as the respect for human life, freedom, justice, or confidentiality (Davis, 1981).

Values are personal beliefs about the truth, beauty, or worth of a thought, object, or behavior (Leach, 1987). *Values clarification* is a process of self-discovery by which people identify their personal values and their value rankings (King, 1984). This process increases awareness about why individuals behave in certain ways. Values clarification is important in nursing to increase understanding about why certain choices and decisions are made over others and how values affect nursing outcomes.

A *right* is that which an individual is entitled (by ethical or moral standards) to have, or to do, or to receive from others within the limits of the law (Goldstein et al, 1989). A right is *absolute* when there is no restriction whatsoever upon the individual's entitlement. A *legal right* is one upon which the society has agreed and formalized into law. Both the National League for Nursing and the American Hospital Association (AHA) have established guidelines of patients' rights. Although these are not considered legal documents, nurses and hospitals are considered responsible for upholding these rights of patients. In certain instances, courts have held a patient's bill of rights to be part of a legally binding contract between hospital and patient (Goldstein et al, 1989). The AHA Patient's Bill of Rights is presented in Table 30.2.

ETHICAL CONSIDERATIONS

Theoretical Perspectives

An *ethical theory* is a moral principle or a set of moral principles that can be used in assessing what is morally right or morally wrong (Ellis & Hartley, 1988). These principles provide guidelines for ethical decision making.

Table 30.2 AMERICAN HOSPITAL ASSOCIATION PATIENT'S BILL OF RIGHTS

1. The patient has the right to considerate and respectful care.

2. The patient has the right to obtain from his physician complete current information concerning his diagnosis, treatment, and prognosis in terms the patient can be reasonably expected to understand. When it is not medically advisable to give such information to the patient, the information should be made available to an appropriate person in his behalf. He has the right to know by name, the physician responsible for coordinating his care.

3. The patient has the right to receive from his physician information necessary to give informed consent prior to the start of any procedure and/or treatment. Except in emergencies, such information for informed consent should include but not necessarily be limited to the specific procedure and/or treatment, the medically significant risks involved, and the probable duration of incapacitation. Where medically significant alternatives for care or treatment exist, or when the patient requests information concerning medical alternatives, the patient has the right to such information. The patient also has the right to know the name of the person responsible for the procedures and/or treatment.

4. The patient has the right to refuse treatment to the extent permitted by law and to be informed of the medical consequences of his action.

5. The patient has the right to every consideration of his privacy concerning his own medical care program. Case discussion, consultation, examination, and treatment are confidential and should be conducted discreetly. Those not directly involved in his care must have the permission of the patient to be present.

6. The patient has the right to expect that all communications and records pertaining to his care should be treated as confidential.

7. The patient has the right to expect that within its capacity a hospital must make reasonable response to the request of a patient for services. The hospital must provide evaluation, service, and/or referral as indicated by the urgency of the case. When medically permissible, a patient may be transferred to another facility only after he has received complete information and explanation concerning the needs for and alternatives to such a transfer. The institution to which the patient is to be transferred must first have accepted the patient for transfer.

8. The patient has the right to obtain information as to any relationship of his hospital to other health care and educational institutions insofar as his care is concerned. The patient has the right to obtain information as to the existence of any professional relationships among individuals, by name, who are treating him.

9. The patient has the right to be advised if the hospital proposes to engage in or perform human experimentation affecting his care or treatment. The patient has the right to refuse to participate in such research projects.

10. The patient has the right to expect reasonable continuity of care. He has the right to know in advance what appointment times and physicians are available and where. The patient has the right to expect that the hospital will provide a mechanism whereby he is informed by his physician or a delegate of the physician of the patient's continuing health care requirements following discharge.

11. The patient has the right to examine and receive an explanation of his bill regardless of source of payment.

12. The patient has the right to know what hospital rules and regulations apply to his conduct as a patient.

Source: AHA (1975).

UTILITARIANISM

The basis of utilitarianism is "the greatest-happiness principle" (Mill, 1957). This principle holds that actions are right in proportion as they tend to promote happiness; wrong as they tend to produce the reverse of happiness. Thus, the "good" is happiness and the "right" is that which promotes the good. Conversely, the "wrongness" of an action is determined by its tendency to bring about unhappiness. An ethical decision based on the utilitarian view would look at the end results of the decision. Action would be taken based on the end results that produced the most good (happiness) for the most people.

KANTIANISM

Named for philosopher Immanuel Kant, this theory is in direct opposition to that of utilitarianism. Kant argued that it is not the consequences or end results that make an action right or wrong, but rather it is the principle upon which the action is based that is the morally decisive factor (Hunt & Arras, 1977). Kantianism suggests that our actions are bound by a sense of duty. This theory is often called *deontology* (from the Greek word *deon*, which means "that which is binding; duty"). Kantian-directed ethical decisions are made out of respect for moral law. For example, "I make this choice because it is morally right and my duty to do so." (not because of consideration for a possible outcome).

CHRISTIAN ETHICS

A basic principle that might be called a Christian philosophy is that which is known as the golden rule: "Do unto others as you would have them do unto you" and, alternatively, "Do not do unto others what you would not have them do unto you." The imperative demand of this principle is to treat others as moral equals and to recognize the equality of other persons by permitting them to act as we do when they occupy a position similar to ours (Hunt & Arras, 1977).

NATURAL-LAW THEORIES

The most general moral precept of the natural-law theory is "do good and avoid evil" (Hunt & Arras, 1977). Natural-law theorists contend, then, that ethics must be grounded in a concern for the human good. Although the nature of this "human good" is not expounded upon, Hunt and Arras (1977) correlate it with the Catholic theologians' view of natural law, that is, that natural law is the law inscribed by God into the nature of things — as a species of divine law. According to this conception, the Creator endows all things with certain potentialities or tendencies that serve to define their natural end. The fulfillment of a thing's natural tendencies constitutes the specific "good" of that thing. For example, the natural tendency of an acorn is to become an oak. What then is the natural potential, or tendency, of human beings? Natural-law theorists focus on an attribute that is regarded as distinctively human, as separating human beings from the rest of worldly creatures — that is, the ability to live according to the dictates of reason. It is with this ability to reason that humans are able to choose "good" over "evil." In natural law, evil acts are never condoned, even if they are intended to advance the noblest of ends.

ETHICAL EGOISM

This theoretical view espouses that what is "right" and "good" is what is best for the individual making the decision. An individual's actions are determined by what is to his or her own advantage. The action may not be best for anyone else involved, but consideration is only for the individual making the decision.

Ethical Dilemmas

Ethical dilemmas arise when no explicit reasons exist that govern an action. Ethical dilemmas generally create a great deal of emotion. Often the reasons supporting each side of the argument for action are logical and appropriate. The actions associated with both sides are desirable in some respects and undesirable in others (Phipps et al, 1987).

Beauchamp and Childress (1983) state:

> "Ethical dilemmas arise when on the basis of moral considerations an appeal can be made for taking each of two opposing courses of action."

Phipps et al (1987) offer the following steps leading to an ethical dilemma:

1. Some evidence indicates that act 'X' is morally right and some evidence indicates that act 'X' is morally wrong.
2. Evidence on both sides is inconclusive.
3. The individual perceives that he or she ought and ought not to perform the act.
4. Some action must be taken.
5. An ethical dilemma exists.

In most situations, *taking no action is considered an action taken.*

Ethical Principles

Ethical principles are fundamental guidelines that influence decision making. The ethical principles of *autonomy, beneficence, nonmaleficence,* and *justice* are helpful and used frequently by health-care workers to assist with ethical decision making (Laufman, 1989; Hunt & Arras, 1977). These principles apply largely to the deontological (Kantianism) ethical theory, in which decisions are made out of a sense of duty.

AUTONOMY

The principle of *autonomy* arises out of the Kantian duty of respect for persons as rational agents (Hunt & Arras, 1977). This viewpoint emphasizes the status of persons as autonomous moral agents whose right to determine their destinies should always be respected. This presumes that individuals are always capable of making independent choices for themselves. Health-care workers know this is not always the case. Children, the comatose patient, and the seriously mentally ill are examples of patients who are not capable of making informed choices. In these instances, a representative of the individual is usually asked to intervene with consent. However, health-care workers must ensure that respect for an individual's autonomy is not disregarded in favor of what another person may view as best for the patient.

BENEFICENCE

Beneficience refers to one's duty to benefit or promote the good of others. Health-care workers who act in their patients' interests are beneficent, provided their actions really do serve the patient's best interest (Beauchamp & Childress, 1983). In fact, some duties do seem to take preference over other duties. For example, the duty to respect the autonomy of an individual may be overridden when that individual has been deemed harmful to self or others.

NONMALEFICENCE

Nonmaleficence involves abstaining from negative acts toward anther, including acting carefully to avoid harm (Laufman, 1989). Some philosophers suggest that this principle is more important than beneficence; that is, they support the notion that it is more important to avoid doing harm than it is to do good (Jameton, 1984). In any event, ethical dilemmas often arise when a conflict exists between an individual's rights (the duty to promote good) and what is thought to best represent the welfare of the individual (the duty to do no harm).

JUSTICE

This principle has been referred to as "justice as fairness." The basic premise of this principle is the notion of a hypothetical social contract between free, equal, and rational persons (Rawls, 1971). The concept of justice reflects a duty to treat all individuals equally and fairly. When applied to health care, this principle suggests that all resources within the society (including health-care services) ought to be distributed evenly without respect to socioeconomic status. Thus, this principle would imply that the vast disparity in the quality of care dispensed to the various classes within our society is unjust and should be reformed in favor of a more equitable distribution of care (Hunt & Arras, 1977).

A Model for Making Ethical Decisions

Following is a set of steps that may be employed in making an ethical decision. These steps closely resemble the steps of the nursing process and are adapted from a model suggested by Shelly (1980).

1. *Assessment.* Gather the subjective and objective data about a situation.
2. *Problem identification*—Identify the conflict between two or more alternative actions.
3. Explore the benefits and consequences of each alternative.
4. Consider principles of ethical theories.
5. Select an alternative.
6. Act upon the decision made and communicate decision to others.
7. Evaluate outcomes.

If the outcome is acceptable, action continues in the manner selected. If the outcome is unacceptable, benefits and consequences of the remaining alternatives are re-examined, and steps 3 through 7 are repeated. A schematic of this model is presented in Figure 30.1.

ETHICAL DECISION MAKING— A CASE STUDY

Following is a case study using the decision-making model previously described.

Step 1. Assessment

Tonja is a 17-year-old girl who is currently on the psychiatric unit with a diagnosis of conduct disorder. Tonja reports that she has been sexually active since she was 14. She had an abortion when she was 15, and a second one just 6 weeks ago. She states that her mother told her she has "had her last abortion," and that she has to start taking birth control pills. She asks her nurse, Kimberly, to give her some information about the pills and tell her how to go about getting some. Kimberly believes Tonja desperately needs information about birth control pills, as well as other types of contraceptives, but the psychiatric unit is part of a Catholic hospital, and hospital policy prohibits distributing this type of information.

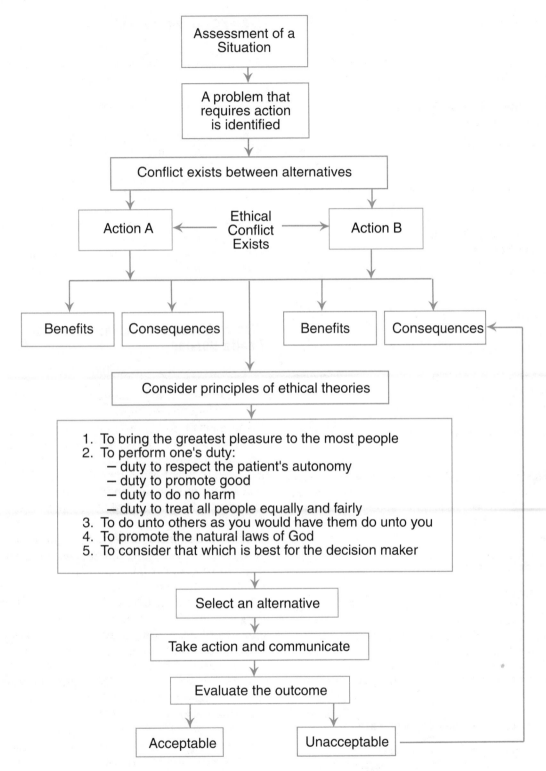

Figure 30.1 Ethical decision-making model.

Step 2. Problem Identification

A conflict exists between the patient's need for information, the nurse's desire to provide that information, and the institution's policy prohibiting the provision of that information.

Step 3. Alternatives — Benefits and Consequences

1. Alternative 1. Give patient information and risk losing job.
2. Alternative 2. Do not give patient information and compromise own values of holistic nursing.
3. Alternative 3. Refer patient to another source outside the hospital and risk reprimand from supervisor.

Step 4. Consider Principles of Ethical Theories

1. Alternative 1. Giving the patient information would certainly respect the patient's autonomy and would benefit the patient by decreasing her chances of becoming pregnant again. It would not be to the best advantage of Kimberly, in that she would likely lose her job. And according to the beliefs of the Catholic hospital, the natural laws of God would be violated.
2. Alternative 2. Withholding information restricts the patient's autonomy. It has the potential for doing harm, in that without the use of contraceptives, the patient may become pregnant again (and she implies that this is not what she wants). Kimberly's Christian ethic is violated in that this action is not what she would want "done unto her."
3. Alternative 3. A referral would respect the patient's autonomy, would promote good, would do no harm (except perhaps to Kimberly's ego from the possible reprimand), and this decision would comply with Kimberly's Christian ethic.

Step 5. Select an Alternative

Alternative 3 is selected based on the ethical theories of utilitarianism (does the most good for the greatest number), Christian ethics (Kimberly's belief of "Do unto others as you would have others do unto you"), and Kantianism (to perform one's duty) and the ethical principles of autonomy, beneficence, and nonmaleficence. The success of this decision depends upon the patient's follow-through with the referral and compliance with use of the contraceptives.

Step 6. Take Action and Communicate

Taking action involves providing information in writing for Tonja, perhaps making a phone call and setting up an appointment for her with Planned Parenthood. Communicating suggests sharing the information with Tonja's mother. Communication also includes documentation of the referral in the patient's chart.

Step 7. Evaluate the Outcome

An acceptable outcome might indicate that Tonja did indeed keep her appointment at Planned Parenthood and is complying with the prescribed contraceptive regimen. It might also include Kimberly's input into the change process in her institution to implement these types of referrals to other patients who request them.

An unacceptable outcome might be indicated by Tonja's lack of follow-through with the appointment at Planned Parenthood or lack of compliance in using the contraceptives, resulting in another pregnancy. Kimberly may also view a reprimand from her supervisor as an unacceptable outcome, particularly if she is told that she must select other alternatives should this situation arise in the future. This may motivate Kimberly to make another decision — that of seeking employment in an institution with a philosophy more consistent with her own.

Ethical Issues in Psychiatric/Mental Health Nursing

THE RIGHT TO REFUSE MEDICATION

The AHA's (1975) Patient's Bill of Rights states, "The patient has the right to refuse treatment to the extent permitted by law, and to be informed of the medical consequences of his action." In psychiatry, refusal of treatment primarily concerns the administration of psychotropic medications. "To the extent permitted by law" may be defined within the Constitution of the United States and several of its amendments (e.g., the First Amendment, which addresses the rights of speech, thought, and expression; the Eighth Amendment, which grants the right to freedom from cruel and unusual punishment; and the Fifth and Fourteenth Amendments, which grant due process of law and equal protection for all). In psychiatry, "the medical consequences of his action" may include such steps as involuntary commitment, a legal competency hearing, or patient discharge from the hospital.

Although many courts are supporting a patient's right to refuse medications in the psychiatric area, some limitations do exist. In one case (*Davis* v. *Hubbard, Ohio*, 1980), a federal district court concluded that no state interest could provide justification for the administration of psychotropic drugs without the consent of a competent patient, *unless the patient presents a danger to self or to others in the institution* (Beis, 1984). In these types of emergency situations, then, it is considered appropriate to medicate forcibly. However, the patient has the right to a hearing as soon as possible.

THE RIGHT TO THE LEAST RESTRICTIVE TREATMENT ALTERNATIVE

Health-care personnel must attempt to provide treatment in a manner that least restricts the freedom of patients (Beis, 1984). The "restrictiveness" of therapy within the psychiatric setting has been described in the context of a continuum, beginning with verbal rehabilitative techniques and moving successively to behavioral techniques, chemical interventions, mechanical restraints, electroconvulsive therapy, and finally, surgical intervention (Winick, 1981).

Psychiatric nurses frequently must make decisions about selection of treatment for patients in emergency situations when there is danger to the patient or others. While attempting to adhere to the principle of least restrictive alternative, harm must be avoided. While physical restraints are the most restrictive form of treatment available to the nurse, this option is sometimes necessary to provide the needed controls, particularly if less restrictive measures have not been effective. Since most institutions have their own policies and procedures associated with the use of restraints, the nurse should be familiar with those of his or her facility.

LEGAL CONSIDERATIONS

In 1980, the 96th Congress of the United States passed the Mental Health Systems Act, which includes a Patient's Bill of Rights for recommendation to the states. An adaptation of these rights is presented in Table 30.3.

Nurse Practice Acts

The legal parameters of professional and practical nursing are defined within each state by the state nurse practice act. These documents are passed by the state legislature and in general are concerned with such provisions as:

1. The definition of important terms, including the definition of nursing and the various types of nurses recognized.
2. A statement of the educational and other

Table 30.3 BILL OF RIGHTS FOR PSYCHIATRIC PATIENTS

1. The right to appropriate treatment and related services in the setting that is most supportive and least restrictive to personal freedom.
2. The right to an individualized, written treatment or service plan; the right to treatment based on such plan; and the right to periodic review and revision of the plan based on treatment needs.
3. The right, consistent with one's capabilities, to participate in and receive a reasonable explanation of the care and treatment process.
4. The right to refuse treatment except in an emergency situation or as permitted by law.
5. The right not to participate in experimentation in the absence of informed, voluntary, written consent.
6. The right to freedom from restraint or seclusion except in an emergency situation.
7. The right to a humane treatment environment that affords reasonable protection from harm and appropriate privacy.
8. The right to confidentiality of medical records (also applicable following patient's discharge).
9. The right of access to medical records except information received from third parties under promise of confidentiality, and when access would be detrimental to the patient's health (also applicable following patient's discharge).
10. The right of access to use of the telephone, personal mail, and visitors, unless deemed inappropriate for treatment purposes.
11. The right to be informed of these rights in comprehensible language.
12. The right to assert grievances if rights are infringed.
13. The right to referral as appropriate to other providers of mental health services upon discharge.

Source: Mental Health Systems Act (1980).

---

training or requirements for licensure and reciprocity.
3. A statement as to permitted nursing practices or acts (e.g., medical diagnosis) that may *not* be performed by a nurse.
4. Conditions under which a nurse's license may be suspended or revoked.
5. The general authority and powers of the state licensing agency having jurisdiction over nurses (Goldstein et al, 1989).

Most nurse practice acts are very general in their terminology and do not provide specific guidelines for practice. Nurses must understand the scope of practice that is protected by their license and should therefore seek assistance from legal counsel if unsure about the proper interpretation of a nurse practice act.

Types of Law

There are two general categories or types of law that are of most concern to nurses: statutory law and common law. These laws are identified by their source or origin.

STATUTORY LAW

Statutory laws are those that have been enacted by legislative bodies, such as a county or city council, state legislature, or the Congress of the United States. An example of statutory law would be the nurse practice acts.

COMMON LAW

Common laws are derived from decisions made in previous cases. These laws apply to a body of principles that evolve from court decisions resolving various controversies. Because common law in the United States has been developed on a state basis, the law on specific subjects may differ from state to state (Beis, 1984). An example of a common law might be how different states deal with a nurse's refusal to provide care for a specific patient.

Classifications Within Statutory and Common Law

Broadly speaking, there are two kinds of unlawful acts: civil and criminal (Willig, 1971). Both statutory law and common law have civil and criminal components.

CIVIL LAW

Civil law protects the private and property rights of individuals and businesses. Private individuals or groups may bring a legal action to court for breach of civil law. These legal actions are of two basic types: torts and contracts.

Torts A *tort* is a violation of a civil law in which an individual has been wronged. In a tort action, one party asserts that wrongful conduct on the part of the other has caused harm, and compensation

for harm suffered is sought. A tort may be *intentional or unintentional*. Examples of unintentional torts are malpractice and negligence actions (Beis, 1984). An example of an intentional tort is the touching of another person without consent. Intentional touching (e.g., a medical treatment) without the patient's consent can result in a charge of "battery," an intentional tort (Beis, 1984).

Contracts In a contract action, one party asserts that the other party has, in failing to fulfill an obligation, breached the contract, and either compensation or performance of the obligation is sought as remedy. An example might be an action by a mental health professional whose clinical privileges have been reduced or terminated in violation of an implied contract between the professional and a hospital (Beis, 1984).

CRIMINAL LAW

Criminal law provides protection from conduct deemed injurious to the public welfare. It provides for punishment of those found to have engaged in such conduct. This commonly includes imprisonment, parole conditions, a loss of privilege (such as license), a fine, or any combination of these (Ellis & Hartley, 1988). An example of a violation of criminal law is the theft by a hospital employee of supplies or drugs.

Legal Issues in Psychiatric/Mental Health Nursing

CONFIDENTIALITY AND RIGHT TO PRIVACY

An individual's privacy is protected by the Fourth, Fifth, and Fourteenth Amendments to the Constitution of the United States. Forty-eight of the fifty states have statutes protecting the confidentiality of patient records and communications. The only individuals who have a right to observe a patient or have access to medical information are those involved in his or her medical care (Goldstein et al, 1989).

Pertinent medical information may be released in a life-threatening situation without consent. If information is released in an emergency, the following information must be recorded in the patient's record: date of disclosure, person to whom information was disclosed, reason for disclosure, reason written consent could not be obtained, and the specific information disclosed (Beis, 1984).

Most states have statutes that pertain to the *doctrine of privileged communication*. Although the codes differ markedly from state to state, most grant certain professionals privileges under which they may refuse to reveal information about and communications with patients. In most states, the doctrine of privileged communication applies to psychiatrists and attorneys; in some instances, psychologists, clergy, and nurses are also included.

In certain instances, nurses may be called upon to testify in cases in which the medical record is used as evidence. In most states, the right to privacy of these records is exempted in civil or criminal proceedings. It is therefore very important that nurses document with these possibilities in mind. Strict record keeping, using statements that are objective and nonjudgmental; care plans that are specific in their prescriptive interventions; and documentation that describes those interventions and their subsequent evaluation all serve the best interests of the patient, the nurse, and the institution should questions regarding care arise. Documentation very often weighs heavily in malpractice case decisions.

The right of confidentiality is a basic one, especially in psychiatry. Even though societal attitudes are improving, individuals have been discriminated against in the past for no other reason than having a history of emotional illness. Nurses working in psychiatry must guard the privacy of their patients with great diligence.

INFORMED CONSENT

According to law, all persons have the right to decide whether to accept or reject treatment (Goldstein et al, 1989). A health-care provider can be charged with assault and battery for providing life-sustaining treatment to a patient when the patient has not agreed to it. The rationale for the doctrine of informed consent is the preservation and protection of individual self-determination (Goldstein et al, 1989).

Informed consent may be defined as permission granted to a physician by a patient to perform a therapeutic procedure, prior to which information about the procedure has been presented to the patient with adequate time given for consideration about the pros and cons. The patient should receive information such as what treatment alternatives are available; why the physician believes this treatment is most appropriate; the possible outcomes, risks, adverse effects; the possible outcome should the patient select another treatment alternative; and the possible outcome should the patient choose to have no treatment.

Goldstein and associates (1989) state that informed consent should be obtained:

". . . any time there is an inherent risk of death or serious bodily injury that the patient might not know about, or when the probability of success in a medical procedure is low. The rule applies equally to administration of investigational drugs, the performance of diagnostic tests, and the performance of major or minor surgical procedures."

An example of a treatment in the psychiatric area that requires informed consent is electroconvulsive therapy.

There are some conditions under which treatment may be performed without obtaining informed consent. A patient's refusal to accept treatment may be challenged under the following circumstances:

1. When a patient is mentally incompetent to make a decision and treatment is necessary to preserve life or avoid serious harm
2. When refusing treatment endangers the life or health of another
3. An emergency where a patient is in no condition to exercise judgment (Beis, 1984; Goldstein et al, 1989).

Although most patients in psychiatric/mental health facilities are competent and capable of giving informed consent, those with severe psychiatric illness will not possess the cognitive ability to do so. If an individual has been legally determined as mentally incompetent, consent is obtained from the legal guardian. The area of difficulty arises when there has been no legal determination made, but the individual's mental state at the present time prohibits informed decision making (e.g., the psychotic person, the unconscious person, the inebriated person). In these instances, informed consent is usually obtained from the individual's nearest relative, or if none exist and time permits, the physician may ask the court to appoint a conservator or guardian. When time does not permit court intervention, permission may even be sought from the hospital administrator.

A patient always has the right to withdraw consent after it has been given. When this occurs, the physician should inform (or reinform) the patient about the consequences of refusing treatment. If treatment has already been initiated, the physician should terminate treatment in a way least likely to cause injury to the patient and inform the patient of the risks associated with interrupted treatment (Goldstein et al, 1989).

The nurse's role in obtaining informed consent is usually defined by agency policy. A nurse may sign the consent form as witness for the patient's signature. However, legal liability for informed consent lies with the physician. The nurse acts as patient advocate to ensure that the three major elements of informed consent have been addressed:

1. Knowledge — that the patient has received adequate information on which to base his or her decision
2. Competency — that the individual's cognition is not impaired to an extent that would interfere with decision making or, if so, that the individual has a legal representative
3. Free will — that the individual has given consent voluntarily without pressure or coercion from others.

RESTRAINTS AND SECLUSION

An individual's privacy and personal security is protected by the U.S. Constitution and supported by the Mental Health Systems Act of 1980, out of which was conceived a Bill of Rights for psychiatric patients. These include "the right to freedom from restraint or seclusion except in an emergency situation."

The Joint Commission on Accreditation of Health Organizations states:

"The use of restraint or seclusion shall require clinical justification and shall be employed only to prevent a patient from injuring himself or others, or to prevent serious disruption of the therapeutic environment. Restraint or seclusion shall not be employed as punishment or for the convenience of staff. [In deciding to restrain or seclude a patient, the] inadequacy of less restrictive intervention techniques must be addressed."

In psychiatry, the term *restraints* generally refers to a set of leather straps that are used to restrain the extremities of an individual whose behavior is out of control and who poses a threat of harm to self or others. Less restrictive measures to decrease agitation, such as "talking down" (verbal intervention) and chemical restraints (tranquilizing medication), are usually tried initially. When these interventions are ineffective, mechanical restraints may be instituted.

In an emergency, where a patient threatens harm to self or others, restraint or seclusion may be implemented without a physician's written order. However, the written order of the physician who is responsible for the patient's medical care is obtained no more than 8 hours after initial employment of the restraint or seclusion. Orders are time limited and vary from state to state. This limited time allows for periodic review and assessment by the physician before orders are renewed.

Patients in restraints or seclusion must be observed and assessed every 10 to 15 minutes with regard to circulation, respiration, nutrition, hydration, and elimination. Such attention should be documented in the patient's record. Periodic (usually every 2 hours) release from restraints or seclusion is recommended (Goldstein et al, 1989).

False imprisonment is the deliberate and unauthorized confinement of a person within fixed limits by the use of threat or force (Willig, 1971). With regard to patients who have sought hospital admission voluntarily, health-care workers may be charged with false imprisonment for restraining or secluding them against their wishes. Should a voluntarily admitted patient decompensate to a point that required restraint or seclusion for protection of self or others, court intervention to determine competency and involuntary commitment would be required to preserve the patient's rights to privacy and freedom.

COMMITMENT ISSUES

Voluntary Admission The general standard or criterion for voluntary admission is whether a person is mentally ill and suitable for treatment (Beis, 1984). Most psychiatric admissions are voluntary. To be admitted voluntarily, an individual makes direct application to the institution for services and may stay as long as treatment is deemed necessary.

He or she may sign out of the hospital at any time, unless following a mental status examination the health-care professional determines that the patient may be harmful to self or others and recommends that the admission status be changed form voluntary to involuntary.

Involuntary Commitment   Because involuntary hospitalization results in substantial restrictions of the rights of an individual, the admission process is subject to the guarantee of the Fourteenth Amendment to the U.S. Constitution that no state may "deprive any person of life, liberty, or property, without due process of law; nor deny to any person within its jurisdiction the equal protection of the laws" (Beis, 1984). Involuntary commitments are made for various reasons. Most states commonly cite the following criteria:

1. In an emergency situation (for the patient who is dangerous to self or others)
2. For observation and treatment of mentally ill persons
3. When an individual is unable to take care of basic personal needs (the "gravely disabled")

Under the Fourth Amendment, individuals are protected from unlawful searches and seizures without probable cause. Therefore, the individual seeking the involuntary commitment must show probable cause why the patient should be hospitalized against his or her wishes — that is, to show that there is cause to believe that the person would be dangerous to self or others, is mentally ill and in need of treatment, or is gravely disabled.

Emergency Commitments   Emergency commitments are sought when an individual manifests behavior that is clearly and imminently dangerous to self or others. These admissions are generally instigated by relatives or friends of the individual, police officers, the court, or a health-care professional. Emergency commitments are time-limited, and a court hearing for the individual will be scheduled, usually within a 72-hour period. At this time, the court may decide that the patient may be discharged, or, if deemed necessary, an additional period of involuntary commitment may be ordered. In most instances, another hearing will be scheduled for a specified time (usually 7 to 21 days).

The "Mentally Ill" Patient in Need of Treatment   A second type of involuntary commitment is for the observation and treatment of mentally ill persons in need of treatment. Most states have established definitions of what constitutes "mentally ill," for purposes of state involuntary admission statutes. Some examples include (Beis, 1984):

1. In Colorado: "Mentally ill person" means a person who is of such mental condition that he is in need of medical supervision, treatment, care, or restraint.
2. In Kansas: "Mentally ill person" is any person who:
   a. is suffering from a severe mental disorder to the extent that such a person is in need of treatment.
   b. lacks capacity to make an informed decision concerning treatment.
   c. is likely too cause harm to self or others.
3. In Oregon: "Mentally ill person" means a person who, because of a mental disorder, is either:
   a. dangerous to himself or others
   b. unable to provide for his basic personal needs and is not receiving such care as is necessary for his health and safety

In determining whether or not commitment is required, the court will look for substantial evidence of abnormal conduct – evidence that cannot be explained as the result of a physical cause. There must be "clear and convincing evidence" as well as "probable cause" to substantiate the need for involuntary commitment to ensure that an individual's rights under the Constitution are protected. The U.S. Supreme Court in *O'Connor* v. *Donaldson* held that the existence of mental illness alone does not justify involuntary hospitalization. State standards require a specific impact or consequence to flow from the mental illness that involves dangerousness or an inability to care for one's own needs (Beis, 1984). These patients are entitled to court hearings with representation, at which time determination of commitment and length of stay are considered. Legislative statutes governing involuntary commitments vary from state to state.

The Gravely Disabled Patient   A number of states have statutes that specifically define the "gravely disabled" patient. For those that do not use this label, the description of the individual who, because of mental illness, is unable to take care of basic personal needs is very similar.

Gravely disabled is generally defined as a condition in which an individual, as a result of mental illness, is in danger of serious physical harm resulting from inability to provide for basic needs such as food, clothing, shelter, medical care, and personal safety. Inability to care for oneself cannot be established by showing that an individual lacks the resources to provide the necessities of life. Rather, it is the inability to make use of available resources (Beis, 1984).

Should it be determined that an individual is gravely disabled, a guardian, conservator, or committee will be appointed by the court to ensure the management of the person and his or her estate. To legally restore competency would then require another court hearing to reverse the previous ruling. The individual whose competency is being determined has the right to be represented by an attorney.

Nursing Liability

Mental health practitioners — psychiatrists, psychologists, psychiatric nurses and social workers — have a duty to provide appropriate care based on the standards of their professions and the standards set by law (Beis, 1984). The standards of care for psychiatric/mental health nursing are presented in Chapter 6 of this text (see Table 6.6).

MALPRACTICE AND NEGLIGENCE

The terms *malpractice* and *negligence* are often used interchangeably. Negligence has been defined as,

"... the failure to do something which a reasonable person, guided by those ordinary considerations which ordinarily regulate human affairs, would do, or doing something which a prudent and reasonable person would not do" (Black, 1979).

Any person may be negligent. In contrast, malpractice is a specialized form of negligence applicable only to professionals. In *Matthews* v. *Walker* (Ohio, 1973) malpractice was defined as:

"The failure of one rendering professional services to exercise that degree of skill and learning commonly applied under all the circumstances in the community by the average prudent reputable member of the profession with the result of injury, loss, or damage to the recipient of those services or to those entitled to rely upon them" (Beis, 1984).

In the absence of any state statutes, common law is the basis of liability for injuries to patients caused by acts of malpractice and negligence of individual practitioners (Beis, 1984). In other words, most decisions of negligence in the professional setting are based on legal precedent (decisions that have previously been made about similar cases) rather than any specific action taken by the legislature.

To summarize, then, when the breach of duty is characterized as malpractice, the action is weighted against the professional standard. When it is brought forth as negligence, action is contrasted with what a reasonably prudent professional would have done in the same or similar circumstances.

Goldstein et al. (1989) state that every nursing malpractice suit must include the following basic elements:

1. A claim that the nurse owed the patient a special duty of care
2. A claim that the nurse was required to meet a specific standard of care in carrying out the nursing act or function in question
3. A claim that the nurse failed to meet the required standard of care
4. A claim that harm or injury resulted, for which compensation is sought

For the patient to prevail in a malpractice claim, each of these elements must be proved. Juries' decisions are generally based on the testimony of expert witnesses, since members of the jury are laymen and cannot be expected to know what nursing interventions should have been carried out. Without the testimony of expert witnesses, a favorable verdict usually goes to the defendant nurse.

TYPES OF LAWSUITS THAT OCCUR IN PSYCHIATRIC NURSING

Most malpractice suits against nurses are civil actions — that is, they are considered breach of conduct actions between private individuals. The nurse in the psychiatric setting should be aware of the types of behaviors that may result in charges of malpractice.

Basic to the psychiatric patient's hospitalization is his or her right to confidentiality and privacy. A nurse may be charged with *breach of confidentiality* for revealing aspects about a patient's case, or even for revealing that an individual has been hospitalized, if that person can show that making this information known resulted in harm.

When shared information is detrimental to the patient's reputation, the person sharing the information may be liable for *defamation of character.* When the information is in writing, the action is called *libel.* Oral defamation is called *slander.* Defamation of character involves communication that is malicious and false (Ellis & Hartley, 1988). Occasionally, libel arises out of critical, judgmental statements written in the patient's medical record. Nurses need to be very objective in their charting, backing up all statements with factual evidence.

Invasion of privacy is a charge that may result when a patient is searched without probable cause. Many institutions conduct body searches on mental patients as a routine intervention. In these cases, a physician's order and written rationale should show probable cause for the intervention. Many institutions are re-examining their policies regarding this procedure.

Assault is an act that results in a person's genuine fear and apprehension that he or she will be touched without consent. *Battery* is the unconsented touching of another person. These charges can result when a treatment is administered to a patient against his or her wishes and outside of an emergency situation. Harm or injury need not have occurred for these charges to be legitimate.

For confining a patient against his or her wishes, and outside of an emergency situation, the nurse may be charged with *false imprisonment.* Examples of actions that may invoke these charges include locking an individual in a room; taking a patient's clothes for purposes of detainment against his or her will; and retaining in mechanical restraints a competent voluntary patient who demands to be released.

AVOIDING LIABILITY

Goldstein et al (1989) suggest the following guidelines for avoiding liability:

1. Practice within the scope of the nurse practice act.
2. Observe the hospital's and department's policy manuals.
3. Measure up to established practice standards.
4. Always put the patient's rights and welfare first.
5. Develop and maintain a good interpersonal relationship with each patient and his or her family.

This final item is an extremely important guideline to follow. Some patients appear to be more *suit prone* than others. Suit-prone patients are often very critical, complaining, uncooperative, and even hostile. A natural response by the staff to these patients is to become defensive or withdrawn. Either of these behaviors increases the likelihood of a lawsuit should an unfavorable event occur (Ellis & Hartley, 1988). Regardless of the nurse's high degree of technical competence and skill, insensitivity to a patient's complaints and failure to meet the patient's emotional needs are important issues that often influence whether or not a lawsuit is generated. A great deal depends upon the psychosocial skills of the health-care professional.

SUMMARY

This chapter examined some of the ethical and legal issues relevant to psychiatric/mental health nursing in an effort to promote enhancement of quality of patient care as well as provide protection to the nurse within the parameters of legal accountability. Ethics is a branch of philosophy that deals with values related to human conduct, to the rightness and wrongness of certain actions, and to the goodness and badness of the motives and ends of such actions.

Patients have certain rights that are afforded them under the Constitution of the United States. Patients' rights have also been set forth by the AHA, National League for Nursing, American Civil Liberties Union, and the Mental Health Systems Act. Nurse practice acts and standards of professional practice guide the scope within which a nurse may legally practice. The ANA has established a Code for Nurses under which guidelines the professional nurse is expected to practice ethical nursing.

Ethical theories and principles are foundational guidelines that influence decision making. Ethical theories include utilitarianism, Kantianism, Christian ethics, natural-law theories, and ethical egoism. Ethical principles include autonomy, beneficence, nonmaleficence, and justice. An individual's ethical philosophy affects his or her decision making and ultimately the outcomes of those decisions.

Ethical issues in psychiatric/mental health nursing include the right to refuse medication and the right to the least restrictive treatment alternative. An ethical decision-making model was presented, along with a case study for application of the process.

Statutory laws are those that have been enacted by legislative bodies, and common laws are derived from decisions made in previous cases. Civil law protects the private and property rights of individuals and businesses, and criminal law provides protection from conduct deemed injurious to the public welfare. Both statutory law and common law have civil and criminal components.

Legal issues in psychiatric/mental health nursing center around confidentiality and the right to privacy, informed consent, restraints and seclusion, and commitment issues. Nurses are accountable for their own actions in relation to these issues, and violation can result in malpractice lawsuits against the physician, the hospital, and the nurse. Nurses must be aware of the kinds of behaviors that place them at risk for malpractice action. Developing and maintaining a good interpersonal relationship with the patient and his or her family appears to be a positive factor when the question of malpractice is being considered.

REVIEW QUESTIONS
Self-Examination/Learning Exercise

Match the following decision-making examples with the appropriate ethical theory:

_____ 1. Carol decides to go against family wishes and tell the patient of his terminal status because that is what she would want if she were the patient.

_____ 2. Carol decides to respect family wishes and not tell the patient of his terminal status because that would bring the most happiness to the most people.

_____ 3. Carol decides not to tell the patient about his terminal status because it would be too uncomfortable for her to do so.

_____ 4. Carol decides to tell the patient of his terminal status because her reasoning tells her that to do otherwise would be an evil act.

_____ 5. Carol decides to tell the patient of his terminal status because she believes it is her duty to do so.

a. Utilitarianism

b. Kantianism

c. Christian ethics

d. Natural-law theories

e. Ethical egoism

Match the following nursing actions with the possible legal action with which the nurse may be charged:

_____ 6. The nurse assists the physician with electroconvulsive therapy on his patient, who has refused to give consent.

_____ 7. When the local newspaper calls to inquire why the mayor has been admitted to the hospital, the nurse replies, "He's here because he is an alcoholic."

_____ 8. A competent, voluntary patient has stated he wants to leave the hospital. The nurse hides his clothes in an effort to keep him from leaving.

_____ 9. Jack recently lost his wife and is very depressed. He is running for re-election to the Senate and asks the staff to keep his hospitalization confidential. The nurse is excited about having a senator on the unit and tells her boyfriend about the admission, which soon becomes common knowledge. Jack loses the election.

_____ 10. Joe is very restless and is pacing a lot. The nurse says to Joe, "If you don't sit down in the chair and be still, I'm going to put you in restraints!"

a. Breach of confidentiality

b. Defamation of character

c. Assault

d. Battery

e. False imprisonment

REFERENCES

American Hospital Association. (1975). *A Patient's Bill of Rights.* Chicago: American Hospital Association, 1975.

American Nurses' Association. (1985). *Code of ethics with interpretive statements.* Kansas City, MO: ANA.

Beauchamp, T. L. & Childress, J. F. (1983). *Principles of biomedical ethics* (2nd ed.). New York: Oxford University Press.

Beis, E. B. (1984). *Mental health and the law.* Rockville, MD: Aspen Systems Corp.

Black, H. *Black's law dictionary* (5th ed.). (1979). St. Paul, MN: West Publishing Co.

Davis C. M. (1981). Affective education for the health professions. *Phys Ther 61*(11), 1587–1593.

Ellis, J. R. & Hartley, C. L. (1988). *Nursing in today's world: Challenges, issues, and trends* (3rd ed.). Philadelphia: JP Lippincott.

Goldstein, A. S., Perdew, S., & Pruitt, S. S. (1989). *The nurse's legal advisor: Your guide to legally safe practice.* Philadelphia: JB Lippincott.

Hunt, R. & Arras, J. (1977). Ethical theory in the medical context. In R. Hunt & J. Arras (Eds.), *Ethical Issues in modern medicine.* Palo Alto, CA: Mayfield Publishing.

Jameton, A. (1984). *Nursing practice: The ethical issues.* Englewood Cliffs, NJ: Prentice-Hall.

King, E. C. (1984). *Affective education in nursing: A guide to teaching and assessment.* Rockville, MD: Aspen Systems Corp.

Laufman, J. K. (1989). Aids, ethics, and the truth. *Am J Nurs, 89*(7), 924–930.

Leach, A. M. (1987). Legal and ethical issues. In J. Haber, A. M. Leach, S. M. Schudy, & B. F. Sidelaw (Eds.), *Comprehensive psychiatric nursing* (3rd ed.). New York: McGraw-Hill.

McGovern, T. F. (1991). Foreword. In P. J. Barker & S. Baldwin (Eds.), *Ethical issues in mental health.* London: Chapman & Hall.

Mental Health Systems Act. P. L. 96-398, Title V, Sect. 501.94 Stat. 1598, October 7, 1980.

Mill, J. S. (1957). *Utilitarianism.* New York: The Liberal Arts Press.

Phipps, W. J., Long, B. C., & Woods, N. F. (1987). *Medical-surgical nursing: Concepts and clinical practice* (3rd ed.). St. Louis: CV Mosby.

Rawls, J. (1971). *Theory of justice.* Cambridge: Harvard University Press.

Shelly, J. A. (1980). *Dilemma: A nurses' guide for making ethical decisions.* Downers Grove, IL: Inter-Varsity.

Willig, S. (1971). Nursing and the law. In D. E. Orem (Ed.), *Nursing: Concepts of practice.* New York: McGraw-Hill.

Winick, B. (1981). Legal limitations on correctional therapy and research. *Minn L Rev, 65,* 331.

BIBLIOGRAPHY

American Nurses' Association. (1988). *Ethics in nursing: position statements and guidelines.* Kansas City, MO: ANA.

Bailey, D. S., Cooper, S. O., & Bailey, D. R. (1984). *Therapeutic approaches to the care of the mentally ill* (2nd ed.). Philadelphia: FA Davis.

Bandman, E. L. & Bandman, B. (Eds.). (1978). *Bioethics and human rights.* Boston: Little, Brown and Co.

Barker, P. J. & Baldwin, S. (Eds.). (1991). *Ethical issues in mental health.* London: Chapman and Hall.

Eth, S. & Mills, M. J. (1989). Ethical and legal considerations. In H. I. Kaplan & B. J. Sadock (Eds.), *Comprehensive textbook of psychiatry,* Vol. I (5th ed.). Baltimore: Williams & Wilkins.

Joint Commission on Accreditation of Health Organizations. (1981). *Consolidated standards manual for child, adolescent, and adult psychiatric, alcoholism, and drug abuse facilities.* Chicago: Joint Commission on Accreditation of Health Organizations.

Murphy, C. P. & Hunter, H. (1983). *Ethical problems in the nurse-patient relationship.* Boston: Allyn and Bacon.

Pavelka, R. (1992). *A summary of the rights of persons with mental illness in Kansas.* Manhattan, KS: Kansas Advocacy and Protective Services.

Appendix A: Answers to Chapter Review Questions

CHAPTER 1

1. Dr. Hans Selye
2. **Eye:** Pupils dilate; increased secretion from the lacrimal glands
   Respiratory system: bronchioles and pulmonary blood vessels dilate; increased respiratory rate
   Cardiovascular system: increase in the following:
   - Force of cardiac contraction
   - Cardiac output
   - Heart rate
   - Blood pressure

   Gastrointestinal system: Overall slowdown. Decreased motility and secretions.
   Liver: increased serum glucose
   Urinary system: Increased sensation for urination (bladder muscle contracts; sphincter relaxes)
3. Glucocorticoids:
   - Increased glucose
   - Decreased immune response
   - Decreased inflammatory response

   Mineralocorticoids:
   - Increased sodium and water retention

   Vasopressin:
   - Constricts blood vessels, resulting in increased blood pressure
   - Increased fluid retention

   Growth hormone:
   - Increased serum glucose and free fatty acids

   Thyrotropic hormone:
   - Increased basal metabolic rate

Gonadotropins:

- Initially, increased secretion of sex hormones
- Later, secretion is suppressed, resulting in decreased libido, or impotence

4. Use the following scale to interpret your score:

0–150	No significant possibility of stress-related illness
150–199	Mild life crisis level — 35 percent chance of illness
200–299	Moderate life crisis level — 50 percent chance of illness
300 or more	Major life crisis level — 80 percent chance of illness

5. The three types of predisposing factors are 1) genetic influences, 2) past experiences, and 3) existing conditions.
6. 1. c   3. b
   2. d   4. a
7. 1. d   4. b
   2. a   5. c
   3. e
8. Adaptive coping strategies discussed in the text were:

   - Awareness
   - Relaxation
   - Meditation
   - Interpersonal communication with caring other
   - Problem solving
   - Pets
   - Music

   What other adaptive coping strategies can you describe?

CHAPTER 2

1. Mental health is defined as the successful adaptation to stressors from the internal or external environment, evidenced by thoughts, feelings, and behaviors that are age-appropriate and congruent with local and cultural norms.
2. Mental illness is defined as maladaptive responses to stressors from the internal or external environment, evidenced by thoughts, feelings, and behaviors that are incongruent with the local and cultural norms and interfere with the individual's social, occupational, or physical functioning.
3. Individuals label behaviors in which they are unable to find meaning or comprehensibility as mental illness (the concept of incomprehensibility). Horwitz states that, "Observers attribute labels of mental illness when the rules, conventions, and understandings they use to interpret behavior fail to find any intelligible motivation behind an action." The element of cultural relativity considers that these rules, conventions, and understandings are conceived within an individual's own particular culture. Behavior that is considered "normal" and "abnormal" is defined by one's cultural or societal norms.
4. Mild = b
   Moderate = d
   Severe = a
   Panic = c
5. Compensation = b
   Denial = h
   Displacement = a
   Identification = m
   Intellectualization = n
   Introjection = c
   Isolation = k
   Projection = e
   Rationalization = i
   Reaction formation = f
   Regression = d
   Repression = o
   Sublimation = g
   Suppression = j
   Undoing = l

6. Denial, anger, bargaining, depression, acceptance
7. Anticipatory grieving occurs when a loss is expected. It begins and sometimes is completed prior to occurrence of the loss. It may shorten the grieving response once the loss has occurred.
8. Resolution of the process of mourning is thought to have occurred when an individual can look back on the relationship with the lost entity and accept both the pleasures and the disappointments (both the positive and the negative aspects) of the association. Length of the grief process is influenced by:
   a. Ambivalence and guilt related to one's association with the lost entity (a love–hate relationship)
   b. Whether one has been able to experience anticipatory grieving
   c. Number of recent losses experienced by an individual (bereavement overload)
9. a. Prolonged grief response—an intense preoccupation with memories of the lost entity for many years after the loss has occurred; person fixed in denial/anger
   b. Delayed/inhibited response—emotional pain associated with the loss is not experienced; may be evidence of emotional or physical disorders; person fixed in denial
   c. Distorted response—all the normal behaviors associated with grieving are exaggerated out of proportion to the situation; person fixed in anger; anger is turned inward on the self; person unable to function in normal activities of daily living
10. Anger; distorted

CHAPTER 3

1. Personality is defined as deeply ingrained patterns of behavior, which include the way one relates to, perceives, and thinks about the environment and oneself.
2. a. generativity vs. stagnation
   b. trust vs. mistrust
   c. Mr. J. is socially isolated; darts head from side to side in a continuous scanning of the

area; refuses to eat for fear of "being poisoned"

 d. Level I — stage 2: egocentrism and concern for self

 e. Internalized rage and fear of abandonment by others

 f. Childhood. He has not yet learned to delay gratification

 g. II. Strong id, weak ego, weak superego

3. a. To decrease anxiety and develop trust

CHAPTER 4

1. a. The mother-surrogate
   b. The technician
   c. The manager
   d. The socializing agent
   e. The health teacher
   f. The counselor
2. The counselor
3. It is through establishment of a satisfactory nurse – patient relationship that individuals learn to generalize the ability to achieve satisfactory interpersonal relationships to other aspects of their lives.
4. Most often the goal is directed at learning and growth promotion, in an effort to bring about some type of change in the patient's life. This is accomplished through use of the problem-solving model.
5. The therapeutic use of self
6. a. 4
   b. 1
   c. 5
   d. 2
   e. 3
7. Preinteraction phase:
   a. Obtain information about the patient
   b. Self-exploration
   Orientation (introductory) phase:
   a. Establish trust
   b. Formulate a contract for nursing intervention
   c. Identify nursing diagnoses
   d. Goals are mutually set by nurse and patient
   e. Develop a plan of action

f. Explore feelings of nurse and patient

Working phase:

a. Maintain trust and rapport

b. Use problem-solving model to promote change

c. Overcome resistance behaviors

d. Evaluate progress

Termination phase:

a. Evaluate goal attainment

b. Ensure therapeutic closure

c. Explore feelings of nurse and patient

CHAPTER 5

1. In the transactional model of communication, both persons are participating simultaneously. They are mutually perceiving each other, simultaneously listening to each other, and are mutually and simultaneously engaged in the process of creating meaning in a relationship.
2. a. One's value system
   b. Internalized attitudes and beliefs
   c. Culture or religion
   d. Social status
   e. Gender
   f. Background knowledge and experience
   g. Age or developmental level
   h. Type of environment in which the communication takes place
3. Territoriality is the innate tendency to own space. People "mark" space as their own and feel more comfortable in these spaces. Territoriality affects communication in that an interaction can be more successful if it takes place on "neutral" ground rather than in space "owned" by one or the other of the communicants.
4. Density refers to the number of people within a given environmental space. It may affect communication in that some studies indicate that a correlation exists between prolonged high-density situations and certain behaviors, such as aggression, stress, criminal activity, hostility toward others, and a deterioration of mental and physical health.

5. a. Intimate distance (0–18 in)—kissing or hugging someone
   b. Personal distance (18–40 in)—close conversations with friends or colleagues
   c. Social distance (4–12 ft)—conversations with strangers or acquaintances (e.g., at a cocktail party)
   d. Public distance (>12 ft)—speaking in public
6. a. Physical appearance and dress (e.g., young men who have hair down past their shoulders may convey a message of rebellion against the establishment)
   b. Body movement and posture (e.g., a person with hands on hips standing straight and tall in front of someone seated who must look up to them is conveying a message of power over the seated individual)
   c. Touch (e.g., laying one's hand upon the shoulder of another may convey a message of friendship and caring)
   d. Facial expressions (e.g., wrinkling up of the nose, raising the upper lip, or raising one side of the upper lip conveys a message of disgust for a situation)
   e. Eye behavior (e.g., direct eye contact, accompanied by a smile and nodding of the head, conveys interest in what the other person is saying)
   f. Vocal cues or paralanguage (e.g., a normally soft-spoken individual whose pitch and rate of speaking increases may be perceived as being anxious or tense)
7. S—Sit squarely facing the patient
   O—Observe an open posture
   L—Lean forward toward the patient
   E—Establish eye contact
   R—Relax
8. a. Nontherapeutic technique: disagreeing
   b. The correct answer. Therapeutic technique: voicing doubt
9. a. The correct answer. Therapeutic technique: giving recognition
   b. Nontherapeutic technique: complimenting—a judgment on the part of the nurse
10. a. Nontherapeutic: giving reassurance
    b. Nontherapeutic: giving disapproval
    c. Nontherapeutic: introducing an unrelated topic

d. Nontherapeutic: indicating an external source of power
e. The correct answer. Therapeutic technique: exploring
11. a. Nontherapeutic: requesting an explanation
    b. Nontherapeutic: belittling feelings expressed
    c. Nontherapeutic: rejecting
    d. The correct answer. Therapeutic technique: formulating a plan of action
12. Therapeutic response: "Do *you* think you should tell him?" Technique: reflecting
    Nontherapeutic response: "Yes, you must tell your husband about your affair with your boss." Technique: giving advice
13. a. The correct answer. Therapeutic technique: reflecting
    b. Nontherapeutic: requesting an explanation
    c. Nontherapeutic: indicating an external source of power
    d. Nontherapeutic: giving advice
    e. Nontherapeutic: defending
    f. Nontherapeutic: making stereotyped comments

CHAPTER 6

1. Assessment, analysis, planning, implementation, evaluation
2. a. Implementation
   b. Analysis
   c. Evaluation
   d. Assessment
   e. Planning
3. Nursing diagnoses:
   a. Altered nutrition, less than body requirements
   b. Social isolation
   c. Self-esteem disturbance
   Goals:
   a. Patient will gain 2 lb/wk in next 3 weeks.
   b. Patient will voluntarily spend time with other patients and staff members in group activities on the unit within 7 days.
   c. Patient will verbalize positive aspects about herself (excluding any references to eating or body image) within 2 weeks.

4. Problem-oriented recording (SOAPIE); Focus Charting®; PIE charting

CHAPTER 7

1. A group is a collection of individuals whose association is founded upon shared comonalities of interest, values, norms, or purpose.
2. a. Teaching group
   Laissez-faire leader
   b. Supportive/therapeutic group
   Democratic leader
   c. Task group
   Autocratic leader

3. 1. b 11. c
   2. i
   3. k 4. 1. e
   4. h 2. h
   5. e 3. f
   6. j 4. d
   7. a 5. a
   8. d 6. c
   9. f 7. g
   10. g 8. b

CHAPTER 8

1. A scientific structuring of the environment to effect behavioral changes and to improve the psychological health and functioning of the individual.
2. The goal of milieu therapy/therapeutic community is for the patient to learn adaptive coping, and interaction and relationship skills that can be generalized to other aspects of his or her life.
3. c
4. b
5. a
6. d
7. 1. f 8. e
   2. h 9. c
   3. b 10. k
   4. i 11. m
   5. g 12. l
   6. j 13. d
   7. a

CHAPTER 9

1. c 6. a
2. d 7. d
3. a 8. b
4. b 9. b
5. c 10. d

CHAPTER 10

3a. (1) Anxiety (moderate to severe) related to lack of self-confidence and fear of making errors
(2) Pain (migraine headaches) related to repressed severe anxiety
(3) Sleep pattern disturbance related to anxiety

3b. The deep-breathing exercises would be especially good for Linda because she could perform them as many times as she needed to during the working day to relieve her anxiety. With practice, progressive relaxation techniques and mental imagery could also provide relief from anxiety attacks for Linda. Any of these relaxation techniques may be beneficial at bedtime to help induce relaxation and sleep. Biofeedback may provide assistance for relief from migraine headaches. Physical exercise, either in the early morning or late afternoon after work, may provide Linda with renewed energy and combat chronic fatigue. It also relieves pent-up tension.

3c. Some outcome criteria for Linda might be:
(1) Patient will be able to perform duties on the job while maintaining anxiety at a manageable level by practicing deep-breathing exercises.
(2) Patient will verbalize a reduction in headache pain following progressive relaxation techniques.
(3) Patient is able to fall asleep within 30 minutes of retiring by listening to soft music and performing mental imagery exercises.

CHAPTER 11

1. a. = AS
   b. = PA
   c. = NA
   d. = AG
2. a. = AG
   b. = NA
   c. = PA
   d. = AS
3. a. = NA
   b. = AS
   c. = PA
   d. = AG
4. a. = PA
   b. = AG
   c. = AS
   d. = NA
5. a. = AS
   b. = NA
   c. = PA
   d. = AG

6. a. = NA
   b. = AS
   c. = AG
   d. = PA
7. a. = AS
   b. = PA
   c. = AG
   d. = NA
8. a. = PA
   b. = NA
   c. = AG
   d. = AS
9. a. = AG
   b. = NA
   c. = AS
   d. = PA
10. a. = AS
    b. = NA
    c. = AG
    d. = PA

CHAPTER 12

1. a
2. c
3. d
4. b
5. c

6. b
7. a
8. b
9. c
10. b

CHAPTER 13

1. c
2. b
3. a
4. c
5. d

6. a
7. d
8. b
9. c

CHAPTER 14

1. a
2. a
3. b
4. c

5. a
6. b
7. d
8. f, b, d, a, e, c

CHAPTER 15

1. b
2. c
3. a
4. b
5. d
6. b

7. c
8. d
9. b
10. d
11. b
12. a

CHAPTER 16

1. c
2. d
3. b
4. a
5. b

6. a
7. c
8. b
9. c
10. c

CHAPTER 17

1. b
2. a
3. c
4. c
5. a

6. b
7. b
8. d
9. a
10. c

CHAPTER 18

1. b
2. b
3. c
4. d
5. d

6. a
7. c
8. b
9. c
10. a

CHAPTER 19

1. c
2. b
3. a
4. d
5. c

6. b
7. c
8. d
9. a
10. c

CHAPTER 20

1. d	6. c
2. c	7. b
3. d	8. c
4. a	9. a
5. b	10. d

CHAPTER 21

1. b	6. a
2. d	7. b
3. a	8. d
4. d	9. b
5. c	10. c

CHAPTER 22

1. d	6. c
2. b	7. a
3. a	8. c
4. b	9. a
5. d	10. b

CHAPTER 23

1. b	6. b
2. c	7. d
3. d	8. a
4. a	9. e
5. b	10. c

CHAPTER 24

1. c	6. d
2. b	7. a
3. a	8. b
4. c	9. e
5. d	10. c

CHAPTER 25

1. c	6. f
2. g	7. d
3. a	8. i
4. e	9. b
5. h	10. b

CHAPTER 26

1. d	6. b
2. a	7. c
3. b	8. c
4. d	9. d
5. a	10. b

CHAPTER 27

1. c	6. d
2. d	7. a
3. b	8. a
4. a	9. c
5. c	10. a

CHAPTER 28

1. d	6. d
2. c	7. a
3. a	8. a
4. c	9. b
5. b	10. b

CHAPTER 29

1. b	6. d
2. c	7. a
3. a	8. b
4. d	9. b
5. b	10. d

CHAPTER 30

1. c	6. d
2. a	7. b
3. e	8. e
4. d	9. a
5. b	10. c

Appendix B: The Rights of Persons with Mental Illness in Kansas

The laws that cover the rights of mentally ill individuals vary from state to state. The material described in this appendix is presented as an *example* of the types of laws that exist for the protection of the mentally ill. If a student or practicing nurse has a question about an issue presented in this example, a check with the state statute would clarify the laws governing the specific issue in his or her state.

This information is a summarization of the rights, under Kansas law, of persons who have been deemed to be mentally ill and who are undergoing residential treatment. Other rights may be applicable in certain mental health facilities. This summarization is not a comprehensive discussion of all of the rights of persons with mental illness.

DEFINITIONS

The following terms are defined in the Treatment Act for Mentally Ill Persons:

1. *Mentally ill person*—This is any person who:
   a. is suffering from a severe mental disorder to the extent that such a person is in need of treatment;
   b. lacks capacity to make an informed decision concerning treatment; and
   c. is likely to cause harm to self or others.
2. *Treatment facility*—This means any mental health center or clinic, psychiatric unit of a medical care facility, psychologist, physician, or other institution or individual authorized or licensed by law to provide either inpatient or outpatient treatment to any person.

This summary of rights was prepared by Ron Pavelka, Coordinator, Protection and Advocacy for Individuals with Mental Illness Program, Kansas Advocacy and Protective Services, July 1992. Used with permission.

3. *Participating mental health center*—This is a mental health center that has contracted with the Department of Social and Rehabilitation Services to provide screening, evaluations, and other treatment services consistent with the terms of the Mental Health Reform Act.
4. *Qualified mental health professional*—This refers, in essence, to professional persons (physicians, psychologists, social workers, registered nurses) who have achieved certain levels of training and who are employed by or under contract to a participating mental health center.

RIGHTS PRIOR TO COMMITMENT

In 1990, the Kansas legislature passed the Mental Health Reform Act. Under this act, the law requires that in areas of the state where there is a "participating mental health center," no person can be sent to a state hospital for evaluation or treatment unless the person has been evaluated by a qualified mental health professional at the mental health center.

Emergency Observation

For some persons, the first contact that they have with the mental health treatment system is through a period of emergency observation. A person may be placed under emergency observation after an application is filed with a treatment facility by either a police officer or any other individual. The application must include a statement that the police officer or other individual believes the person is mentally ill and is likely to cause harm to self or others if not confined.

Emergency observation is only appropriate

under certain circumstances. First of all, the staff of the treatment facility must agree that the potential patient needs to be hospitalized. Another prerequisite is that the application for emergency observation must state that the applicant will also be requesting an Order of Protective Custody. If the applicant is someone other than a police officer, he or she must also provide a written statement from a physician or psychologist confirming the potential patient's condition.

Emergency observation can last for just a short period. Unless the treatment facility receives a court order, the person being observed must be released by 5:00 PM on the first day after the hospitalization that the local district court is open for business.

Under some circumstances, the staff of a treatment facility to which a person is brought may decide not to admit the person for observation, even though it is thought that the person is a mentally ill person. In such cases, in areas in which participating mental health centers are located, no person with a mental illness is to be placed in a nonmedical facility used for the detention of persons charged with or convicted of a crime.

While a person is subject to emergency observation, he or she has some additional specific rights:

1. The person must be informed of the right to immediately contact his or her legal counsel, next of kin, or both.
2. The person must be provided a copy of the application completed by the police officer or other individual.
3. The person is entitled to communicate by reasonable means with a reasonable number of persons. This includes private consultations with an attorney, a personal physician or psychologist, a minister, and at least one family member or a guardian.
4. Unless a particular medication or therapy is necessary to sustain life or protect the person or others, the treatment facility may not administer to the person any medication or therapy that will adversely affect his or her judgment.

Order of Protective Custody

The second way in which a person may officially be brought within the mental health treatment system in Kansas is through an Order of Protective Custody. Such an order may be applied to someone who is already under emergency observation or to someone who is not being confined at all.

Anyone can ask a district court to issue an Order of Protective Custody. A request for such an order must be accompanied by an application to determine whether a proposed patient is a mentally ill person. Under some circumstances, which are similar to those that are the basis for holding a person under emergency observation, an Order of Protective Custody can be issued without a hearing. An order obtained without a hearing is valid only until 5:00 PM of the second full day after its issuance that the local district court is open for business. A second successive order may not be obtained without a hearing.

An Order of Protective Custody may also be issued after a hearing. For the order to be issued, the court must have found probable cause to believe that the person who was the subject of the hearing is a mentally ill person.

The person with respect to whom the application for an Order of Protective Custody was filed is, in general, entitled to be present at the hearing. This is the case even though Kansas law provides that under some circumstances, the presence of the proposed patient may be waived. The law goes on to state, however, that if the person requests, in writing, to attend the hearing, his or her presence cannot be waived.

A person who is potentially subject to an Order of Protective Custody has a right to be represented by a lawyer at the probable cause hearing. The court will appoint a lawyer to represent the person at no cost to that person if he or she does not already have a lawyer. The person must also be given an opportunity to testify at the hearing and to present and cross-examine witnesses.

Before either form of Order of Protective Custody, the one obtained without a hearing and the other issued subsequent to a hearing, can be made, the requirements of the Mental Health Reform Act apply. The district court must obtain from a qualified mental health professional a written recommendation for such an admission to a state hospital.

If an Order of Protective Custody is issued, it is effective until completion of the hearing on whether the person to whom it applies is a mentally ill person. During the time prior to the mental illness hearing, the person must be housed in a designated treatment facility or other suitable place. He or she should not be confined in a jail or correctional setting unless no other facilities are available.

The rights listed earlier under "Emergency Observation"—the right to contact legal counsel or family members, the right to communicate with other people, and the prohibition on medication that would alter one's mental state—all apply to persons who are being held under an Order of Protective Custody.

Order for Treatment

The third legally defined manner in which a person may involuntarily come within the influence of the mental health system is through an Order for Treatment. Such an order is issued if it is found, after a hearing, by clear and convincing evidence, that a proposed patient is a mentally ill person. This means that all three of the elements in the definition of a mentally ill person, which was included earlier, have been established.

Before a mental illness hearing can be held, several preliminary steps should have been taken. The first of these is that an application to determine whether a person is a mentally ill person must have been filed. Anyone can file this application, in the district court of the county in which the person lives or is present.

Unless it includes a statement to the effect that the proposed patient has refused to submit to an evaluation, the application must be accompanied by a signed statement from a physician, psychologist, or someone designated by the head of a treatment facility. This statement should provide the results of an evaluation of the proposed patient.

Once an application for a determination of mental illness is filed, several preliminary orders must be issued by the court:

1. An order setting the time and place for the hearing on the application. The hearing may take place in a courtroom, at a treatment facility, or at some other suitable place. The hearing should be held from 7 to 14 days after the application is filed, but, in some circumstances, a longer time is allowed.
2. There must also be an order that the proposed patient be present at the hearing. Under certain conditions, a proposed patient's presence at the hearing can be waived, but if the patient, in writing, asks to be allowed to attend the

hearing, his or her presence cannot be waived.
3. An attorney must be appointed to represent the proposed patient at all stages of the proceedings and until all orders resulting from the case have expired. This must be done through a judge's order.
4. In addition, there must be an order that the proposed patient meet with his or her court-appointed attorney. This should be at least 5 days before the mental illness hearing.

Another order that is issued after an application for determination of mental illness is filed is an Order of Mental Evaluation. Basically, this order requires the proposed patient to undergo a psychological evaluation. In areas in which there is a participating mental health center, this evaluation must not be administered at a state hospital unless the court has been notified in writing that the evaluation cannot be conducted at the center.

A proposed patient who is not subject to an Order of Protective Custody has the right to refuse to submit to an evaluation. This right lasts until a separate hearing is held, and the court finds that there is probable cause to believe that the proposed patient is a mentally ill person. If no probable cause is found, the patient need not submit to an evaluation, and the entire proceeding is ended.

The proposed patient has a right to be notified of the fact that an application for determination of mental illness is pending. In particular, the notice provided to the patient must state:

1. That an application requesting court-ordered treatment has been filed
2. The time and place of the hearing
3. The name of the attorney who has been appointed to represent the patient and the place where the patient will need the attorney
4. That the proposed patient has the right to a trial before a jury

In addition to the prohibition on medication of a person under Orders of Protective Custody, Kansas law contains a specific limitation on the administration of medication prior to the hearing. If a particular medication or therapy will alter the patient's mental state so as to adversely affect his or her judgment, or to impair his or her ability to prepare for or participate in the hearing, it may not be administered within 48 hours prior to the hearing. The only exception to this limitation is if the medication or therapy is necessary to sustain life or protect the patient or others.

As was mentioned earlier, the proposed patient is entitled to a hearing before a jury. To exercise that right, however, the proposed patient must, in writing, request that the hearing be held before a jury. This written request must be submitted at least 4 days before the time of the hearing.

During the course of the mental illness hearing, the proposed patient has several specific rights. The patient must have an opportunity to appear at the hearing, to testify, and to present and cross-examine witnesses.

At the conclusion of the hearing, the court or jury must find by clear and convincing evidence that the proposed patient is a mentally ill individual before an Order for Treatment can be made. If that occurs, the court orders treatment for the patient at a treatment facility. The term *treatment facility* includes more than state hospitals. With the exception of state hospitals, however, an order of treatment at a particular facility depends on the consent of that facility.

Under the requirements of the Mental Health Reform Act, in areas of the state in which there is a participating mental health center, a patient may not be ordered to a state hospital for treatment unless the court has received a written recommendation for such treatment from a qualified mental health professional.

In addition, under certain circumstances, a patient may be ordered to take part in outpatient treatment. This can be done if the court concludes that the person undergoing outpatient treatment will not be potentially dangerous to the community and that the patient is not likely to cause harm to self or others while in the community.

Unlike other treatment facilities, when the order for outpatient treatment is to a participating mental health center, that order cannot be refused.

An order for outpatient treatment normally lists some specific conditions with which the patient is required to comply. If the patient fails to substantially comply with those conditions, however, a process resulting in the hospitalization of the patient could be initiated.

RIGHTS AFTER HOSPITALIZATION

As soon as a person becomes a patient in a treatment facility, that person acquires an additional series of rather specific legal rights. In fact, under Kansas law, a section of the law has come to be known as a Patient's Bill of Rights. This section indicates that patients have the following rights:

1. To wear one's own clothes, to keep and use one's own personal possessions, and to keep and be allowed to spend one's own money
2. To communicate by phone, including making and receiving confidential calls, and to communicate by letter, both sending and receiving unopened letters
3. To visit privately with a husband or wife, if facilities are available
4. To receive visitors every day
5. To refuse involuntary labor and to be paid for any work done other than cleaning one's own bedroom and bathroom
6. To not be subject to procedures such as psychosurgery, electroconvulsive therapy, experimental medication, aversion therapy, or hazardous treatment procedures without the written consent of the patient and, if appropriate, the written consent of the patient's parent or legal guardian
7. To have explained the nature of all medications prescribed, the reason for the prescription, and the most common side effects, and if requested, the nature of any other treatment ordered
8. To prompt uncensored written communication with the Secretary of Social and Rehabilitation Services, the head of the treatment facility, and any court, physician, psychologist, minister, or attorney
9. To be visited by one's physician, psychologist, minister, or attorney at any time
10. Upon admission to a treatment facility, to be informed both orally and in writing about these rights

For good cause only, some of the patient's rights can be restricted by the head of the treatment facility. The rights listed under Numbers 5 through 10 and the right to mail any correspondence that does not violate postal regulations may not, however, be restricted under any circumstances.

If one of the patient's rights is restricted, a written explanation of the restriction must be promptly included in the patient's medical record. Copies of the explanation are to be made available to the patient, his or her parent(s) or guardian(s), and attorney. If the right to receive unopened correspondence is restricted, such correspondence must be opened and read in the presence of the patient.

In addition to those rights listed in the Patient's Bill of Rights, Kansas law also provides for the rights of patients in certain other areas. Among those areas are:

1. *Restraints and seclusion*—Restraints or seclusion are not to be used unless either the head of a treatment facility, a physician, or a psychologist decides that such a form of treatment is necessary to prevent substantial bodily injury to a patient or others. The use of restraints or seclusion should not exceed 3 hours without medical re-evaluation, except that between 12:00 midnight and 8:00 AM re-evaluation is not mandatory. Whenever restraints or seclusion are used, the patient's condition must be monitored, at a minimum, or an hourly basis, and a record of this monitoring should be made. The head of the treatment facility, a physician, or a psychologist is required to sign a statement describing why each use of seclusion or restraints was necessary. This statement should be included in the patient's treatment records. An exception to this procedure is included in Kansas law. To prevent physical injury, restraints may be used for a period no longer than 2 hours without the approval of the head of the facility, a physician, or a psychologist.

2. *Court review*—Every 90 days during the first 6 months of involuntary treatment and every 180 days after that point, a patient is entitled to request a hearing. The purpose of the hearing is to determine whether the patient is still, by clear and convincing evidence, a mentally ill person. A written request for the hearing must be filed in the district court that has jurisdiction in the patient's case. In most instances, this will be the court in which the original commitment hearing was held. The hearing should be scheduled as soon as it is reasonably possible, but in any case, it must take place no more than 10 days after the written request was filed. The review hearing should be conducted in the same way as a commitment hearing, with the exception that the patient is not entitled to ask for a jury.

3. *Administration of medication*—A specific section of Kansas law provides that if a patient objects to a particular medication,

those objections must be included in the patient's treatment record. Within 5 days of the objections, they must be submitted to administrative review by the head of the treatment facility or by a designated psychiatrist. After an explanation of the medication, it may be administered over the patient's objections. The medication, however, may be continued only if approved by the administrative reviewer. The responsible physician is required to regularly review the medications being prescribed for each patient, with particular attention to be paid to the symptoms of harmful side effects.

4. *Access to records*—As a general rule, any patient of a treatment facility is entitled to obtain copies of his or her records. The only exception to this rule is that the head of a treatment facility may refuse to disclose portions of the records. To do this, the head of the treatment facility must state in writing that disclosure would be injurious to the welfare of the patient or former patient.

5. *Privilege against identification*—A patient in a treatment facility has a privilege to prevent employees of the facility from acknowledging that the patient is currently receiving or has ever received treatment. Also under this privilege, no one associated with a treatment facility may disclose the contents of any confidential communication made for the purpose of evaluation or treatment. This privilege exists unless the patient has specifically waived it in writing.

6. *Voluntary admission*—Subject to the availability of space and to a conclusion on the part of the treatment facility that the person is in need of treatment, anyone may apply for voluntary admission to a treatment facility. Once admitted on a voluntary basis, a patient may submit a request for discharge. The patient must be discharged no later than 3 working days after the request is submitted. During that 3-day period, however, the treatment facility staff may initiate in the court system an application for determination of mental illness.

7. *Transportation*—Kansas law provides specifically that the "least amount of restraint necessary shall be used . . ." when persons with mental illness are being transported. This means that if a person is calm and coop-

erative, handcuffs or shackles should not be applied to the person. Beyond that, a marked police or sheriff's car should not be used if other means of transportation are available.

8. *Transfers*—Patients may be transferred from one state hospital to another. Unless it is an emergency, the patient's guardian or family should be notified prior to the transfer. In addition, the patient has the option of requesting a hearing on the transfer.

9. *Discharge procedures*—Once a patient is no longer in need of treatment in a treatment facility, that patient is to be discharged from the facility. If there is a participating mental health center in the area in which the patient intends to reside, however, the patient should not be discharged until recommendations are received from the center.

A patient may also be granted a conditional release if a decision is made that the release is in the best interests of the patient and if facility staff believe the patient is not likely to cause harm to self or others while participating in a treatment plan in the community. Failure to comply with the terms of the treatment plan may result in readmission to the treatment facility.

10. *Humane treatment*—Under Kansas law, every patient has a right to receive humane treatment that is consistent with accepted ethics and practices. Kansas law also defines mistreatment of a confined person as a criminal offense.

Appendix C: Glossary

A

abreaction "Remembering with feeling." Bringing into conscious awareness painful events that have been repressed and re-experiencing the emotions that were associated with the events.

abuse Use of psychoactive drugs that pose significant hazards to health and interfere with social, occupational, psychological, or physical functioning.

acquired immunodeficiency syndrome (AIDS) A condition in which the immune system becomes deficient in its efforts to prevent opportunistic infections, malignancies, and neurologic disease. It is caused by the HIV, which is passed from one individual to another through body fluids.

adaptation Restoration of the body to homeostasis following a physiological or psychological response to stress.

adjustment disorder A maladaptive reaction to an identifiable psychosocial stressor that occurs within 3 months after onset of the stressor. The individual shows impairment in social and occupational functioning or exhibits symptoms that are in excess of a normal and expectable reaction to the stressor.

aggression Harsh physical or verbal actions intended (either consciously or unconsciously) to harm or injure another.

aggressiveness Behavior that defends an individual's own basic rights by violating the basic rights of others (as contrasted with assertiveness).

agoraphobia The fear of being in places or situations from which escape might be difficult (or embarrassing) or in which help might not be available in the event of a panic attack.

agranulocytosis Extremely low levels of white blood cells. Symptoms include sore throat, fever, and malaise. May be a side effect of long-term therapy with some antipsychotic medications.

AIDS dementia complex (ADC) A neuropathological syndrome, possibly caused by chronic HIV encephalitis and myelitis, and manifested by cognitive, behavioral, and motor symptoms that become more severe with progression of the disease.

AIDS-related complex (ARC) Identifies individuals with HIV infection who have persistent generalized lymph-adenopathy, oral candidiasis, single or multidermatomal herpes zoster, biopsy-proven hairy leukoplakia, persistent fever, and diarrhea. This diagnosis is no longer used clinically.

akathesia Restlessness; an urgent need for movement. A type of extrapyramidal side effect associated with some antipsychotic medications.

akinesia Muscular weakness; a loss or partial loss of muscle movement. A type of extrapyramidal side effect associated with some antipsychotic medications.

Alcoholics Anonymous (AA) A major self-help organization for the treatment of alcoholism. It is based on a 12-step program to help members attain and maintain sobriety. Once individuals have achieved sobriety, they in turn are expected to help other alcoholic persons.

altruism One curative factor of group therapy (identified by Yalom) in which individuals gain self-esteem through mutual sharing and concern. Providing assistance and support to others creates a positive self-image and promotes self-growth.

amenorrhea Cessation of menses. May be a side effect of some antipsychotic medications.

amnesia A sudden inability to recall important personal information that is too extensive to be explained by ordinary forgetfulness.

amnesia, continuous The inability to recall events occurring after a specific time up to and including the present.

amnesia, generalized The inability to recall anything that has happened during the individual's entire lifetime.

amnesia, localized The inability to recall all incidents associated with a traumatic event for a specific time following the event (usually a few hours to a few days).

amnesia, selective The inability to recall only certain incidents associated with a traumatic event for a specific time following the event.

anhedonia The inability to experience or even imagine any pleasant emotion.

anorgasmia Inability to achieve orgasm.

anosmia Inability to smell.

anticipatory grief A subjective state of emotional, physical, and social responses to an anticipated loss of a valued entity. The response is repeated once the loss actually occurs; however, it may not be as intense as it might have been if anticipatory grieving has not occurred.

antisocial personality disorder A pattern of socially irresponsible, exploitative, and guiltless behavior evident in the tendency to fail to conform to the law and to sustain consistent employment as well as the tendency to exploit and manipulate others for personal gain, to deceive, and to fail to develop stable relationships.

anxiety Diffuse apprehension that is vague in nature and is associated with feelings of uncertainty and helplessness.

aphasia Inability to communicate through speech, writing, or signs due to dysfunction of brain centers.

aphonia Inability to speak.

apraxia Inability to carry out motor activities despite intact motor function.

ascites Excessive accumulation of serous fluid in the abdominal cavity. Occurs in response to portal hypertension caused by cirrhosis of the liver.

assault An act that results in a person's genuine fear and apprehension that he or she will be touched without consent. Nurses may be guilty of assault for threatening to place an individual in restraints against his or her will.

assertiveness Behavior that enables individuals to act in their own best interests, to stand up for themselves without undue anxiety, to express their honest feelings comfortably, or to exercise their own rights without denying the rights of others.

associative looseness Sometimes called loose associations. A thinking process characterized by speech in which ideas shift from one unrelated subject to another. The individual is unaware that the topics are unconnected.

attachment theory The hypothesis that individuals who maintain close relationships with others into old age are more likely to remain independent and less likely to be institutionalized than those who do not.

autism A focus inward on a fantasy world, while distorting or excluding the external environment. Common in schizophrenia.

autistic disorder The withdrawal of an infant or child into the self and into a fantasy world of his or own creation. Characteristics of autism include marked impairment in interpersonal functioning and communication, and in imaginative play. Activities and interests are restricted and may be considered somewhat bizarre.

autocratic A leadership style in which the leader makes all decisions for the group. Productivity is very high with this type of leadership, but morale is often low as a result of lack of member input and creativity.

autoimmune A condition in which the body produces a disordered immunological response against itself. In this situation, the body fails to differentiate between what is normal and what is a foreign substance. When this occurs, the body produces antibodies against normal parts of the body to such an extent as to cause tissue injury.

autonomy Independence; self-governance. An ethical principle that emphasizes the status of persons as autonomous moral agents whose right to determine their destinies should always be respected.

aversive stimulus A stimulus that follows a behavioral response and decreases the probability that the behavior will recur. Also called punishment.

azidothymidine (AZT) An antiviral agent used to treat individuals with AIDS.

B

battering A pattern of repeated physical abuse, usually of a woman by her spouse or intimate partner. Men are also battered, although the incidence is much less frequent.

battery The touching of another person without consent. Nurses may be charged with battery should they participate in the treatment of a patient without his or her consent and outside of an emergency situation.

behavior modification A treatment modality aimed at changing undesirable behaviors that uses a system of reinforcements to bring about the modifications desired.

beneficence An ethical principle that refers to one's duty to benefit or promote the good of others.

bereavement overload An accumulation of grief that occurs when an individual experiences many losses over a short period and is unable to resolve one before another is experienced. This phenomenon is common among the elderly.

binge and purge A syndrome associated with eating disorders, especially bulimia, in which an individual consumes thousands of calories of food in one sitting, followed by self-induced vomiting.

bioethics The term used for ethical principles that refer to concepts within the scope of medicine, nursing, and allied health.

biofeedback The use of instrumentation to become aware of processes in the body that usually go unnoticed (e.g., blood pressure, pulse) and to bring them under voluntary control. Used as a method of stress reduction.

bipolar disorder A disorder characterized by mood swings from profound depression to extreme euphoria (mania), with intervening periods of normalcy. Psychotic symptoms may or may not be present.

body image One's perception of one's own body. May also be how one believes others perceive one's body.

borderline personality disorder A disorder characterized by a pattern of intense and chaotic relationships, with affective instability, fluctuating and extreme attitudes regarding other people, impulsivity, direct and indirect self-destructive behavior, and lack of a clear or certain sense of identity, life plan, or values.

C

cachexia A state of ill health, malnutrition, and wasting. Extreme emaciation.

cannabis The dried flowering tops of the hemp plant. Produces euphoric effects when ingested or smoked. Commonly used as marijuana or hashish.

carcinogen Any substance or agent that produces or increases the risk of developing cancer in humans or lower animals.

case management A health-care delivery process the goals of which are to provide quality health care, decrease fragmentation, enhance the patient's quality of life, and contain costs (ANA, 1988). A case manager coordinates the patient's care from admission to discharge and sometimes following discharge. Critical pathways are the tools used to provide care in a case management system.

catatonia A type of schizophrenia that is characterized by stupor or excitement. In catatonic stupor, there is extreme psychomotor retardation, mutism, negativism, and posturing. Catatonic excitement is characterized by psychomotor agitation, in which the movements are frenzied and purposeless.

catharsis One curative factor of group therapy (identified by Yalom) in which members within a group are able to express both positive and negative feelings in a nonthreatening atmosphere.

child sexual abuse Any sexual act, such as indecent exposure or improper touching to penetration (sexual intercourse), that is carried out with a child.

Christian ethics The ethical philosophy that states one should treat others as moral equals and recognize the equality of other persons by permitting them to act as we do when they occupy a position similar to ours. Sometimes referred to as "the ethic of the golden rule."

circumstantiality In speaking, an individual is delayed in reaching the point of a communication owing to unnecessary and tedious details.

civil law Law that protects the private and property rights of individuals and businesses.

clang associations A pattern of speech in which the choice of words is governed by sounds. Clang associations often take the form of rhyming.

classical conditioning A type of learning that occurs when an unconditioned stimulus (UCS) that produces an unconditioned response (UCR) is paired with a conditioned stimulus (CS), until the CS alone produces the same response, which is then called a conditioned response (CR). Pavlov's example: food (UCS) causes salivation (UCR); ringing bell (CS) with food (UCS) causes salivation (UCR); ringing bell (CS) causes salivation (CR).

co-dependency An exaggerated dependent pattern of learned behaviors, beliefs, and feelings that make life painful. It is a dependence on people and things outside the self, along with neglect of the self to the point of having little self-identity.

cognition Mental operations that relate to logic, awareness, intellect, memory, language, and reasoning powers.

cognitive therapy A type of therapy in which the individual is taught to control thought distortions that are considered to be a factor in the development and maintenance of emotional disorders.

common law Laws that are derived from decisions made in previous cases.

compensation Covering up a real or perceived weakness by emphasizing a trait one considers more desirable.

compounded rape reaction Symptoms that are in addition to the typical rape response of physical complaints, rage, humiliation, fear, and sleep disturbances. They include depression, suicide, substance abuse, and even psychotic behaviors.

concrete thinking Thought processes are focused on specifics rather than generalities and immediate issues rather than eventual outcomes. Individuals who are experiencing concrete thinking are unable to comprehend abstract terminology.

confidentiality The right of an individual to the assurance that his or her case will not be discussed outside the boundaries of the health-care team.

contingency contracting A written contract between individuals used to modify behavior. Benefits and consequences for fulfilling the terms of the contract are delineated.

controlled response pattern The response to rape in which feelings are masked or hidden, and a calm, composed, or subdued affect is seen.

countertransference In psychoanalytic theory, the development by the therapist of emotional feelings toward the patient.

covert sensitization An aversion technique used to modify behavior that relies on the individual's imagination to produce unpleasant symptoms. When the individual is about to succumb to undesirable behavior, he or she visualizes something that is offensive or even nauseating in an effort to block the behavior.

criminal law Law that provides protection from conduct deemed injurious to the public welfare. It provides for punishment of those found to have engaged in such conduct.

crisis Psychological disequilibrium in a person who confronts a hazardous circumstance that constitutes an important problem which for the time he or she can neither escape nor solve with usual problem-solving resources.

crisis intervention An emergency type of assistance in which the intervener becomes a part of the individual's life situation. The focus is to provide guidance and support to help mobilize the resources needed to resolve the crisis and restore or generate an improvement in previous level of functioning. Usually lasts no longer than 6 to 8 weeks.

critical pathways of care An abbreviated plan of care that provides outcome-based guidelines for goal achievement within a designated length of stay.

cycle of battering Three phases of predictable behaviors that are repeated over time in a relationship between a batterer and a victim. These phases include the tension-building phase, the acute battering incident, and the calm, loving respite (honeymoon) phase.

cyclothymia A chronic mood disturbance involving numerous episodes of hypomania and depressed mood of insufficient severity or duration to meet the criteria for bipolar disorder.

D

date rape A term applied to situations in which the rapist is known to the victim. They may be dating, just acquaintances, or schoolmates.

defamation of character An individual may be liable for defamation of character by sharing with others information about a person that is detrimental to his or her reputation.

delirium A state of mental confusion and excitement characterized by disorientation for time and place, often with hallucinations, incoherent speech, and a continual state of aimless physical activity.

delusions False personal beliefs, not consistent with a person's intelligence or cultural background. The individual continues to have the belief in spite of obvious proof that it is false or irrational.

dementia Global impairment of cognitive functioning that is progressive and interferes with social and occupational abilities.

denial Refusal to acknowledge the existence of a real situation or the feelings associated with it.

density Density refers to the number of people within a given environmental space and has been shown to influence interpersonal interaction.

dependence *Physical* dependence is identified by the inability to stop using a substance despite attempts to do so; a continual use of the substance despite adverse consequences; a developing tolerance; and the development of withdrawal symptoms upon cessation or decreased intake. *Psychological* dependence is said to

exist when a substance is perceived by the user to be necessary to maintain an optimal state of personal well-being, interpersonal relations, or skill performance.

depersonalization An alteration in the perception or experience of the self so that the feeling of one's own reality is temporarily lost (APA, 1987).

derealization An alteration in the perception of one's surroundings so that a sense of the reality of the external world is lost (APA, 1987).

diagnosis-related group (DRG) A system used to determine prospective payment rates for reimbursement of hospital care based on the patient's diagnosis.

Diagnostic and Statistical Manual of Mental Disorders, 3rd ed., Revised (DSM-III-R) Standard nomenclature of emotional illness published by the American Psychiatric Association and used by all health-care practitioners. It classifies mental illnesses and presents guidelines and diagnostic criteria for various mental disorders.

directed association A technique used to help patients bring into consciousness events that have been repressed. Specific thoughts are guided and directed by the psychoanalyst.

discriminative stimulus A stimulus that precedes a behavioral response and predicts that a particular reinforcement will occur. Individuals learn to discriminate between various stimuli that will produce the responses they desire.

disengagement theory The hypothesis that there is a process of mutual withdrawal of aging persons and society from each other that is correlated with successful aging. This theory has been challenged by many investigators.

displacement Feelings are transferred from one target to another that is considered less threatening or neutral.

disulfiram A drug that is administered to individuals who abuse alcohol as a deterrent to drinking. Ingestion of alcohol while disulfiram is in the body results in a syndrome of symptoms that can produce a great deal of discomfort and can even result in death if the blood alcohol level is high.

double-bind communication Communication described as contradictory that places an individual in a "double bind." It occurs when a statement is made and succeeded by a contradictory statement or when a statement is made accompanied by nonverbal expression that is inconsistent with the verbal communication.

dyspareunia The occurrence of pain during sexual intercourse.

dysthymia A depressive neurosis. The symptoms are similar to, if somewhat milder than, those ascribed to major depression. There is no loss of contact with reality.

dystonia Involuntary muscular movements (spasms) of the face, arms, legs, and neck. May occur as an extrapyramidal side effect of some antipsychotic medications.

E

echolalia An individual with loose ego boundaries attempts to identify with the person speaking by repeating words he or she hears.

echopraxia An individual with loose ego boundaries attempts to identify with another person by imitating movements that the other person makes.

ego One of the three elements of the personality identified by Freud as the rational self or "reality principle." The ego seeks to maintain harmony between the external world, the id, and the superego.

ego defense mechanisms Strategies employed by the ego for protection in the face of threat to biological or psychological integrity (see individual defense mechanisms).

electroconvulsive therapy (ECT) A type of somatic treatment in which electric current is applied to the brain through electrodes placed on the temples. A grand mal seizure produces the desired effect. Used with severely depressed patients refractory to antidepressant medications.

emotional injury A pattern of behavior on the part of a parent or caretaker that results in serious impairment of a child's social, emotional, or intellectual functioning.

emotional neglect A chronic failure by a parent or caretaker to provide a child with the hope, love, and support necessary for the development of a sound, healthy personality.

empathy The ability to see beyond outward behavior and sense accurately another's inner experiencing. With empathy, one is able to accurately perceive and understand the meaning and relevance in the thoughts and feelings of another.

esophageal varices Veins in the esophagus that have become distended due to excessive pressure from defective blood flow through a cirrhotic liver.

essential hypertension Persistent elevation of blood pressure for which there is no apparent cause or associated underlying disease.

ethical dilemma A situation that arises when, on the basis of moral considerations, an appeal can be made for taking each of two opposing courses of action.

ethical egoism An ethical theory espousing that what is "right" and "good" is what is best for the individual making the decision.

ethics A branch of philosophy dealing with values related to human conduct, to the rightness and wrongness of certain actions, and to the goodness and badness of the motives and ends of such actions.

exhibitionism A paraphilic disorder characterized by a recurrent urge to expose one's genitals to a stranger.

expressed response pattern The victim of rape expresses feelings of fear, anger, and anxiety through such behavior as crying, sobbing, smiling, restlessness, and tenseness. This is in contrast to the rape victim who withholds feelings in the controlled response pattern.

extinction The gradual decrease in frequency or disappearance of a response when the positive reinforcement is withheld.

extrapyramidal symptoms (EPS) A variety of symptomatology that occurs outside the pyramidal tracts and in the basal ganglion of the brain. Symptoms may include tremors, chorea, dystonia, akinesia, akathisia, and others. May occur as a side effect of some antipsychotic medications.

F

false imprisonment The deliberate and unauthorized confinement of a person within fixed limits by the use of threat or force. A nurse may be charged with false imprisonment by placing a patient in restraints against his or her will in a nonemergency situation.

family therapy A type of therapy in which the focus is on relationships within the family. The family is viewed as a system in which the members are interdependent and a change in one creates change in all.

fetishism A paraphilic disorder characterized by recurrent sexual urges and sexually arousing fantasies involving the use of nonliving objects.

fight or flight A syndrome of physical symptoms that result from an individual's real or perceived perception that harm or danger is imminent.

flooding Sometimes called implosive therapy, this technique is used to desensitize individuals to phobic stimuli. The individual is "flooded" with a continuous presentation (usually through mental imagery) of the phobic stimulus until it no longer elicits anxiety.

Focus Charting® A type of documentation that follows a data, action, and response (DAR) format. The main perspective is a patient "focus," which can be a nursing diagnosis, a patient concern, change in status, or significant event in the patient's therapy. The focus cannot be a medical diagnosis (Lampe, 1985).

free association A technique used to assist an individual to bring to consciousness material that has been repressed. The individual is encouraged to verbalize whatever comes into his or her mind, drifting naturally from one thought to another.

frotteurism A paraphilic disorder characterized by the recurrent preoccupation with intense sexual urges or fantasies involving touching or rubbing against a non-consenting person.

fugue Sudden, unexpected travel away from home or customary work locale with assumption of a new identity and an inability to recall one's previous identity. Usually occurs in response to severe psychosocial stress.

G

gains The reinforcements an individual receives for somaticizing.

gains, primary An individual receives positive reinforcement for somaticizing through added attention, sympathy, and nurturing.

gains, secondary An individual receives positive reinforcement for somaticizing by being able to avoid difficult situations because of physical complaint.

gains, tertiary An individual receives positive reinforcement for somaticizing by causing the focus of the family to switch to him or her and away from conflict that may be occurring within the family.

Gamblers Anonymous (GA) An organization of inspirational group therapy, modeled after Alcoholics Anonymous, for individuals who desire to, but cannot, stop gambling.

gender identity disorder A sense of discomfort associated with an incongruence between biologically assigned gender and subjectively experienced gender.

generalized anxiety disorder A disorder that is characterized by chronic (at least 6 months), unrealistic, and excessive anxiety and worry.

genogram A graphic representation of a family system. It may cover several generations. Emphasis is on family roles and emotional relatedness between members. Facilitates recognition of areas requiring change.

genuineness The ability to be open, honest, and "real" in interactions with others. The awareness of what one is experiencing internally and the ability to project the quality of this inner experiencing in a relationship.

geriatrics The branch of clinical medicine specializing in the care of the elderly and psychopathology of the elderly.

gerontology The study of normal aging.

geropsychiatry The branch of clinical medicine specializing in psychopathology of the elderly.

gonorrhea A sexually transmitted disease caused by the bacterium *Neisseria gonorrhoeae* and resulting in inflammation of the genital mucosa. Treatment is with antibiotics, particularly penicillin. Serious complications can result if it is left untreated.

"granny bashing" Media-generated slang term for abuse of the elderly.

"granny dumping" Media-generated slang term for abandoning elderly individuals at emergency departments, nursing homes, or other facilities—literally leaving them in the hands of others when the strain of caregiving becomes intolerable.

grief A subjective state of emotional, physical, and social responses to the real or perceived loss of a valued entity. Change and failure can also be perceived as losses. The grief response consists of a set of relatively predictable behaviors that describe the subjective state that accompanies mourning.

grief, exaggerated A reaction in which all of the symptoms associated with normal grieving are exaggerated out of proportion. Pathological depression is a type of exaggerated grief.

grief, inhibited The absence of evidence of grief when it ordinarily would be expected.

grief, prolonged The situation that exists when there has been no resumption of normal activities of daily living within 4 to 8 weeks of a loss.

group therapy A therapy group, founded in a specific theoretical framework, and led by a person with an advanced degree in psychology, social work, nursing, or medicine. The goal is to encourage improvement in interpersonal functioning.

gynecomastia Enlargement of the breasts in men. May be a side effect of some antipsychotic medications.

H

hallucinations False sensory perceptions not associated with real external stimuli. Hallucinations may involve any of the five senses.

hepatic encephalopathy A brain disorder resulting from the inability of the cirrhotic liver to convert ammonia to urea for excretion. The continued rise in serum ammonia results in progressively impaired mental functioning, apathy, euphoria or depression, sleep disturbances, increasing confusion, and progression to coma and eventual death.

histrionic personality disorder Conscious or unconscious overly dramatic behavior for the purpose of drawing attention to one's self.

HIV wasting syndrome An absence of concurrent illness other than HIV infection, and presence of the following symptoms: fever, weakness, weight loss, and chronic diarrhea.

homosexuality A sexual preference for persons of the same sex.

hospice A program that provides palliative and supportive care to meet the special needs arising out of the physical, psychosocial, spiritual, social, and economic stresses that are experienced during the final stages of illness and during bereavement.

human immunodeficiency virus (HIV) The virus that is the etiologic agent that produces the immunosuppression resulting in AIDS.

hypertensive crisis A potentially life-threatening syndrome that results when an individual taking monoamine oxidase inhibitors eats a product high in tyramine. Symptoms include severe occipital headache, palpitations, nausea and vomiting, nuchal rigidity, fever, sweating, marked increase in blood pressure, chest pain, and coma. Foods with tyramine include aged cheeses or other aged, overripe, and fermented foods; broad beans; pickled herring; beef or chicken liver; preserved meats; beer and wine; yeast products; chocolate; caffeinated drinks; canned figs; sour cream; yogurt; soy sauce; and over-the-counter cold medications and diet pills.

hypnosis A treatment for disorders brought on by repressed anxiety. The individual is directed into a state of subconsciousness and assisted, through suggestions, to recall certain events that he or she is not able to recall in the conscious state.

hypochondriasis Unrealistic preoccupation with fear of having a serious illness.

hypomania A mild form of mania. Symptoms are excessive hyperactivity but not severe enough to cause marked impairment in social or occupational functioning or to require hospitalization.

hysteria A polysymptomatic disorder that is characterized by recurrent, multiple somatic complaints often described dramatically.

I

id One of the three components of the personality identified by Freud as the "pleasure principle." The id is the locus of instinctual drives; is present at birth; and compels the infant to satisfy needs and seek immediate gratification.

identification An attempt to increase self-worth by acquiring certain attributes and characteristics of an individual one admires.

illusion A misperception of a real external stimulus.

implosion therapy See flooding.

incest Sexual exploitation of a child younger than 18 years of age by a relative or nonrelative who holds a position of trust in the family.

informed consent Permission granted to a physician by a patient to perform a therapeutic procedure, prior to which information about the procedure has been presented to the patient with adequate time given for consideration about the pros and cons.

insulin coma therapy The induction of a hypoglycemic coma aimed at alleviating psychotic symptoms. A dangerous procedure, questionably effective, and no longer used in psychiatry.

integration The process used with individuals with multiple personality disorder in an effort to bring all the personalities together into one. Usually achieved through hypnosis.

intellectualization An attempt to avoid expressing actual emotions associated with a stressful situation by using the intellectual processes of logic, reasoning, and analysis.

interdisciplinary care A concept of providing care for a patient in which members of various disciplines work together with common goals and shared responsibilities for meeting those goals.

intimate distance The closest distance that individuals will allow between themselves and others. In the United States, this distance is 0 to 18 inches.

introjection The beliefs and values of another individual are internalized and symbolically become a part of the self to the extent that the feeling of separateness or distinctness is lost.

isolation The separation of a thought or a memory from the feeling tone or emotions associated with it (sometimes called emotional isolation).

J

justice An ethical principle reflecting that all individuals should be treated equally and fairly.

K

Kantianism The ethical principle espousing that decisions should be made and actions should be taken out of a sense of duty.

Kaposi's sarcoma Malignant areas of cell proliferation initially in the skin and eventually in other body sites. Thought to be related to the immunocompromised state that accompanies AIDS.

kleptomania A recurrent failure to resist impulses to steal objects not needed for personal use or their monetary value.

Korsakoff's psychosis A syndrome of confusion, loss of recent memory, and confabulation in alcoholics due to a deficiency of thiamine. Often occurs together with Wernicke's encephalopathy and may be termed Wernicke-Korsakoff's syndrome.

L

la belle indifference A French term that describes a symptom of conversion disorder in which there is a relative lack of concern that is out of keeping with the severity of the impairment.

laissez-faire A leadership style in which the leader allows group members to do as they please. There is no direction from the leader. Member productivity and morale may be low due to frustration from lack of direction.

lesbian A female homosexual.

libel Action with which an individual may be charged for sharing *in writing* information that is detrimental to a person's reputation.

libido Freud's term for psychic energy used to fulfill basic physiological needs or instinctual drives, such as hunger, thirst, and sex.

long-term memory Memory for remote events or those events that occurred many years ago. The type of memory that is preserved in the elderly individual.

M

magical thinking A primitive form of thinking in which an individual believes that thinking about a possible occurrence can make it happen.

maladaptation A failure of the body to return to homeostasis following a physiological or psychological response to stress, resulting in the disruption of the integrity of the individual.

malpractice The failure of one rendering professional services to exercise that degree of skill and learning commonly applied under all the circumstances in the community by the average prudent, reputable member of the profession, with the result of injury, loss, or damage to the recipient of those services or to those entitled to rely upon them.

mania A type of bipolar disorder in which the predominant mood is elevated, expansive, or irritable. Motor activity is frenzied and excessive. Psychotic features may or may not be present.

mania, delirious A grave form of mania characterized by severe clouding of consciousness and representing an intensification of the symptoms associated with mania. The symptoms of delirious mania have become relatively rare since the availability of antipsychotic medications.

marital rape Sexual violence directed at a marital partner against that person's will.

masochism Sexual stimulation derived from being humiliated, beaten, bound, or otherwise made to suffer.

Medicaid A system established by the federal government to provide medical care benefits for indigent Americans. Medicaid funds are matched by the states, and coverage varies significantly from state to state.

Medicare A system established by the federal government to provide medical care benefits for elderly Americans.

meditation A method of relaxation in which an individual sits in a quiet place and focuses total concentration on an object, word, or thought.

melancholia A severe form of major depressive episode. Symptoms are exaggerated, and there is a loss of interest or pleasure in virtually all activities.

menopause The period that marks the permanent cessa-tion of menstrual activity. Occurs at approximately 48 to 51 years of age.

mental imagery A method of stress reduction that employs the imagination. The individual focuses imagination on a scenario that is particularly relaxing to him or her (e.g., a scene on a quiet seashore, a mountain atmosphere, or floating through the air on a fluffy white cloud).

migraine personality Personality characteristics that have been attributed to the migraine-prone person. These individuals are perfectionistic, overly conscientious, somewhat inflexible, neat and tidy, compulsive, hard working, intelligent, exacting, and place a very high premium on success, setting high (sometimes unrealistic) expectations on self and others.

milieu A French word meaning "middle." The English translation is "surroundings or environment."

milieu therapy Also called therapeutic community or therapeutic environment, this type of therapy consists of a scientific structuring of the environment to effect behavioral changes and to improve the psychological health and functioning of the individual.

modeling The learning of new behaviors by imitating the behavior of others.

mood An individual's sustained emotional tone, which significantly influences behavior, personality, and perception.

moral behavior Conduct that results from serious critical thinking about how individuals ought to treat others. Reflects respect for human life, freedom, justice, or confidentiality.

mourning The psychological process (or stages) through which the individual passes on the way to successful adaptation to the loss of a valued object.

multidisciplinary care A concept of providing care for a patient in which individual disciplines provide specific services for the patient without formal arrangement for interaction between the disciplines.

N

narcissistic personality disorder Individuals with this disorder have an exaggerated sense of self-worth. They lack empathy and are hypersensitive to the evaluation of others.

natural-law theory The ethical theory that has as its moral precept to "do good and avoid evil" at all costs. Natural-law ethics are grounded in a concern for the human good that is based on humanity's ability to live according to the dictates of reason.

negative reinforcement. Increasing the probability that a behavior will recur by removal of an undesirable reinforcing stimulus.

negativism Strong resistance to suggestions or directions. Exhibiting behaviors contrary to what is expected.

negligence The failure to do something that a reasonable person, guided by those considerations that ordinarily regulate human affairs, would do or doing something that a prudent and reasonable person would not do.

neologism New words that a psychotic individual invents that are meaningless to others but have symbolic meaning to that person.

neuroleptic Antipsychotic medications that are used to prevent or control psychotic symptoms.

neuroleptic malignant syndrome (NMS) A rare, but potentially fatal, complication of treatment with neuroleptic drugs. Symptoms include severe muscle rigidity, high fever, tachycardia, fluctuations in blood pressure, diaphoresis, and rapid deterioration of mental status to stupor and coma.

neurotic disorder A psychiatric disturbance characterized by excessive anxiety or depression, disrupted bodily functions, unsatisfying interpersonal relationships, and behaviors that interfere with routine functioning. There is no loss of contact with reality.

nonassertiveness Individuals who are nonassertive (sometimes called passive) seek to please others at the expense of denying their own basic human rights.

nonmaleficence The ethical principle that espouses abstaining from negative acts toward another, including acting carefully to avoid harm.

nursing diagnosis A clinical judgment about individual, family or community responses to actual and potential health problems/life processes. Nursing diagnoses provide the basis for selection of nursing interventions to achieve outcomes for which the nurse is accountable (NANDA, 1990).

nursing process A dynamic, systematic process by which nurses assess, analyze, plan, implement, and evaluate nursing care. It has been called "nursing's scientific methodology." Nursing process gives order and consistency to nursing intervention.

O

object constancy The phase in the separation/individuation process in which the child learns to relate to objects in an effective, constant manner. A sense of separateness is established, and the child is able to internalize a sustained image of the loved object/person when out of sight.

obsessive-compulsive disorder Recurrent thoughts or ideas (obsessions) that an individual is unable to put out of his or her mind and actions that an individual is unable to refrain from performing (compulsions). The obsessions and compulsions are severe enough to interfere with social and occupational functioning.

oculogyric crisis An attack of involuntary deviation and fixation of the eyeballs, usually in the upward position. May last for several minutes or hours. May occur as an extrapyramidal side effect of some antipsychotic medications.

operant conditioning The learning of a particular action or type of behavior that is followed by a reinforcement.

opportunistic infection Infections with any organism, but especially fungi and bacteria, that occur owing to the opportunity afforded by the altered physiological state of the host. Opportunistic infections have long been a defining characteristic of AIDS.

orgasm A peaking of sexual pleasure, with release of sexual tension and rhythmic contraction of the perineal muscles and pelvic reproductive organs.

osteoporosis A reduction in the mass of bone per unit of volume that interferes with the mechanical support function of bone. This process occurs as a result of demineralization of the bones and is escalated in menopausal women.

overt sensitization A type of aversion therapy that produces unpleasant consequences for undesirable behavior. An example is the use of disulfiram therapy with alcoholics, which induces an undesirable physical response if the individual has consumed any alcohol.

P

panic disorder A disorder characterized by recurrent panic attacks, the onset of which are unpredictable, and manifested by intense apprehension, fear, or terror, often associated with feelings of impending doom, and accompanied by intense physical discomfort.

paralanguage The gestural component of the spoken word. It consists of pitch, tone, and loudness of spoken messages, the rate of speaking, expressively placed pauses, and emphasis assigned to certain words.

paranoia A term that implies extreme suspiciousness. Paranoid schizophrenia is characterized by persecutory delusions and hallucinations of a threatening nature.

paraphilias Repetitive behaviors or fantasies that involve nonhuman objects, real or simulated suffering or humiliation, or nonconsenting partners.

passive-aggressive behavior Behavior that defends an individual's own basic rights by expressing resistance to social and occupational demands. Sometimes called indirect aggression, this behavior takes the form of sly, devious, and undermining actions that express the opposite of what they are really feeling.

pathological gambling A failure to resist impulses to gamble and gambling behavior that compromises, disrupts, or damages personal, family, or vocational pursuits.

pedophilia Recurrent urges and sexually arousing fantasies involving sexual activity with a prepubescent child.

peer assistance programs A program established by the American Nurses' Association to provide assistance to impaired nurses. The individuals who administer these efforts are nurse members of the state associations as well as nurses who are in recovery themselves.

perseveration Persistent repetition of the same word or idea in response to different questions.

persistent generalized lymphadenopathy (PGL) A condition common in HIV-infected individuals in which there are lymph nodes greater than 1 cm in diameter at two extrainguinal sites persisting for 3 months or longer, not attributed to other causes and not associated with other substantial constitutional symptoms.

personal distance The distance between individuals who are having interactions of a personal nature, such as a close conversation. In the United States, personal distance is approximately 18 to 40 inches.

personality Deeply ingrained patterns of behavior, which include the way one relates to, perceives, and thinks about the environment and oneself.

pharmacoconvulsive therapy The chemical induction of a convulsion used in the past for the reduction of psychotic symptoms. This type of therapy is no longer used in psychiatry.

phencyclidine An anesthetic used in veterinary medicine. It is used illegally as a hallucinogen and referred to as PCP or angel dust.

phobia An irrational fear.

phobia, simple A persistent fear of a specific object or situation, other than the fear or being unable to escape from a situation (agoraphobia) or the fear of being humiliated in social situations (social phobia).

phobia, social The fear of being humiliated in social situations.

physical neglect The failure on the part of a parent or caregiver to provide for a child's basic needs, such as food, clothing, shelter, medical/dental care, and supervision.

PIE charting More specifically called APIE, this method of documentation has an assessment, problem, intervention, and evaluation (APIE) format. It is a problem-oriented system that is used to document nursing process.

Pneumocystis carinii **pneumonia (PCP)** The most common, life-threatening opportunistic infection seen in patients with AIDS. Symptoms include fever, exertional dyspnea, and nonproductive cough.

positive reinforcement A reinforcement stimulus that increases the probability that the behavior will recur.

postpartum depression Depression that occurs during the postpartum period. It may be related to hormonal changes, tryptophan metabolism, or alterations in membrane transport during the early postpartum pe-

riod. Other predisposing factors may also be influential.

posttraumatic stress disorder (PTSD) A syndrome of symptoms that develops following a psychologically distressing event that is outside the range of usual human experience (e.g., rape, war). The individual is unable to put the experience out of his or her mind and has nightmares, flashbacks, and panic attacks.

posturing The voluntary assumption of inappropriate or bizarre postures.

precipitating event A stimulus arising from the internal or external environment that is perceived by an individual as taxing or exceeding his or her resources and endangering his or her well-being.

predisposing factors A variety of elements that influence how an individual perceives and responds to a stressful event. Types of predisposing factors include genetic influences, past experiences, and existing conditions.

Premack principle This principle states that a frequently occurring response (R_1) can serve as a positive reinforcement for a response (R_2) that occurs less frequently. For example, a girl may talk to her friends on the phone (R_2) only if she does her homework (R_1).

premature ejaculation Ejaculation that occurs with minimal sexual stimulation or before, upon, or shortly after penetration and before the person wishes it.

presenile pertaining to premature old age as judged by mental or physical condition. In presenile-onset dementia, initial symptoms appear at age 65 or younger.

priapism Prolonged, painful penile erection. May occur as an adverse effect of some antidepressant medications, particularly trazodone.

privileged communication A doctrine common to most states that grants certain professionals privileges under which they may refuse to reveal information about and communications with patients.

problem-oriented recording (POR) A system of documentation that follows a subjective, objective, assessment, plan, implementation, and evaluation (SOAPIE) format. It has as its basis a list of identified patient problems to which each entry is directed.

progressive relaxation A method of deep muscle relaxation in which each muscle group is alternately tensed and relaxed in a systematic order, with the person concentrating on the contrast of sensations experienced from tensing and relaxing.

projection Feelings or impulses unacceptable to one's self are attributed to another person.

pseudocyesis A condition in which an individual has nearly all the signs and symptoms of pregnancy, but is not pregnant. A conversion reaction.

psychodrama A specialized type of group therapy that employs a dramatic approach in which patients become "actors" in life-situation scenarios. The goal is to resolve interpersonal conflicts in a less threatening atmosphere than the real-life situation would present.

psychomotor retardation Extreme slowdown of physical movements. Posture slumps, speech is slowed, and digestion becomes sluggish. Common in severe depression.

psychophysiological Responses in which it has been determined that psychological factors contribute to the initiation or exacerbation of the physical condition. Either demonstrable organic pathology or a known pathophysiological process is involved.

psychosomatic See psychophysiological.

psychotic disorder A serious psychiatric disorder in which there is a gross disorganization of the personality, a marked disturbance in reality testing, and the impairment of interpersonal functioning and relationship to the external world.

public distance Appropriate interactional distance for speaking in public or yelling to someone some distance away. U.S. culture defines this distance as 12 feet or more.

pyromania The inability to resist the impulse to set fires.

R

rape The expression of power and dominance by means of sexual violence, most commonly by men over women, although men may also be rape victims. Rape is an act of aggression, not passion.

rapport The development of special feelings in a relationship on the part of two people, based on mutual acceptance, warmth, friendliness, common interest, a sense of trust, and a nonjudgmental attitude.

rationalization Attempting to make excuses or formulate logical reasons to justify unacceptable feelings or behaviors.

reaction formation Preventing unacceptable or undesirable thoughts or behaviors from being expressed by exaggerating opposite thoughts or types of behaviors.

reciprocal inhibition Also called counterconditioning, this technique serves to decrease or eliminate a behavior by introducing a more adaptive behavior, but one that is incompatible with the unacceptable behavior. For example, introduce relaxation techniques to the anxious person. Relaxation and anxiety are incompatible behaviors.

regression A retreat to an earlier level of development and the comfort measures associated with that level of functioning.

religiosity Excessive demonstration of or obsession with religious ideas and behavior. Common in schizophrenia.

repression The involuntary blocking of unpleasant feelings and experiences from one's awareness.

retarded ejaculation Delayed or absent ejaculation, even

though the man has a firm erection and has had more than adequate stimulation.

retrograde ejaculation Ejaculation of the seminal fluid backward into the bladder. May occur as a side effect of some antipsychotic medications.

right That which an individual is entitled (by ethical or moral standards) to have, or to do, or to receive from others within the limits of the law.

ritualistic behavior Purposeless activities that an individual performs repeatedly in an effort to decrease anxiety. Example: hand washing. Common in obsessive-compulsive disorder.

S

sadism Recurrent urges and sexually arousing fantasies involving acts (real, not simulated) in which the psychological or physical suffering (including humiliation) of the victim is sexually exciting.

safe house or shelter An establishment set up by many cities to provide protection for battered women and their children.

schizoid personality disorder A profound defect in the ability to form personal relationships or to respond to others in any meaningful, emotional way.

schizotypal personality disorder An individual with this disorder exhibits behavior that is odd and eccentric but does not decompensate to the level of schizophrenia.

senile Pertaining to old age and the mental or physical weakness with which it is sometimes associated. In senile-onset dementia, first symptoms appear after age 65.

sensate focus A therapeutic technique developed by Masters and Johnson that is used to treat individuals and couples with sexual dysfunction. The technique involves touching and being touched by another and focusing attention on physical sensations. The couple gradually moves through various levels of sensate focus that progress from nongenital touching to touching that includes the breasts and genitals; touching that is done in a simultaneous, mutual format rather than by one person at a time; and touching that extends to and allows eventually for the possibility of intercourse.

seroconversion The development of evidence of antibody response to a disease or vaccine. The time at which antibodies may be detected in the blood.

sexual exploitation of a child The coercion of a child to engage in sexually explicit conduct for the purpose of promoting any performance (e.g., child pornography).

shaping In learning, one shapes the behavior of another by giving reinforcements for increasingly closer approximations to the desired behavior.

short-term memory The ability to remember events that

occurred very recently. This ability deteriorates with age.

silent rape reaction The response of a rape victim in which he or she tells no one about the assault.

slander An action with which an individual may be charged for *orally* sharing information that is detrimental to a person's reputation.

social distance The distance considered acceptable in interactions with strangers or acquaintances, such as at a cocktail party or in a public building. American culture defines this distance as 4 to 12 feet.

social skills training Educational opportunities through role play for the person with schizophrenia to learn appropriate social interaction skills and functional skills that are relevant to daily living.

somatization A method of coping with psychosocial stress by developing physical symptoms.

splitting A primitive ego defense mechanism in which persons are unable to integrate and accept both positive and negative feelings. In their view, people—including themselves—and life situations are either all good or all bad. Common in borderline personality disorder.

statutory law Laws that have been enacted by legislative bodies, such as a county or city council, state legislature, or the Congress of the United States.

statutory rape Unlawful intercourse between a man older than age 16 and a woman younger than the age of consent. The man can be arrested for statutory rape even when the interaction has occurred between consenting individuals.

stimulus generalization The process by which a conditioned response is elicited from all stimuli *similar* to the one from which the response was learned.

stress A state of disequilibrium that occurs when there is a disharmony between demands occurring within an individual's internal or external environment and his or her ability to cope with those demands.

stress management Various methods used by individuals to reduce tension and other maladaptive responses to stress in their lives. Includes relaxation exercises, physical exercise, music, mental imagery, or any other technique that is successful for a person.

stressor A demand from within an individual's internal or external environment that elicits a physiological or psychological response.

sublimation The rechanneling of drives or impulses that are personally or socially unacceptable into activities that are more tolerable and constructive.

suicide, altruistic In the sociological theory of suicide, this type occurs out of allegiance to the cultural group.

suicide, anomic In the sociological theory of suicide, this type occurs in response to changes that occur in an individual's life that disrupt feelings of relatedness to the group.

suicide, egoistic In the sociological theory of suicide, this type occurs because the individual felt separate and apart from the mainstream of society.

superego One of the three elements of the personality identified by Freud that represents the conscience and the culturally determined restrictions that are placed on an individual.

suppression The voluntary blocking of unpleasant feelings and experiences from one's awareness.

symbiotic relationship A type of "psychic fusion" occurs between two people that is unhealthy in that severe anxiety is generated in either or both if separation is indicated. A symbiotic relationship is normal between infant and mother.

sympathy The actual sharing of another's thoughts and behaviors. It differs from empathy, in that with empathy one experiences an objective understanding of what another is feeling rather than actually sharing those feelings.

syphilis A sexually transmitted disorder caused by the spirochete *Treponema pallidum* and resulting in a chancre on the skin or mucous membranes of the sexual organs. If left untreated, it may go systemic. End-stage disease can have profound effects, such as blindness or insanity.

systematic desensitization A treatment for phobias in which the individual is taught to relax and then asked to imagine various components of the phobic stimulus on a graded hierarchy, moving from that which produces the least fear to that which produces the most.

T

T4 lymphocyte The white blood cell that is the primary target of the HIV virus. These cells are destroyed by the virus, causing the striking depletion of T4 cells associated with HIV infection.

tangentiality The inability to get to the point of a story. The speaker introduces many unrelated topics until the original discussion is lost.

tardive dyskinesia Syndrome of symptoms characterized by bizarre facial and tongue movements, stiff neck, and difficulty swallowing. May occur as an adverse effect of long-term therapy with some antipsychotic medications.

temperament Inborn personality characteristics that influence an individual's manner of reacting to the environment and ultimately influence his or her developmental progression.

territoriality The innate tendency of individuals to own space. Individuals lay claim to areas around them as their own. This phenomenon can have an influence on interpersonal communication.

therapeutic groups Differs from group therapy due to lesser degree of theoretical foundation. Focus is on group relations, interactions between group members, and the consideration of a selected issue. Leaders of therapeutic groups do not require the degree of educational preparation required of group therapy leaders.

thought-stopping techniques A self-taught technique that an individual employs each time he or she wishes to eliminate intrusive or negative, unwanted thoughts from awareness.

time out An aversive stimulus or punishment during which the patient is removed from the environment where the unacceptable behavior is being exhibited.

token economy In behavior modification, a type of contracting in which the reinforcers for desired behaviors are presented in the form of tokens, which may then be exchanged for designated privileges.

tort The violation of a civil law in which an individual has been wronged. In a tort action, one party asserts that wrongful conduct on the part of the other has caused harm, and compensation for harm suffered is sought.

transference In psychoanalytic theory, the mental process by which the patient transfers feelings and behaviors that had previously been directed toward important figures, such as parents or siblings, to the therapist.

transsexualism A disorder of gender identity or gender dysphoria (unhappiness or dissatisfaction with one's gender) of the most extreme variety. The individual, despite having the anatomical characteristics of a given gender, has the self-perception of being of the opposite gender, and may seek to have gender changed through surgical intervention.

transvestic fetishism Recurrent urges and sexually arousing fantasies involving dressing in the clothes of the opposite gender.

trichotillomania The recurrent failure to resist impulses to pull out one's own hair.

type A personality The term used to describe personality characteristics attributed to individuals prone to coronary heart disease. Includes characteristics such as excessive competitive drive, chronic sense of time urgency, being easily angered, very aggressive, very ambitious, and unable to enjoy leisure time.

type B personality The term used to describe personality characteristics attributed to individuals who are *not* prone to coronary heart disease. Includes characteristics such as ability to perform, even under pressure, but without the competitive drive and constant sense of time urgency experienced by the type A personality. Type Bs are able to enjoy their leisure time without

feeling guilty, and they are much less impulsive than type A individuals. That is, they think things through before making decisions.

type C personality The term used to describe personality characteristics attributed to the cancer-prone individual. Includes characteristics such as suppressing anger, being calm and passive, putting the needs of others before one's own, but holding resentment toward others for perceived "wrongs."

tyramine An amino acid found in aged cheeses or other aged, overripe, and fermented foods; broad beans; pickled herring; beef or chicken liver; preserved meats; beer and wine; yeast products; chocolate; caffeinated drinks; canned figs; sour cream; yogurt; soy sauce; and over-the-counter cold medications and diet pills. If foods high in tyramine content are consumed while an individual is taking monoamine oxidase inhibitors, a potentially life-threatening syndrome called hypertensive crisis can result.

U

unconditional positive regard Carl Rogers's term for the respect and dignity of an individual regardless of his or her unacceptable behavior.

undoing A mechanism that is used to symbolically negate or cancel out a previous action or experience that one finds intolerable.

universality One curative factor of groups (identified by Yalom) in which individuals come to realize that they are not alone in a problem, and the thoughts and feelings they are experiencing. Anxiety is relieved by the support and understanding of others in the group who share similar experiences.

universal precautions Guidelines established by the Centers for Disease Control in which special barrier precautions (e.g., gloves, mask, eye protection) should be used with ALL patients with whom there is a risk of blood or body-fluid exposure.

utilitarianism The ethical theory that espouses "the greatest happiness for the greatest number." Under this theory, action would be taken based on the end results that produced the most good (happiness) for the most people.

V

vaginismus Involuntary constriction of the outer one third of the vagina that prevents penile insertion and intercourse.

values Personal beliefs about the truth, beauty, or worth of a thought, object, or behavior.

values clarification A process of self-discovery by which people identify their personal values and their value rankings. This process increases awareness about why individuals behave in certain ways.

voyeurism Recurrent urges and sexually arousing fantasies involving the act of observing unsuspecting people, usually strangers, who are either naked, in the process of disrobing, or engaging in sexual activity.

W

waxy flexibility A condition by which the schizophrenic patient passively yields all moveable parts of the body to any efforts made at placing them in certain positions.

Wernicke's encephalopathy A brain disorder caused by thiamine deficiency and characterized by visual disturbances; ataxia; somnolence; stupor; and, without thiamine replacement, death.

word salad A group of words that are put together in a random fashion, without any logical connection.

Index

Numbers followed by an "f" indicate figures; numbers followed by a "t" indicate tables.

Methamphetamine;
Methylphenidate
Spiritual care, 651
Spiritual distress (nursing
diagnosis), in depression,
361, 363t
"Splash." *See* Amphetamine sulfate
Splitting, in borderline personality
disorder, 578
Spouse abuse, 663
Staff support, for hospice care
personnel, 652
Stage, in psychodrama, 105
Staring behavior, 70
Status epilepticus, 162
Statutory law, 690
Statutory rape, 668
STD. *See* Sexually transmitted
disease
Stealing. *See* Kleptomania
Stereotyped comment, 74t
Steroid therapy, 368
"Stick." *See* Marijuana
Stimulant(s)
general cellular, 280–282
historical aspects of use of, 282
profile of substances, 280
psychomotor, 280–282
use/abuse of, 280–284, 291t
effects on body, 283–284
patterns of, 282–283
withdrawal from, 262
Stimulus, 192–194, 194t
STP. *See* 2,5-Dimethoxy-4-
methylamphetamine
Stress
as biological response, 4, 5t
definition of, 4
elder abuse and, 614
as environmental event, 6, 6t
precipitating event, 7
individual's perception of, 7
predisposing factors in, 7–8, 136
psychological adaptation to,
19–25
anxiety, 19–24
grief, 24–25
schizophrenia and, 317
as transaction between
individual and
environment, 7–8
transactional model of
stress/adaptation, 7–8, 9f,
124, 125f
vulnerability to, 136, 137–138t

Stress appraisal
challenging, 7, 9f
harm/loss, 7, 9f
threatening, 7, 9f
Stress management, 8–10. *See
also* Coping strategy
awareness, 8
communication with caring
other, 8
meditation, 8
music, 10
pets, 10
problem solving, 8–10
relaxation therapy. *See*
Relaxation therapy
Stress response
neurotic, 539
normal, 539
psychophysiological, 539
psychotic, 539
Sublimation, 22, 26f
Substance use disorder. *See*
Psychoactive substance use
disorder
Substitution therapy, in alcohol
withdrawal, 261–262
Succinylcholine (Anectine), 185
"Sugar." *See* Lysergic acid
diethylamide
Suicidal act, 384
Suicidal crisis
life-stages issues in, 384
precipitating stressor in, 384
relevant history in, 384
Suicidal idea, 384
Suicidal individual, 128
Suicide
in adolescent, 357, 382
in AIDS, 639
altruistic, 383
anomic, 383
application of nursing process
to, 383–386
assessment of suicidal patient,
383–384
in borderline personality
disorder, 578
egoistic, 383
in elderly, 358, 607, 614–615
epidemiological factors in, 381
evaluation of care in, 385–386
facts and fables about, 382
planning/implementation of
care for suicidal patient,
384–385

psychoanalytic theory of, 383
risk factors for, 381–383
sociological theory of, 383
Sulfasalazine, 557
Sumatriptin, 555
Superego, 39
conscience, 39
ego-ideal, 39
Support group, 100, 377
Suppression, 22, 26f
Surmontil. *See* Trimipramine
Survival stage, in recovery from
co-dependency, 301
Sweating
decreased, drug-related, 173
in "fight or flight syndrome," 5t
"Sweet Lucy." *See* Hashish
Symbiotic phase, in theory of
object relations, 46, 46t
Symmetrel. *See* Amantadine
Sympathy, 59
Syphilis, 508t
"Syrup." *See* Codeine
Systematic desensitization, 196,
420–422
Systemic lupus erythematosus, 354

T helper cell(s). *See* T4
lymphocyte(s)
T4 lymphocyte(s), 631–633
"T's." *See* Pentazocine
Tachycardia, drug-related, 165, 173
Tactile hallucination, 323
Talwin. *See* Pentazocine
Tangentiality, 323
Taphaphobia, 402t
"Tar." *See* Opium
Taractan. *See* Chlorprothixene
Tardive dyskinesia, 171, 379
Task group, 100–101
Taste, in elderly, 605
Tea, 282, 283t
Teaching group, 101
Tegretol. *See* Carbamazepine
Temazepam (Restoril), 177, 261,
278
Temperament, 38, 136
in anxiety disorders of
childhood or adolescence,
222
in conduct disorder, 216
phobias and, 403
Temporal lobe lesion, 255
Tension headache, 23, 539t